Abrams' Urodynamics

Abrams' Urodynamics

Fourth Edition

Edited by

Marcus Drake, MA BM BCh DM FRCS(Urol)

Professor of Physiological Urology and Honorary Consultant Urologist
Translational Health Sciences, Bristol Medical School
Southmead Hospital
Bristol, UK

Hashim Hashim, MB BS MD FEBU FRCS(Urol)

Consultant Urological Surgeon & Honorary Professor of Urology
Bristol Urological Institute, Southmead Hospital
Bristol, UK

Andrew Gammie, MA CEng MIET CSci MIPEM

Clinical Engineer
Bristol Urological Institute
Southmead Hospital
Bristol, UK

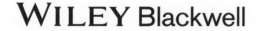

This edition first published 2021
© 2021 John Wiley & Sons Ltd

Edition History
Urodynamics, Springer-Verlag London (3e, 2006)

Registered Offices
John Wiley & Sons, Inc., 111 River Street, Hoboken, NJ 07030, USA
John Wiley & Sons Ltd, The Atrium, Southern Gate, Chichester, West Sussex, PO19 8SQ, UK

Editorial Office
9600 Garsington Road, Oxford, OX4 2DQ, UK
For details of our global editorial offices, customer services, and more information about Wiley products, visit us at www.wiley.com.
Wiley also publishes its books in a variety of electronic formats and by print-on-demand. Some content that appears in standard print versions of this book may not be available in other formats.

Library of Congress Cataloging-in-Publication Data

Names: Drake, Marcus, editor. | Hashim, Hashim, editor. | Gammie, Andrew, editor. | Abrams, Paul, Urodynamics.
Title: Abrams' urodynamics / edited by Marcus Drake, Hashim Hashim, Andrew Gammie.
Other titles: Urodynamics
Description: Fourth edition. | Hoboken, NJ : Wiley-Blackwell, 2021. | Preceded by Urodynamics / Paul Abrams. 3rd ed. c2006. | Includes bibliographical references and index.
Identifiers: LCCN 2020040344 (print) | LCCN 2020040345 (ebook) | ISBN 9781118844717 (paperback) | ISBN 9781118844724 (Adobe pdf) | ISBN 9781118844731 (epub)
Subjects: MESH: Urodynamics | Urologic Diseases–diagnosis
Classification: LCC RC874 (print) | LCC RC874 (ebook) | NLM WJ 102 | DDC 616.6/075–dc23
LC record available at https://lccn.loc.gov/2020040344
LC ebook record available at https://lccn.loc.gov/2020040345

Cover Design: Wiley
Cover Images: © Marcus Drake

Set in 9.5/12.5pt STIXTwoText by SPi Global, Pondicherry, India
Printed and bound by CPI Group (UK) Ltd, Croydon, CR0 4YY

C9781118844717_190824

Contents

Abbreviations

ACh	Acetyl-choline	DRE	Digital rectal examination
		DSD	Detrusor sphincter dyssynergia
AD	Autonomic dysreflexia	DUA	Detrusor underactivity
ADH	Anti-diuretic hormone	ED	Erectile dysfunction
AFC	Air-filled catheter	EBRT	External beam radiotherapy
ANP	Atrial natriuretic peptide	EMG	Electromyogram
AP	Antero-posterior	EUS	External urethral sphincter
ARM	Anorectal manometry	FDA	Food and Drug administration
ATP	Adenosine Triphosphate	FFR	Free flow rate
AUDS	Ambulatory urodynamics	Fr	French
AUS	Artificial urinary sphincter	FSF	First sensation of filling
BCI	Bladder contractility index	FUTURE	Female Urgency, Trial of Urodynamics
BMI	Body mass index		as Routine Evaluation
BOO	Bladder outlet obstruction	FVC	Frequency/volume chart
BOOI	Bladder outlet obstruction index	GI	Gastrointestinal
BPE	Benign prostate enlargement	GUP	Good Urodynamic Practices
BPH	Benign prostatic hyperplasia	HR-ARM	High resolution anorectal manometry
BPS	Bladder pain syndrome	HRM	High resolution manometry
BNI	Bladder neck incision	IAS	Internal anal sphincter
BNO	Bladder neck obstruction	IC	Intermittent catheterisation
BNP	Brain natriuretic peptide	ICI	International Consultation on
BPO	Benign prostatic obstruction		Incontinence
BTX	Onabotulinum toxin-A	ICIQ	International Consultation on
BWT	Bladder wall thickness		Incontinence Questionnaire
BVE	Bladder voiding efficiency	ICIQ-B	International Consultation on
CC	Cystometric capacity		Incontinence Questionnaire-Bowel
CEPNL	Cauda equina and peripheral nerves		symptoms
	lesion (infrasacral)	ICIQ-FLUTS	International Consultation on
CFS	Clinical Frailty Scale		Incontinence Questionnaire-Female
CKD	Chronic kidney disease		LUTS
CLPP	Cough leak point pressure	ICIQ-MLUTS	International Consultation on
CNS	Central nervous system		Incontinence Questionnaire-Male
CPAP	Continuous positive airway pressure		LUTS
CSF	Cerebrospinal fluid	ICCS	International Children's Continence
CSU	Catheter specimen of urine		Society
CT	Computed tomography	ICS	International Continence Society
CVA	Cerebro-vascular accident	IR(ME)R	Ionising Radiation (Medical Exposure)
DLPP	Detrusor leak point pressure		Regulations
DLPV	Detrusor Leak Point Volume	ISC	Intermittent self-catheterisation
DO	Detrusor overactivity	ISD	Intrinsic sphincter deficiency
DOI	Detrusor overactivity incontinence	IVU	Intravenous urogram

LUTD	Lower Urinary Tract Dysfunction	PRIMUS	PRImary care Management of lower Urinary tract Symptoms
LUTS	Lower Urinary Tract Symptoms		
M	Muscarinic	PRO	Patient-reported outcomes
MCUG	Micturating cystourethrogram	PSA	Prostate-specific antigen
MRI	Magnetic resonance imaging	PTNS	Percutaneous tibial nerve stimulation
MS	Multiple sclerosis	p_{ura}	Urethral pressure
MSA	Multiple system atrophy	PUV	Posterior urethral valves
MSU	Mid-stream urine	p_{ves}	Vesical pressure
MUCP	Maximum urethral closure pressure	PVR	Post-void residual
MUI	Mixed urinary incontinence	Q_{max}	Maximum flow rate
MUP	Maximum urethral pressure	RAIR	Recto Anal Inhibitory Reflex
MUT	Midurethral tape	SBO	Spina bifida occulta
MVV	Maximum voided volume	SCI	Spinal cord injury
NIRS	Near infrared spectroscopy	SDV	Strong desire to void
NLUTD	Neurogenic Lower Urinary Tract Dysfunction	SPL	Suprapontine lesion
		SSCL	Sacral Spinal Cord lesion
NDV	Normal desire to void	SSL	Suprasacral spinal cord/pontine lesion
NICE	National Institute for Health and Clinical Excellence	SNM	Sacral neuromodulation
		SNS	Sympathetic nervous system
NP	Nocturnal polyuria	SUI	Stress urinary incontinence
NPH	Normal pressure hydrocephalus	TURP	Transurethral resection of the prostate
NPi	Nocturnal polyuria index	TVT	Transvaginal tape
NUV	Nocturnal urine volume	TWOC	Trial without catheter
OAB	Overactive bladder	UAB	Underactive bladder
OSA	Obstructive sleep apnoea	UDS	Urodynamics
PA	Postero-anterior	UPP	Urethral pressure profile
p_{abd}	Abdominal pressure	UPSTREAM	Urodynamics for Prostate Surgery: Randomised Evaluation of Assessment Methods
PAG	Periaqueductal grey		
PCR	Penile compression-release		
PD	Parkinson's disease	USI	Urodynamic stress incontinence
p_{det}	Detrusor pressure	UTI	Urinary tract infection
$p_{detQmax}$	Detrusor pressure at maximum flow rate	UUI	Urgency urinary incontinence
		UUT	Upper urinary tract
PFC	Prefrontal cortex	VLPP	Valsalva leak point pressure
PFME	Pelvic floor muscle exercises	VUDS	Video-urodynamics
PFS	Pressure-flow studies	VUJ	Vesicoureteric junction
PMC	Pontine micturition centre	VUR	Vesicoureteric reflux
PMD	Post-micturition dribble	VV	Voided volume
PNS	Parasympathetic nervous system	VVF	Vesico-vaginal fistula
POP	Pelvic organ prolapse		
POP-Q	Pelvic organ prolapse quantification	WFC	Water-filled catheter
PPI	Post-prostatectomy incontinence		

Contributors

Abdelmageed Abdelrahman, MBBCh, BAO, DIPM, DFSRH, MRCOG, MSc
Subspecialty Trainee in Urogynaecology,
Liverpool Women's Hospital NHS Foundation Trust,
Crown Street, Liverpool, UK

Wael Agur, MB, BCh, MSc, MD(res), FRCOG
Subspecialist Consultant Urogynaecologist,
NHS Ayrshire & Arran University Hospital Crosshouse,
Kilmarnock, UK

Alexandra Bacon, MSc
Clinical Scientist,
Urodynamics & Gastrointestinal Physiology, Southmead
    Hospital,
Bristol, UK

Mohammed Belal, MA, MB, BChir, FRCS(Urol)
Consultant Urological Surgeon,
Department of Urology, University Hospitals
    Birmingham,
Mindelsohn Way, Edgbaston, Birmingham, UK

Wendy Bevan
Registered Nurse, Senior Urodynamic Nurse (Ret'd),
Urodynamics Department,
Bristol Urological Institute, North Bristol NHS Trust,
    Southmead Hospital,
Bristol, UK

Christopher Blake, FRCS(Urol) MD
Consultant Urological Surgeon,
Royal Cornwall Hospital,
Treliske, Truro, Cornwall, UK

Alison Bray, BSc, PhD
Northern Medical Physics and Clinical Engineering
    Department,
The Newcastle upon Tyne Hospitals NHS Foundation
    Trust, Royal Victoria Infirmary,
Newcastle upon Tyne, UK

Connie Chew, RGN
Senior Urodynamic Nurse,
Urodynamics Department,
Bristol Urological Institute, North Bristol NHS Trust,
    Southmead Hospital,
Bristol, UK

Nikki Cotterill, PhD, BSc(Hons), RN
Associate Professor in Continence Care,
University of the West of England, Bristol Urological
    Institute, Learning and Research, Southmead Hospital,
Bristol, UK

Devang Desai, MB BS, MS, FRACS(Urology)
Associate Professor of Urology,
University of Queensland, Toowoomba Base Hospital,
Queensland, Australia

Julie Ellis-Jones, DPhil, MSc, RN, RNT
Senior Lecturer in Adult Nursing,
University of the West of England,
Bristol, UK

Jonathan S. Ellison, MD
Assistant Professor,
Urology Dept., Children's Hospital of Wisconsin &
    Medical College of Wisconsin,
Children's Corporate Center Suite 330,
Milwaukee, WI, USA

Arturo García-Mora, MD
Head of Functional Urology and Urodynamics,
Instituto Nacional de Ciencias Médicas y Nutrición
    "Salvador Zubirán",
Hospital Médica Sur Mexico City, México

C. K. Harding, MA, MB, BChir, MD, FRCS(Urol)
Consultant Urological Surgeon,
Freeman Hospital, Newcastle upon Tyne Hospitals NHS
    Foundation Trust, Freeman Rd, High Heaton, Newcastle
    upon Tyne, UK

Emily Henderson, MB, ChB, MRCP, PhD
Consultant Senior Lecturer, Honorary Consultant
  Geriatrician,
Population Health Sciences, Bristol Medical School,
  University of Bristol,
Senate House, Tyndall Ave, Bristol, UK

Dharmesh Kapoor, MB, BS, MD, FRCOG
Consultant Gynaecologist and Subspecialist in
  Urogynaecology,
Mumbai, India

George Kasyan, MD, PhD
Professor of Urology,
Urology Department, Moscow State University of
  Medicine and Dentistry,
Moscow, Russian Federation

Su-Min Lee PhD, MBChB, MRCS
Urology Registrar,
Department of Urology, Royal United Hospital,
Combe Park, Bath,
Somerset, United Kingdom, UK

Chendrimada Madhu, MD, MA, MRCOG, FHEA
Consultant Gynaecologist, Subspecialist in Urogynaecology,
Department of Women's Health, The Chilterns,
Southmead Hospital, Bristol, UK

Kathryn McCarthy MB, BS, MD, MRCS, FRCS(Gen Surg)
Consultant in Colorectal Surgery,
Department of General Surgery, Southmead Hospital,
Bristol, UK

Amit Mevcha, MBBS, MRCS, FRCS (Urol)
Consultant Urologist,
Royal Bournemouth Hospital,
Bournemouth, UK

Richard Napier-Hemy, MB, ChB, FRCS(Urol)
Consultant Urological Surgeon,
Manchester Royal Infirmary,
Manchester, UK

Jeremy Nettleton, MBBS, Bsc (Hons), FRCS(Urol)
Consultant Urological Surgeon,
Cheltenham General Hospital, Gloucestershire Hospitals
  NHS Foundation Trust, Sandford Rd, Cheltenham, UK

Guy Nicholls, BSc, MD, FRCS (Paeds)
Consultant Paediatric Surgeon and Urologist,
Bristol Royal Hospital for Children,
Upper Maudlin Street, Bristol, UK

Michelle Ong, MBBS (Hons)
Resident in Urology,
Toowoomba Base Hospital, South Toowoomba,
  Queensland, Australia

Antonín Prouza, MD
Senior Clinical Fellow in Female and Functional
  Urology,
Bristol Urological Institute, Southmead Hospital,
Bristol, UK

Joanne Sheen
Senior Administrator,
Bristol Urological Institute, Southmead Hospital,
Bristol, UK

Eskinder Solomon, MSc, MEng
Consultant Clinical Scientist,
Department of Urology, Guy's and St Thomas' Hospital
  and Department of Paediatric Nephro-Urology, Evelina
  Children's Hospital,
London, UK

Laura Thomas, MSc
Clinical Scientist,
Urodynamics & Gastrointestinal Physiology, Southmead
  Hospital,
Bristol, UK

Rachel Tindle, MSc
Clinical Scientist,
Urodynamics & Gastrointestinal Physiology, Southmead
  Hospital,
Bristol, UK

Ruben Trochez, MBBS, MRCOG
Consultant Urogynaecologist,
Liverpool Women's Hospital NHS Foundation Trust,
Crown Street, Liverpool, UK

Alan Uren, BSc(Hons), MPH
Specialist Clinical Researcher,
Bristol Urological Institute, Southmead Hospital,
Bristol, UK

Mark Woodward, MD, FRCS (Paed Surg)
Consultant Paediatric Urologist,
Bristol Royal Hospital for Children,
Upper Maudlin Street, Bristol, UK

Michel Wyndaele, MD, PhD, FEBU
Urology Consultant,
Division of Surgical Specialties, Department of Urology,
    University Medical Center Utrecht,
Heidelberglaan 100, The Netherlands

Musaab Yassin
Consultant Urologist,
Oxford University Hospitals NHS Foundation Trust,
    Churchill Hospital, Oxford, UK

Sharon Yeo, MBBS, MRCS (Glasg), MMed (Surgery), FAMS (Urology)
Senior Consultant and Head
Department of Urology, Tan Tock Seng Hospital
11 Jalan Tan Tock Seng, Singapore

Preface

Lower urinary tract dysfunction (LUTD) produces a large burden on sufferers in particular, and on society in general. Lower urinary tract symptoms (LUTS) are very prevalent; 5% of children aged 10 years wet the bed. In all, 15% of women and 7% of men have troublesome incontinence. In elderly men of 75 years, benign prostatic hyperplasia occurs in more than 80% of individuals, with benign prostatic enlargement coexisting in up to half this group and half of these having bladder outlet obstruction. Most people with a neurological disease have some form of LUTD.

Urodynamics is invaluable in assessing people with LUTD. The need to support the clinical assessment with objective measurement is accepted by most clinicians specialising in the care of patients with LUTS. Since the first edition of this book in 1983, urodynamics has become more widely accepted. The number of urodynamic units worldwide has increased to enable access to this important testing modality. Almost every hospital of any significance embraces urodynamic investigations as an essential part of the diagnostic pathway for urology and gynaecology departments. Further, specialists in geriatrics, paediatrics and neurology recognise the importance of urodynamics in the investigation of a significant minority of their patients. The expertise involved in assessing neurogenic LUTD by urodynamicists can help neurologists refine their insights into the neurological deficit in individual patients. However, the take-up is not universal, especially worldwide. This may result from the perceived cost to the healthcare unit, the presumed unpleasantness to the patient, and the varied expertise in functional urology.

The objective of this book is to deliver a definitive manual of practical urodynamics, showing how urodynamic investigation contributes to the management of patients and describing the tests clearly and comprehensively. To do this means not only discussing the tests but also showing in which clinical areas they help management and those where urodynamic tests are largely pointless. It means concentrating on the common clinical problems and on the presenting symptom complexes, while pointing out any limitations and possible artefacts of investigation.

The Bristol Urological Institute (BUI) serves a large patient population in South West England and has developed skills in urodynamics and functional urology over several decades. It runs educational courses (the Basic Urodynamics course, the Certificate of Urodynamics, and the Expert Urodynamics course) which take place in the UK and several places globally, and also online. This makes the BUI one of the world-renowned leading units in female and functional urology generally, and urodynamics specifically, that is visited by healthcare professionals from all over the world. Professor Paul Abrams was not the only individual responsible for this strength, but his contributions to Urology in Bristol and worldwide are truly impressive. They include the development of the Abrams-Griffiths nomogram [1], which was adopted by the International Continence Society (ICS) as the Bladder Outlet Obstruction Index. He was a major promoter of the ICS Standardisations of Terminology in Lower urinary tract function, including being the first author on the paper which has been more widely quoted from urology than any other [2]. He also serves as one of the Chairs of the International Consultations on Incontinence. When he wrote the preceding editions of this book, his aim was to help a clinician with no previous experience in urodynamics to appreciate both the value and limitations of the subject and give the necessary practical advice on the use of the appropriate equipment in the correct situations. This was delivered with characteristic wit and imagination (see figure). One of the principal reasons for producing the 3rd edition was the publication of the ICS terminology report and the 'Good Urodynamic Practices' document [3]. With the updating of Good Urodynamic Practices [4], and now the 'Fundamentals of Urodynamic Practice' document [5], it is timely to continue Professor Abrams' achievements in this fourth edition, the first to become an eponymous *Abrams' Urodynamics*. In it, we have aimed to stay true to the importance of the practical application of urodynamic tests, we draw on the latest scientific evidence, have sourced an extensive new tranche of illustrations, and have revisited the ICS Standardisations to reflect their revisions in recent years. In doing so, we wish to record our personal appreciation of and debt to Paul Abrams' inspiration, leadership, and support of us and countless others in this field.

Marcus Drake, Hashim Hashim,
Andrew Gammie, 2020
Bristol Urological Institute
and University of Bristol

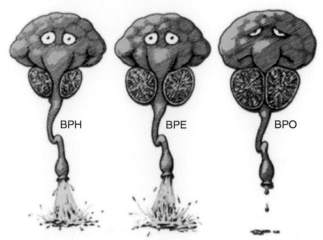

Figure A classic picture of the fundamental insights on the implications of prostate pathology for the male lower urinary tract, showing the relationships between benign prostate hyperplasia (BPH), benign prostate enlargement (BPE), and benign prostate obstruction (BPO). *Source*: Drawn by Alex James from a sketch by Paul Abrams in 1993.

References

1 Abrams, P.H. and Griffiths, D.J. (1979). The assessment of prostatic obstruction from urodynamic measurements and from residual urine. *Br. J. Urol.* 51 (2): 129–134.

2 Abrams, P., Cardozo, L., Fall, M. et al. (2002). The standardisation of terminology of lower urinary tract function: report from the Standardisation Sub-committee of the International Continence Society. *Neurourol. Urodyn.* 21 (2): 167–178.

3 Schafer, W., Abrams, P., Liao, L. et al. (2002). Good urodynamic practices: uroflowmetry, filling cystometry, and pressure-flow studies. *Neurourol. Urodyn.* 21 (3): 261–274.

4 Rosier, P., Schaefer, W., Lose, G. et al. (2017). International Continence Society Good Urodynamic Practices and Terms 2016: Urodynamics, uroflowmetry, cystometry, and pressure-flow study. *Neurourol. Urodyn.* 36 (5): 1243–1260.

5 Drake, M.J., Doumouchtsis, S.K., Hashim, H., and Gammie, A. (2018). Fundamentals of Urodynamic Practice, based on International Continence Society Good Urodynamic Practices recommendations. *Neurourol. Urodyn.* 37 (S6): S50–S60.

First Foreword

I feel honoured and humbled to find my name attached to this new edition, but need to set the record straight!

After graduating from Sheffield, I arrived in Bristol in 1972 to begin my surgical training. The surgical registrar (resident) was Michael Torrens, who was a neurosurgical resident, and about to become Roger Feneley's new research fellow in the newly founded urodynamic unit. Mike was going to use urodynamics to evaluate sacral neurectomy in women with intractable detrusor overactivity, then called 'detrusor instability'. After six months of general surgery, I rotated to the urology department and got interested in the older men coming for TURP for their 'prostatism'. Even then I was an annoying and inquisitive individual who constantly asked, 'Why .... ?'. Mike suggested that I approach Roger to see whether I could start to assess these men, initially by urine flow measurement. I describe these beginnings of my urological life, as they were determined by serendipity. The opportunities I was given, and those I worked with, in that first year in Bristol determined the rest of my professional career. Mike's early encouragement and advice, and Roger's mentorship throughout, have been the bedrock of my professional development. Roger provided the environment where all young, naive but enthusiastic clinicians could speak without fear, knowing that their unanswered questions could be pursued in an academically sound manner according to the null hypothesis.

It has been my privilege and pleasure to work in academic and clinical teams that have been devoted to patient care, and free of rancour and division. The stability of the urodynamic team in Bristol was anchored by Roger initially, then by Angela Shepherd, followed by Lucy Swithinbank and now by Hashim Hashim. The technical side of urodynamics is also of paramount importance to the quality of service. From the beginning, Pat Lewis and then Sue Howell ensured that Bristol Urodynamics adhered to high technical standards, and the clinicians were kept on the 'straight and narrow': any upstart doctor was reminded who were the most important members of

staff! We have continued to be most fortunate in having excellent scientific colleagues. Andrew Gammie is our first clinical engineer, and Laura Thomas is our first clinical scientist. With their involvement, not only has our urodynamic quality advanced, but our teaching activity too has been able to improve in quality.

I owe great debts to many others. I met and worked with Derek Griffiths, then in the physics department at Exeter. He was my urodynamic and scientific mentor, and he taught me 'intellectual honesty' – what I knew from what I thought I knew. We collaborated for many years, even after he moved to Holland and then to North America. Early on, I met Alan Wein and Linda Cardozo, who have both been very important in developing functional urology worldwide, and together we have worked closely with the International Continence Society (ICS) and in developing the International Consultation on Incontinence (ICI), and from that the ICI Research Society. Saad Khoury has been another valued mentor who made the ICI possible and has been an important and wise counsel for many years. The camaraderie of these old friends has been very important to me.

Urodynamics remains a controversial subject to the 'non-believers', and there remains much to be achieved in identifying its exact place in the evaluation of lower urinary tract dysfunction (LUTD). What is clear is that the *a priori* argument remains: the bladder, urethra and sphincter are, in engineering terms, a reservoir, outlet and valve, and therefore must be studied by pressure and flow measurements. The United Kingdom Continence Society (UKCS) has led the way in determining how urodynamics can improve and reach the quality standards of other physiological measurement units. Another of the fundamental problems, in managing patients' problems, is that the LUT is connected to the brain. Of course, this is essential, but it leads to enormous problems, as the nervous system is so incompletely understood. In any urodynamic team, there has to be a basic science including neurophysiological input, and Marcus Drake has added that dimension to our work. Advances will not come until we develop our understanding of the interactions between the nervous system and the LUT. Marcus, like many other members of the urodynamic team, has completed his training in other centres, and this cross-fertilisation by ideas is essential for creative thinking. I am proud that I have had a part in appointing colleagues who will develop a wider range of skills than I have had. This is never a threat, only an opportunity.

We all have the duty to educate, and I hope this book will support that effort. Finally, I must thank my wife Kirsten and my children, the members of 'my crew', who ground me when necessary, and are ever tolerant and supportive. They have certainly become familiar with the basics of lower urinary tract function! So, in addition to developing the science of urodynamics, we have to help all people, as well as patients, to better understand their bladder function so that they can preserve their bladder health and help themselves when it 'plays up'.

Thank you, Marcus, Andrew and Hashim, for your collaboration in science and clinical work and for your friendship.

Professor Paul Abrams, Bristol
December 2020

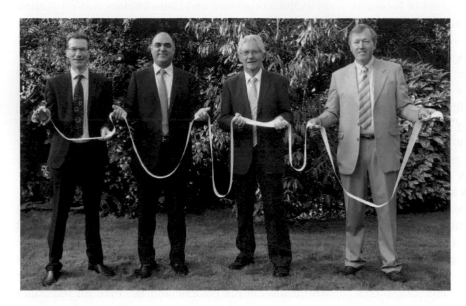

Figure Marcus Drake, Hashim Hashim, Paul Abrams, and Andrew Gammie holding an extremely long flowmetry printout that exemplifies slow flow and terminal dribble. Bristol, September 2020.

Second Foreword

The name 'Paul Abrams' has been synonymous with expertise in many subjects associated with normal function and lower urinary tract dysfunction (LUTD), but none more so than the science, performance, interpretation and clinical utility of urodynamics of the LUT. I thought that I was a good organiser of subject material and a good and succinct writer when I picked up the first edition of *Urodynamics* in 1983, but I had to tip my hat to Paul. The 229 pages of this text rapidly became the 'gold standard', and the charts, tables and diagrams quickly became a part of my own presentations on the subject (properly referenced, of course!). I found the organisation of the subject, which included the science necessary to understand what happens during filling/storage and emptying/voiding, and how to properly measure and categorise the findings, to 'make sense' and enable understanding of where these straightforwardly explained techniques fit into the overall evaluation of LUTD. The notes on management were a bonus.

Subsequent editions (I am looking at the third now - 331 pages) have expanded the concepts and techniques that have occurred parallel to the advances in the related scientific disciplines, just as the terminology has evolved (please do not ever say 'urge incontinence' as opposed to 'urgency incontinence' in Paul's presence!). It is only fitting that the title of this book, the most complete text on the science and practice of urodynamics, now be preceded by Paul's name and carried on by members of the department that he developed.

Paul, congratulations on having the text renamed *Abrams' Urodynamics*, an honour well deserved!

Alan J. Wein, MD, PhD(hon), FACS
Professor with Tenure and Emeritus Chief of Urology
Perelman School of Medicine at the
University of Pennsylvania
Penn Medicine
Philadelphia, Pennsylvania, USA

Part I

Basic Principles

1

Basic Urodynamics and Fundamental Issues

Marcus Drake[1], Andrew Gammie[2], Laura Thomas[3], Arturo García-Mora[4], and Hashim Hashim[2]

[1] *Translational Health Sciences, Bristol Medical School, Southmead Hospital, Bristol, UK*
[2] *Bristol Urological Institute, Southmead Hospital, Bristol, UK*
[3] *Urodynamics & Gastrointestinal Physiology, Southmead Hospital, Bristol, UK*
[4] *Instituto Nacional de Ciencias Médicas y Nutrición "Salvador Zubirán", Hospital Médica Sur, Mexico City, México*

CONTENTS

Introduction to Urodynamics

Urodynamics has two basic aims:

- **To reproduce the patient's symptomatic complaints while making key observations**
- **To provide a pathophysiological explanation by correlating the patient's symptoms with the urodynamic findings**

These two basic aims are crucial to the purpose of urodynamics – essentially, it is a diagnostic test that will aid in the management of patients. The need to make urodynamic observations reflects the fact that the patient's symptoms are important, but they might be somewhat misleading. Most patients with lower urinary tract dysfunction (LUTD) present to their doctor with symptoms. However, lower urinary tract symptoms (LUTS – Table 1.1) should not simply be taken at face value, since a range of differing mechanisms may result in rather similar symptomatic presentations. The statement 'the bladder is an unreliable witness' [2] reflects how symptoms are the starting point but do not actually identify the ultimate explanation. Since treatment should

correct the underlying cause, it is necessary to identify mechanisms, avoiding assumption or prejudice coming from taking symptoms at face value. An excellent example of this is voiding LUTS in men, where the cause on urodynamic testing may prove to be bladder outlet obstruction (BOO) and/or detrusor underactivity (DUA); BOO should respond fully to surgery to relieve obstruction such as transurethral resection of prostate (TURP), while such surgery is potentially not helpful in the second [3]. Voiding LUTS in males are of unreliable diagnostic value, and only slow stream and hesitancy show any correlation with the urodynamic findings of BOO [4–6]. Even with flow rate assessment, one cannot be sure whether BOO is present (Figure 1.1). The difficulty of assessing LUTD by symptoms alone is the uncertainty about establishing truly what is going on in the individual describing them.

For women diagnosed by their symptoms as having stress urinary incontinence (SUI), only 50–68% have urodynamic stress incontinence (USI) [7, 8]. These studies also looked at patients with apparent overactive bladder (OAB) symptoms presumed to be the result of detrusor overactivity (DO), and here, the correspondence was

---

Table 1.1 Classification of lower urinary tract symptoms (LUTS) [1].

Storage	Voiding	Post-micturition
Urgency	Slow stream	Post-micturition dribbling
Urinary incontinence	Splitting/spraying	Feeling of incomplete emptying
Increased daytime frequency	Intermittency	
Nocturia	Hesitancy	
Pain	Straining	
	Terminal dribbling	

Note: Do NOT forget to enquire about Pelvic Organ Prolapse in Women and Erectile Dysfunction in Men. *Source*: Modified from Abrams et al. [1].

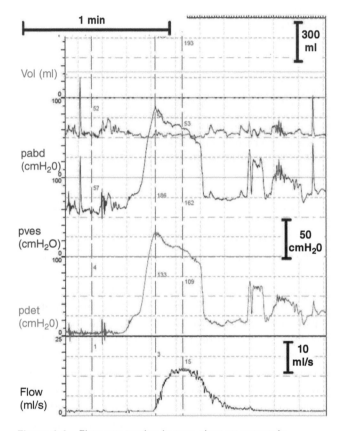

Figure 1.1 Flow rate testing in men gives an uncertain understanding. This man had previously done a free flow rate test which showed a reasonable maximum flow rate of 16 ml/s; taken alone, this might suggest he does not have bladder outlet obstruction (BOO). However, when he attended for urodynamics (see the pressure-flow study illustrated above), his flow rate was 15 ml/s as shown, but the pressure needed to achieve this was high, indicating BOO is present (see Chapter 14 for more details on assessing BOO in men).

33–51%. A key factor is the link to coughing, often used as a question to elicit a history of SUI; if a woman says 'I leak when I cough', it sounds like SUI. However, a cough can be a trigger to set off an overactive detrusor contraction, leading to detrusor overactivity incontinence (DOI) (Figure 1.2).

Thus, the history may suggest that SUI treatment is needed, but for some of these women, the urodynamic observation identifies that DO treatment is the appropriate choice.

Accordingly, in both men and women, there is potential mismatch between reported LUTS and the LUTD identified by detailed investigation. This issue is particularly prominent in people with neurological conditions and children. In neurological disease, it is common for sensation to be absent or abnormal, making LUTS even more difficult to interpret. Children may find it difficult to describe their symptoms in any setting and particularly in a healthcare environment. Because symptoms have been shown to lack diagnostic specificity in the key clinical groups, it is not surprising to find that when surgery was based on symptoms alone, the results could be unsatisfactory. Urodynamic studies provide explanations for many symptoms based on mechanism and accordingly provide better support for therapy selection.

There is a well-recognised and substantial placebo effect for therapy in patients with LUTS. The symptoms of men with proven BOO, secondary to benign prostatic enlargement (BPE), can be improved in 40–60% of men in the placebo arm of drug studies. Such an effect can be surmised in men undergoing prostate surgery, but usually it is not sustained and in due course will be counterbalanced by the other effects of surgery, notably impairment of sexual function. Some patients submitted for surgery without objective confirmation of their condition potentially can do badly; this might reflect a poor-quality operation, or it may be that the problem lay in the preceding assessment. Urodynamics in modern practice gives greater insight into each patient's LUTD and hence helps advise patients on potential benefit and risks for intervention, to support their expectations of informed decision-making.

Ultimately, a successful urodynamics test is a clinically relevant investigation which seeks:

- to reproduce the patient's symptoms,
- to define bladder and urethral function,
- to provide precise diagnoses,

standards, and how to deal with challenges that may be encountered.

The Urodynamic History and Examination

When meeting a new patient with LUTS, it is important to establish a rapport. The LUTS present must be captured systematically, identifying the severity of individual symptoms and the bother each causes to the patient, preferably by using a symptom score completed before the appointment. There are several developed by the International Consultation on Incontinence Questionnaires group [9] which can suit a wide range of patients. They have the advantage of efficiently capturing both severity and bother for each symptom.

The history needs to cover several influences, for example:

- previous urological treatments,
- urinary tract infections (UTIs) – confirmed or suspected,
- obstetric and gynaecological background (in women),
- bowel function,
- sexual problems, including sexual trauma in the past, or recent emergence of sexual dysfunction,
- medical problems and medications, and
- the possibility of an underlying neurological condition.

Malignancy and neurological disease are key considerations. Undiagnosed cancer, such as bladder, prostate, gynaecological, or pelvic malignancy, must also be considered and is potentially at the back of the patient's mind, even if they don't say so [10]. Most patients with neurological disease have been diagnosed as such before coming to have LUTS assessed. However, some conditions can cause LUTS early on in the disease process. In these patients, it is possible that no one has yet realised the situation. Urological clinics sometimes encounter LUTS which turn, on investigation, to have been caused by a neurological problem that has not yet been diagnosed – 'occult neurology' [11]; the main conditions which can cause this sort of situation are described in the last part of this chapter.

Patients referred for urodynamics will have been examined in a general way, either in the hospital clinic from which the referral originated, or by the patient's general practitioner (primary care physician). Hence, the urodynamic staff should concentrate efforts on a physical examination relevant to the symptomatic complaints and the possible underlying pathophysiological processes, for example:

- features suggestive of wider problems, such as neurological disease (e.g. slurred speech, altered gait, and tremor),

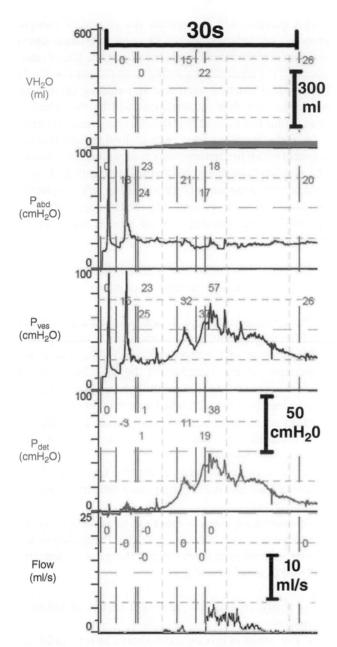

Figure 1.2 A woman who reported leakage with coughing in her history, suggestive of stress urinary incontinence (SUI). Her urodynamic test showed cough-provoked detrusor overactivity (DO) incontinence, and she described this as representative of her presenting complaint. Hence, this is not urodynamic stress incontinence, but effort-provoked detrusor overactivity incontinence; the symptomatic presentation was misleading and could have led to inappropriate surgery for SUI (see Chapter 13 for more details on assessing incontinence in women).

- to define the most significant abnormality,
- to allow selection of most appropriate treatment, and
- to predict post-operative problems.

This book describes how these can be achieved across a wide range of settings, complying with modern practice

- abdominal examination to identify scars from previous surgery, or a distended palpable bladder, and
- internal examination to assess pelvic floor tone and contraction, pelvic organ prolapse, or formal prostate evaluation.

Urine examination should be performed in all patients, in the form of a urine dipstick to help rule out obvious causes for the LUTS. Other tests, such as blood tests (e.g. renal function and prostate-specific antigen), radiology, and endoscopy, have their indications and may need to be conducted alongside the ongoing LUTD assessment in accordance with the applicable clinical guidelines.

Invasive urodynamic studies are generally not indicated early in the pathway. They follow on once

1) careful investigations have been performed to exclude other pathologies that might mimic LUTD,
2) a bladder diary has been completed,
3) urinary free flow rate test and post-void residual (PVR) have been done, and
4) conservative treatment, which may include testing out response to medications, has been undertaken for a sufficient duration.

The Aims and Considerations of Urodynamics

A urodynamic test has several aims:

- To reproduce the patient's symptoms
- To define bladder and urethral function
- To provide precise diagnoses
- To define the most significant abnormality
- To allow selection of most appropriate treatment
- To predict potential post-operative problems
- To assess the results of treatment

The prelude to a urodynamic test is to identify the information needed, which can be described as 'formulating the urodynamic question'. The needs of the patient are fundamentally to resolve bothersome symptoms and reduce possible future problems. The history, symptom score, and bladder diary will help specify the situation. It follows that the needs of the clinician are to help suitable therapy selection and ensure avoidance of harm by identifying causative mechanisms. The urodynamicist should be considering 'what do I want to know about this patient?' It can be considered in terms of the micturition cycle ('What is wrong with storage, what is wrong with voiding?') and in terms of the lower urinary tract organs ('What is wrong with the bladder, what is wrong with the bladder outlet?'). In this way, the urodynamicist is in a position to consider 'Which urodynamic investigations need to be performed to define this patient's problems?'

This question will concentrate the clinician's thought processes on undertaking only those investigations which can help to make the diagnosis or indicate the line of management. For example, if a young male patient previously had urethral stricture treatment and voiding LUTS have returned, urine flow measurement will be the principal urodynamic test to identify if stricture recurrence is likely.

Once the questions have been defined, it will become apparent which urodynamic tests to do, as discussed below. The next question should be: 'Is the investigation likely to be of benefit to the patient?' This question reflects how the increased knowledge generated by the test might influence the clinical management. Several aspects are relevant, including:

1) *Individual considerations*: Is there therapy available, and is the patient healthy enough to tolerate the therapy?
2) *Disease knowledge*: In a difficult clinical area without effective treatment, urodynamic insights may facilitate introduction of treatment options in the future. An example is the introduction by the International Continence Society (ICS) of the concept of underactive bladder syndrome [12], which currently has no specific effective treatment but which will stand a better chance of future therapy development now that a terminology framework is in place.
3) *Financial cost and risks of testing*: The incidence of UTI after a UDS test is 2–3%, and some discomfort may be experienced.
4) *Potential harm the tests could do*: In particular, 'Is the urodynamic unit able to make a reliable diagnosis?' with erroneous diagnosis being the greatest concern. Three factors are crucial:

- The urodynamic technique should be free of technical artefacts.
  - The results of investigations should be reproducible.
  - The clinician should be properly trained and able to interpret the results of the urodynamics (Figure 1.3).

From a technical point of view, the tests must be carried out in a careful way, continuously monitoring during the test and eliminating artefacts (see Chapters 18 and 19). The clinician needs to allow for variation in LUTS from day to day and symptomatic progression over longer timescales. At the end of the urodynamic tests, it is pertinent to ask 'Did the urodynamic studies reproduce the patient's complaints and did the complaints correlate with known urodynamic features?' Answers to this question would be yes, no, or partially.

In the Bristol unit, we believe the presence of the clinician, or an experienced practitioner who is aware of the therapeutic possibilities of subsequent treatment, is very beneficial during tests. This individual can then consider

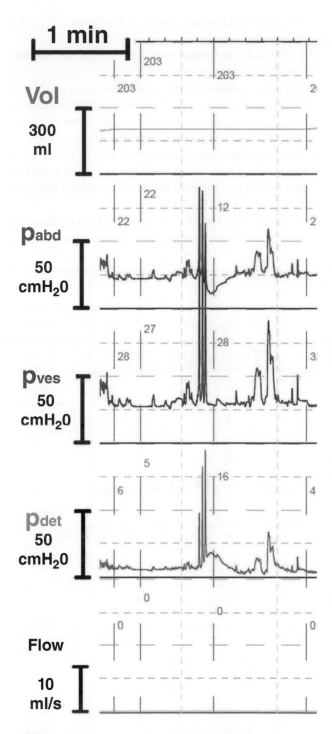

Figure 1.3 The importance of training and interpretation. This trace shows a brief moment from a filling cystometry. It illustrates a transient rise in detrusor pressure after a cough (green tracing), which resembles the detrusor overactivity (DO) seen in Figure 1.2 (but with no associated incontinence). Inspection of the bladder pressure trace (blue tracing) shows there was no bladder contraction associated with the detrusor pressure change, so this is not DO- despite the appearance. The actual explanation is that the cough caused the rectal catheter to shift, causing the recorded drop in abdominal pressure (red tracing) – an entirely different process from an involuntary bladder contraction. Proper training and interpretation will ensure that a mistaken diagnosis of DO is avoided.

whether the sensations felt by the patient during testing fit with the patient's reported everyday experiences and how they may relate to the urodynamic observations. Occasionally, during urodynamic studies, the patient may complain of a symptom they do not generally experience in everyday life, for example, urgency. Alternatively, a urodynamic abnormality may be noted which does not correlate with the patient's symptoms. These discrepancies can be detected and put into perspective if the clinician is present. However, if the urodynamics is delegated to someone with minimal urodynamic experience, the matching of LUTS to observations which underpins therapy selection is less direct. They may likely develop a basic test report which is observational and does not have the clinical interpretations at its heart. This report is of huge importance in therapy decision-making, with potentially life-long implications for the patient. Accordingly, a surgeon making decisions based on a basic report must consider: 'Does the report make sense in the context of the patient's symptoms and preceding tests?' and 'Can the features mentioned in the report be identified on the plotted traces, and is anything visible on the traces not mentioned in the report?'

In some instances, more than one abnormality is detected, so it is important to ask: 'Can urodynamics decide which abnormality is the most significant, if more than one is detected?' Multiple abnormalities are commonly seen in patients with neurogenic LUTD. They also occur in non-neurological patients, such as in women with mixed urinary incontinence. Treatment should be directed to the most significant and/or troublesome abnormality. Hence, the correspondence between the patient's symptomatic complaint and the urodynamic findings is important and needs to be documented in the report.

As well as seeking answers to the above questions, the urodynamicist needs to define the goals of the invasive urodynamic investigation, and these can be listed as follows:

- To **increase diagnostic accuracy** above that which can be achieved by non-urodynamic means.
- To **make a diagnosis on which a management plan can be based**. OAB is usually treated empirically; if a patient fails conservative and medical therapy, urodynamic proof of DO is appropriate prior to invasive surgery.
- If there are coexisting abnormalities, to **provide evidence to determine which abnormality should be treated first**. In a female patient with mixed urinary incontinence, it is usually possible to decide which is the main problem and so establish the treatment priority by careful assessment during urodynamics.
- To **define the current situation as a baseline for future surveillance**. In spinal cord trauma, it is usual to perform urodynamics after spinal shock has resolved. These baseline urodynamics establish whether there is a detrusor contraction in reaction to bladder filling and

whether or not detrusor-sphincter-dyssynergia (DSD) has developed. DSD is a potentially dangerous condition, as discussed in Chapter 16.

- To **predict problems that may follow treatment interventions**. Elderly men with BOO and coexisting DO should be warned that whilst their urine flows and other voiding symptoms should be improved by TURP, OAB symptoms due to DO may persist and in fact leakage due to the DO may occur.
- To **provide evidence that decides the timing of treatment**. In patients with neurological disease (e.g. meningomyelocele) being treated by antimuscarinics, ultrasound may show the development of upper tract dilatation. Urodynamics are vital to confirm whether or

not poor bladder compliance is the cause, such that intervention is needed.

- To **exclude abnormalities which might interfere with the management**. For example, in patients with SUI being considered for an artificial urinary sphincter (AUS), demonstration of DO or poor bladder compliance would indicate the need for extra treatment to ensure that the additional problem is resolved (Figure 1.4).
- To **assess the natural history of** LUTD. Our unit, by investigating men and women studied many years ago, provided important evidence as to the natural history of LUT dysfunction [3, 13, 14].
- To **assess the results of treatments**. Simple urodynamics tests, such as urine flow studies, should be used

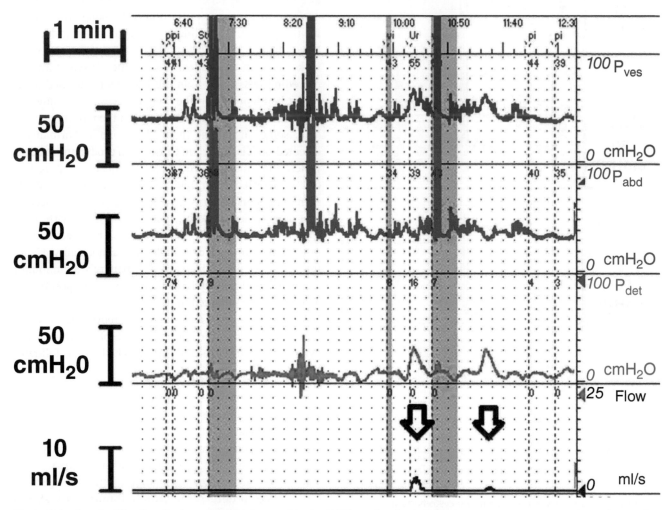

Figure 1.4 A man with a functioning artificial urinary sphincter (AUS) previously placed to treat post-prostatectomy incontinence; he subsequently complained of painful urgency incontinence. This illustration shows a small section of the filling phase, with a series of forceful coughs (stress testing) that did not cause leakage; a fully active AUS can resist 61–70 cmH₂O pressure. While he did not experience stress incontinence despite several forceful coughs, he did experience leakage with low amplitude of detrusor overactivity (DO) (black arrows), and it is hard to explain how forceful coughs did not cause leakage yet low amplitude DO did – we speculate this was due to the sustained nature of the DO pressure change, allowing greater effect on the pressure in the urethra. Indeed, pressure building up in his proximal urethra may have been responsible for the discomfort he described with his urgency incontinence. Note, this trace is not displayed with the correct sequence of traces; the bladder pressure should not be at the top for 'logistical' reasons, notably for the fact that some of the trace may go off the top of the page, as in this case.

Figure 1.5 Urodynamics pathway in Bristol UDS Unit.

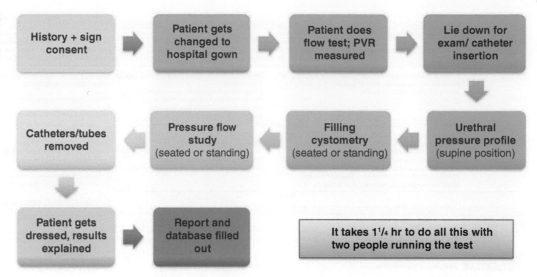

History + sign consent → Patient gets changed to hospital gown → Patient does flow test; PVR measured → Lie down for exam/ catheter insertion

Catheters/tubes removed ← Pressure flow study (seated or standing) ← Filling cystometry (seated or standing) ← Urethral pressure profile (supine position)

Patient gets dressed, results explained → Report and database filled out

It takes 1¼ hr to do all this with two people running the test

to evaluate outcomes of surgery, for example, after optical urethrotomy for urethral stricture.

This book will help readers understand the scientific basis of LUTD and urodynamic evaluation. It takes a therapy-led approach to framing urodynamic questions in a wide range of contexts. One of the great advantages of the Bristol unit is that adequate time is given for close questioning, the relevant physical examination, a calm urodynamic investigation, and practical advice, usually including the therapeutic recommendation and counselling, generating a report, and filling out the urodynamics database. Generally, we allow 75 minutes for each case, though shorter time is possible in clear-cut straightforward cases (Figure 1.5). This approach is worth emulating in all units, since the insight into each patient's needs and expectations, and ability to help their understanding as they make important decisions, is profoundly beneficial.

The prospect of having this type of clinical investigation causes anxiety for some individuals. Hence, beforehand, it is essential to give proper information, and a leaflet designed in conjunction with patients is probably the most practical and effective way to do this; the one we use in Bristol is included in the Appendix C.2 of this book. Patients should be introduced to the clinicians present and informed of their role, with agreement sought for the involvement of trainees in the procedure [10]. A written consent form needs to be signed. During urodynamic practice, efforts should be made to limit the number of staff present in the assessment room and ensure maximum possible privacy is maintained. After the test, patients should be allowed to get dressed in their normal clothes before the concluding discussions. It is important to discuss side-effects with patients and what to do if they experience any problems. Clinicians and patients will

ideally discuss the results of urodynamic testing on the same day as the test or shortly after, with the detail and depth of the explanation in line with the patient's personal preference [10]. This assimilates the patient's medical background, previous therapy, and treatment preferences and goals to guide the therapeutic pathway to a suitable culmination (Figure 1.6).

Basics of Urodynamics

This section describes a starting point for anyone new to urodynamics. It gives a brief summary of what the test is about for starting practice, with directions to help find more details on the key points elsewhere in the book. It should be read alongside the ICS 'Fundamentals' documents for LUTS [15], flow rate testing [16], and urodynamics [17], which are given in the Appendix B.1. Once people have become familiar with basic testing, the extensive experience described in detail in the book will help readers respond to the numerous situations that can arise in real-life practice.

What Is Urodynamics?

Urodynamics is the umbrella term that covers investigations of lower urinary tract function. The term includes uroflowmetry and cystometry, which are the basic tests, along with the advanced tests such as video urodynamics, urethral pressure profilometry, and ambulatory urodynamics. Standard cystometry is the commonest investigation assessing storage function (filling cystometry) and voiding (pressure-flow study [PFS]). Both are normally performed as part of every investigation, unless the patient is unable

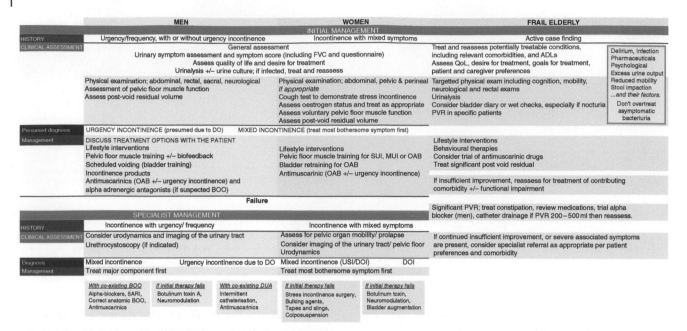

	MEN	WOMEN	FRAIL ELDERLY	
		INITIAL MANAGEMENT		
HISTORY	Urgency/frequency, with or without urgency incontinence	Incontinence with mixed symptoms	Active case finding	
CLINICAL ASSESSMENT	General assessment Urinary symptom assessment and symptom score (including FVC and questionnaire) Assess quality of life and desire for treatment Urinalysis +/– urine culture; if infected, treat and reassess		Treat and reassess potentially treatable conditions, including relevant comorbidities, and ADLs Assess QoL, desire for treatment, goals for treatment, patient and caregiver preferences	Delirium, Infection Pharmaceuticals Psychological Excess urine output Reduced mobility Stool impaction ...and their factors. Don't overtreat asymptomatic bacteriuria
	Physical examination; abdominal, rectal, sacral, neurological Assessment of pelvic floor muscle function Assess post-void residual volume	Physical examination; abdominal, pelvic & perineal *If appropriate* Cough test to demonstrate stress incontinence Assess oestrogen status and treat as appropriate Assess voluntary pelvic floor muscle function Assess post-void residual volume	Targetted physical exam including cognition, mobility, neurological and rectal exams Urinalysis Consider bladder diary or wet checks, especially if nocturia PVR in specific patients	
Presumed diagnosis	URGENCY INCONTINENCE (presumed due to DO)	MIXED INCONTINENCE (treat most bothersome symptom first)		
Management	DISCUSS TREATMENT OPTIONS WITH THE PATIENT Lifestyle interventions Pelvic floor muscle training +/– biofeedback Scheduled voiding (bladder training) Incontinence products Antimuscarinics (OAB +/– urgency incontinence) and alpha adrenergic antagonists (if suspected BOO)	Lifestyle interventions Pelvic floor muscle training for SUI, MUI or OAB Bladder retraining for OAB Antimuscarinic (OAB +/– urgency incontinence)	Lifestyle interventions Behavioural therapies Consider trial of antimuscarinic drugs Treat significant post void residual If insufficient improvement, reassess for treatment of contributing comorbidity +/– functional impairment	
		Failure		
	SPECIALIST MANAGEMENT		Significant PVR; treat constipation, review medications, trial alpha blocker (men), catheter drainage if PVR 200–500 ml then reassess.	
HISTORY	Incontinence with urgency/ frequency	Incontinence with mixed symptoms		
CLINICAL ASSESSMENT	Consider urodynamics and imaging of the urinary tract Urethrocystoscopy (if indicated)	Assess for pelvic organ mobility/ prolapse Consider imaging of the urinary tract/ pelvic floor Urodynamics	If continued insufficient improvement, or severe associated symptoms are present, consider specialist referral as appropriate per patient preferences and comorbidity	
Diagnosis	Mixed incontinence Urgency incontinence due to DO	Mixed incontinence (USI/DOI) DOI		
Management	Treat major component first	Treat most bothersome symptom first		

With co-existing BOO	*If initial therapy fails*	*With co-existing DUA*	*If initial therapy fails*	*If initial therapy fails*
Alpha-blockers, 5ARI, Correct anatomic BOO, Antimuscarinics	Botulinum toxin A, Neuromodulation	Intermittent catheterisation, Antimuscarinics	Stress incontinence surgery, Bulking agents, Tapes and slings, Colposuspension	Botulinum toxin, Neuromodulation, Bladder augmentation

Figure 1.6 The diagnostic and therapeutic pathways for important patient groups seeking treatment of lower urinary tract symptoms (LUTS), summarising key points from the International Consultation on Incontinence algorithms. 5ARI: 5-alpha reductase inhibitor; BOO: bladder outlet obstruction; DO(I): detrusor overactivity (incontinence); DUA: detrusor underactivity; FVC: frequency volume chart; MUI: mixed urinary incontinence; OAB: overactive bladder; PVR: post-void residual; SUI: stress urinary incontinence; ADLs: Activities of daily living

to void (in which case filling cystometry alone would be carried out). Cystometry aims to reproduce a patient's symptoms and, by means of pressure measurements, provide a pathophysiological explanation for them.

During cystometry, there is a constant dialogue between the investigator and the patient so that any symptoms experienced during the test can be related to urodynamic findings. A full report is produced following a urodynamic investigation, which will normally include history, examination, urodynamic findings, and suggestions concerning management. The report should state whether the patient's symptoms were reproduced and whether voiding was felt to be representative.

What Is Measured?

Detrusor pressure is measured indirectly from bladder and abdominal pressures (respectively, referred to as p_{ves} and p_{abd}) using the formula: $p_{ves} - p_{abd} = p_{det}$. Abdominal pressure is measured because the bladder is an abdominal organ, so it is necessary to allow for the effect of increases in abdominal pressure, for example, straining, on vesical pressure. Pressure can be measured as the height of a column of fluid. To describe pressure, you simply need to specify what the fluid is and the height to which it goes. In urodynamics, the unit of pressure has been standardised as if we are measuring the height of a column of water in centimetres (cmH_2O). There are usually two pressure

transducers associated with urodynamic equipment. One to measure p_{ves} and one to measure p_{abd}. The pressure generated by the detrusor smooth muscle, p_{det}, is derived by the urodynamic equipment electronically subtracting p_{abd} from p_{ves}.

Pressure transducers are not perfect instruments; therefore, it is important to regularly check their calibration to ensure that accurate pressure measurements are always made. In most urodynamics, the transducers are attached to the urodynamic equipment and are remote from the patient. Pressures inside the patient are transmitted to the pressure transducers via water-filled pressure catheters. To ensure appropriate pressure measurements, there must be:

1) no bubbles of air in the water connection between the patient and the transducer,
2) no water leaks, and
3) a good connection between the transducer dome and the diaphragm of the transducer if using non-disposable transducers.

A simple check of calibration for external pressure transducers (before connection to the patient) is to move the end of the filled pressure line through a known vertical distance (e.g. 20 cm) above the transducer dome and the pressure reading on the urodynamic equipment should change by the same amount (i.e. 20 cmH_2O). For air-filled or catheter tip transducers, calibration can be checked, if necessary, by submerging the catheter tip in a known depth of

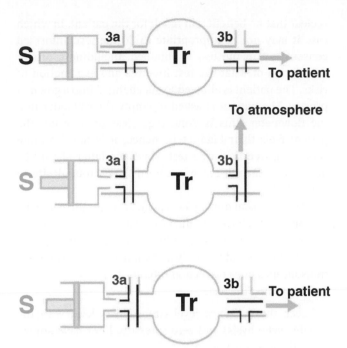

Figure 1.7 A schematic diagram of the set-up of three-way taps to enable key steps in urodynamics for pressure recording from the bladder (the same arrangements are also used for the abdominal pressure recording). The p_{ves} transducer (Tr) has a three-way tap '3a' connecting it to a syringe (S) and another to the patient '3b'. In the top diagram, both 3a and 3b are open, so this is the setting where the syringe can be used to flush air out of the transducer, connection tubing, and catheter. 3a is shut in the other two set-ups, so it is is closed to the transducer (indicated by red colour). In the middle set-up, 3b is open to the air (indicated by blue colour), so this the setting where the zero button can be pressed to set the reference value as atmospheric pressure. The bottom diagram is the set-up used when running the test, with 3b connecting the transducer to the bladder via the connection tubing and catheter.

sterile water. Again, the pressure reading on the equipment should change by the value of that depth.

Good urodynamics is carried out by making pressure measurements relative to atmospheric pressure. This is achieved in a water-filled system by zeroing the equipment with the transducers closed off to the patient and open to the atmosphere. Pressure measurements may also be made in urodynamics by using air-filled catheters. With these, there is a practically weightless connection between the patient and the external transducer. This means that the system is simpler to use compared to the external water-filled devices because there is no need to flush air from the system nor is there any need to place anything at a reference level. However, it is still important to set the baseline pressure of these devices to atmospheric pressure, and these catheters are not yet fully validated (see Chapter 7).

For uroflowmetry and for PFSs, urine flow rate in urodynamics is measured using a flowmeter which can either be mounted on a stand or in a commode. Urine is usually directed into the flow sensor by a funnel. The electronics of the flowmeter converts the changes of volume with time into urine flow rate (Q), which is measured in the units of millilitres per second (ml/s). Flowmeters (and other less common ones) will measure flow rate accurately, but it is important to examine the flow trace after it has been produced in order to correct for any artefacts that have occurred during voiding:

1) Knocking the flowmeter may produce 'spikes' on the trace which need to be ignored.
2) Moving the urinary stream relative to the flow-meter will produce artefactual fluctuations in the flow trace.

Setting Up the Equipment

For external, water-filled transducers, the disposables required are syringes, three-way taps, domes, manometer tubing/catheter to patient, and sterile water or physiological saline. The lines to the patient need to be primed with sterile water to remove air bubbles, and thus create a continuous column of water between patient and transducer. This can be done before the start of the test. The use of two three-way taps either side of the dome makes it easier for troubleshooting (checking zero and flushing) before and during the test (Figure 1.7), without introducing unnecessary air into the system. These allow completion of the important steps of basic urodynamics:

- Prime system: Flush sterile water through the whole system, with both three-way taps open before the domes are attached to the external transducers. A small flush after attachment is also advised.
- Zero to atmosphere: Position the taps so that the transducer is open to the atmosphere and closed to the patient and syringe. The 'zero' or 'balance' option on the urodynamic equipment is then selected. Pressures will now be read relative to atmospheric pressure.
- Set reference height: The pressure transducers need to be placed at the upper edge of the symphysis pubis to avoid artefactual pressure measurements due to the hydrostatic pressure effect. If the patient changes position during the test, the height of the transducers should be changed to the new level of the upper border of the symphysis pubis.
- For recording: The tap to the syringe remains off. The other tap is open to the transducer and the patient, but off to atmosphere. A cough test can now be performed. If the height of one cough peak is less than 70% of the other, the line with the lower value should be flushed with water and the cough test repeated.

If air-filled catheters are used, they need to be connected to their individual pressure transducer units. This can be done with the catheters already inside the patient. The switches on the transducer units are turned to the 'open' position, and the 'zero' or 'balance' option on the urodynamic equipment is then selected. The switches on the transducer units are then moved to the 'charge' position, and the catheters will record pressures inside the patient relative to atmospheric pressure. 'Zero' should not be done when patient pressures are being read, as these pressures are never truly zero.

Running the Test

Before their appointment, an information leaflet (an example is provided in the Appendix C.2) and suitable description should be provided so that the patient knows what to expect. A considerate attitude is needed, since the patient will generally be anxious.

The clinical requirement is to identify the 'urodynamic question', i.e. to clarify what symptoms experienced by this patient we are trying to observe during the urodynamic test. If we are able to reproduce the symptom during the test, the urodynamic features present at that time may provide the explanation for the symptom. Hence, urodynamics is preceded by a full clinical assessment:

1) History
   - Symptoms; best captured with a symptom score
     - Duration
     - Stress/urgency/other incontinence
   - Degree of leakage
     - Pad usage
   - Voiding difficulties
   - Quality of life
   - Past medical history
   - Medication e.g. anticholinergics
   - Allergies (latex)
   - Parity (where relevant!)

2) Frequency/volume chart (bladder diary)
   - Fluid intake – caffeine/alcohol
   - Voided volumes (VVs)
   - Voiding frequency
   - Nocturia?

3) Flow rate test
   - Maximum flow rate (Q_{max})
   - Shape of the flow trace
   - VV
   - PVR

This information is used to make the urodynamic test specific for the patient's clinical need. A decision is needed whether they actually need the test; sometimes, it is clear that no benefit will result for the patient, in which case it may not be appropriate to do the test. Informed consent to run the test is obtained, including a proper description of what the test involves and explanation of risks. The patient is allowed to get changed into a gown in privacy. The patient is asked to empty their bladder into the flowmeter (this is done regardless of how full the patient feels their bladder is; hence, it is not the quite same as a free flow rate test, since the latter should be done when the patient has a normal or strong desire to void [SDV]).

All staff present during the test must be introduced to the patient, and their role should be explained. Physical examination is undertaken. The catheters for recording p_{ves} and p_{abd} are then placed carefully and connected to the relevant transducers using connection tubing.

Before starting the test:

- Check the reference level (transducers level with the pubic symphysis) and zero (pressure lines have atmospheric pressure as zero)
- Check that the vesical and abdominal pressures are in the normal range
- Initial cough to test both lines are picking up rapid pressure changes promptly and equally

If any problems are identified, delay starting the test until the problem has been fully dealt with.

When running the test:

- Run the test in the position the patient usually adopts to pass urine (generally seated for women and standing for men)
- Use annotation marks to record aspects such as sensations reported by the patient, provocation tests, and urodynamic observations
- Monitor recording quality

  - Presence of physiological signals (e.g. if the patient moves, some change in the pressure lines is apparent)
  - Ask for coughs/deep exhalations regularly

- Understand other influences on the pressure recording

  - Drift of one of the baseline pressures may indicate a loose connection
  - Position changes will affect the resting pressure and require the urodynamicist to move the pressure transducers to lie level with the new height of the patient's pubis
  - Rectal contractions will cause a phasic rise in rectal pressure seen in the p_{abd} trace
  - Tube artefacts: knocks on the catheter or connection tubing will cause a clear disturbance in the pressure trace
  - Pump artefact is seen as disturbance in one of the pressure traces (usually p_{ves}) when the pump is running

- Tailor to the individual patient
  - ○ Expected cystometric capacity can be estimated from the largest VV on the bladder diary but should be adjusted according to the patient's actual experience during the test.
  - ○ Adjust filling speed if the patient develops urgency or DO is seen. Sometimes, it is necessary to change to filling in the supine position if overactivity is so prominent that it prevents reaching an adequate volume for reliable assessment of stress incontinence or voiding.
  - ○ Do provocation tests to try to elicit issues, e.g. stress testing with a rapid sequence of coughs, or a Valsalva, to try to see USI. The sound of gently trickling water may help provoke DO.

- Once cystometric capacity is reached:
  - ○ Do a cough to check pressure recording
  - ○ Explain to the patient that urine will pass around the catheter and may land on the floor, but to void as naturally as can be managed in the circumstances
  - ○ Give a clear 'permission to void' to initiate the PFS
  - ○ Do another cough check after voiding has concluded

After the test:

- Remove the catheters and allow the patient to change back to normal clothing and wash their hands
- Explain the preliminary findings and what the next steps will be
- Describe what to look out for as the initial signs of a UTI and how to deal with it

After the patient has departed, clinical waste should be disposed of safely, and the equipment should be cleaned and set up for the next test.

Writing a report:

- Summarise the history, examination, and bladder diary findings
- Summarise the process followed (e.g. type of catheter, patient position, filling rate, and provocation tests) and report any problems encountered
- Describe the urodynamic observations and how they corresponded with sensations described by the patient. Clarify whether the patient's everyday symptoms were reproduced
- Describe any incontinence seen specifically
- Note whether the voiding in the PFS was typical, both from what the patient described and by comparing with the free flow rate test(s) done previously. Was there a PVR?
- Conclude with the summary of urodynamic observations and management suggestions.

Troubleshooting

Troubleshooting is a form of problem solving, defined by Wikipedia as 'the systematic search for the source of a problem so that it can be solved'. Troubleshooting is necessary if there are concerns about the quality of a urodynamic test while it is in progress. There is little that can be done to correct poor traces retrospectively, so quality control checks should be performed both before and during the investigation. Any problems with quality control should be addressed as soon as they are noted; the test can be paused while troubleshooting is performed.

The following information provides only a guide to common problems that are encountered during setting up and running a test, when quality control is not satisfactory. The unexpected can always happen, but problems can be solved if troubleshooting is performed in a systematic manner.

1) Baseline pressure readings outside acceptable ranges: Vesical and abdominal pressure measurements should both be within the range of 5–20 cmH$_2$O if measured with the patient supine, 15–40 cmH$_2$O if sitting, and 30–50 cmH$_2$O if standing. If pressures are outside the acceptable range:
   - If vesical and abdominal pressures are similar, but outside the acceptable range: check the height of the transducers – they should be level with the upper edge of the symphysis pubis
   - If only one pressure is outside the acceptable range:
     - ○ Flush the relevant catheter
     - ○ Check that zero has been set correctly on the relevant transducer
     - ○ Consider re-siting the affected catheter
2) If there is unequal transmission of pressure between vesical and abdominal lines, before or during the test
   - Flush the line which is giving the smaller response
   - Check whether there is any air in the dome over the external transducer
   - Check the three-way taps are in the correct positions
   - Consider re-siting catheter
3) During the test, if there is a fall in pressure of the vesical or the abdominal line during filling
   - Flush the affected line – this may be enough to restore pressure
   - If pressures continue to fall, check for leaks in a systematic manner
     - ○ Check taps and all connections have been adequately tightened
     - ○ Check lines (connection tubes and catheters) – occasionally, there may be a manufacturing fault
4) If lines stop recording and the pressures drop dramatically

This is probably because one of the catheters has fallen out or become compressed

- Reposition or re-site the affected catheter
- If the vesical catheter has fallen out before Q_{max}, consider refilling and repeating the PFS.

5) Troubleshooting with air-filled catheters where a problem arises with quality control:

- Try 'opening' them and 'recharging' the catheters, ensuring that the patient coughs between charges
- While 'open', the zero level can be checked
- Try moving the catheter position, in case the balloon has become trapped or compressed
- If these fail, the catheter will need to be changed.

Fundamentals

Anyone working in urodynamics needs to remain vigilant and ensure high quality of practice. In this section, we describe some issues which are not covered specifically elsewhere in the book, but which nonetheless are important for all practitioners to bear in mind.

'Occult' Neurological Disease

A rare but vital situation a urodynamicist needs to look for in everyday practice is the possibility that someone has been referred for LUTS assessment where a neurological disease is the cause, but it has not yet been recognised by anyone. For some neurological conditions, LUTS can characteristically be an early feature in the disease [11]. LUTS may constitute the sole initial complaint in up to 15% of multiple sclerosis (MS) patients [18], so acute urinary retention of unknown aetiology or an acute onset of urgency and frequency in young adults should be carefully assessed. Every year we pick up some patients in this situation, and the urodynamic unit might be an excellent opportunity to identify these 'occult' cases. Note that the features are subtle (because if they were obvious, the diagnosis would have been made previously). Since urodynamicists may not be particularly confident in neurological examination, it means that they may have to act on suspicion or 'a hunch' that there may be something neurological going on. A vague suspicion and hard-to-explain severe LUTS is sufficient justification to make a neurology referral. No neurologist would object to a referral that turned out not to be neurological after all. On the contrary, failing to refer someone where neurology is later identified and an avoidable complication or progression occurs is a disaster for the affected person.

Occult neurology is especially relevant for people experiencing sudden onset rather severe LUTS, especially in younger age groups. Obviously, straightforward explanations like uncomplicated UTI must be excluded. Accordingly, urodynamicists need to be able to identify particular presentations where additional consideration to exclude an undiagnosed neurological disease is needed. Identifying a neurological mechanism where present is important for several reasons:

- To avoid adverse outcomes of urological intervention
- To minimise progression of the neurological condition by obtaining specialist input to disease management
- To enable patients to adapt their life according to prognosis.

The following conditions may present for LUTS assessment before a neurological condition has been recognised, because LUTS are potentially an early feature in the disease course:

1) MS, which is the most common progressive neurological disease affecting younger people, produces demyelination of the nerve fibres. Because any part of the neuro-axis may be affected, the exact pattern of LUTS and the associated non-urological features is potentially diverse. An important trigger to pick up is a history of transient blindness in one eye (optic neuritis). Suggestive features include weakness or sensory changes in the upper or lower limbs, loss of balance, coordination or falls, or visual symptoms (vision loss and double vision).

2) Parkinson's disease (PD) is a movement disorder with prominent non-motor symptoms, including LUTD. In its early stages, PD can cause storage and voiding LUTS, and motor symptoms may be mild. Important symptoms include a unilateral tremor; rather than the classic 'pill-rolling' tremor, early PD can have a unilateral tremor at a low frequency (approximately 2 Hz). Stiffness, bradykinesia, balance problems (presenting as falls), loss of smell, and urinary incontinence may be relevant.

3) Multiple system atrophy (MSA) is a PD-like problem causing chronic progressive neurodegeneration in the brainstem and cerebellum. This often affects people in their late 40s, with a male predominance. For men, erectile dysfunction (ED) [11] is commonly an earlier feature than LUTS; the reviewing doctor considering this possibility needs to enquire about ED, since men commonly do not volunteer the symptom without prompting. Archetypal symptoms include ED, slow movements, tremor, stiffness, reduced coordination, changes in voice, orthostatic hypotension, and urinary incontinence.

4) Normal pressure hydrocephalus (NPH) is a dilation of the cerebral ventricles, associated with stretching of

white matter tracts in the brain. The classic triad is abnormal gait, urinary incontinence, and dementia.

5) Alzheimer's disease and other forms of dementia are neurodegenerative conditions with wide-ranging effects on memory, cognition, and personality. Although LUTS generally increase in incidence with age, they are also more common in demented than non-demented patients. LUTS can be an early feature of dementia, in particular with Lewy body dementia. The archetypal symptoms are short-term memory loss; difficulty in performing familiar tasks; problems with language; disorientation in time and place, poor or decreased judgement; and changes in mood, behaviour, or personality.

6) Spinal cord conditions. This is a mixed group of potential causes due to direct or indirect effects on the spinal cord. There may be little in the way of indicative or localising symptoms. The archetypal condition is spina bifida occulta (SBO) and tethered cord, in which a developmental abnormality fixes the lower part of the spinal cord, placing it at risk by stretching and distortion as the person grows. Tumours (spinal or vertebral) can have this

effect. Spinal stenosis (narrowing of the vertebral spinal canal), leading to claudication (leg pain with exercise) and LUTS, is another potential consideration.

The following symptoms should mandate a more careful neurological assessment in the urodynamic clinic: (i) enuresis, (ii) voiding dysregulation, e.g. voiding in socially inappropriate settings, (iii) involuntary voiding, and (iv) evidence of LUT muscle weakness, e.g. abdominal straining for voiding (bladder weakness), SUI (sphincter weakness), or retrograde ejaculation (bladder neck weakness), or (v) altered perineal sensation. Changes to one or more of the following non-urological features could suggest neurological impairment: gait, speech, cognition, memory, dexterity, vision, balance, or new headache. Some patients may volunteer new and/or sudden focal neurological changes. Furthermore, practitioners should stay alert, and if they feel there is something unusual about the current presentation, they should act on their intuition. On this basis, both urological and neurological examinations should be completed (see

Figure 1.8 Additional evaluation to undertake in the event that a patient has presentation features that might suggest an undiagnosed underlying neurological condition. *Source*: Roy et al. [44]. © 2020 John Wiley & Sons.

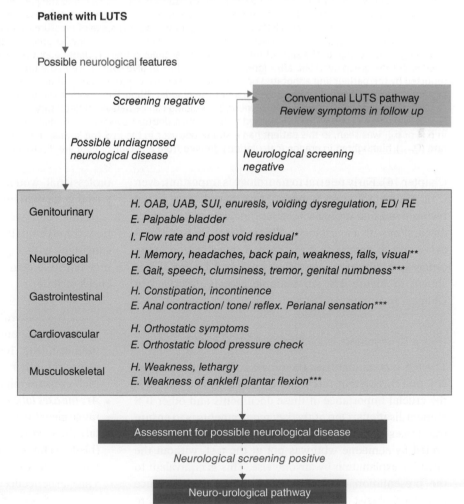

Patient with LUTS

Possible neurological features

Screening negative → Conventional LUTS pathway / *Review symptoms in follow up*

Possible undiagnosed neurological disease

Neurological screening negative

Genitourinary	*H. OAB, UAB, SUI, enuresis, voiding dysregulation, ED/ RE*
	E. Palpable bladder
	I. Flow rate and post void residual*
Neurological	*H. Memory, headaches, back pain, weakness, falls, visual***
	E. Gait, speech, clumsiness, tremor, genital numbness***
Gastrointestinal	*H. Constipation, incontinence*
	E. Anal contraction/ tone/ reflex. Perianal sensation***
Cardiovascular	*H. Orthostatic symptoms*
	E. Orthostatic blood pressure check
Musculoskeletal	*H. Weakness, lethargy*
	E. Weakness of anklefl plantar flexion***

Assessment for possible neurological disease

Neurological screening positive

Neuro-urological pathway

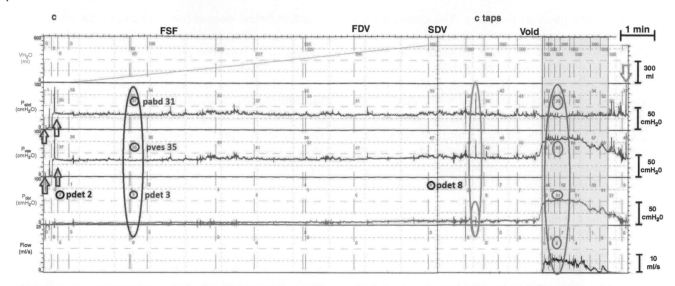

Figure 1.9 Features to look out for when looking at a complete trace done by someone else. The record shows continuous tracings recorded from a male patient aged 55 years, displayed in a manner consistent with International Continence Society recommendations. The abdominal pressure p_{abd} is shown in red and the vesical bladder pressure p_{ves} in blue. These are continuously subtracted ($p_{ves} - p_{abd}$) to give the detrusor p_{det}, in green. Also shown are the volume instilled in orange and flow rate in black. The sequence of the traces is appropriate, with p_{ves}, p_{det}, and flow in the lower half. Axes, units, and timescale are shown. Filling cystometry precedes permission to void (indicated with 'void'), and the pressure-flow study (PFS) follows it. The zero reference point is atmospheric pressure (purple arrows), so when the transducers are connected to the patient (blue arrows), there is an obvious rise in p_{abd} and p_{ves}, referred to as 'resting pressures' – the blue oval indicates the resting pressures for this patient at one timepoint. Coughs (indicated with 'c') are used to check that p_{abd} and p_{ves} detect a short spike of pressure (larger green oval) and that the p_{det} has a deflection which is equal above and below the line, the biphasic artefact (smaller green oval). It is important to check pressure recording with a cough at the start of filling and at other times if there is doubt about recording quality during filling. A cough is also needed before (green oval) and after (green arrow) the PFS to give confidence in the pressures recorded when voiding. Sensations are reported by the patient and annotated on the trace. First sensation of bladder filling (FSF) is the feeling the patient has, during filling cystometry, when he/she first becomes aware of the bladder filling. First desire to void (FDV) is the feeling that would lead the patient to pass urine at the next convenient moment, but voiding can be delayed if necessary. SDV is a persistent desire to void without the fear of leakage. A provocation was applied to try to elicit detrusor overactivity by making the sound of running water 'taps'; no change in p_{ves} or p_{det} was seen, so this patient had a stable detrusor. In the PFS, the key parameters derive from the time of maximum flow rate (Q_{max}), highlighted in orange (calculations derived from this type of data are discussed in Chapter 14). *Source*: Drake [15].

Chapter 16). Early referral to neurology is important, even if no concrete finding is made. Most neurologists do *not* recommend that urologists request imaging without prior discussion with a neurologist. This is due to the additional delay and to ensure that the correct investigation(s) are ordered. A summary algorithm produced by the ICS is shown in Figure 1.8. An example case is described in Chapter 16 (Figure 16.26).

How a Urodynamic Trace Should Be Presented

The ICS has standardised the process of urodynamics [19, 20], and throughout this book, we will repeatedly refer to the crucial importance of these documents and other ICS Standardisations. One of the key requirements is to ensure that traces are displayed in a way that they can be interpreted by someone who was not at the test, without the need for explanation by anyone else. This is equivalent to the presentation of an electrocardiogram (ECG), since any cardiologist or appropriately trained healthcare professional would expect a standardised presentation, enabling them to interpret the traces.

In this book, we try to comply with ICS recommendations throughout. In general, we display traces in a manner consistent with Figure 1.9, though older example traces may not fully comply. Some of the most useful things to check include:

- *What is displayed?* Typically, this will be two recorded pressures, p_{abd} and p_{ves}, a calculated p_{det}, flow and volume instilled. The p_{ves} and p_{det} traces should be plotted below the others (since they are most important, and high pressure might disappear off the top of the page).
- *Are the axes labelled?* Are the units stated and the volume range clear? We try to colour code our traces, so red (rectal) lines correspond to abdominal pressure and blue (bladder) lines correspond to vesical pressure.
- *Was the test set-up with zero set at atmospheric pressure?* This can be deduced if the pressures in p_{ves} and p_{abd} are zero and flat if opened to atmosphere (because atmospheric

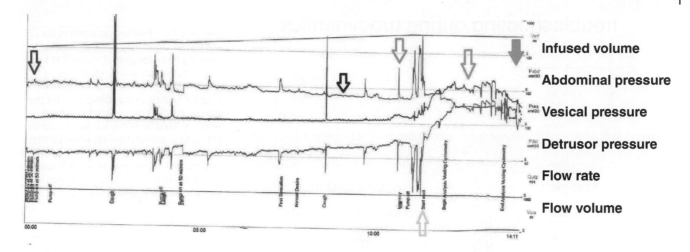

Figure 1.10 Examples of some of the quality control issues that need to be identified during urodynamics. Purple arrow: pressures set to zero while recording from patient, not to atmosphere. Black arrow: downward pressure drift in abdominal pressure. Blue arrows, open arrow: cough before void which is only picked up in the abdominal pressure; closed arrow: lack of cough test after conclusion of the void. Yellow arrow: start of void. Green arrow: drop in abdominal pressure during void. Vesical pressure shows a lack of fine detail and poor cough spikes, without a flush through needed to attempt remedial action. *Source*: Aiello et al. [21].

pressure fluctuates very little). If recording was not started before zeroing, the pressures in p_{ves} and p_{abd} should begin within the normal resting pressure range.

- Once recording from the patient starts, is there movement in the lines as expected, due to the patient breathing, speaking, and moving?
- *Are there annotations?* These are crucial, indicating when events such as provocation tests, sensations, and instructions happened. Without these, the test is uninterpretable. For example, if 'permission to void' is not annotated, a detrusor pressure change accompanied by flow could be either DO incontinence or voiding.
- *Are there checks of recording reliability?* Coughs done during the course of filling, and before and after voiding, help confirm that the recorded pressures can be trusted; the spike associated with a cough should be similar in amplitude in both the p_{ves} and p_{abd} lines, and measures should be taken to resolve them if not (usually a flush through of the transducer and catheter with the smaller spike).
- *Are there provocation tests aimed at reproducing symptoms?* For example, a sequence of high amplitude coughs in quick succession is a means of eliciting USI.

If part of a trace is selectively shown to illustrate a point in this book, we describe the circumstances so that the reader can appreciate what has occurred.

Adhering to High Standards

Disappointingly, the urodynamic community often fails to meet the expectations of the ICS standards [21]. The issues are discussed extensively throughout this book. As described in the preceding section, it is important to ensure that traces are presented in such a way that they can be verified by someone not present at the test. Any major errors must be identified (Figure 1.10). Failure to do this in some centres has led to a deeply unsatisfactory situation that many surgeons simply accept the urodynamic report at face value. This ultimately means that the urodynamic technician can have considerable influence on treatment choice, without necessarily realising it. One particularly problematic issue is failure to identify for an artefact affecting the maximum flow rate (Q_{max}) value, and using this uncorrected value to calculate important information like the BOO index, thus coming up with a wrong value. The urodynamicist _must_ look at the trace, and if an artefact is present, the cursor must be moved so that the values (Q_{max}, and hence $p_{detQmax}$) are taken from a spot not affected by spurious influences (see Chapter 6). This is often not done in many established units [21], and the result potentially can mean a wrong diagnosis and consequently a risk of inappropriate surgery.

Many units actually have a very poor understanding of urodynamic techniques, quality control, and interpretation [21]. One extraordinary weakness is a substantial lack of understanding of DUA; the majority of sites get this wrong or fail to comment on it at all (Table 1.2). This gives a risk of misdiagnosis and consequently the potential that some people could undergo surgery inappropriately.

The responsibility placed on the urodynamicist to achieve a meaningful test has a couple of implications for how to practice:

Troubleshooting during urodynamics

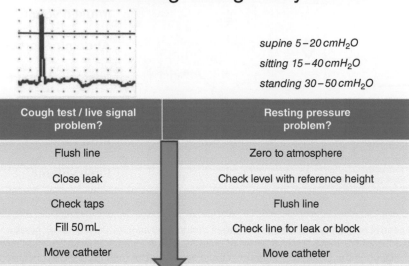

supine 5–20 cmH$_2$O

sitting 15–40 cmH$_2$O

standing 30–50 cmH$_2$O

Cough test / live signal problem?	Resting pressure problem?
Flush line	Zero to atmosphere
Close leak	Check level with reference height
Check taps	Flush line
Fill 50 mL	Check line for leak or block
Move catheter	Move catheter
Change catheter	Change catheter

Figure 1.11 Two key parameters are scrutinised routinely throughout the running of a urodynamic study. The first is the resting pressures, which are affected by the position of the patient (supine, seated, or standing). Second, the pressure spikes generated by a cough, which should be of similar amplitude in the vesical and abdominal lines. Spotting when things are not recording properly is crucial, and a sequence of steps taken to deal with issues in either parameter is illustrated. More details are given in Chapter 19.

1) During the test, the traces must constantly be reviewed so that any problems can be identified and dealt with on the spot. We refer to this as 'troubleshooting'. It is described in detail in Chapter 19, and a brief summary is given in Figure 1.11.
2) If, despite best efforts, the test does not proceed smoothly, or the patient's symptoms were not reproduced during the test, then that must be stated clearly in the report. This can happen in any unit, and willingness to concede a test was unsuccessful is a vital protection for the patient.

It is always necessary to stay alert. First, even experienced urodynamics practitioners can make unexpected mistakes from a lapse in concentration, as exemplified in Figure 1.12. Second, unexpected challenges can crop

Table 1.2 Prevalence rates of the urodynamic observation of DO and pressure-flow diagnosis of BOO and DU, comparing categorisations by hospitals ('sites') with central expert review.

	Categorisation by central review			Categorisation by sites		
Observation/diagnosis	Prevalence	Correct (*n*)	Correct (%)	Incorrect (*n*)	Uncategorised (*n*)	Non-correct (%)
DO present	46/99 (46.4%)	26/46	57	1/46	19/46	43
DO absent	53/99 (53.6%)	27/53	51	2/53	24/53	49
BOO present (BOOI >40)	55/107 (51.4%)	39/55	71	1/55	15/55	29
BOO equivocal (BOOI 20–40)	14/107 (13.1%)	11/14	79	3/14[a]	0/14	21
Unobstructed (BOOI <40)	19/107 (15.9%)	8/19	42	6/19	5/19	58
Unable to derive BOOI	19/107 (15.9%)	N/A	N/A	15/19[b]	4/19	1
DU present (BCI <100)	27/107 (25.2%)	14/27	52	2/27	11/27	48
DU absent (BCI >100)	59/107 (55.1%)	18/59	31	1/59	40/59	69
Unable to derive BCI	21/107 (19.6%)	N/A	N/A	4/19[c]	15/19	1

Abbreviations: BCI: Bladder Contractility Index; BOO: bladder outlet obstruction; BOOI: BOO Index; DO: detrusor overactivity; DU: detrusor underactivity; N/A: not applicable.

Note: 'Uncategorised' indicates that the site provided the trace but did not make a comment on diagnosis.

The 'non-correct' column indicates what proportion of diagnoses the hospital got wrong ('incorrect') or failed to comment on ('uncategorised').

[a] Categorised as obstructed in two, unobstructed in one.

[b] Categorised as obstructed in 10.

[c] Categorised as DU in two. *Source*: Reproduced with permission from [21].

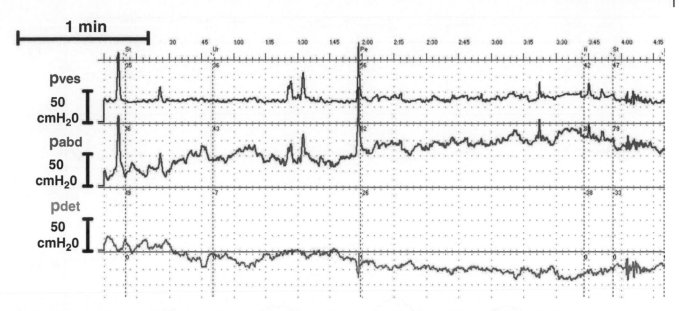

Figure 1.12 An unusual error (fortunately) is to connect the filling pump to the rectal catheter. When the healthcare practitioner asked the patient if she felt her bladder filling, the reply was 'no, but I really want to open my bowels'. The steady climbing p_{abd} is clear, and it is responsible for the falling p_{det} over the time illustrated. This is an old trace; modern traces do not have p_{ves} placed at the top.

up, for which adaptations will need to be made (Figure 1.13).

Safety of the Urodynamics Staff

The Covid-19 pandemic of 2020 highlights a potential for communication of respiratory-transmitted illness from patient to practitioner, or vice versa. Alterations across the entire healthcare system became necessary. Urodynamics is affected, since physical proximity and use of coughs to check pressure recording or provoke symptoms could increase the risk of respiratory pathogen transmission. We have therefore adapted practice to mitigate some of these concerns (Figure 1.14) [22]. Single-use surgical face masks and eye protection are recommended for both patients and staff, in addition to the normal use of single-use gloves and aprons by the urodynamicist. There is no need for patients to wear gloves, but patients will either use hand-gel or wash their hands for 20 seconds before entering and leaving the urodynamics room. Local and national guidelines should be followed with regard to personal protective equipment (PPE). Wherever possible, a distance of 2 m should be maintained between staff and patient. Clearly, for procedures such as catheterisation and examination of the patient, this is impossible. Precautions must, therefore, be taken in the form of PPE as above and adjusting elements of the test to allow observation from a distance of at least 2 m. Where urinary leakage needs to be observed, especially in women, the patient could be asked to stand or squat over a pad on the floor, rather than sit on the flowmeter, in order that leakage can be seen from further away.

During video-urodynamics, fluoroscopic screening can provide evidence of urethral leakage and will be sufficient for a diagnosis of USI. Coughing should be kept to an absolute minimum and always with a mask in place. Quality control can be carried out effectively by a Valsalva manoeuvre or even by gentle external pressure on the abdomen by the patient. Valsalva manoeuvre or other physical provocations can be attempted first, and only after that, all other provocations having failed, would the patient be asked to cough,. In that case, the cough must be directed away from others in the room and shielded by an elbow or by a hand-held tissue that is then discarded, since the mask itself must not be touched during use. A period for cleaning the room is needed between each patient.

A Brief History of Urodynamics

Interest in the hydrodynamics of micturition started with the early cystometric studies of the nineteenth century, but it was the advent of electronics that acted as the catalyst for modern urodynamic studies. In 1956, von Garrelts described a simple practical apparatus, using a pressure transducer, to record the volume of urine voided as a function of time. By differentiation, urine flow rates could be calculated. His work stimulated a revival of interest in cystometry because it was then possible to record the bladder pressure and the urine flow rate simultaneously during voiding. As a result, normal and obstructed micturition could be defined in terms of these measurements [23], and a formula was applied to express urethral resistance [24].

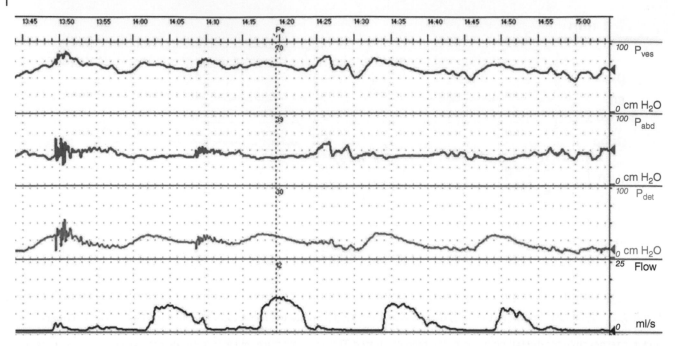

Figure 1.13 This pressure-flow study of a male patient shows a grossly abnormal interrupted flow pattern, yet his pre-urodynamics flow test showed a normal flow pattern and good flow rate. The problem was a consequence of his p_{ves} catheter; as he passed urine, some of it tracked along the catheter so that it was carried beyond the rim of the funnel. When it fell off the catheter, his foot happened to be underneath, which was very distracting for him, causing him to inhibit his voiding contraction. Each time he restarted voiding, the same happened, leading to repeated interruptions. Since this event, we have been careful with routing the p_{ves} catheter. (This is another old trace with p_{ves} placed at the top.)

Enhorning [25] measured bladder and urethral pressures simultaneously with a specially designed catheter, and he termed the pressure difference between them the 'urethral closure pressure'. He demonstrated that a reduction of intraurethral pressure occurred several seconds prior to detrusor contraction at the initiation of voiding. This appeared to relate to the relaxation of the pelvic floor, consistent with the electromyogram (EMG) studies of Franksson and Peterson [26].

Application of urodynamic investigations in the clinical field soon followed. Radiological studies of the lower urinary tract, using the image intensifier and cine or videotape recordings, were already established, and their value in the assessment of micturition disorders had been described [27]. It was a relatively simple step to combine cystourethrography with pressure-flow measurements [2]. Sophisticated techniques followed, for example, using EMG recordings of the pelvic floor, particularly for neurogenic bladder problems [28]. These clinical studies during the 1970s emphasised the need to investigate the function as well as the anatomical structure of the lower urinary tract, when evaluating micturition disorders. Urodynamics was becoming established as a necessary service rather than a research tool.

As these technical developments progressed, there was an increasing awareness of the clinical problem of urinary incontinence. Caldwell [29], working in Exeter in the UK, initiated considerable interest in the subject because he approached the treatment of incontinent patients with electronic implants. In his sphincter research unit, a small receiver was developed that could be placed subcutaneously in the abdominal wall and activated by a small external radio-frequency transmitter. Platinum iridium electrodes led down to the pelvic floor muscles, which could be stimulated. Other new techniques advocated at this time included pelvic floor stimulation, including use of a variety of external electronic devices which could be placed in the anal canal or vagina to stimulate pelvic floor contraction [30, 31].

Both technique and terminology should be standardised, to allow for interpretation of findings and so that others may understand and interpret the results from any urodynamic unit. To facilitate this, the ICS in 1973 set up a Standardisation Committee, which has produced reports on the terminology of lower urinary tract function. The first six reports were collated in 1988 and comprehensively rewritten. Undoubtedly, two key documents published in 2002 which served as a platform in the development of

Figure 1.14 Adaptations to urodynamic practice in response to the Coronavirus pandemic. PPE: Personal Protective Equipment. UDS: Urodynamics. *Source*: Hashim et al. [22].

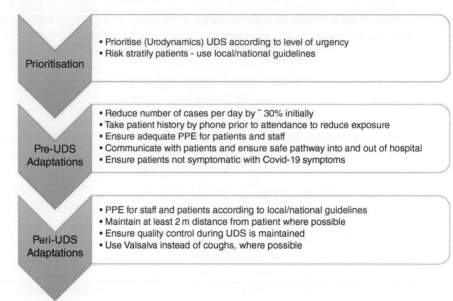

Prioritisation
- Prioritise (Urodynamics) UDS according to level of urgency
- Risk stratify patients - use local/national guidelines

Pre-UDS Adaptations
- Reduce number of cases per day by ˜ 30% initially
- Take patient history by phone prior to attendance to reduce exposure
- Ensure adequate PPE for patients and staff
- Communicate with patients and ensure safe pathway into and out of hospital
- Ensure patients not symptomatic with Covid-19 symptoms

Peri-UDS Adaptations
- PPE for staff and patients according to local/national guidelines
- Maintain at least 2 m distance from patient where possible
- Ensure quality control during UDS is maintained
- Use Valsalva instead of coughs, where possible

professional terminology and practice were the Standardisation of Lower Urinary Tract Function [32] and Good Urodynamic Practices [19]. The latter document has been extended and updated [20]. In addition, the International Children's Continence Society (ICCS) has published standards for the paediatric population [33–35].

In recent years, the importance of modern-day governance led to the ICS placing the standardisation process under a Steering Committee, which oversees independent working groups and follows clear governance procedures and an evidence-based approach [36]. Subsequently, the Standardisation documents now undergo a process of iterative and ongoing review and development, including documents for chronic pelvic pain [37], neurogenic LUTD [38], female LUTS [39], pelvic organ prolapse [40, 41], nocturia [42], and urodynamic equipment [43].

These ICS and ICCS Standards aim to facilitate comparison of results by investigators who use urodynamic methods. Written publications are expected to acknowledge the use of these standards by stating: 'Methods, definitions and units conform to the standards proposed by the International Continence Society except where specifically noted'. This book applies the ICS Standardisations throughout.

Summary

In the basic assessment, the following are important:

- Establish a rapport with the patient
- Look at the symptom score
- Review previous treatments
- Consider bowel, gynaecological, and sexual function
- Identify medical problems and medications
- Consider possibility of neurological disease or malignancy
- General examination
- Examination features suggestive of wider problems, e.g. occult neurology or malignancy
- Focussed lower urinary tract examination, abdominal and internal

This comprehensive evaluation allows the investigator to formulate their urodynamic questions:

1) 'What do I want to know about this patient?'
    a) 'What is wrong with storage, what is wrong with voiding?'
    b) 'What is wrong with the bladder, what is wrong with the bladder outlet?'
2) 'Which urodynamic investigations need to be performed to define this patient's problems?'
3) 'Is the investigation likely to be of benefit to the patient?'
4) 'Is urodynamics able to make a reliable diagnosis?'

Having run the test, the report should be written in detail, mentioning full aspects of the technical procedure, but also answering the following:

- Did the urodynamic studies reproduce the patient's complaints, and did the complaints correlate with known urodynamic features?
- Does the report make sense in the context of the patient's symptoms and preceding tests?

- Can urodynamics decide which abnormality is the most significant if more than one is detected?

- Can the features mentioned in the report be identified on the plotted traces, and is anything visible on the traces not mentioned in the report?

References

1. Abrams, P., Cardozo, L., Fall, M. et al. Standardisation Sub-committee of the International Continence, S (2002). The standardisation of terminology of lower urinary tract function: report from the standardisation sub-committee of the International Continence Society. *Neurourol. Urodyn.* 21: 167–178.
2. Bates, C.P., Whiteside, C.G., and Turner-Warwick, R. (1970). Synchronous cine-pressure-flow-cysto-urethrography with special reference to stress and urge incontinence. *Br. J. Urol.* 42: 714–723.
3. Thomas, A.W., Cannon, A., Bartlett, E. et al. (2004). The natural history of lower urinary tract dysfunction in men: the influence of detrusor underactivity on the outcome after transurethral resection of the prostate with a minimum 10-year urodynamic follow-up. *BJU Int.* 93: 745–750.
4. Reynard, J., Lim, C., and Abrams, P. (1996). Significance of intermittency in men with lower urinary tract symptoms. *Urology* 47: 491–496.
5. Reynard, J.M., Lim, C., Peters, T.J., and Abrams, P. (1996). The significance of terminal dribbling in men with lower urinary tract symptoms. *Br. J. Urol.* 77: 705–710.
6. Andersen, J.T., Nordling, J., and Walter, S. (1979). Prostatism. I. The correlation between symptoms, cystometric and urodynamic findings. *Scand. J. Urol. Nephrol.* 13: 229–236.
7. Jarvis, G.J., Hall, S., Stamp, S. et al. (1980). An assessment of urodynamic examination in incontinent women. *Br. J. Obstet. Gynaecol.* 87: 893–896.
8. Powell, P.H., Shepherd, A.M., Lewis, P., and Feneley, R.C. (1981). The accuracy of clinical diagnoses assessed urodynamically. *Prog. Clin. Biol. Res.* 78: 201–203.
9. Abrams, P., Avery, K., Gardener, N., and Donovan, J. (2006). The international consultation on incontinence modular questionnaire: www.iciq.net. *J. Urol.* 175: 1063–1066; discussion 1066.
10. Selman, L.E., Ochieng, C.A., Lewis, A.L. et al. (2019). Recommendations for conducting invasive urodynamics for men with lower urinary tract symptoms: qualitative interview findings from a large randomized controlled trial (UPSTREAM). *Neurourol. Urodyn.* 38: 320–329.
11. Wei, D.Y. and Drake, M.J. (2016). Undiagnosed neurological disease as a potential cause of male lower urinary tract symptoms. *Curr. Opin. Urol.* 26: 11–16.
12. Chapple, C.R., Osman, N.I., Birder, L. et al. (2018). Terminology report from the International Continence Society (ICS) working group on underactive bladder (UAB). *Neurourol. Urodyn.* 37 (8): 2928–2931.
13. Garnett, S., Swithinbank, L., Ellis-Jones, J., and Abrams, P. (2009). The long-term natural history of overactive bladder symptoms due to idiopathic detrusor overactivity in women. *BJU Int.* 104 (7): 948–953.
14. Thomas, A.W., Cannon, A., Bartlett, E. et al. (2005). The natural history of lower urinary tract dysfunction in men: minimum 10-year urodynamic followup of transurethral resection of prostate for bladder outlet obstruction. *J. Urol.* 174: 1887–1891.
15. Drake, M.J. (2018). Fundamentals of terminology in lower urinary tract function. *Neurourol. Urodyn.* 37: S13–S19.
16. Gammie, A. and Drake, M.J. (2018). The fundamentals of uroflowmetry practice, based on International Continence Society good urodynamic practices recommendations. *Neurourol. Urodyn.* 37: S44–S49.
17. Drake, M.J., Doumouchtsis, S.K., Hashim, H., and Gammie, A. (2018). Fundamentals of urodynamic practice, based on International Continence Society good urodynamic practices recommendations. *Neurourol. Urodyn.* 37: S50–S60.
18. De Ridder, D., Van Der Aa, F., Debruyne, J. et al. (2013). Consensus guidelines on the neurologist's role in the management of neurogenic lower urinary tract dysfunction in multiple sclerosis. *Clin. Neurol. Neurosurg.* 115: 2033–2040.
19. Schafer, W., Abrams, P., Liao, L. et al. (2002). Good urodynamic practices: uroflowmetry, filling cystometry, and pressure-flow studies. *Neurourol. Urodyn.* 21: 261–274.
20. Rosier, P., Schaefer, W., Lose, G. et al. (2017). International Continence Society good urodynamic practices and terms 2016: urodynamics, uroflowmetry, cystometry, and pressure-flow study. *Neurourol. Urodyn.* 36: 1243–1260.
21. Aiello, M., Jelski, J., Lewis, A. et al. (2020). Quality control of uroflowmetry and urodynamic data from two large multicenter studies of male lower urinary tract symptoms. *Neurourol. Urodyn.* 39 (4): 1170–1177.

22. Hashim, H., Thomas, L., Gammie, A. et al. (2020). Good urodynamic practice adaptations during the COVID-19 pandemic. *Neurourol. Urodyn.* 39 (6): 1897–1901.

23. Claridge, M. (1966). Analyses of obstructed micturition. *Ann. R. Coll. Surg. Engl.* 39: 30–53.

24. Smith, J.C. (1968). Urethral resistance to micturition. *Br. J. Urol.* 40: 125–156.

25. Enhorning, G. (1961). Simultaneous recording of intravesical and intra-urethral pressure. A study on urethral closure in normal and stress incontinent women. *Acta Chir. Scand. Suppl.* (Suppl. 276): 1–68.

26. Franksson, C. and Petersen, I. (1955). Electromyographic investigation of disturbances in the striated muscle of the urethral sphincter. *Br. J. Urol.* 27: 154–161.

27. Turner-Warwick, R. and Whiteside, C.G. (1970). Investigation and management of bladder neck dysfunction. In: Modern Trends in Urology 3 (ed. E. Riches), 295–311. London: Butterworth.

28. Thomas, D.G., Smallwood, R., and Graham, D. (1975). Urodynamic observations following spinal trauma. *Br. J. Urol.* 47: 161–175.

29. Caldwell, K.P. (1967). The treatment of incontinence by electronic implants. Hunterian lecture delivered at the Royal College of Surgeons of England on 8th December 1966. *Ann. R. Coll. Surg. Engl.* 41: 447–459.

30. Alexander, S. and Rowan, D. (1968). An electric pessary for stress incontinence. *Lancet* 1: 728.

31. Hopkinson, B.R. and Lightwood, R. (1967). Electrical treatment of incontinence. *Br. J. Surg.* 54: 802–805.

32. Abrams, P., Cardozo, L., Fall, M. et al. (2002). The standardisation of terminology of lower urinary tract function: report from the standardisation sub-committee of the International Continence Society. *Neurourol. Urodyn.* 21: 167–178.

33. Bauer, S.B., Nijman, R.J., Drzewiecki, B.A. et al. International Children's Continence Society Standardization, S (2015). International children's continence society standardization report on urodynamic studies of the lower urinary tract in children. *Neurourol. Urodyn.* 34: 640–647.

34. Austin, P.F., Bauer, S.B., Bower, W. et al. (2016). The standardization of terminology of lower urinary tract function in children and adolescents: update report from the standardization committee of the international Children's continence society. *Neurourol. Urodyn.* 35: 471–481.

35. Neveus, T., von Gontard, A., Hoebeke, P. et al. (2006). The standardization of terminology of lower urinary tract function in children and adolescents: report from the Standardisation Committee of the International Children's Continence Society. *J. Urol.* 176: 314–324.

36. Rosier, P.F., de Ridder, D., Meijlink, J. et al. (2012). Developing evidence-based standards for diagnosis and management of lower urinary tract or pelvic floor dysfunction. *Neurourol. Urodyn.* 31: 621–624.

37. Doggweiler, R., Whitmore, K.E., Meijlink, J.M. et al. (2016). A standard for terminology in chronic pelvic pain syndromes: a report from the chronic pelvic pain working group of the International Continence Society. *Neurourol. Urodyn.* 36 (4): 984–1008.

38. Gajewski, J.B., Schurch, B., Hamid, R. et al. (2017). An International Continence Society (ICS) report on the terminology for adult neurogenic lower urinary tract dysfunction (ANLUTD). *Neurourol. Urodyn.* 37 (3): 1152–1161.

39. Haylen, B.T., de Ridder, D., Freeman, R.M. et al. (2010). An International Urogynecological Association (IUGA)/International Continence Society (ICS) joint report on the terminology for female pelvic floor dysfunction. *Neurourol. Urodyn.* 29: 4–20.

40. Haylen, B.T., Maher, C.F., Barber, M.D. et al. (2016). An International Urogynecological Association (IUGA)/International Continence Society (ICS) joint report on the terminology for female pelvic organ prolapse (POP). *Neurourol. Urodyn.* 35: 137–168.

41. Toozs-Hobson, P., Freeman, R., Barber, M. et al. International Urogynecological, A. and International Continence, S (2012). An International Urogynecological Association (IUGA)/International Continence Society (ICS) joint report on the terminology for reporting outcomes of surgical procedures for pelvic organ prolapse. *Neurourol. Urodyn.* 31: 415–421.

42. Hashim, H., Blanker, M.H., Drake, M.J. et al. (2019). Wein A: International Continence Society (ICS) report on the terminology for nocturia and nocturnal lower urinary tract function. *Neurourol. Urodyn.* 38 (2): 499–508.

43. Gammie, A., Clarkson, B., Constantinou, C. et al. (2014). International Continence Society guidelines on urodynamic equipment performance. *Neurourol. Urodyn.* 33: 370–379.

44. Roy, H.A., Nettleton, J., Blain, C. et al. (2020). Assessment of patients with lower urinary tract symptoms where an undiagnosed neurological disease is suspected: a report from an International Continence Society consensus working group. *Neurourol. Urodyn.* 39 (8): 2535–2543.

2

Applied Anatomy and Physiology

Chendrimada Madhu[1] and Marcus Drake[2]

[1] *Department of Women's Health, The Chilterns, Southmead Hospital, Bristol, UK*
[2] *Translational Health Sciences, Bristol Medical School, Southmead Hospital, Bristol, UK*

CONTENTS

Introduction

Urodynamic investigations developed because of dissatisfaction with the assessment of patients and treatment results when management was based on examination of anatomical abnormalities. Urodynamics attempts to relate physiology to anatomy so that both function and structure are considered alongside each other. A sound knowledge of anatomy and physiology form the basis for the effective assessment and treatment of patients. In addition, this knowledge can be used to evaluate the role of urodynamic studies critically in assessing patients with lower urinary tract symptoms (LUTS). The lower urinary tract comprises the urinary structures of the bladder and bladder outlet (Figure 2.1).

In men, the close relationship to genital structures also makes the phrase 'genitourinary tract' appropriate (Figure 2.2). Although the bladder and urethra are described separately below, it should be remembered that they normally act as a functional unit. During urine storage, the bladder is quiescent, and the urethra contracted, and vice versa when voiding. This co-operative function is imposed by the central nervous system (CNS) control, ensuring synergy of the lower urinary tract.

Upper Urinary Tract

The upper urinary tract comprises the kidneys and ureters (Figure 2.3). Kidneys are excretory organs which have a vital role in homeostasis. They ensure appropriate salt and water levels, control acid–base balance, and eliminate water-soluble toxins. This is achieved by varying the composition and volume of urine to reflect overall body requirements when healthy. Water elimination is known as diuresis, and there is typically a production of urine at a rate of at least 0.5 ml/kg body weight every hour. 'Forced diuresis', i.e. absolute maximum rate of urine production to get rid of a large overload of water, is about 900 ml/hour [1]. Elimination of excess salt is known as natriuresis, and this will also increase urine production rate because the salt requires water to dissolve it. The control of how fast urine

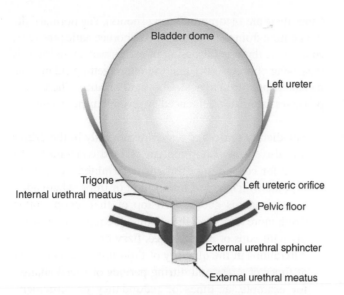

Figure 2.1 The lower urinary tract joins the upper urinary tract at the ureteric orifices. Its main structures are the bladder and the bladder outlet. The trigone sits in the bladder base, demarcated by the ureteric orifices and the internal urethral meatus. The bladder outlet is the urethra, which runs from the internal to the external urethral meatus. The external urethral sphincter in women is a horseshoe-shaped structure, mainly sitting dorsally.

is produced is determined by key hormones, notably anti-diuretic hormone (ADH), which is responsible for retaining water if a person is dehydrated. ADH levels are reduced where someone has surplus water to eliminate. Atrial natriuretic peptide (ANP) and brain natriuretic peptide (BNP) are present when there is excess salt to dispose of, a process that increases rate of urine production like diuresis.

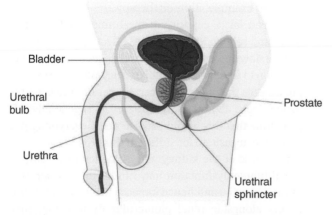

Figure 2.2 The male genitourinary tract. Key differences from the lower urinary tract in women include the entry points of the ejaculatory ducts (see Figure 2.12), the presence of the prostate between the internal meatus and the external urethral sphincter, the circular structure of the sphincter, and the substantially longer urethra.

Where there is kidney disease, rate of production of urine may be altered, depending on which part of the kidney is affected. The glomeruli are the structures in the kidney responsible for filtering the blood, so if they are diseased (reduced glomerular filtration rate), water will be retained (leading to body swelling and increased weight), toxins will accumulate (increased serum creatinine and urea levels), and rate of urine production will be reduced. The kidney tubules reabsorb water and nutrients from filtered urine. In diseases selectively affecting the kidney tubules, failure of reabsorption leads to water loss and hence increased urine production. This can result in dehydration (so the person may compensate by increasing their fluid intake), but serum creatinine is normal (or low). Chronic kidney disease (CKD) generally affects both glomeruli and tubules, so it will have features of both problems. Patients with CKD or tubular disease will have a high rate of urine production (and compensate for this by increasing fluid intake). This can also happen if the tubules become insensitive to ADH (nephrogenic diabetes insipidus), which can be a feature of treatment of psychiatric conditions with lithium. Central diabetes insipidus is another cause of water loss, in this case, due to impaired production of ADH.

Natriuresis can be severe when asleep in patients with obstructive sleep apnoea (OSA), due to high production of ANP; this is a major cause of nocturia. If someone is losing water or salt and presents for treatment of increased voiding frequency, it is not appropriate to advise fluid restriction, since they could become dangerously dehydrated. Drinking due to a constant feeling of thirst is the key point to ascertain in the history. Other notable medical factors include fluid and salt retention, leading to ankle swelling, as is seen in heart failure in particular, as this retained fluid may be excreted when the patient lies down.

Osmotic diuresis is a process of water loss as a result of high amounts of solutes in the urine. An important example is poorly controlled diabetes mellitus, in which very high sugar levels spill over into the urine and, consequently, increase the volume passed. This is rarely a cause of nocturia, but it could happen if someone is on a treatment schedule which is insufficient to control their overnight sugar levels. A spot test of daytime sugar levels would not necessarily identify that, but a glycosylated haemoglobin blood test would probably be abnormal.

These influences on urine production are fundamental factors determining voiding frequency, along with increased awareness (see below) and reduced bladder storage capacity (discussed throughout this book). A schematic summary is given in Figure 2.4.

Most people have two kidneys (1% are born with one kidney), which drain into the urinary bladder along the ureters

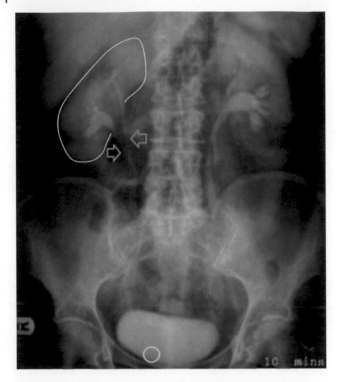

Figure 2.3 The upper urinary tract comprises the kidneys and ureters. In this intravenous urogram (IVU), the right kidney is outlined in white. On both sides, the ureter is partially duplicated, and the two duplex parts for the right ureter are indicated by green arrows. The majority of people have one ureter on each side, but duplication can happen to one or both sides and ranges from partial to complete. The lower limit of the upper urinary tract is the vesicoureteric junction (VUJ). In this IVU, the VUJs cannot be seen as they are hidden by contrast in the bladder, but the approximate location of the right VUJ is indicated by the green circle. This film was taken 10 minutes after contrast injection and shows just how quickly the bladder can fill in a well-hydrated patient receiving a diuretic injection prior to administration of the contrast. *Source*: Marcus Drake.

(usually one on each side). The ureters enter the wall of the urinary bladder obliquely for about 2 cm and open by slit-like apertures at the lateral angles of the trigone. This oblique course through the bladder musculature helps the terminal ureters to occlude, thus acting like a one-way valve, the vesicoureteric junction (VUJ). The VUJ allows urine to enter the bladder and prevents backwards return of urine (vesicoureteric reflux, or VUR). VUR can be a result of various pathologies, notably embryological problems, surgical damage, and high bladder pressures. When VUR is severe, it prevents efficient drainage of the kidney, which can lead to CKD.

Alterations in Fluid Excretion

Commonly, 24-hour urine output lies between 1 and 3 l, and 1.5 l (i.e. 1500 ml) is a perfectly healthy value for most people. This equates to an average output of about 1 ml per minute

(since there are 1440 minutes per 24 hours). The normal daily fluid output from the kidneys reflects homeostatic processes, comprising diuresis (disposing of excess water), natriuresis (disposing of excess salt), and excretion (getting rid of toxic metabolic products) to achieve overall balance. These basic processes are hugely influenced by several further factors:

1) The dietary sources of water are not only in the drinks but also in the water content of food consumed. The need for consuming drinks is determined by osmoreceptors, which trigger a sensation of thirst where additional water is needed. On top of that, people often drink more than their thirst-guided requirements, notably with cups of tea or coffee, fizzy drinks, or alcohol. Alterations in the quantity of fluid imbibed may occur at times of stress and during periods of social change, for example, at times of redundancy or retirement. Many people follow spurious trends like 'drinking more is healthier', but some drink more specifically because of advice to do so (notably those with a history of kidney stones or urinary tract infections [UTIs]).

2) Allowance is also needed for the loss of water elsewhere from the body, notably sweating, in the faeces, and water vapour in breath.

3) Overnight, there is normally a reduction in the rate of urine output due to circadian hormonal control (increased ADH secretion overnight). Approximately 80% of the 24 hour volume is excreted during the waking hours, and this nocturnal reduction therefore means it is not necessary to empty the bladder at night in the normal condition. Abnormalities of the normal circadian rhythm may be induced primarily by relevant diseases, such as renal failure or heart failure, or be secondary to drugs used in the treatment of such conditions, for example, diuretic therapy.

4) There is a lot of capacity in the human body to store water and salt, and the processes affecting their balance may be slow and unpredictable. Consequently, it is rather common to find the bladder diary suggests the urine output exceeds the intake for a certain period. Provided the patient looks appropriately hydrated, it is generally safe to assume that this would balance out if everything was accurately measured for sufficient duration.

5) Any disease of the kidney will influence urine output. Renal tubule dysfunction may hinder the reabsorption of filtered urine and hence increase urine output. If this occurs alongside renal glomerular dysfunction, then the renal disease will show up in standard renal blood tests. However, some problems affecting the tubules are not associated with glomerular disease, notably diabetes insipidus. Here, the renal fluid handling may be abnormal, yet with normal renal function blood tests.

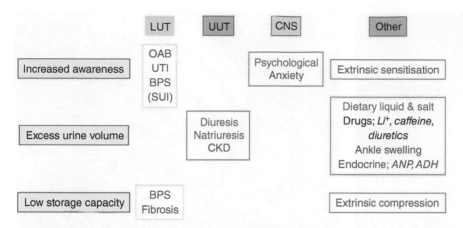

Figure 2.4 Influences on voiding frequency; how often someone passes urine is determined by amount of urine, storage capacity, and awareness, which are affected by normal functions (green text) and medical causes (red text), in a wide range of organ systems. Overactive bladder (OAB) and urinary tract infection (UTI) increase urinary tract sensation via bladder afferents (A-delta) and stress urinary incontinence (SUI) via urethral afferents. The bladder afferents can be sensitised by extrinsic inflammation, such as diverticular disease or gynaecological inflammation. Bladder pain syndrome (BPS) can do so via bladder afferents (gamma) and by reducing storage capacity. Chronic kidney disease (CKD) affects the ability of renal tubules to reabsorb filtered urine. Several hormones are relevant, notably atrial natriuretic peptide (ANP) which triggers salt loss (natriuresis) and anti-diuretic hormone (ADH) which controls water loss. Li+: Lithium. Extrinsic compression relates to the space-occupying effect of nearby organs; in the constrained space of the pelvis, this means less room for the bladder (see Figure 2.5). CNS: central nervous system; UUT: upper urinary tract.

6) Many medical conditions away from the urinary tract affect urine output due to effects on water or salt balance or endocrine function. Nocturnal polyuria in elderly men might reflect subclinical cardiac failure, leading to increased ANP released at night. ANP is also released in OSA, again causing severe nocturnal polyuria, and reversed by treating the patient's OSA with a continuous positive airway pressure (CPAP) machine.

7) Medications can be relevant, notably anything with a diuretic effect, e.g. furosemide or bumetanide. Lithium can cause nephrogenic diabetes insipidus.

8) The bladder may be a 'mirror of the mind', and psychological influences occasionally manifest themselves initially as urological symptoms. Such voiding patterns are often 'diagnoses of exclusion' following persistently negative urological studies. The frequency/volume chart (FVC) may show a high voiding frequency and sometimes nocturia, occurring at times of social and mental stress. Sometimes, nocturia is absent, despite high frequency during the day. Completing the bladder diary may lead the patient to recognise such influences.

The Urinary Bladder

The urinary bladder is a musculomembranous organ located in the bony pelvis (Figure 2.5) and acts as a reservoir of urine. The fundus of the empty bladder, which is entirely located in the front part of the pelvis, is separated from the rectum (posteriorly in the pelvis) by the rectovesical fascia in men or the vagina, cervix, and uterus in women. The superior surface of the bladder is covered with peritoneum. The inferior surface is in contact with the fascia covering the levator ani and obturator internus muscles. When distended, the upper part of the bladder rises up above the pubis (Figures 2.5 and 2.6) and lies between the peritoneum and the back wall of the rectus abdominis muscles (meaning that a suprapubic catheter can enter into the bladder without traversing the peritoneum). The bladder in the newborn infant is largely abdominal, and it gradually moves to the adult pelvic position by about nine years.

Within the bladder, there is an area of the base referred to as the trigone (Figure 2.1), which is the space between the two ureteric orifices and the internal urethral meatus. Here, the trigonal epithelium is firmly attached to the muscular layer. Two bands of oblique muscle fibres originating from the two VUJs, converging to the back of the prostate, are thought to help retain the oblique direction of the ureters with voiding, thus preventing VUR.

Elsewhere, in the greater part of the bladder, the urothelium is rather loosely attached with a submucosal layer comprising loose areolar tissue. This can make the urothelium sufficiently mobile that it can drift into the eyehole of a catheter and block it, interfering with drainage (urinary catheters) and pressure recording (urodynamic catheters). The urothelium is a non-glandular transitional epithelium,

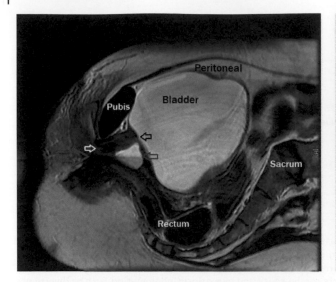
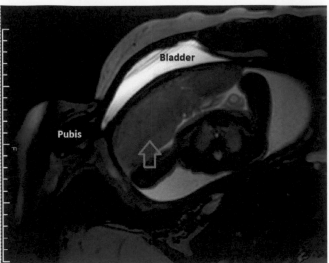

Figure 2.5 Anatomical relationships of the bladder scanned with magnetic resonance imaging (MRI) in the supine position in two women, one with a urethral diverticulum (left) and another with an augmented bladder during pregnancy. The pubis is in front of the lower part of the bladder and the urethra. When full, the bladder dome rises into the abdomen, with the top part (indicated by 'peritoneal') related to the peritoneal cavity. The non-peritoneal part is where a suprapubic catheter would normally be targeted (indicated by a green line). Black arrow: internal urethral meatus; white arrow: external urethral meatus, located in the vaginal vestibule (purple arrow). The blue arrow indicates the urethral diverticulum (containing a fluid level). Behind the urethra and bladder lies the vagina, which has the cervix and uterus superiorly. Space in the lesser pelvis, between pubis and sacrum, is constrained. Hence, any bulky tissue (fibroids, pregnancy) or fluid collection will compress and distort the bladder and could reduce capacity, as illustrated on the right. This woman has a bladder augmentation, so the bladder is tethered by the previous surgery. She will need a caesarean section, and the bladder lies directly in line with the access to the uterine lower segment, so specialist expertise will be needed to avoid catastrophic bladder damage. The placenta is indicated by the orange arrow. *Source*: Marcus Drake.

configured to be able to expand sufficiently to maintain waterproof lining properties so that it can protect the inside of the bladder over the wide range of volumes it routinely encounters. When empty, the loose attachment of the urothelium permits it to fold. The luminal aspect of the bladder is protected by a glycosaminoglycan layer attached to the superficial umbrella cells of the urothelium. This helps with the barrier properties and also gives some resistance to bacterial adhesion. Alongside its barrier role preventing water and toxins from reaching inner layers, the urothelium is metabolically active and able to release a range of active molecules, notably adenosine triphosphate (ATP) [2]. Since there are numerous afferent nerves just under the urothelium, the compounds released from it may influence sensory reporting from the bladder.

The muscular layer comprises smooth muscle, known as the detrusor (short for detrusor vesicae). In humans, it forms an interlacing meshwork of bundles, with fine nerve fibres interspersed throughout (Figure 2.7). These nerve fibres express acetylcholine (ACh) as their main transmitter, but they also contain other possible transmitters, notably ATP and peptides [4]. The role of these other transmitters is not fully understood, but the number of nerve fibres and the range of transmitters they express are markedly reduced in neurological disease (Figure 2.7) [4].

The detrusor and suburothelial layer have large numbers of a metabolically active cell type known as the 'interstitial cells'. These may mediate some aspects of neuromuscular transmission, sensory transduction (i.e. the process of turning a stimulus into nerve impulses), and muscle excitation [5].

The nerve fibres branch out within the connective tissue planes between the muscle bundles, from which they enter the bundles (Figure 2.8) in order to gain close access to the detrusor, which ensures the entire bundle can contract effectively in response to command from the spinal cord.

Notably, the role of the innervation is not solely for making the detrusor contract for voiding. It is also needed for suppressing spontaneous muscle activity. Once the nerve supply is removed, there is considerable movement evident in detrusor. This is very clear in the laboratory setting, where strips of muscle and isolated whole bladders show intriguing micromotions – localised contractions and elongations [6]. The micromotion activity is an important property for normal bladder function [7] and also provides a measure of compensation which can compensate for a small amount of denervation [8]. It may also explain why some people can get substantial urgency even if they do not have an associated change in bladder pressure (Figure 2.9). Overall, denervation may explain why some people experience both

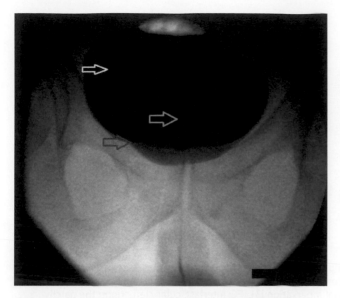

Figure 2.6 Relationship of the bladder to the pubis; X-ray taken during video urodynamics in a man in the standing position. The purple arrow indicates the top of the pubis. The green arrow is where a suprapubic catheter could be placed safely in someone slim who has not previously had abdominal surgery (ultrasound confirmation to ensure no bowel is in the way can be used to check safety of this location in other patients). The yellow arrow indicates an estimation of where the peritoneum crosses from the top of the bladder to the back of the rectus muscles; there is no indicator on an X-ray image to indicate exactly where this occurs. *Source*: Marcus Drake.

overactive bladder (OAB) (urgency during the storage phase due to increased micromotions) and underactive bladder (weak voiding, as the reduced innervation is insufficient to generate adequate overall bladder contraction) [8].

The Male Urethra

The male urethra averages 16–20 cm in length (Table 2.1) and can be considered in four portions (Figure 2.10):

1) Prostatic urethra: from bladder neck to prostate apex. The bladder neck constricts the internal urethral meatus and stays shut at all times except when voiding. This

Table 2.1 Comparison of male and female lower urinary tract.

Female	Male
3–4 cm straight urethra	15–20 cm 'S'-shaped urethra
Wide diameter outlet	Narrow diameter outlet
Sphincter 'horseshoe'	Sphincter 'circular'
Laminar flow	Turbulent flow
Voiding 'low pressure'	Voiding 'high pressure'

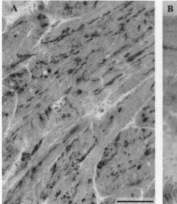
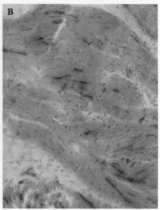

Figure 2.7 Thick muscle of the detrusor (light grey). On the left, the muscle has normal cholinergic innervation density, shown by the numerous black fibres (nerves viewed from the side) and black dots (nerves cut transversely). On the right, a person with spinal cord injury, shown to have partial denervation (far fewer black fibres and dots). *Source*: Reproduced with permission from [3].

well-defined muscle represents the 'genital sphincter' designed to prevent reflux of ejaculate at the time of orgasm. Below the bladder neck, the prostatic urethra is surrounded by the prostate gland and hence is at risk of any nodular enlargement of the gland intruding into the lumen, leading to benign prostate obstruction. The posterior aspect of the prostate is palpable from the rectum (Figure 2.11). This part of the urethra is about 3 cm long and it receives the ejaculatory ducts (Figure 2.12). It is horseshoe shaped on transverse section, with the convexity upwards. The smooth muscle of the prostatic urethra in males is histochemically distinct from that of the detrusor and from urethral muscle in females. This muscle also forms the prostatic capsule. It is richly provided with noradrenergic (norepinephric) nerve terminals, and little acetylcholinesterase has been found. Changes in pressure can occur in this part of the urethra during penile erection, and these changes do not seem to occur during any part of the micturition cycle unless there is erection.

2) Membranous urethra: the part which traverses the pelvic floor, closed by the urinary sphincter in the storage phase. The membranous portion is the shortest portion of the urethra at 2 cm and is the least dilatable. It perforates the pelvic diaphragm behind the bottom end of the pubic symphysis (viewed with the man standing) (Figure 2.10). The male external urethral sphincter is circular, and it works by concentric constriction of the lumen. It applies a constant sustained (tonic) squeeze, supplemented by an enhanced squeeze (phasic) which is reflexly applied prior to and during physical exertion. Additional enhancement of the sphincter squeeze can be exerted deliberately by the person. Voluntary contraction of the

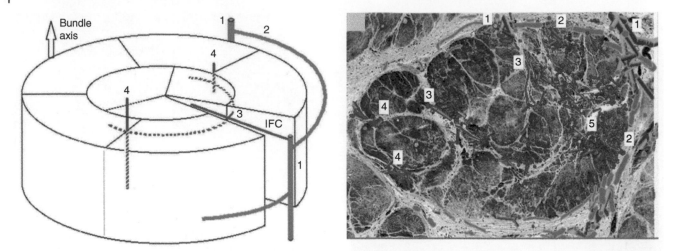

Figure 2.8 Left: a schematic representation of the midpoint of a muscle bundle, made up of eight fascicles separated by connective tissue planes. 1: longitudinal peribundle nerve trunk (green); 2: circumferential peribundle nerve branch; 3: transverse interfascicular branch (orange); 4: axial interfascicular branch, source of the terminal innervation [3]. IFC: interfascicular cleft. Right: the patchy nature of denervation in spinal cord injury. *Source*: Reproduced with permission from [3].

relaxed sphincter is probably the way that most people interrupt the urinary stream, should they choose to do so when voiding. The sphincter stays shut at all times, except when voiding and during ejaculation. The opening of the sphincter during ejaculation does not usually lead to any urinary incontinence due to the maintained closure of the bladder neck. However, previous damage to the bladder neck (e.g. prostatic resection) or loss of its nerve supply (e.g. retroperitoneal lymph node dissection to treat testicular cancer metastases, or neurological disease of the thoracolumbar spinal cord) may lead to reporting of incontinence with ejaculation ('climacturia') and/or dry orgasm (retrograde ejaculation).

3) Bulbar urethra: from below the sphincter to the penoscrotal junction. This is the fleshy part of the male urethra palpable from outside just in front of the anus, an area which can pool urine after voiding in men and hence be responsible for post-micturition dribble (Figure 2.13). It lies close to the attachments (crura) of the corpora cavernosa on the ischiopubic rami. This part receives ducts of urethral glands. The proximal part of the bulb has some skeletal muscle on its ventral side, the bulbospongiosus; this muscle contributes to expelling semen during ejaculation.

4) Penile urethra: extends to the external meatus. This section may be responsible for the spiral nature of the urine stream when it leaves the external meatus. This effect may help prevent spraying and allow accurate direction of the stream. It is perhaps equivalent to the spin of a rifle bullet introduced by spiral 'rifling' grooves inside the barrel, which keeps the bullet stable in flight. If this effect is lost, due to scarring or damage anywhere along the urethra, the resulting turbulence is experienced as a splitting and spraying stream.

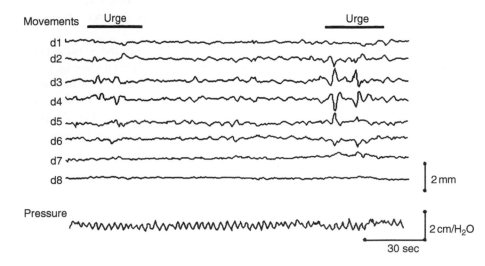

Figure 2.9 Detrusor muscle can show localised contractions which distort the bladder sufficiently to cause urgency sensations but do not cause sufficient pressure change to be detectable by urodynamic equipment recording at conventional sensitivity settings. Pressure is shown at the bottom, while d1–d8 plots the separation of points in different parts of the bladder. Picture reproduced with permission from [9]. 'Urge' indicates the moments at which the patient experienced urinary urgency. *Source*: Drake et al. [9].

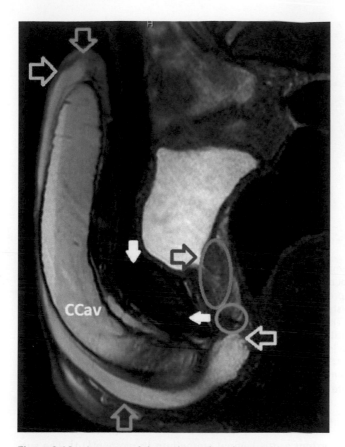

Figure 2.10 Anatomy of the male urethra shown with a magnetic resonance imaging (MRI) scan (sagittal view). White arrows indicate the top and bottom of the pubic bone (which shows up dark in these MRI settings). Purple arrow: bladder neck. Orange circle: the prostate – the prostatic urethra cannot be seen as it is empty during the storage phase of the micturition cycle. Green circle: membranous urethra, lying level with the bottom of the pubis. The membranous urethra is also not actually visible on MRI at these settings during the storage phase. Yellow arrow: start of the bulbar urethra. Blue arrows: penile urethra running from the bulbar urethra alongside the penile crura (anchor point of the erectile mechanism) to the external urethral meatus just beyond the right corpus cavernosum (CCav; erectile mechanism). The pink arrow indicates a dilation in the distal urethra known as the navicular fossa, which can sometimes cause awkwardness when trying to catheterise. *Source*: Marcus Drake.

The male urethra is well supported due to its relationships to the prostate, pelvic floor, and crura of the corpora cavernosa. The curvatures of the male urethra are worth considering, since they have to be negotiated for placing vesical catheters. Holding the penis vertically when the man is lying supine means that the main curve is where the bulb joins the membranous urethra just in front of the anus (Figure 2.10). This is approximately a right angle. Once past the membranous urethra, the prostatic urethra represents a slight upwards curve, which basically continues the preceding bulbar-membranous curve so that the overall effect is greater than a right angle – almost a hairpin bend.

At the proximal end of the prostatic urethra, the bladder neck can provide a lip against which the tip of the catheter can bump, preventing entry into the bladder when virtually there. This can very easily be overcome with a catheter possessing a slight angulation at the end (Coudé or Tiemann-tipped catheter [Figure 2.14]); should the catheter tip bump against an obstruction at the bladder neck (or indeed anywhere along the urethra), rotating the catheter while trying to advance it will usually allow the angle to find the lumen very easily. This is occasionally necessary at the distal end of the penile urethra, level with the rim of the glans, as this can have a bit of a lip at the start of the navicular fossa (Figure 2.9), which can cause a bit of awkwardness to find the lumen. In this area, there can sometimes be a blind pit which looks like the urethra (Figure 15.10). It is then necessary to inspect carefully with a good light available and try passing the catheter at various angles in the anterior-posterior plane until the lumen becomes evident.

The Female Urethra

The female urethra is membranous canal, approximately 4 cm long, which extends from the internal to the external urethral meatus (Table 2.1). It is placed behind the pubic symphysis (Figure 2.5) and obliquely traverses the anterior wall of the vagina. When a woman is lying supine, the urethra is roughly horizontal.

The smooth muscle of the female urethra is arranged longitudinally so that when it contracts, the urethra becomes a bit shorter and wider, which facilitates voiding. When passing urine, the urinary stream for a woman does not spiral (as it does for a man); the flow is described as 'laminar', with the inner part of the stream moving quickest, and the outer part slowest, due to the slight friction drag against the epithelium. Another big difference from the male is the configuration of the sphincter, which is asymmetric, being much thicker on the dorsal side (on top of the urethra when the woman is lying supine) [11]. Consequently, the sphincter in women does not constrict, it presses in to cause a 'kink'. This is an efficient way of occluding flow, and a similar approach is used by gardeners to stop flow along a hosepipe by bending it, as opposed to constricting it. The other muscles of the pelvic floor also contribute to this effect.

The female urethra could be considered in segments: intramural, midurethra, membranous (in the urogenital diaphragm), and distal [12]. The maximum urethral pressure (MUP) at rest is in the region of the 40th and 54th percentile along the total urethral length. This peak occurs within the area of the rhabdosphincter and the circular

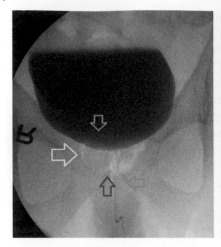
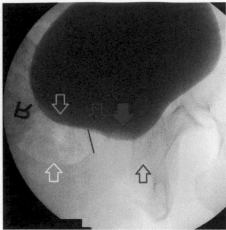
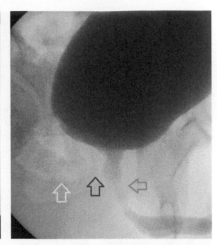

Figure 2.11 In the postero-anterior (PA) view (left), an object resembling the prostate is indicated by the yellow arrow (compare with Figure 8.19). This object extends distally to the level of the external urethral sphincter (green arrows), as expected of the prostate. However, the oblique views during filling cystometry (middle) and pressure flow study (right) show the object is too posterior to be prostate, and it is in fact a hard bolus of faeces in the rectum, consistent with a reported history of constipation. The prostate is indicated by purple arrows (open for posterior, closed for anterior). The red arrows are included to show the bottom of the pubic arch, as this is the only indicator of the likely level of the external urethral sphincter during filling cystometry, and its appearance on oblique view needs familiarisation. The blue arrows are included to indicate the absence of any intrusion of the faecal mass into the bladder, despite the presence of a reasonably large amount of firm faeces. This rather suggests that a widely held assumption that constipation reduces bladder capacity by taking up excessive space in the pelvis is hard to support in reality, in contrast to the potentially substantial effect of uterine anatomy illustrated in Figure 2.5. *Source*: Marcus Drake.

smooth muscle of the urethra. This high-pressure zone is located proximal to the urogenital diaphragm [13]. Voluntary contraction of the rhabdosphincter and the pelvic floor muscles increases the MUP in this area and can be demonstrated by asking the patient to contract their pelvic floor, with the urethral catheter at this area. This can also be used as a biofeedback tool in educating patients whilst performing urethral pressure profile studies. Pathologies affecting these muscles affect the MUP.

The muscle is of a 'slow twitch' type, adapted to maintain contraction over a relatively long period of time. The pelvic floor is separated from the urethra by a layer of connective tissue and is histochemically and histologically different from the intraurethral striated sphincter. It is important in providing an effective platform for sphincter function, including reinforcing contraction when undertaking physical exertion. This solid platform is particularly important for function reliant on an asymmetric sphincter, as contraction of the sphincter could otherwise simply push the urethra away without generating the necessary kink. Hence, healthy pelvic floor muscles, and the associated ligamentous supports, are particularly important for urinary continence in women.

The epithelial lining of the urethra is organised into longitudinal folds that give the urethral lumen a stellate appearance when closed. When opened (as in voiding), this arrangement ensures considerable distensibility so that the urethra does not restrict the channel for urine flow.

Oestrogen receptors are noted in the urethra to a similar extent as the vaginal epithelium in women [14]. The submucosal layer below the epithelium is a vascular plexus. Zinner et al. [15] discussed the role of this layer in relation to inner urethral wall softness. He suggested that the submucosa acts in a passive plastic way to 'fill in' between the folds of mucosa as the urethra closes and hence improves the efficiency of the closure of the urethral lumen. The contribution of this vascular closure may explain the presence of urethral pressure changes synchronous with the arterial pulse (Figure 2.15). Following menopause, oestrogen deficiency may reduce turgor of the vascular plexus and could be one factor in the increased prevalence of LUTS.

Overall, maintenance of high intraurethral pressure, and hence continence, can be considered to have three contributors [16]. Striated muscle (rhabdosphincter) of the urethra and pelvic floor is responsible for some of the total intraurethral pressure. The vascular plexus of the urethra contributes as well, and the remaining part could be attributed to the smooth muscle and connective tissues in the urethra. The integral theory is an anatomical framework for understanding pelvic function and dysfunction. 'Restoration of the form (structure) leads to restoration of function' is the main principle of the integral theory [17]. According to the theory, the pelvic muscles, connective tissue (endopelvic fascia and its condensations), and nerve components are crucial in the support and functioning of the pelvic organs like the lower urinary tract, vagina, and

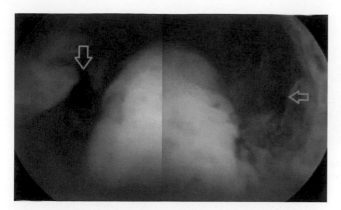

Figure 2.12 Urethroscopy showing the prostatic urethra, to illustrate the entry points of the ejaculatory ducts on the right (blue arrow) and left (green). The pink mound between the arrows is known as the verumontanum, an anatomical landmark for surgeons, as just below it is the external sphincter (not shown). *Source*: Marcus Drake.

the anorectal canal. The suspension bridge analogy explains the pelvic structure, and the trampoline analogy explains the function. This theory formed the basis for the development of the midurethral sling operation in managing stress urinary incontinence [17].

In women with stress urinary incontinence, imaging can find changes related to the urethral sphincter deficiency

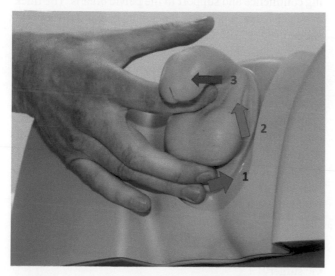

Figure 2.13 The location of the urethral bulb, and how knowledge of this area is important when teaching men how to get rid of drops of urine caught here after voiding, which later on dribble out into the underwear (post-micturition dribble). Instructions given to patients: '1. Press upwards gently but firmly, between the anus and scrotum. 2. Gently keeping the pressure on, ease your fingers forwards, so the urine can be eased forwards towards the penis. 3. You can shake the last drops from the penis'. Instruction 1 relates to compressing the urethral bulb. Figure reproduced with permission from the TRIUMPH (TReatIng Urinary symptoms in Men in Primary Healthcare) study (protocol [10]). *Source*: Marcus Drake.

and defects of the urethral support ligaments and urethral hypermobility. These include a small urethral muscle volume or a short urethra, defects in the urethral sphincter, funnelling at the bladder neck, distortion of the urethral support ligaments, cystocele, an asymmetric pubococcygeus muscle, abnormal shape of the vagina, enlargement of the retropubic space, and an increased vesicourethral angle [18].

The Pelvis

The Bones

The pelvis forms embryologically from the pubis (in front), the ischium (below), and ilium (behind) and is completed by the sacral part of the spinal column. This provides a solid framework for the lower urinary tract and nearby structures and, being radio-opaque, shows up clearly on X-ray. Interpreting the 3D framework in 2D images is an important step for understanding video urodynamics (the subject of Chapter 8) (Figure 2.16).

The Pelvic Floor

The levator ani (pubococcygeus, puborectalis, and the iliococcygeus) and the coccygeus muscles run in the anterior-posterior plane. In the midline, they diverge around the anus and urethra, and vagina in women, as they leave the abdominal cavity on to the perineum. This muscular diaphragm thus supports the pelvic viscera and hence is referred to as the pelvic floor. It curves downwards slightly when relaxed, and contraction of the muscles flattens the curvature, lifting up the pelvic organs. This also compresses the medial edges of the levator muscles together. The elevation and compression can be felt by internal examination during a voluntary pelvic floor squeeze. Elongation of the muscle or damage to its ligamentous support makes both the elevation and the compression more difficult to achieve so that organs are less well supported (prolapse risk) and the asymmetric sphincter contraction is less able to compress the urethra (in women). Some of the predisposing factors that can contribute to this include:

- myopathy,
- denervation,
- ligamentous damage (notably caused by childbirth),
- chronic straining,
- postural problems, and
- bony malformations, e.g. pubic diastasis or sacral anomalies.

Older people are at greater risk of accumulating some of these problems.

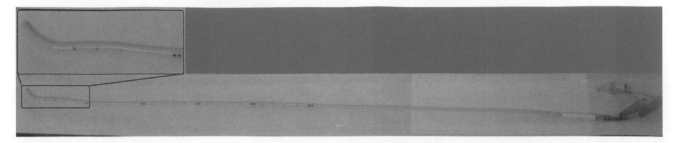

Figure 2.14 Coudé catheter. Gently rotating the catheter during the insertion often facilitates placement, overcoming awkward curves in the male urethra. It can sometimes be helpful for catheterising women as well. *Source*: Marcus Drake.

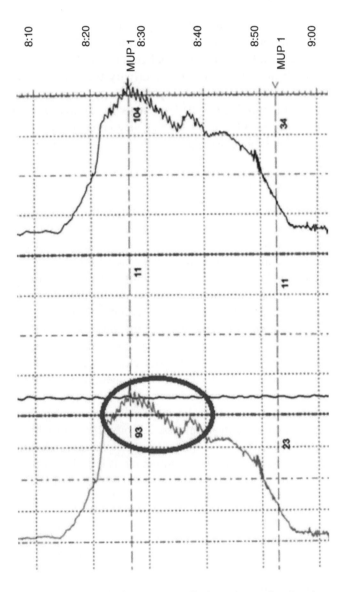

Figure 2.15 Urethral pressure profile in a woman showing the small pulsations on top of the high-pressure part of the profile (purple oval), synchronous with the pulse, known as vascular pulsations. The vascular plexus under the epithelium of the female urethra is prominent and may be a contributor to maintaining continence.

Endopelvic Fascia

The connective tissue (collagen, elastin, and smooth muscles) covering the pelvic organs and sidewalls is referred to as the endopelvic fascia and has an important role in supporting and functioning of the pelvic organs. A distinctive band of connective tissues extends from the lower pubic symphysis to the ischial spine on either side of the pelvic side wall, over the upper fascia (perineal membrane), and the levator ani. This condensation of the endopelvic fascia is referred to as the arcus tendineus fascia pelvis or 'the white line'. There are lateral attachments to the white line which support the pelvic organs. Some of the attachments can be distinctively observed and have a role in maintaining continence and support to the pelvic organs. The thickened pelvic fascia between the pubic bone and the anterior vaginal wall (prostatic tissue in males) is called the pubourethral ligament. This supports the urethra and bladder and has a role in continence. Any damage to the pubourethral ligament in women is clinically observed as urethral hypermobility and can be demonstrated on speculum examination and by asking the woman to strain or bear down. There are lateral (Mackenrodt's or cardinal ligaments) and posterior (uterosacral ligaments) fascial attachments to the cervix and the upper vagina, which provide important supports. Any trauma to these structures may result in pelvic organ prolapse. It is also important to recognise that the endopelvic fascia (loose connective tissue) carries much of the vascular, lymphatic, and nervous supply to the pelvic viscera and could be damaged during pelvic surgery.

Nervous System Control of the Lower Urinary Tract

The Peripheral Motor Nerves; 'The Efferents'

Excitatory efferents are the nerve fibres that go to the muscle and cause it to contract. Damage to these nerves will lead to paralysis, meaning that the muscle will not contract

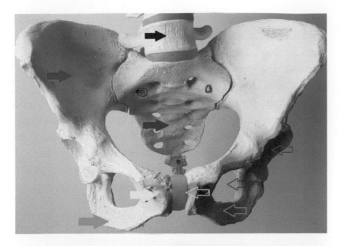

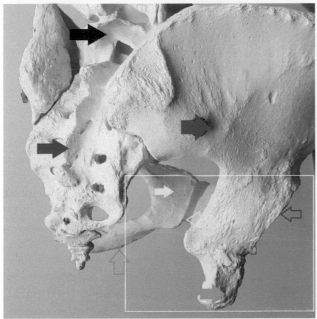

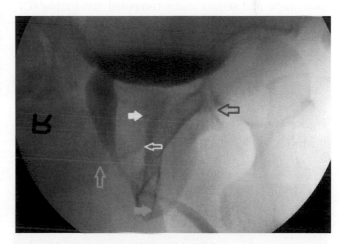

Figure 2.16 The bones of the pelvis, seen straight on (top) and obliquely; the pubis (solid yellow arrow), ischium (solid green arrow), and ilium (solid red arrow). Open yellow arrow indicates the pubic symphysis; open green arrow is the ischiopubic ramus; open blue arrow is the obturator foramen; open red arrow is the acetabulum (the hip socket). Bones of the spinal column; the sacrum (solid purple arrow) and fifth lumbar vertebra (solid black arrow). In the oblique view, the white rectangle gives the approximate area of an X-ray image taking during voiding in a man undergoing video-urodynamics. Illustrated on the right. *Source*: Marcus Drake.

when the person wishes, or a reflex relying on the muscle is triggered. For the bladder, the excitatory efferents are a network ('plexus') of fine fibres running over the other pelvic organs. As a consequence, they may be affected in diseases or surgery to the nearby organs, most notably gynaecological and colorectal operations. In the past, radical surgery (as needed in some cancer operations) to either of these organs could damage the plexus of bladder nerves so much that the bladder became acontractile. Modern-day surgical techniques have been designed to reduce the potential impact on the bladder. Nonetheless, there is likely to be some damage to a few of the nerves; the effect will usually be subsymptomatic, but a patient with extensive past background of pelvic operations could be at risk of impaired voiding function as a result of the accumulation of multiple low-level damage events.

Inhibitory efferents are also present in the plexus of nerves running to the bladder. These suppress spontaneous muscle 'non-voiding microcontractions', which are an innate feature of uninhibited detrusor muscle. The presence of an inhibitory innervation is needed to ensure the quiescence of the detrusor generally applying during filling. Nonetheless, microcontractions can sometimes emerge in normal function, indicating that the detrusor inhibition by inhibitory efferents is probably varied physiologically; allowing some microcontraction activity may be relevant to maintaining tone [8, 19]. Likewise, the localised movements would potentially stimulate afferents even in the absence of any associated effect on intravesical pressure. Consequently, such a mechanism could help report state of bladder filling or may explain 'latchkey urgency' (the strong desire to void when returning home, signifying a safe environment) (Figure 2.9). Excessive or widespread emergence of microcontractions, perhaps because of dysfunction of the inhibitory efferents, would be a factor in detrusor overactivity [8], and the consequent activation of afferents would generate urgency (OAB) [8, 9].

The sphincter is supplied by the pudendal nerve, a clearly identified structure (unlike the plexus supplying the bladder), which runs on the inner side of the ischium. Here, there is a ligamentous/bone channel known as 'Alcock's canal' (Figure 2.17). The nerve can get compressed in the canal, for example, during labour, or from fibrous narrowing, leading to pain affecting the perineum and genitalia. This location can be targeted by interventional radiologists, injecting local anaesthetic and steroid under computed tomography (CT) guidance (Figure 2.17). The relevant fibres then run up the ischiopubic ramus, so they can be damaged when a person fractures their pelvis. The pudendal nerve contains nerve fibres which the person can control voluntarily ('somatic'), enabling deliberate tightening of the sphincter. In addition, the nerve contains autonomic nervous system input comprising involuntary 'visceral' fibres, ensuring the sphincter is held shut without the person having to think about it. This

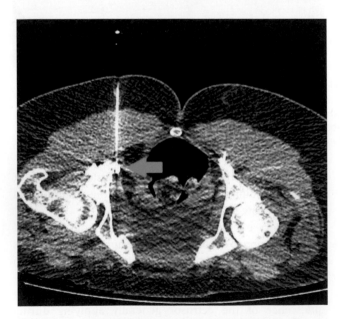

Figure 2.17 Computed tomography-guided placement of a needle for injection of local anaesthetic and steroid adjacent to the pudendal nerve in Alcock's canal (green arrow) in a woman with pudendal neuralgia. She is lying in the prone position. *Source*: Marcus Drake.

direct combination of somatic and visceral components is highly unusual in the human body. Note that the bladder is a visceral structure; people cannot directly make the bladder contract, they can only elicit a bladder contraction indirectly by setting off the voiding reflex.

The bladder neck in men is supplied by the sympathetic nerves (excitatory efferents), which are partly plexiform, but they have some thicker nerve bundles, referred to as hypogastric nerves. If there is a problem with these nerves, paralysis of the bladder neck means it is open during the storage phase – a readily observed feature in video urodynamics (Figure 2.18).

Neuromuscular Transmitters and Their Receptors

Much recent effort has been directed towards the analysis of receptors in the urinary tract, and the following are fairly well-established observations:

- Alpha-adrenergic receptors, causing smooth muscle contraction when stimulated, are present in the bladder neck and the proximal urethra principally in men. Alpha-adrenergic antagonists ('alpha-blockers'), such as tamsulosin, are used to treat voiding LUTS in men.
- Beta-adrenergic receptors are present in the detrusor. The beta-3 subtype has the effect of eliciting detrusor relaxation, and this is exploited using beta-3 agonists to treat OAB and detrusor overactivity.
- ACh is the major efferent neuromuscular transmitter (cholinergic transmission) generating the detrusor contraction for voiding, acting via muscarinic receptors (M2 and M3). The bladder contains acetylcholinesterase enzymes which break down ACh and shorten its duration of effect. Deficiency in these enzymes might be a factor in detrusor overactivity. Even during the storage phase, there is a very low level of ACh release within the bladder, partly from the nerves, partly from the urothelium. While this may seem counterintuitive, in fact the bladder keeps some 'tone' during filling, which is probably why people can generally void however much (or little) is in their bladder. It is probably this low-level release that is blocked by the comparatively small doses of anticholinergic medications used to treat OAB and detrusor overactivity. These small doses are easily overcome by the substantial surge of ACh seen during voiding, which is why these drugs generally do not cause urinary retention.
- ATP is often released as a co-transmitter (purinergic transmission), and this is especially significant at low-frequency nerve firing and possibly in pathophysiology, such as detrusor overactivity. No medication has been developed to exploit this clinically as yet.

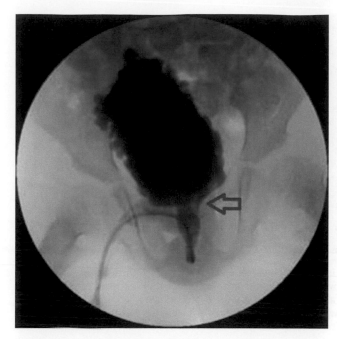

Figure 2.18 Open bladder neck in the storage phase (purple arrow) caused by neurological lower urinary tract dysfunction in a young male. The roughened bladder wall is caused by thickened muscle (trabeculation) and little pockets of urothelium (diverticulation) pushed out by high bladder pressures. *Source*: Marcus Drake.

Several other active compounds are present in nerves, such as nitric oxide and peptides. Their roles are not properly understood, but they do reflect potential interest for physiological understanding and therapeutic potential. For example, fewer of these compounds are present in neurological disease [4]. Nitric oxide is interesting as it may not influence the muscle directly, but instead alter function of the interstitial cells.

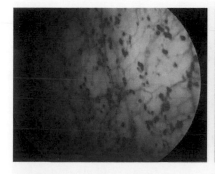

Figure 2.19 Cystoscopic appearance of inflammation in bladder pain syndrome. On the left, the blood spots referred to as 'glomerulations', seen when filling the bladder under general anaesthetic. These are generally seen only during general anaesthetic cystoscopy, as the patient demands the test be discontinued if still awake due to the significant level of discomfort. On the right, a different patient where the inflammatory glomerulations are so superficial they lead to bleeding. *Source*: Marcus Drake.

Peripheral Sensory Nerves; 'The Afferents'

Afferents translate a stimulus into a nerve firing pattern which reports to the spinal cord. From the bladder, there are two main classes of afferents. Some report bladder wall distension and distortion, so they become more active if the bladder is fuller. The sensory reporting from the bladder is delivered by afferents located under the urothelium or in the detrusor layer, and the traffic is probably carried along a similar peripheral pathway to the parasympathetic motor nerves. They report continuously, providing a graded nerve traffic proportionate to how full the bladder is. Note that people are not normally aware of this sensory information most of the time, i.e. it is reporting subconsciously. The conscious sensations derived from this information (sensation of filling or desire to void) are only experienced sporadically (see below). The nerve fibres carrying this type of information are mainly myelinated (A-) and small diameter (A-δ).

Another bladder afferent group becomes active only at very high volumes, beyond the point at which the person would have a very strong desire to pass urine. Consequently, they are rarely active, since the person will take steps to pass urine before the threshold volume for these afferents is reached. If activated, they give rise to an unpleasant/painful sensation ('nociception'). These afferents run with the sympathetic nerves. There are some patients who have lost function of the usual A-δ bladder sensory nerves and describe low abdominal pain and a large mass due to over-distension becoming sufficient to reach the nociceptive afferent threshold volume. These fibres are unmyelinated (γ), so they transmit slowly.

The amount of information coming from the urinary tract can be sensitised, i.e. more afferent nerve 'traffic' is carried for the same bladder volume. The increased sensory information due to bladder inflammation is an important sensitiser in the clinical setting. UTI or other forms of bladder inflammation lead to a stimulation of the afferents in the bladder wall (affecting both the usual sensory nerves and the noxious painful nerves). As a result, people have both increased sensation and an unpleasant 'noxious' feeling, leading to increased urinary frequency, and discomfort which persists after voiding. Characteristically, there will be leukocytes in the urine, and the bladder will appear inflamed if viewed cystoscopically; this might be a factor in bladder pain syndrome (Figure 2.19).

Sensitisation can also result from inflammation present anywhere along the track of the peripheral nerves. This might be a result of gynaecological inflammation, such as pelvic inflammatory disease or endometriosis. Alternatively, there might be an inflamed colonic diverticulum close to the bladder. The result is increased sensory

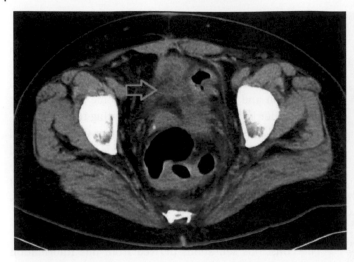
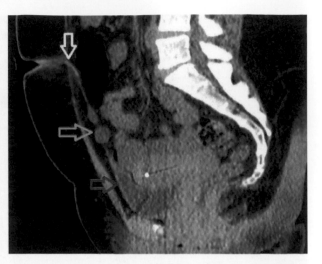

Figure 2.20 Computed tomography scans in people with extrinsic inflammation of bladder afferents, which the affected patients described in such a way that a UTI was suspected, but urinalysis showed no leukocytes. Imaging revealed the cause in each case. Left: inflamed colonic diverticular mass stuck to the bladder dome (blue arrow). Right: urachal cysts (blue arrow) which had become infected. The urachus is a structure joining the bladder (purple arrow) to the umbilicus (yellow arrow) in the foetus, which can persist into childhood giving rise to cysts and sometimes even allowing urine to escape from the umbilicus. *Source*: Marcus Drake.

information, both normal and noxious (as for the inflamed bladder), but without leucocytes in the urine. In these cases, history of gynaecological or colonic symptoms, and CT imaging to look for an inflammatory mass, may be informative (Figure 2.20). Should colonic diverticular disease progress, it can eventually lead to a colovesical fistula, where the urinalysis findings are strongly suggestive of UTI. However, this is not an ordinary case of cystitis, but actually a consequence of the bladder communicating with the colon. For this reason, it is vital to understand the possible significance if a patient describes gas in the urine or 'bubbly urine' (properly known as pneumaturia), faecal matter in the urine, or urinary diarrhoea (Figure 2.21).

Urethral receptors are an important group of afferents, which serve to detect flow. They are thus only occasionally perceived by the person (since there should be no flow during storage). However, they are extremely important in voiding. When urine is flowing, the resulting stimulation of the urethral afferents reports to the pontine micturition centre (PMC; see below). The presence of urine in the urethra indicates to the CNS that bladder emptying is not yet complete, and this sustains the drive maintaining detrusor contraction. Once the bladder has emptied, the urethral afferents stop reporting urine flow; at this point, the voiding reflex terminates. Thus, the reduced urethral afferent traffic is a key contributor to concluding the voiding contraction.

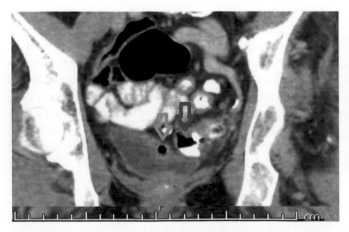
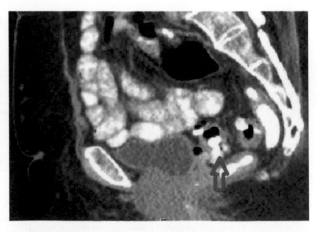

Figure 2.21 Abdominal computed tomography scan (left: antero-posterior view; right: lateral view) of a woman with diverticular disease which has stuck to the bladder and penetrated the bladder wall. It has caused a colovesical fistula so that gas is present not only in the colon (red arrow) but also in the bladder (blue arrow), leading to pneumaturia. *Source*: Marcus Drake.

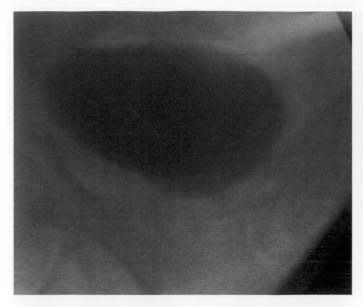
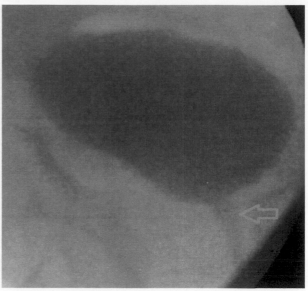

Figure 2.22   Urethral receptors can cause urgency. In this man undergoing video-urodynamics, urgency was reported when his prostatic urethra was stimulated by entry of liquid from the bladder into the prostatic urethra (blue arrow, right-hand image). There was no detrusor overactivity. He previously had had a bladder neck incision. *Source*: Marcus Drake.

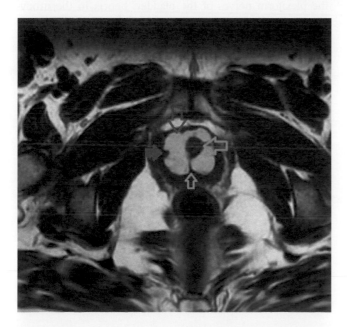

Figure 2.23   Structural changes related to the urethra can lead to lower urinary tract symptoms (LUTS). In this case, a large urethral diverticulum (UD) in a woman was associated with both storage and voiding symptoms. The storage symptoms could result from inflammation in the trapped contents of the diverticulum, while voiding LUTS could be a direct compressive effect on the urethra. The image is from magnetic resonance imaging, with a UD (open red arrow) fully surrounding the urethra (green arrow). The closed red arrow indicates a small lump in the UD; this will need interval scanning, as malignant change in a UD is occasionally reported. The blue arrow indicates the meeting point where the two arms of the UD make contact with each other behind the urethra. *Source*: Marcus Drake.

A couple of interesting clinical observations can be understood by appreciating the contribution of these receptors:

1) If by chance they get stimulated during the storage phase, they give an extremely strong sensation, perceived by the patient as powerful urgency and concern that leakage is imminent (Figure 2.22). This is a factor in the urgency experienced by some people with stress incontinence. Inflammation close to the urethra (e.g. a urethral diverticulum [Figure 2.23]) can also cause increased sensation.

2) Men who have had bladder outlet surgery usually lose bladder neck function. They still have external sphincter function, so they are not incontinent. However, the fact that urine can now stimulate the prostatic urethral receptors means they get a strong urgency feeling and worry that they are about to leak (Figure 2.22).

3) People who have lost urethral afferents do not know when flow is happening and so can only detect it indirectly. For example, when reported by skin afferents of the thigh/perineum, auditory (sound of water hitting the toilet bowl), or by looking at the flow emerging from the external urethral meatus.

In summary, the peripheral innervation of the LUT has several components with distinct functional roles. Selective loss of the fibres or the associated spinal centres has associated effects that can be derived logically and sometimes can be discerned clinically (Table 2.2).

Table 2.2 Matching specific LUT functions to subpopulations of LUT nerves.

Problem	Implication	Clinical manifestation
Loss of bladder excitatory efferents	Impaired voiding contraction	Underactive bladder/detrusor, retention
Loss of bladder inhibitory efferents	Storage microcontractions	Overactive bladder, detrusor overactivity
Loss of bladder afferents	No normal sensation. Overdistention	Person palpates full bladder. Noxious sensation if very full
Bladder afferent sensitisation (intrinsic/extrinsic)	Increased afferent traffic	Increased filling sensation
Loss of urethral afferents	No feedback of urine flow	Person listens or visualises to detect when flow happens
Loss of pudendal nerve (sphincter efferents and perineal afferents)	Sphincter weakness and lack of genital sensation	Stress/continuous incontinence. Difficulty achieving orgasm
Loss of bladder sympathetic innervation	Storage microcontractions	Overactive bladder, detrusor overactivity
Loss of bladder neck sympathetic nerves (male)	Bladder neck paralysis	Retrograde ejaculation (if sexual function preserved). Feeling of leakage (if urethral afferents preserved)

Spinal Centres

The CNS plays a major part in lower urinary tract and genitourinary function at all levels (Figure 2.24). The sacral spinal cord (segments S2–4) is crucial, as it contains the cell bodies giving rise to the nerve fibres that head to the detrusor and the external urethral sphincter, gathered together in groups known as 'nuclei'. The parasympathetic nucleus is in the intermediolateral (autonomic) horn, which is the source of the plexiform nerves of the bladder; hence, in the urodynamic context, it is sometimes referred to as the 'detrusor nucleus', even though it controls more than just the bladder. Onuf's nucleus is also in S2–4, in the anterior horn, and is the source of the nerves supplying the urinary and anal sphinc-

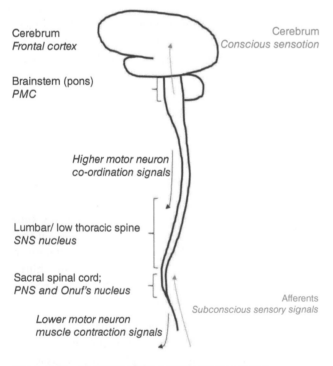

Figure 2.24 Key parts of the central nervous system responsible for lower urinary tract function. The sensory pathway is shown in green, and the motor pathway is shown in red. PMC: pontine micturition centre; PNS: parasympathetic nervous system; SNS: sympathetic nervous system.

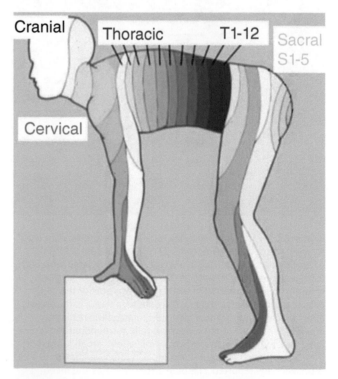

Figure 2.25 The dermatomes are the areas of skin supplied by the various spinal cord segments. These are easiest to appreciate when viewed from the evolutionary perspective of originating from a four-legged configuration.

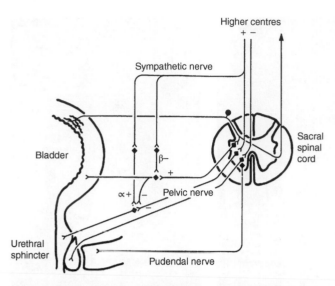

Figure 2.26 A wiring diagram summarising sacral spinal centres and their interactions with the lower urinary tract organs.

ters, carried in the pudendal nerve. Onuf's nucleus has somatic inputs, enabling people to squeeze their sphincters voluntarily. It also has visceral inputs underpinning reflex sphincter contraction (e.g. the guarding reflex, which is an anticipatory contraction just before lifting a heavy object).

Most of the sensory nerves of the lower urinary tract enter the spinal cord at this level, including the bladder afferents reporting filling state. The urethral afferents and the dermatomal (skin) sensation of the perineum and genitals also enter at this part of the spinal cord (Figure 2.245). However, the nociceptive afferents enter the spinal cord in the lumbar spinal cord. This anatomical variation in the afferent nerve course means that selective nerve loss, such as trauma or surgical damage, can occur. Hence, some people never experience normal bladder or urethral sensation but may report unpleasant/painful sensations once their bladder overdistends, indicating that the main bladder afferents have been damaged but the nociceptive nerves have not.

In the thoracolumbar spinal cord, the intermediolateral (autonomic) horn is the sympathetic nucleus. This structure controls the bladder neck and is also responsible in part for keeping the bladder quiescent during the storage phase. Furthermore, This nucleus controls the blood vessels and hence is crucial for maintaining a healthy blood pressure through regulation of vascular tone. Damage to sympathetic nucleus results in:

- low blood pressure at rest (due to loss of resting vascular tone) and postural hypotension (due to loss of reflex vascular tone adjustment);
- a paralysed bladder neck in men, visible as an open bladder neck in the filling phase of video-urodynamics (Figure 2.18); and

- overactive detrusor, due to loss of sympathetic inhibitory influence.

If the sympathetic nucleus is preserved but the inputs from the PMC are damaged, as in spinal cord injury (SCI), there is a risk of autonomic dysreflexia. This is a rapid elevation of blood pressure due to marked vasoconstriction of blood vessels of the gut and lower limbs, which is triggered by traffic in the nociceptive afferents coming up to this level of the spinal cord. Urethral catheterisation is a classic trigger for this, so urodynamics units need to be aware of this risk of testing people with SCI. It applies in patients with SCI at the level of T6 or higher, since this allows enough of the sympathetic nucleus to be preserved to result in dangerous potential for hypertension. These interactions from the sacral spinal cord to the periphery and back again are summarised in Figure 2.26.

The cervical spinal cord does not contain any specific centres responsible for lower urinary tract function. Nonetheless, it is traversed by the ascending sensory pathway in the white matter and the descending motor pathways. The entire spinal cord is the route by which afferent information ascends to the brain, and motor instructions come down from higher centres. Significant damage to the spinal cord at any point means the person may not experience conscious sensation derived from the sensory information carried in those afferents. Nonetheless, the afferent traffic is still present in the spinal cord (subconsciously), hence the potential to trigger autonomic dysreflexia. In addition, these people will have uncoordinated muscle function, notably detrusor sphincter dyssynergia (DSD; see below) since the higher centres cannot communicate the co-ordination instructions to the motor nuclei in the spinal cord.

Dysreflexia and DSD reflect failure of co-ordination of spinal cord centres, but they do not happen if considerable lengths of the spinal cord have been killed, meaning that the nuclei are actually dead. This can happen in major trauma, or a blockage of the anterior spinal artery, which is the dominant blood supply of the lower spinal cord. The resulting 'spinal stroke' leads to flaccid paralysis of all the muscle groups in the lower urinary tract, along with the other organs and the lower limbs.

An important anatomical point to bear in mind is that the segments of the spinal cord are numbered according to the vertebrae which they develop adjacent to in the embryo. By the time a person reaches adulthood, there has been considerable difference in growth, with the vertebrae growing substantially more than the spinal cord. As a consequence, whilst the cervical spinal cord segments are close by the original vertebrae, they develop next to, this does not apply in the sacral segments, which actually lie adjacent to, the upper lumbar vertebrae (Figure 2.27). Hence, if some-

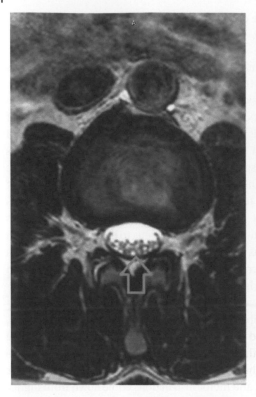
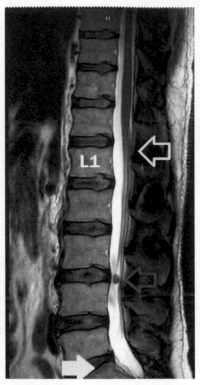
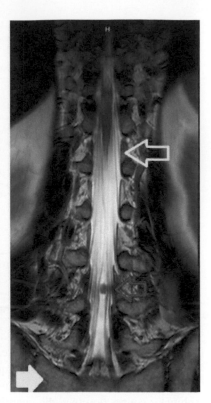

Figure 2.27 Magnetic resonance imaging of the lower spine and spinal cord. The top of the sacrum (closed yellow arrow) is anatomically at a considerable distance from the lowest sacral segment of the spinal cord (open yellow arrow), which is level with the first lumbar vertebra. In order to reach the foramina in the sacrum, the sacral nerve roots travel alongside each other (green arrow); this structure is the cauda equina. Hence, a lumbar prolapsed intervertebral disc, lumbar infection, or metastasis causes sacral nerve root dysfunction. This patient had a resolving abscess in the spinal canal (red arrow), which was responsible for cauda equina syndrome. *Source*: Marcus Drake.

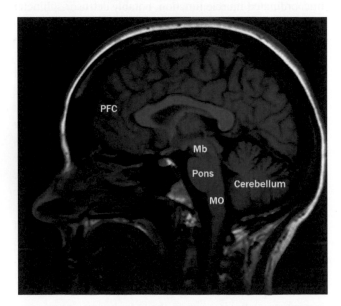

Figure 2.28 Key centres in the higher regions of the central nervous system. The hindbrain includes the pons, near to the location of the pontine micturition centre, and the medulla oblongata (MO). The midbrain (Mb) is the location of the periaqueductal grey. The front part of the cerebral hemispheres is the prefrontal cortex (PFC). *Source*: Marcus Drake.

body is unlucky enough to develop a central prolapsed intervertebral disc, the disc affected will be numbered according to its vertebrae, but the effect of the disc as it enters the spinal canal will be to compress a different spinal cord segment. L1 is the lowest vertebral segment at which the spinal canal contains spinal cord (Figure 2.27), so a disc prolapse between vertebrae L2 and L3 will affect the cauda equina (the nerves spreading out from the sacral spinal cord into the sacrum).

Brain Centres

The brain is divided into three parts anatomically: the forebrain, the midbrain, and the hindbrain. Each of these has direct relevance to LUT function (Figure 2.28).

The hindbrain comprises the pons and the medulla oblongata and is particularly important in the motor control of the LUT. The pons contains the PMC, which regulates many vegetative functions including storage and voiding. For men, the urethra is also part of the genital tract, so the PMC additionally co-ordinates semen emission and ejaculation. By default, the LUT is held in the storage phase, and this is generated by PMC signals sustaining inhibition of the detrusor

Table 2.3 Synergic actions of lower urinary tract nuclei determined by the PMC.

Phase	PNS nucleus *Bladder*	Onuf's nucleus *External sphincter*	SNS nucleus *Bladder neck (male)*
Voiding	Active	Relaxed	Relaxed
Storage	Inhibited/Not inhibited[a]	Contracted	Contracted
Ejaculation (men)	Inhibited	Relaxed	Contracted

PNS: parasympathetic nervous system; SNS: sympathetic nervous system.

[a] The extent to which the PMC inhibits the bladder may vary, with greater inhibition when away from home ('unsafe') and reduction when returning to the safety of home.

nucleus and excitation of Onuf's nucleus. In response to a permissive signal from the prefrontal cortex (PFC; see below), the PMC switches the activity of the two nuclei, ensuring that bladder pressure rises, the sphincter relaxes, and voiding can happen. Thus, the PMC is an upper motor neuron complex that imposes synergic behaviour on the LUT lower motor neurones (Table 2.3).

The midbrain includes the periaqueductal grey (PAG), which receives afferents from widely dispersed parts of the body, including from the lower urinary tract. This convergence of afferents is an integration point to ensure balanced control with related organ systems working appropriately together, without conscious effort. From the PAG, subconscious information is relayed upwards, where the cerebral hemispheres can use it to establish conscious sensations. At any given time, a person is conscious of only a modest number of inward signals, even though the range of afferent information transmitted from the body is enormous. Consequently, there must be an extremely selective relaying of this information. There appears to be two ways by which traffic from a particular group of afferents is selected for relay to the cerebrum. One is an upwards 'push', in which a very strong sensory signal is likely to dominate and therefore be relayed. In terms of the bladder, this could be the strong signal generated when the bladder is getting full and hence approaching the need to pass urine. Such a sensory push would be exaggerated if the afferents are very active (as in detrusor overactivity), sensitised (as in UTI), or involve a nociceptive component. The other possibility is a sensory 'pull', in which the cerebral cortex specifically interrogates certain functions, in a function known as 'sampling'. For example, most people are able to estimate the state of their bladder filling by briefly giving it some consideration and tuning into the sensory traffic coming up from the LUT. This is a useful feature which enables them to keep track of the progress of their bladder filling.

An important time for someone to respond to bladder signals is whenever the organ starts to get full whilst the person is asleep. This may be mediated by collateral effects on the reticular formation, which is a network in the brainstem with widespread influences. One of these is to regu-

late conscious state/wakefulness (the 'reticular activating system'). Hence, bladder filling can wake a person up by interaction in the midbrain with the reticular activating system. Failure of this interaction (either failure of maturation when growing up, or loss of function in adulthood) could mean voiding whilst asleep (enuresis).

The midbrain and brainstem sit in the midst of several nerve structures which are essential for life. Consequently, it is rare to see a patient surviving with a lesion of either of these structures. However, a brainstem stroke is sometimes survivable, and focal lesions may affect part of the brainstem. If there is a deficit in the PMC, it can affect the top-down inhibition of the detrusor, allowing detrusor overactivity to emerge. Sometimes, there may be dysregulation of the sacral motor centres resulting in DSD. However, those two features are much more likely to be seen as a result of the interruption of the descending pathways from the PMC, such as in SCI (where lesions are more likely to be survivable). These processes are described in more detail in Chapter 16.

The forebrain is dominated by the cerebral hemispheres, which have a huge range of functions, including planning, social awareness, and consciousness. For the LUT, these functions mean that people can weigh up the current and anticipated status of their lower urinary tract, i.e. 'how full is my bladder, and how soon am I likely to want the toilet?' This internal scrutiny can then be corresponded with upcoming commitments, such as a meeting or a journey, to make sure that plans are made for appropriate timing to go to the toilet. As the seat of consciousness, it is in the cerebral hemispheres that subconscious sensory information from lower down is turned into conscious sensation. A crucial part of the forebrain for the LUT is the PFC, which is fundamental for social function and planning. The PFC maintains the LUT in its default storage mode, doing so by regulating the PMC. The PFC regulatory control is so tight that it is almost impossible to try to overrule, as can be easily appreciated by imagining passing urine in socially inappropriate circumstances (e.g. when fully dressed and having a conversation with someone). It is generally only switched off when a person perceives themselves to be in a suitable situation for toilet use (in the right location and with clothes out of the way). Hence, passing urine requires suitable circumstances, so the person can switch off PFC inhibition of the PMC and, hence, instigate the micturition reflex. Cerebral control of the lower urinary tract is thus indirect but extremely strong. In addition to the PFC, the primary motor cortex (the rearmost part of the frontal cortex) has an area whose activities tightly correlate with the onset of urination, at least in mice during territorial marking [20].

When someone has cerebral dysfunction, the tight regulation by the PFC can be affected. This may occur in dementia, a stroke affecting the frontal cortex, or severe alcohol intoxication. The result is that the person may initiate voiding, or be unable to prevent the initiation of voiding, under socially inappropriate circumstances. This is known as voiding dysregulation [21], which is basically a normal micturition reflex but in an abnormal situation. This is not the same as urgency urinary incontinence (UUI), though many people with voiding dysregulation also experience UUI. Enuresis (bedwetting) may be a form of voiding dysregulation. Presumably, a lesion of a cortical area responsible for initiating voiding (such as the primary motor cortex area described in mice above) would prevent voiding and so put the affected individual into retention.

References

1. Noakes, T.D., Wilson, G., Gray, D.A. et al. (2001). Peak rates of diuresis in healthy humans during oral fluid overload. *S. Afr. Med. J.* 91 (10): 852–857.
2. Birder, L. and Andersson, K.E. (2013). Urothelial signaling. *Physiol. Rev.* 93 (2): 653–680.
3. Drake, M.J., Gardner, B.P., and Brading, A.F. (2003). Innervation of the detrusor muscle bundle in neurogenic detrusor overactivity. *BJU Int.* 91 (7): 702–710.
4. Drake, M.J., Hedlund, P., Mills, I.W. et al. (2000). Structural and functional denervation of human detrusor after spinal cord injury. *Lab. Invest.* 80 (10): 1491–1499.
5. Fry, C.H. and McCloskey, K.D. (2019). Spontaneous activity and the urinary bladder. *Adv. Exp. Med. Biol.* 1124: 121–147.
6. Parsons, B.A., Drake, M.J., Gammie, A. et al. (2012). The validation of a functional, isolated pig bladder model for physiological experimentation. *Front. Pharmacol.* 3: 52.
7. Drake, M.J., Mills, I.W., and Gillespie, J.I. (2001). Model of peripheral autonomous modules and a myovesical plexus in normal and overactive bladder function. *Lancet* 358 (9279): 401–403.
8. Drake, M.J., Kanai, A., Bijos, D.A. et al. (2017). The potential role of unregulated autonomous bladder micromotions in urinary storage and voiding dysfunction; overactive bladder and detrusor underactivity. *BJU Int.* 119 (1): 22–29.
9. Drake, M.J., Harvey, I.J., Gillespie, J.I., and Van Duyl, W.A. (2005). Localized contractions in the normal human bladder and in urinary urgency. *BJU Int.* 95 (7): 1002–1005.
10. Frost, J., Lane, J.A., Cotterill, N. et al. (2019). TReatIng urinary symptoms in men in primary healthcare using non-pharmacological and non-surgical interventions (TRIUMPH) compared with usual care: study protocol for a cluster randomised controlled trial. *Trials* 20 (1): 546.
11. Ho, K.M., Ny, L., McMurray, G. et al. (1999). Co-localization of carbon monoxide and nitric oxide synthesizing enzymes in the human urethral sphincter. *J. Urol.* 161 (6): 1968–1972.
12. DeLancey, J.O. (1986). Correlative study of paraurethral anatomy. *Obstet. Gynecol.* 68 (1): 91–97.
13. Westby, M., Asmussen, M., and Ulmsten, U. (1982). Location of maximum intraurethral pressure related to urogenital diaphragm in the female subject as studied by simultaneous urethrocystometry and voiding urethrocystography. *Am. J. Obstet. Gynecol.* 144 (4): 408–412.
14. Elia, G. and Bergman, A. (1993). Estrogen effects on the urethra: beneficial effects in women with genuine stress incontinence. *Obstet. Gynecol. Surv.* 48 (7): 509–517.
15. Zinner, N.R., Sterling, A.M., and Ritter, R.C. (1980). Role of inner urethral softness in urinary continence. *Urology* 16 (1): 115–117.
16. Rud, T., Andersson, K.E., Asmussen, M. et al. (1980). Factors maintaining the intraurethral pressure in women. *Investig. Urol.* 17 (4): 343–347.
17. Petros, P.E. and Ulmsten, U.I. (1990). An integral theory of female urinary incontinence. Experimental and clinical considerations. *Acta Obstet. Gynecol. Scand. Suppl.* 153: 7–31.
18. Macura, K.J., Genadry, R.R., and Bluemke, D.A. (2006). MR imaging of the female urethra and supporting ligaments in assessment of urinary incontinence: spectrum of abnormalities. *Radiographics* 26 (4): 1135–1149.
19. Drake, M.J. (2007). The integrative physiology of the bladder. *Ann. R. Coll. Surg. Engl.* 89 (6): 580–585.
20. Yao, J., Zhang, Q., Liao, X. et al. (2018). A corticopontine circuit for initiation of urination. *Nat. Neurosci.* 21: 1541–1550.
21. Gajewski, J.B., Schurch, B., Hamid, R. et al. (2018). An International Continence Society (ICS) report on the terminology for adult neurogenic lower urinary tract dysfunction (ANLUTD). *Neurourol. Urodyn.* 37 (3): 1152–1161.

3

The Physics of Urodynamic Measurements

Andrew Gammie

Bristol Urological Institute, Southmead Hospital, Bristol, UK

CONTENTS

Measurement of Pressure

The principles and practice discussed below apply to the measurement of pressure at any site, be it the bladder, the urethra, or the rectum. If a balloon filled with water is connected to a tube, any pressure in the balloon will be able to support a column of liquid in the tube, as shown in Figure 3.1. More pressure in the balloon enables a taller column to be supported. Thus, pressure can be measured by the height of this column of liquid.

A number of features of this system will not change the height of the liquid column. For instance, variations in atmospheric pressure will not change the column, since this pressure acts equally on the whole system. More significantly, the tube diameter does not change the height of the column. We know this from personal experience from going underwater to a depth of say 1 m in either a swimming pool or the sea – the pressure sensed by our ears will be the same in all cases, regardless of the width of the body of water. This is because it is the weight of the water above us, not beside us, that causes the water pressure, due to gravity. Since gravity acts vertically, and sideways pressures in static fluids equalise and become stable, only the vertical height of fluid above a pressure sensor will change the pressure, not the horizontal width of fluid surrounding it. However, if the liquid in the system is changed, the height of liquid column that can be supported by a given pressure will be altered according to its density. A dense liquid, such as mercury or X-ray contrast medium, will mean a shorter height of liquid than the water column, and a low-density liquid, for example, alcohol, will give a taller height, for the same pressure underneath. Accordingly, pressure needs to be stated in terms of the vertical height of liquid column and also the type of liquid used. Healthcare professionals are familiar with the concept of mmHg used in blood pressure recording, i.e. the amount of pressure in the bloodstream required to support a given vertical height of a mercury column. Since in urodynamics we generally use water, pressure is measured in cmH_2O.

A rudimentary way to measure pressure within the bladder could be to connect a water column to a catheter. This is shown in Figure 3.1, with the height of the water column in centimetres giving the pressure within the bladder, measured in cmH_2O. However, such a rudimentary system is poor for infection control and for recording data, and impractical when we need the patient to undertake provocation tests, so modern urodynamic systems utilise transducers for the accurate measurement of pressure.

Measuring Pressure in Urodynamics

A pressure transducer is a device which converts (transduces) a change in pressure into a change in electrical

---

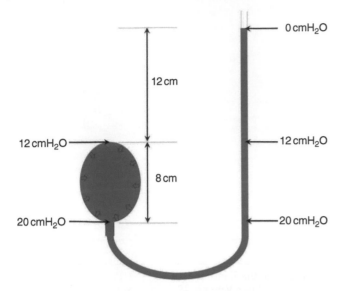

Figure 3.1 The pressures in the bladder can be appreciated by connecting the fluid in the bladder to a graduated column, allowing a visual understanding of the concept of 'centimetres of water' (cmH$_2$O) as a unit of pressure. In this illustration, the additional pressure generated by the bladder on the water gives a force able to lift the height of the water column an extra 12 cm; hence, the pressure at the top of the balloon is quantified as 12 cmH$_2$O. Note how the pressures at the same height within the water system are equal.

signal. This change can then be magnified (amplified) until it is large enough for a computer to record the signal. Transducers should be able to measure in the range −20 to +250 cmH$_2$O with an accuracy of ±1 cmH$_2$O [1]. If using catheter-tip transducers, it is not necessary to be able to record pressure readings below zero.

Systems vary in how the transducer is connected to the organ from which pressure is being recorded.

1) External transducer. The most common arrangement for urodynamics is a water-filled system, which uses water (or saline) filled connection tubing and an external strain gauge transducer. The water-filled tube carries any pressure change to the transducer, where it bends a thin metal diaphragm (Figure 3.2). On the back of the diaphragm is a strain gauge manufactured from a metal alloy which, when bent, changes its electrical resistance. A pressure change produces a movement of the transducer diaphragm, which bends the strain gauge, producing a change in the electrical signal (Figure 3.3). This type of transducer is normally reusable, robust, and easy to handle. However, the water-filled tube by which it is linked to the patient can introduce artefacts (see Chapter 19).

2) Catheter-tip sensing. By detecting the pressure change directly at the tip of the catheter, instead of needing

water-filled tubing to carry the pressure signals to an external transducer, there is less chance of encountering artefacts and no flushing of tubing is required.

a) Microtip transducers. Transducers can be made small enough to be placed inside the patient (Figure 3.4). The cable on which the strain gauge is mounted under a layer of protective silicone rubber contains the wires that carry the electrical signal to the amplifier. These transducers, also called 'solid-state' transducers, are reusable and are useful if rapid changes in pressure need to be measured, for example, during stress urethral profilometry. Unfortunately, internal transducers are expensive, fragile, and difficult to sterilise, so they are now not in general use.

b) Air-filled catheters. A small balloon at the catheter tip filled with air (Figure 3.5) is used to sense the pressure and is connected to an external transducer by an air-filled catheter. Since the air is almost weightless, the pressure sensed at the position of the balloon is passed along the air column to the transducer without being affected by the relative positions of the balloon and transducer. Also, as air is compressible, fast changes in pressure tend to be dampened by the time they reach the strain gauge, but the speed of response is adequate for most applications in urodynamics. The balloons and tubes are disposable, but the transducers are reusable.

c) Optical transducers. These measure the change in light reflected by a diaphragm at the catheter tip, rather than using a strain gauge. As the pressure bends the diaphragm, the characteristics of the light in the connect-

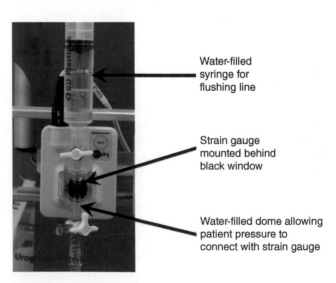

Water-filled syringe for flushing line

Strain gauge mounted behind black window

Water-filled dome allowing patient pressure to connect with strain gauge

Figure 3.2 External transducer. The most common arrangement for urodynamics is a water-filled system, which uses water (or saline) filled connection tubing and an external strain gauge transducer. *Source*: Marcus Drake.

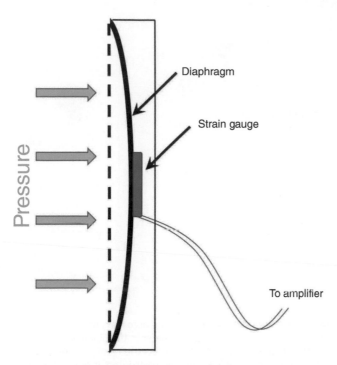

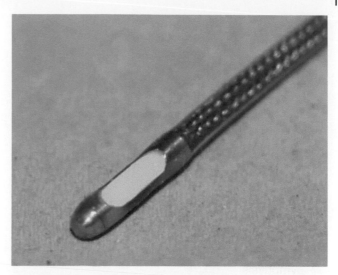

Figure 3.4 Microtip transducer. The white silicone covers the strain gauge, which can therefore be used within the patient. This reusable catheter is approximately 2 mm in diameter. *Source*: Marcus Drake.

Figure 3.3 A pressure change produces a movement of the transducer diaphragm, which bends the strain gauge, producing a change in the electrical signal.

ing fibreoptic cable can be sensed. The catheters can be smaller than other tip-sensing types and are reusable.

A water-filled system registers the pressure within the body at the level of the external transducer. When recording from the bladder, for instance, the measurement at the transducer of p_{ves} depends on the vertical level of the transducer relative to the bladder (Figure 3.6). If we fix the vertical level of the transducer by using the pubic symphysis as a useful anatomical landmark for the bladder, we can thus be confident about consistent measurement of p_{ves} with a water-filled system. The pressure measured by a catheter-tip sensor depends on the position of the tip *within* the bladder (Figure 3.6). Since we cannot actually see in the bladder to identify the location of the tip (which may move during the test), it leads to some uncertainty in the reading. This is one of the reasons why the International Continence Society (ICS) recommends the use of water-filled systems for urodynamics.

Measuring Pressure Correctly; Setting Zero (Reference) Pressure and Calibrating

Setting Zero

It is important to realise that pressure is always measured relative to a known reference or zero point. The ICS recom-

mends that *zero pressure is the surrounding atmospheric pressure*. Atmospheric pressure is readily available and does not fluctuate much (certainly not to an extent that causes a problem in clinical measurement). So, a standard approach at the start of any test is to measure from the atmosphere and 'set zero' while doing so [2, 3]; this then defines zero on the urodynamic plot so that when recording from the patient is started, it is the pressures of the organs above atmospheric pressure that are being plotted. Bladder and abdominal pressures are always higher than atmospheric pressure, since they are both within the pelvic cavity, and consequently compressed by other organs, notably the liver and gut resting on them. The zero is *never* set with the transducer exposed to intravesical pressure after the catheter is passed into the bladder since the pressure registered in that case is unknown and variable and is certainly not zero (Figure 3.7).

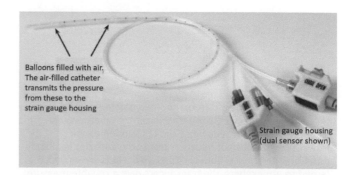

Balloons filled with air. The air-filled catheter transmits the pressure from these to the strain gauge housing

Strain gauge housing (dual sensor shown)

Figure 3.5 Air-filled catheter system. A dual sensor catheter is shown, with two balloons mounted on separate air-filled tubes. The balloons are therefore positioned within the patient. Source: Marcus Drake.

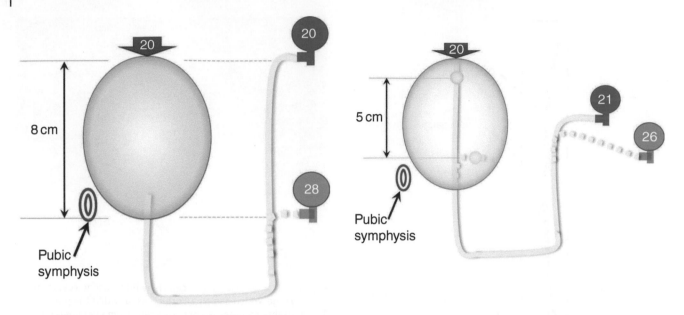

Figure 3.6 External pressure transducers with water-filled tubing (left-hand diagram) measure pressure according to their height relative to the patient (using the pubic symphysis as a landmark), so the position of the end of the catheter in the bladder does not change the pressure measurement. The position of the transducer outside the patient, however, does affect the reading displayed, as the transducer 8 cm lower than the other has 8 cm additional height of water resting on it. Catheter-tip transducers (right-hand diagram) measure pressure according to the position of the tip within the bladder. Thus, if the position of the tip is different (normally the exact position is not known for certain), then the reading will reflect the different height of water above the tip, here 5 cm more for the lower catheter tip.

With a water-filled system, the reference height needs to be set, since the height of the connecting column of liquid will affect the pressure registered at the transducer (see Figure 3.6). The ICS has defined the reference level (or height) for external transducers with water-filled catheters

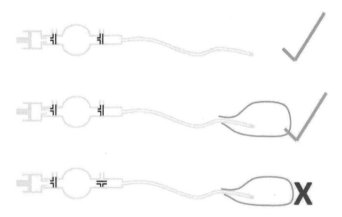

Figure 3.7 Setting zero. In the top two diagrams, the three-way tap on the right connects the transducer to the atmosphere, so it is appropriate to set zero. Since the tap is open to the atmosphere, it does not matter whether the catheter is already in the bladder; hence, both the top two options are correct. Zeroed to atmosphere, the transducers give a reliable measure of patient resting pressures. In the lowest option, the transducer is connected to the patient, so zeroing in this configuration is incorrect. More information about the three-way taps is given in Chapter 7 (see Figure 7.7).

as the symphysis pubis (specifically its superior edge). Hence, it is required to place the transducers in the same horizontal plane as the pubis (Figure 3.6). Water-filled systems cannot measure large values of negative pressure, so moving transducers to the reference height is especially important if the patient moves below the level of the transducer. Transducers measuring pressure at the catheter tip do not need a reference level in this way.

In a water-filled system, three-way taps can be used to switch efficiently between the key functions needed to run a urodynamic test, namely:

- setting the zero pressure as atmospheric pressure for p_{ves} and p_{abd},
- flushing out air bubbles and checking for leaks with a water-filled syringe, and
- recording from the patient for the test, or for calibrating.

For a catheter-tip system, the arrangement for setting zero is described in Figure 3.8. The pressure sensing point should be exposed to atmospheric pressure when zero is set.

Calibrating the Transducer

Calibration is the process of ensuring that the measuring equipment accurately measures a known quantity. Most urodynamic systems have the facility for calibration of the

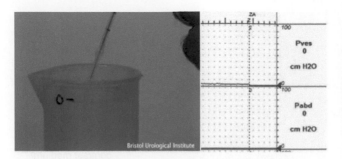

Figure 3.8 Setting zero with a catheter-tip sensor. Note that the balloon is not submerged but is surrounded by atmosphere when setting zero. The transducer is also exposed to atmosphere when the switch on the connector housing is set to 'Open', so zero can properly be set in that situation too. Source: Marcus Drake.

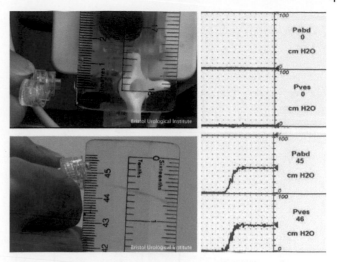

Figure 3.9 Manual checking of transducer calibration is easy. For a water-filled system, simply place the open end of the manometer tubing at two different heights and check whether the transducers display the height difference accurately (to the nearest $1-2\,cmH_2O$). Place the open ends of both water-filled tubes at the level of the tap used for zeroing to atmosphere and check whether the display on the computer screen indicates zero. Then, raise the ends of both tubes to a known height above that, e.g. to 45 cm. Check whether the screen display matches the new height, e.g. if held at 45 cm, then the reading on both lines should be $45\,cmH_2O$. Source: Marcus Drake.

pressure transducers. However, the accuracy of calibration must be checked regularly. This is very easy to do (Figures 3.9 and 3.10). If any reading is inaccurate by more than $1-2\,cmH_2O$ (in fact by >3% [1]), recalibration is recommended – a process that is likely to benefit from the input of Medical Physics or Clinical Engineering.

Measuring Infused Volume

Although gravity-fed systems have been used to infuse fluid into the bladder, it is normal to use a peristaltic pump for this purpose, as the rate of infusion can be precisely controlled (Figure 3.11). Knowing the volume of fluid infused is an important feature of urodynamic testing. This can be measured by using a weight transducer from which the infusion bag is suspended so that the reduction in weight in mg can be assumed to match the volume of fluid in ml, if a density of 1 mg/ml is assumed. Care needs to be taken with this method that movement or replacement of the bag is taken into account, as these will change the weight sensed by the transducer. Another method is to calibrate the pump, such that a given number of revolutions corresponds to a given volume of fluid infused. The urodynamic machine will have a software routine to do this calibration for the user. With this method, errors can occur if the tube clamp is inadvertently left closed so that pump revolutions do not result in fluid movement. The drip chamber must also be partly filled prior to starting the pump so that airlocks do not form.

For video-urodynamics, contrast medium is used that has a density greater than water, normally 16% greater. This difference in density will affect the measurement made from bag weight loss and also from voided fluid weight. The machine's software must be set to reflect this, and, again, modern urodynamic machines make this easy to do.

Measuring Flow Rate

Uroflowmetry involves measuring the speed of urine flow and the volume that is passed. It is carried out either as a stand-alone test (free uroflowmetry) or in combination with catheters measuring internal pressure (pressure-flow studies). The measurement of urine flow can be carried out in a number of ways, but there are two main methods (Figure 3.12). For details of the clinical application of uroflowmetry, see Chapter 6.

a) *Weight transducer flowmeter.* This weighs the urine voided, thereby measuring the volume of urine. By continuously measuring changes in urine volume, it calculates the urine flow rate by differentiation with respect to time.

b) *Rotating-disc flowmeter.* This has a spinning disc on which the urine falls. The disc is kept rotating at the same speed by a servo-motor, in spite of changes in the urine flow rate; the weight of the urine tends to slow the rotation of the disc. The differing power needed to keep disc rotation constant is proportional to the urine flow rate. The flow signal is electronically integrated to record the volume voided.

Calibration of flowmeters is normally carried out by pouring a precise volume of water at a steady, reasonably

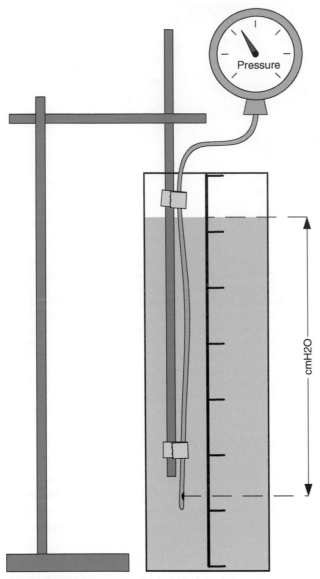

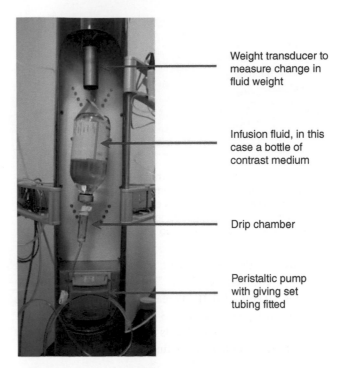

Weight transducer to measure change in fluid weight

Infusion fluid, in this case a bottle of contrast medium

Drip chamber

Peristaltic pump with giving set tubing fitted

Figure 3.11 Arrangement for infusion of fluid into the bladder. In this case, a weight transducer is used to measure the amount of contrast medium pump from the bottle. Source: Marcus Drake.

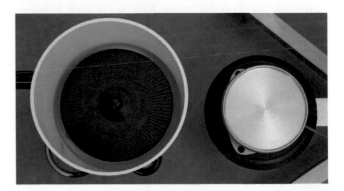

Figure 3.12 Urine flowmeters; rotating disc type on the left, weight transducer type on the right. See also Figure 6.18. *Source*: Marcus Drake.

Figure 3.10 Catheter-tip sensing systems can be calibrated by submerging the catheter tip in a water column of measured depth and checking whether the pressure is registered accurately. Source: Gammie et al. [1].

Figure 3.13 Calibrating a flowmeter with a known volume or weight.

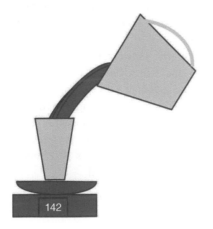

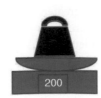

slow rate into the flowmeter (Figure 3.13). The machine can then be programmed to record the actual volume poured and scale the liquid flow rate accordingly. Regular checks should be made by pouring in a known volume and checking the reading concurs. Alternatively, the vol- ume voided can be checked by pouring the urine from the flowmeter collecting jug into a measuring beaker after a flowmetry or urodynamic test.

For further details on specifying, procuring, and checking urodynamic equipment, see Chapter 22.

References

1. Gammie, A., Clarkson, B., Constantinou, C. et al. (2014). International Continence Society guidelines on urodynamic equipment performance. *Neurourol. Urodyn.* 33 (4): 370–379.

2. Schafer, W., Abrams, P., Liao, L. et al. (2002). Good urodynamic practices: uroflowmetry, filling cystometry, and pressure-flow studies. *Neurourol. Urodyn.* 21 (3): 261–274.

3. Rosier, P., Schaefer, W., Lose, G. et al. (2017). International Continence Society Good Urodynamic Practices and Terms 2016: urodynamics, uroflowmetry, cystometry, and pressure-flow study. *Neurourol. Urodyn.* 36 (5): 1243–1260.

Part II

Functional Urology

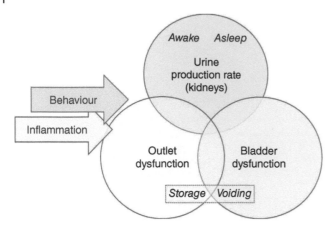

Figure 4.1 Fundamental focus on some underlying factors in lower urinary tract symptoms. Both storage and voiding problems must be considered as potentially resulting from bladder and/or outlet dysfunction. People presenting with symptoms attributed to the lower urinary tract may actually have factors unrelated to the bladder or outlet, such as overproduction of urine or inflammation of another organ irritating the lower urinary tract nerves as they head to the central nervous system.

they intuitively capture the key issues for a comprehensive patient-centred evaluation. Sixteen fully validated questionnaires are available for clinical and academic use covering broad LUTS and specific complexes such as nocturia and overactive bladder (OAB) (see www.iciq.net). The ICIQ has also been investigated for its measurement capability when delivered using an electronic format. Studies undertaken with core LUTS questionnaires have demonstrated that electronic versions measure as well as their paper-based counterparts. Given that consultations are often very short in modern healthcare, questionnaires completed by the patient just before the appointment provide a remarkably efficient way to communicate precisely what symptoms are present. The healthcare professional can take them in rapidly, and this time saved allows them to cover the other relevant influences.

The ICIQ-Male LUTS (MLUTS) and ICIQ-Female LUTS (FLUTS) questionnaires (included in full in the Appendix A), for men and women, respectively, catalogue the storage phase, voiding symptoms, and post-micturition symptoms, each one in terms of both severity and bother. Consequently, each LUTS is linked to the micturition cycle in a logical way, which makes it possible to produce a provisional symptomatic diagnosis. Hence, it is immediately obvious where the main issues lie for the patient. Subsequent tests, such as urodynamics, then become investigations to back up a clinical impression. The feedback from functional urodynamic information helps to improve symptomatic diagnosis.

The full coverage of the potential LUTS achieved by the ICIQ questionnaires highlights problems with the best-known LUTS questionnaire used for assessing men, the International Prostate Symptom Score (IPSS):

1) It does not cover some key symptoms, notably urgency incontinence and post-micturition dribble [1]. These can be a substantial burden to patients and really should not be ignored.
2) The wording of the questions was not derived using modern patient-facing methods, so they may be considered unclear by many patients.
3) Using a global question about quality of life means the specific LUTS driving the quality of life impact need to be asked about separately [1].
4) The name is misleading; it implies that the prostate is the identified cause, whereas that maybe completely wrong for many patients (not least for women, who often report high scores when asked to complete the IPSS).

For these reasons, it is probably best to consider the most efficient and effective tool to use when trying to reach diagnosis. While the IPSS is useful as a research outcome measure, it is not so effective in the context of decision-making for individual LUTS treatment.

FVCs and Bladder Diaries

The volumes and timing of toilet trips are crucial when evaluating the severity of storage LUTS and the contribution of fluid intake. Since it is almost impossible to estimate volumes, and remembering toilet trips for any length of time is doubtful, asking the patient to measure volumes and note them soon afterwards is highly useful [2].

The International Continence Society (ICS) describes three types of such charts [3]:

- *Micturition time chart:* A very simple record of only the times of voiding, kept for at least 24 hours. This provides some useful information and may be all that can be managed by some patients, but it is a limited assessment.
- *FVC:* This records the times and volumes voided day and night, for at least 24 hours.
- *Bladder diary:* This records not only the times and volumes voided but also other relevant information, which may include incontinence episodes, pad usage, fluid intake, the degree of urgency, or indeed anything considered potentially useful. This is the most detailed evaluation and can be tailored to the individual patient.

This record is more reproducible and accurate than relying on the patient's recall. For example, it has been shown that for nocturia, most men are inaccurate in their estimation of the number of episodes per night. It is now largely agreed that a 3-day duration is appropriate for most patients [4]. This is compromise between a sufficient duration to capture the full situation while not being too onerous for most patients. Some patients will be happy to record some information over a longer time frame if the potential benefit is properly explained.

The most robust diary has been developed by the ICIQ (Figure 4.2, Appendix A) [5, 6], developed based on patient and clinician views of importance using the psychometric validation protocol applied to all ICIQ modules. Opinions were sought on diary content, format, and duration using interviews and questionnaires allowing the formation of a draft bladder diary. The ICIQ bladder diary is designed to be versatile enough to accommodate specific requirements that are not included in the generic diary. The bladder sensation scale can be replaced with other scales, such as a pain score, to provide a more tailored evaluation in specific circumstances where alternative outcomes may be anticipated, for example, when evaluating a new treatment. Use of the ICIQ bladder diary is encouraged to standardise this form of assessment and facilitate comparisons between different populations and interventions. The bladder diary is also the most effective way to appreciate maximum and average voided volumes, which are helpful when deciding what volume a patient's bladder should be filled to during cystometry.

These tools are particularly useful when considering the potential range of influences on LUTS and their varying nature. Confidently identifying the specific situation requires a logical approach (Figure 4.3), and doing so can avoid the need for urodynamic investigation.

Importantly, the bladder diary shows behavioural influences effectively, with caffeine intake, alcohol consumption, and fizzy drinks (with their high sodium levels and artificial additives) being obvious factors (Figures 4.4 and 4.5). In particular, it is not appropriate to reach a conclusion on mechanism until these extraneous influences have been addressed. For example, it is not appropriate to assume OAB syndrome and instigate pharmaceutical treatment until it is clear that the patient's fluid intake is a sensible volume and type of fluid.

Certain patterns of FVC completion suggest the possibility of particular types of bladder or urethral pathology and also identify cases where there may be altered renal excretion or circadian rhythms. Abrams and Klevmark developed a classification recognising six basic patterns [2] (Table 4.1). The FVC thus shifts the therapy focus away from the lower urinary tract (which may actually be working pretty well) to the root of the problem (Figure 4.6). Of course, this is absolutely fundamental when nocturia is the dominant symptom [8].

DAY 1 **DATE:** ____/____/____

Time	Drinks		Urine output (mls)	Bladder sensation	Pads
	Amount	Type			
6am					
7am					
8am					
9am					
10am					
11am					
Midday					
1pm					
2pm					
3pm					
4pm					
5pm					
6pm					
7pm					
8pm					
9pm					
10pm					
11pm					
Midnight					
1am					
2am					
3am					
4am					
5am					

Figure 4.2 The International Consultation on Incontinence Questionnaire bladder diary [5]. A single day is shown from the 3-day diary. The diary, including the patient instructions, is given in full in Appendix A. The bladder sensation is scored each time the patient passes urine, using the scale. *0 – If you had no sensation of needing to pass urine but passed urine for 'social reasons', for example, just before going out, or unsure where the next toilet is. 1 – If you had a normal desire to pass urine and no urgency. 2 – If you had urgency, but it had passed away before you went to the toilet. 3 – If you had urgency but managed to get to the toilet, still with urgency, but did not leak urine. 4 – If you had urgency and could not get to the toilet in time so you leaked urine.* Source: Bright et al. [5].

Table 4.1 Frequency-volume chart basic patterns.

Pattern	Description	Significance
Normal volumes, normal frequency	Normal 24-hr urine volume	Normal patients
Normal volumes, increased frequency	Increased 24-hr urine production (polyuria)	Most frequently, this is high fluid intake by choice, but occasionally will indicate a significant pathology such as diabetes insipidus or uncontrolled diabetes mellitus
Reduced fixed volumes	Day and night	Consider an intravesical pathology, such as 'interstitial cystitis' or carcinoma in situ
Reduced variable volumes	Day and night	Suggests detrusor overactivity
Normal early morning void, reduced variable day volumes	Patient sleeps well and voids a normal or even increased volume on rising but passes small, variable amounts during the day	Suggests a psychosomatic cause for frequency
Nocturnal polyuria	Increased frequency at night, with >33% of the 24-hr urine production being passed during the 8 hr of rest	Often idiopathic, but consider congestive cardiac failure or abnormalities of antidiuretic hormone or atrial natriuretic hormone secretion

Source: Adapted from Abrams and Klevmark [2].
Note that there is no clear pattern on a frequency-volume chart to indicate a likely diagnosis of bladder outlet obstruction.

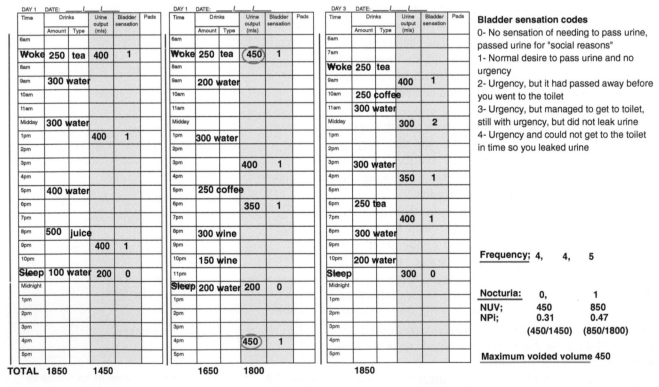

Figure 4.3 Information abstracted from a bladder diary showing some commonplace features. 'Woke' indicates the start of each day; 'sleep' indicates the start of each night. Daytime frequency is the number of voids recorded during waking hours and includes the last void before sleep and the first void after waking and rising in the morning. Frequency was 4–5 over the three complete days of the study period. Twenty-four hour urine production is measured by collecting all urine for 24 hr. This is usually commenced after the first void produced after rising in the morning and is completed by including the first void on rising the following morning. The range in the current example was 1450–1800 ml for the two complete 24 h using this definition. Nocturia (nocturnal frequency) is the number of voids recorded during a night's sleep. It was 0–1 over the two complete nights of the study period. Nocturnal urine volume (NUV) is the total volume of urine passed between the time the individual goes to bed with the intention of sleeping and the time of waking with the intention of rising; it excludes the last void before going to bed but includes the first void after waking. NUV was high on the second night, perhaps due to alcohol consumption in the preceding evening. This also is associated with a high nocturnal polyuria index (NPi, calculated from NPi = NUV/24 h volume) at 0.47. The maximum voided volume was normal (450 ml). Bladder sensation was generally 1 or 0; the only 2 was on day 3 and followed a couple of caffeine drinks. *Source*: Drake [7].

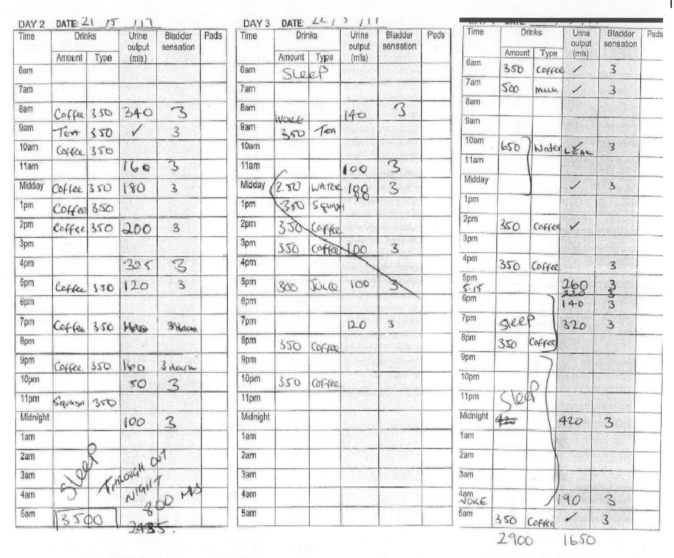

Figure 4.4 A diary which clearly indicates a considerable caffeine intake, indicative of possible contributory mechanism, and a useful visual aid for communicating the issue to the patient. Note, however, that caffeine intake may not be the whole story, since there are voids scored as having significant urgency by the patient on waking in the morning which precede coffee intake (first void on day 2). Hence, this patient needs not only fluid advice on caffeine intake and suitable volumes but also follow-up to check compliance with the advice and confirmation of the extent to which symptoms have improved.

Alterations in Fluid Excretion

Commonly, 24-hr urine output lies between 1 and 3 l, and 1.5 l is a perfectly healthy value for most people. Factors to weigh up include the following:

1) Dietary intake
   a) The dietary sources of water in the drinks and food consumed (foods like salads and pasta have a significant amount of water)
   b) The salt levels (high in many foods and fizzy drinks), since the body excretes salt by increasing urine volumes (natriuresis)
2) Normal water handling by the body
   a) There is a lot of capacity in the body to store water and salt, and the processes affecting their balance may be slow and unpredictable. Consequently, it is rather common to find the bladder diary suggests the urine output exceeds the fluid intake; if measured in detail for sufficient duration, this would balance out.
   b) Loss of water elsewhere from the body: sweating, faeces, and breath.
   c) Overnight, there is normally a reduction in the rate of urine output due to circadian hormonal control.
3) Medical conditions/treatments affecting salt or water handling
   a) Many medical conditions away from the urinary tract affect urine output due to effects on water and/or salt balance, or endocrine function, for example, congestive cardiac failure (Figure 4.7). Poorly con-

Time	Drinks Amount	Type	Urine Output (mls)	Bladder sensation
6am				
7am	SIP	H2O	300	3
8am				
9am				
10am WOKE	CUP	H2O	300	3
11am	CUP	TEA		
Midday	CUP	TEA	200	3
1pm				
2pm	PINT	GUINESS		
3pm	PINT	GUINESS	500	3
4pm			300	3
5pm				
6pm			300	3
7pm	250cL	WINE		
8pm	250 cl	WINE		
9pm	250cl	WINE	100	3
10pm	CUP	TEA		
11pm	SIP	H2O	300	3
Midnight			100	3
1am				
2am	SIP	H2O	200	4
3am				
4am				
5am				

Time	Drinks Amount	Type	Urine Output (mls)	Bladder sensation
6am	SIP	H2O	300	3
7am				
8am				
9am	CUP	H2O	400	3
10am	CUP	TEA		
11am			200	0
Midday			400	3
1pm	GINGER Bd.	300mL		
2pm				
3pm			300	3
4pm				
5pm	CUP	COFFEE		
6pm			200	3
7pm	250cl	WINE		
8pm				3
9pm	250cl	WINE		
10pm	250cl	WINE		
11pm	50cl	BR	200	3
Midnight			100	3
1am				
2am	SIP	H2O		
3am			200	200 3
4am				
5am				

Figure 4.5 Two days from a 3-day diary showing a high alcohol intake, relevant because the drinks contain a high volume of liquid and the alcohol is diuretic.

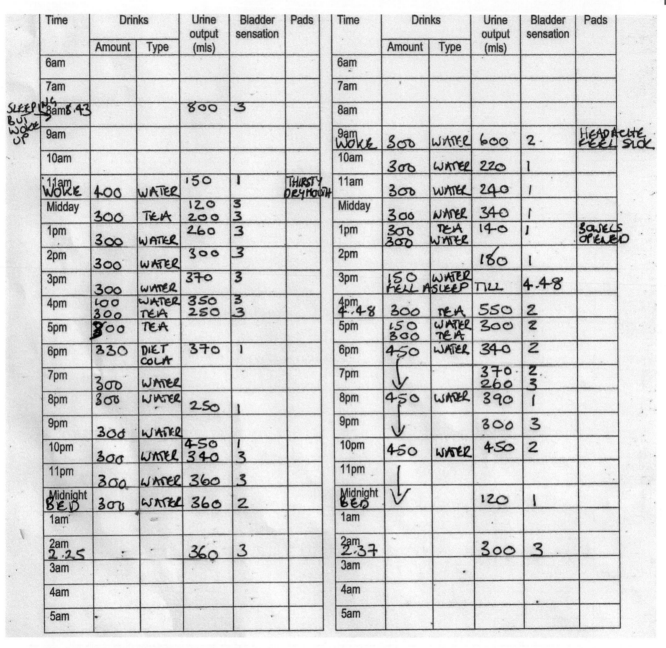

Figure 4.6 A patient with diabetes insipidus, a situation where the kidneys fail to concentrate the urine appropriately, leading to significant water loss. The bladder diary (2 days of a 3-day diary illustrated) shows that there are high fluid intake and urine output volumes. A key indicator is the patient's thirst; they are drinking a lot to make up for the fact they are losing large volumes of water pathologically, and they need to keep up this high fluid intake. This type of patient must not be advised to fluid restrict. (The diary looks like that of someone with a habit of drinking lots of liquid; the latter patient does not experience significant thirst and can safely be advised to restrict their intake).

trolled diabetes mellitus can cause osmotic diuresis (i.e. sufficiently elevated sugar levels to cause sugary urine). This is not common, since most diabetics compliant with modern healthcare are closely monitored and effectively treated.

b) Any disease of the kidney causing renal tubule dysfunction (which hampers water and salt handling by the kidney). The key one is diabetes insipidus (DI) (Figures 4.6 and 4.8).

c) Medications can be relevant, notably anything with a diuretic effect, for example, furosemide, bumetanide and calcium channel blockers. Lithium therapy can cause water loss though nephrogenic DI.

d) Psychological and psychiatric conditions.

DAY 2   DATE: 20/12/18

Time	Drinks		Urine output (mls)	Bladder sensation	Pads
	Amount	Type			
6am					
7am	AWOK		300	1	
8am 30			200	1	
9am	2 MUG TEA				
10am					
11am 30	1 MUG	COFFEE	100	1	
Midday	PINT	WATER			
1pm 30	MUG	TEA	100	1	
2pm					
3pm	1 CUP	COFFEE			
4pm			200	1	
5pm			200	1	
6pm 40	1 GLAS	WINE	225	1	
7pm	1 CUP	COFFEE			
8pm 30			150	1	
9pm					
10pm 15			300	1	
11pm	BED		100	1	
Midnight 30			200	1	
1am			275	1	
2am	SIP	WATER	300	1	
3am 2.20			300	1	
4am 10			400	1	
5am					

DAY 3   DATE: 21/12/18

Time	Drinks		Urine output (mls)	Bladder sensation	Pads
	Amount	Type			
6am					
7am AWOK	SIP	WATER	325	1	
8am					
9am 15	1 MUG	TEA	150	1	
10am					
11am	1 MUG	COFFEE			
Midday 15			200	1	
1pm	1 PINT	WATER			
2pm 30	1 MUG	TEA	150	1	
3pm 30	1 PINT	WATER	200	1	
4pm			275	1	
5pm	GLASS	WINE			
6pm 30			300	1	
7pm					
8pm					
9pm	1 PINT	BEER	250	1	
10pm 45			275	1	
11pm	BED				
Midnight 30			250	1	
1am 30			300	1	
2am					
3am	SIP	WATER	300	1	
4am					
5am			100	1	

Figure 4.7 Two days from a 3-day diary of a man with congestive cardiac failure. He had significant ankle and leg swelling due to water and fluid retention. It caused him to have bothersome nocturia. Attempting to get rid of some of this in the evening by lying on the sofa with his legs elevated above the heart level failed to have any significant impact (the illustrated diary was measured whilst he was attempting evening fluid elevation). There is very little that can be done to alleviate nocturia in this situation; occasionally, afternoon diuretic dosing (6 hours before bedtime) might make a small difference, but it is important not to suggest diuretics will have a curative effect.

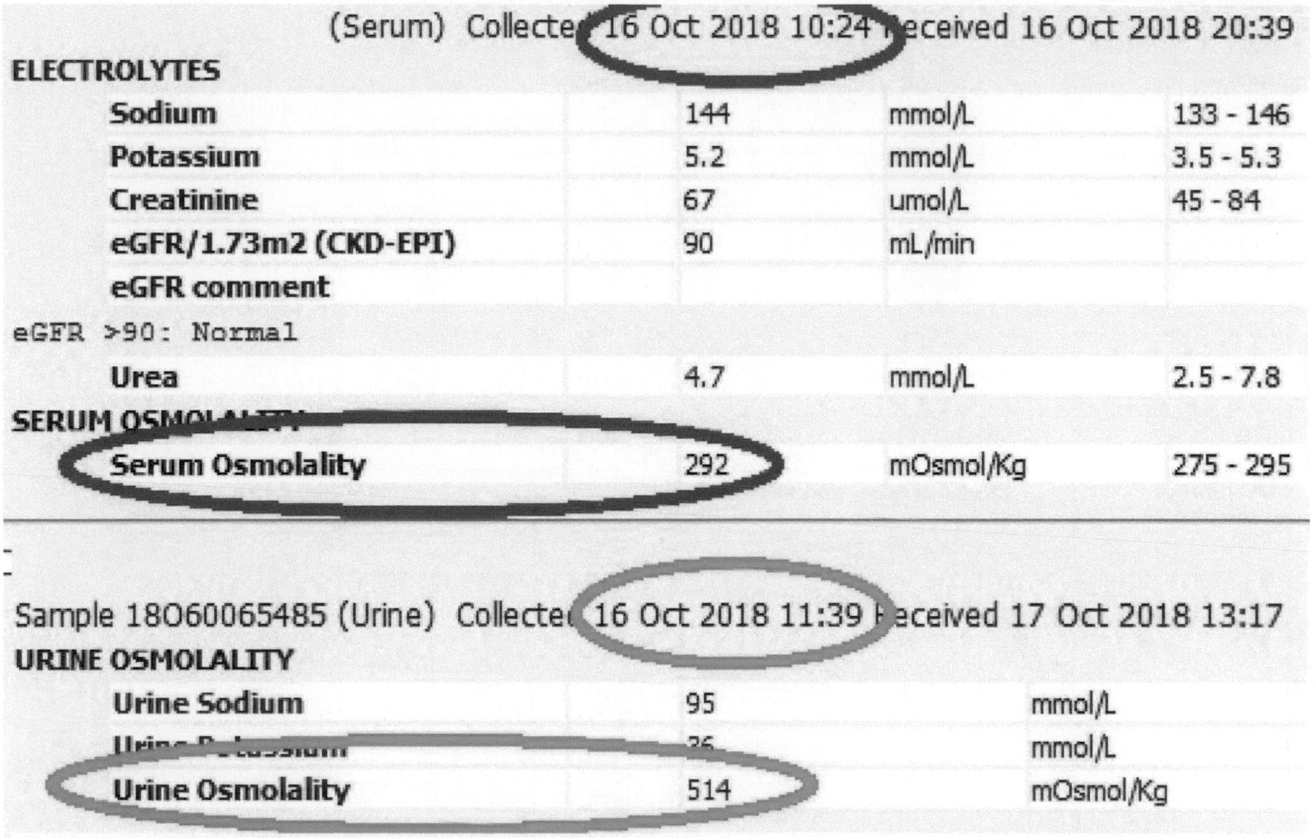

(Serum) Collected 16 Oct 2018 10:24 Received 16 Oct 2018 20:39

ELECTROLYTES			
Sodium	144	mmol/L	133 – 146
Potassium	5.2	mmol/L	3.5 – 5.3
Creatinine	67	umol/L	45 – 84
eGFR/1.73m2 (CKD-EPI)	90	mL/min	
eGFR comment			

eGFR >90: Normal

Urea	4.7	mmol/L	2.5 – 7.8
SERUM OSMOLALITY			
Serum Osmolality	292	mOsmol/Kg	275 – 295

Sample 18060065485 (Urine) Collected 16 Oct 2018 11:39 Received 17 Oct 2018 13:17

URINE OSMOLALITY		
Urine Sodium	95	mmol/L
Urine Potassium	26	mmol/L
Urine Osmolality	514	mOsmol/Kg

Figure 4.8 Urine concentration test; the ability to make concentrated urine indicates someone does not have diabetes insipidus (DI). Here, the rise in urine concentration (osmolality level) before (purple ovals) and after (green) a period of fluid restriction indicates ability to concentrate urine, so screening for DI was negative.

Intravesical Pathology

Inflammation and serious bladder pathology (e.g. infiltrating carcinoma or carcinoma in situ) occasionally may present with the symptoms of increased daytime frequency and nocturia. The bladder diary often shows consistent small voided volumes with persistently frequent voiding all the time, and the urinalysis may show microscopic haematuria and inflammation. For this reason, it is fundamentally important to review a urinalysis for inflammatory cells or haematuria and to act on the results to identify the cause.

OAB Syndrome and Nocturia

OAB is defined as urgency with or without urgency urinary incontinence, usually with increased daytime frequency and nocturia, in the absence of any other pathology [9]. The defining symptom is urgency, so using the ICIQ bladder diary is useful, as it incorporates an urgency scaling the patient applies to each void. Of course, this is highly subjective and some time should be spent establishing exactly what an individual means when they have applied the scaling – ensuring that they have not used a score of 2 or 3 to indicate a strong (but fundamentally normal) desire to void. Having this score cements the confidence in the diagnosis, provided it has been used in the way intended. The timings where urgency is reported can also provide some guidance on treatment timing. Specifically, if urgency seems to be mainly a daytime problem, the timing of any long-acting medication logically can be recommended for morning dosing.

Urgency in some OAB patients can be volume dependent, meaning that they experience it above a certain threshold volume. For these people, voiding frequently can mean they rarely experience urgency (Figure 4.9). Occasionally, they may deny experiencing urgency altogether, in which case technically they do not fit the definition of OAB syndrome. However, a direct question such as 'if you were prevented from passing urine, for example, because no toilet is available when out at the shops, what do you think would happen?' can be used to clarify whether further evaluation for OAB may be considered.

Nocturia in OAB needs specific consideration. While nocturia is mentioned in the description of OAB given above, OAB patients commonly report less severe urgency when lying down. This is one of the reasons that filling

DAY 2   DATE: 17 / 9 / 2019

Time	Drinks		Urine output (mls)	Bladder sensation	Pads
	Amount	Type			
6am					
7am WOKE	150	COFF	200	1	
8am					
9am			100	1	
10am	150	TEA			
11am			150	1	
Midday					
1pm	150	COFF	100	0	
2pm					
3pm	150	TEA	100	0	
4pm CLOSq					
5pm			120	0	
6pm	150	COFF			
7pm			200	1	
8pm					
9pm	150	TEA	150	1	
10pm					
11pm			100	0	
Midnight			200	0	
1am			150	0	
2am BCO			50	1	
3am					
4am					
5am					

DAY 3   DATE: 18 / 9 / 2019

Time	Drinks		Urine output (mls)	Bladder sensation	Pads
	Amount	Type			
6am					
7am WOKE	150	COF	130	1	
8am			100	1	
9am					
10am	150	TEA	130	0	
11am					
Midday	150	COFF	200	1	
1pm					
2pm			100	0	
3pm	150	TEA	155	0	
4pm CLOSq	100				
5pm			200	1	
6pm					
7pm			90	0	
8pm			120	1	
9pm	150	TEA	200	1	
10pm			100	1	
11pm			140	0	
Midnight					
1am BCO			155	0	
2am					
3am			125	1	
4am					
5am					

Bladder sensation codes

Figure 4.9 Two days from a 3-day diary illustrating frequent voiding to prevent urgency happening. This man routinely voided at small bladder volumes and never experienced urgency. This persisted after he complied with fluid advice to reduce caffeine intake, and he went on to trial an antimuscarinic medication, despite which he still remained symptomatic. Subsequent urodynamics identified clear detrusor overactivity, which emerged past a filling volume of 200 ml.

cystometry is done in the upright position during urodynamics so that detrusor overactivity is not missed. Hence, it is common to see lower urgency scores in the overnight voids of an OAB patient (Figure 4.9). If that is the case for an individual, and they complain of bothersome nocturia, it is vital to look for nocturnal polyuria (NP), which is a common issue, especially in older patients. For a patient with OAB and NP, it is vital not to assume that nocturia is going to improve with OAB therapy. The best chance that OAB treatment will improve any nocturia present is for those patients whose nocturia is truly associated with urgency (Figures 4.10 and 4.11).

To gain more detailed insight into patients experiencing bothersome nocturia, the International Consultations on Urological Diseases produced a summary algorithm (Figure 4.12) [10]. Here, the emphasis is on understanding the wide range of influences, including conditions which cause selective urine production during the night, conditions affecting sleep, and conditions which cause a general increase in urine production rate. In fact, the extensive list of potential causative factors means that nocturia cannot be considered a lower urinary tract symptom until these numerous other factors have been considered.

Medical History

General Features

Childhood medical problems and relevant family history should be considered.

Obstetric and Gynaecological History

The incidence of stress urinary incontinence (SUI) increases with the number of pregnancies and the difficulties of parturition. The number of pregnancies, the length of labour, the size of the babies, any episiotomies or tears, and the use of forceps during delivery might all be relevant. The use of post-partum exercises designed to improve pelvic floor tone may help to prevent SUI.

The relationship between the lower urinary tract and hormonal status in a woman is often significant; for example, patients with SUI may report that their symptoms are worse in the week before their period begins. This is probably due to increased progesterone levels and relative tissue laxity. Hence, the menstrual cycle and menopausal status are important.

Gynaecological surgery may interfere with the innervation of the bladder or may lead to distortion of the lower urinary tract. Denervation, more properly termed 'decentralisation', is most likely after radical hysterectomy for neoplasia and may act at both the bladder and urethral levels. Any history of vaginal or suprapubic procedures for prolapse or incontinence may be relevant, because such procedures can produce urethral or bladder neck distortion, scarring, or narrowing. An issue that is now increasingly evident is the potential problem that medical mesh, as used in some pro-

Time	Drinks		Urine output (mls)	Bladder sensation	Pads
	Amount	Type			
6am WOKE	350 M	WATER	150 ML	1	
7am			100 ML / 100 ML	3 / 0	
8am	CUP	COFFEE	✓	0	
9am			✓ / ✓	3 / 3	GOLF
10am	300 ML	WATER	✓	3	ı
11am	cup	COFFEE	✓ / ✓	3 / 3	ıı
Midday			150 ML / 100 ML	3 / 0	
1pm	CUP	TEA	125 ML / 125 ML	3 / 3	
2pm			150 ML	3	
3pm			175 ML	3	
4pm	350 ML	WATER	150 ML / 150 ML	3 / 3	
5pm			150 ML	3	
6pm	350 ML	WATER	100 ML	0	
7pm					
8pm	CUP	COFFEE	✓	0	BAND
9pm	CUP	WATER	✓	0	PRACTICE
10pm	300 ML	WATER	300 ML	4	
11pm	175 ML	RUM& COKE	150 ML / 200 ML	3 / 3	
Midnight BED			150 ML	3	
1am	50 ML	WATER	200 ML	1	
2am					
3am	50 ML	WATER	200 ML	1	
4am					
5am					

Figure 4.10 One day from a 3-day bladder diary for a patient with both overactive bladder (OAB) and nocturnal polyuria. This patient's nocturia probably will not improve with OAB treatment.

lapse or SUI operations, can become infected, leading to very challenging complications (Figure 4.13).

Surgical and Trauma History

Previous urological operations are clearly important. Any endoscopic procedure or catheterisation may lead to a ure-

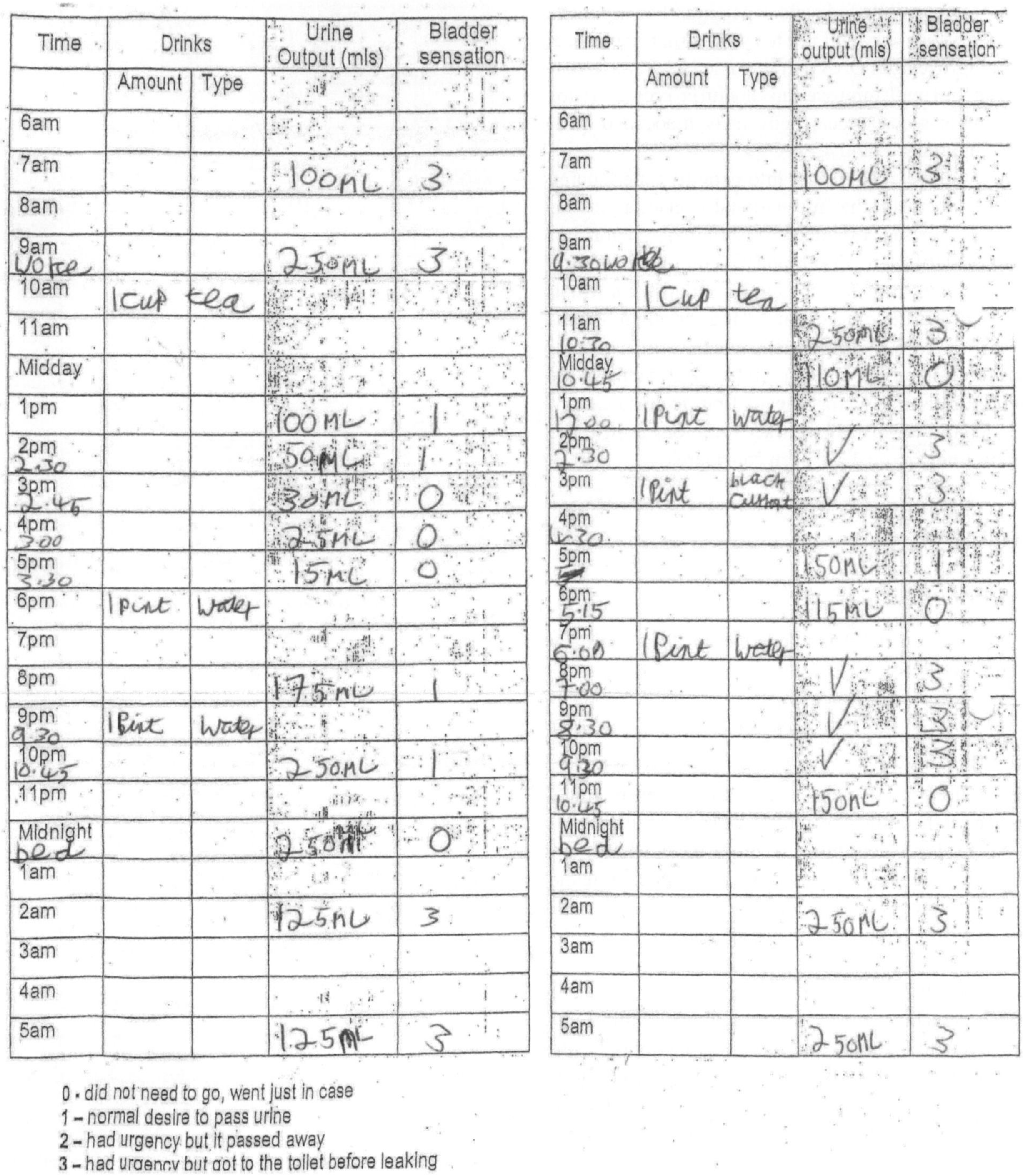

Time	Drinks		Urine Output (mls)	Bladder sensation
	Amount	Type		
6am				
7am			100ML	3
8am				
9am woke			250ML	3
10am	1cup	tea		
11am				
Midday				
1pm			100ML	1
2pm 2.30			50ML	1
3pm 2.45			30ML	0
4pm 3.00			25ML	0
5pm 3.30			15ML	0
6pm	1 pint	Water		
7pm				
8pm			175ML	1
9pm 9.30	1 pint	Water		
10pm 10.45			250ML	1
11pm				
Midnight bed			250ML	0
1am				
2am			125ML	3
3am				
4am				
5am			125ML	3

Time	Drinks		Urine output (mls)	Bladder sensation
	Amount	Type		
6am				
7am			100ML	3
8am				
9am 9.30 woke				
10am	1cup	tea		
11am 10.30			250ML	3
Midday 10.45			110ML	0
1pm 12.00	1 pint	water		
2pm 2.30			√	3
3pm	1 pint	black currant	√	3
4pm 4.30				
5pm 5			150ML	1
6pm 5.15			15ML	0
7pm 6.00	1 pint	water		
8pm 7.00			√	3
9pm 8.30			√	3
10pm 9.30			√	3
11pm 10.45			150ML	0
Midnight bed				
1am				
2am			250ML	3
3am				
4am				
5am			250ML	3

0 - did not need to go, went just in case
1 - normal desire to pass urine
2 - had urgency but it passed away
3 - had urgency but got to the toilet before leaking

Figure 4.11 Nocturia caused by urgency. This patient's nocturia may improve with overactive bladder treatment.

thral stricture. Surgery to relieve obstruction may not fully relieve the blockage. Sphincter damage after radical prostatectomy is a prominent issue. A history of trauma to the urethra should be considered. A fractured pelvis with disruption of the pubic symphysis, the pubis, or the ischiopubic ramus will likely be directly relevant, either by directly traumatising the lower urinary tract or by distorting it

(Figure 4.14). Problems can even follow an apparently trivial perineal injury.

Other operations most relevant to lower urinary tract function are those on the lower large bowel, where dissection at the side wall of the pelvis may result in nerve damage, especially during abdominal-perineal resection of the rectum. Bowel disease can affect the bladder, for example,

Category	LUT dysfunction	Problem of fluid or salt balance	Sleep disturbance
Examples	*OAB syndrome* *Bladder pain* *syndrome* *Neuro-urological*	*Cardiac* *Endocrine* *Neurological* *Pulmonary*	*Anxiety, depression* *Poor sleep habits* *Parasomnias* *Restless legs* *syndrome*
History Medication **Examination**	*LUTS, pain* *Pelvic disease/ cancer/* *surgery.* *Drugs affecting LUT* *Genital/Pelvic* *Neuro-urological*	*Known medical history* *Ankle swelling, shortness of breath* *Snoring/ breathing interruptions.* *Drugs affecting diuresis* *Peripheral edema* *Screening for medical conditions*	*Behavioural, Enuresis,* *Daytime sleepiness,* *Sleepwalking, Nightmares.* *Drugs affecting CNS/ sleep*
Diary **Other tests**	*Abnormal day and night* *Urinalysis* *Free flow rate/ residual* **Specific tests for** **suspected condition**	*Global or nocturnal polyuria* *Renal/liver function tests* **Specific tests for suspected** **condition; Specialist advice**	*Normal daytime pattern* **Polysomnography;** **Specialist advice**

Figure 4.12 Summary diagram for assessment of male nocturia patients based on potential mechanisms. CNS: central nervous system; LUT: lower urinary tract; LUTS: lower urinary tract symptoms; OAB: overactive bladder. *Source*: Marshall et al. [10].

the proximity of an inflamed diverticulum can cause altered bladder sensations through exogenous excitation of the afferent nerves (see Chapter 2). Any operation or situation in which the patient has needed catheterisation can be relevant, since stricture can be a consequence.

Other Significant Conditions

Any neurological condition should be explored, since the lower urinary tract is so dependent on normal nervous con-trol (see Chapter 2). The range of conditions and their effects are described in Chapter 16. Some neurological conditions can actually present with LUTS before the presence of the neurological condition has even been identified (see 'Occult Neurology' in Chapter 1). Hence, the history and physical examination should factor in consideration of the possibility of occult neurology (Figure 4.15).

Diabetes mellitus should be noted, as it can affect fluid balance and peripheral innervation. However, it is generally only when the diabetic control is poor (high haemoglobin

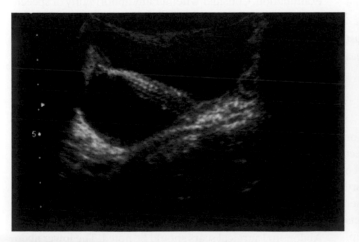
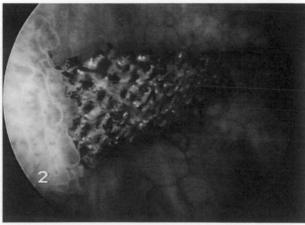

Figure 4.13 Ultrasound and cystoscopy images of a transvaginal tape (TVT) clearly visible in the bladder lumen. Mesh used in vaginal surgery, including tapes used to treat stress urinary incontinence, can later on become exposed within the lumen of one of the urinary tract organs (bladder or urethra), where it can lead to pain or serious infection. This might be due to tissue breakdown of the epithelial lining of the organ following placement. In the illustrated case, the suspicion is that there was an error by the surgeon, who seems to have placed the tape into the bladder at the time of surgery. *Source*: Marcus Drake.

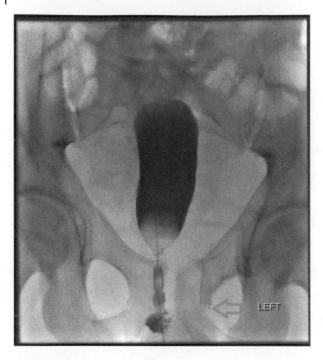

Figure 4.14 The considerably distorted bladder of a man following pelvic trauma, caused by substantial haematomas compressing the bladder and forcing its dome upwards. The urethra is also disrupted. At several points, the bones of the pelvis are broken (the most obvious point being indicated by the green arrow). Once this person has recovered from the trauma, it is likely he will have significant lower urinary tract dysfunction. *Source*: Marcus Drake.

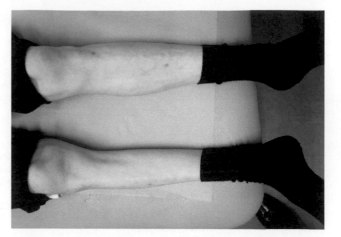

Figure 4.15 On physical examination, this man was noticed to have an abnormal gait. Examining his legs showed unilateral calf wasting. He also had patchy reduction of perianal skin sensation. He was later found to have a tumour compressing his sacral nerve roots (plantar flexion is controlled by the S1 part of the spinal cord, while perineal and perianal skin sensation are sacral dermatomes). *Source*: Marcus Drake.

A1c [HbA1c] levels) or there is peripheral neuropathy that this really applies. For many diabetics, their condition actually has minimal effect on LUT function.

Pelvic radiotherapy may produce a post-irradiation cystitis with limitation of the bladder capacity, together with increased frequency and sometimes bladder pain. Mucosal telangiectasia following radiotherapy may occasionally cause haematuria.

Infections such as tuberculosis and schistosomiasis must be remembered, so it is prudent to ask about travel to areas where these conditions are endemic.

Drug Therapy

Enquiries should be made as to any drugs the patient is or has been taking, and whether these drugs have any effect on bladder function or produce side effects. Drugs may be taken intentionally to modify urinary function, or urinary symptoms may be a side effect of a drug taken for another purpose. All drugs with enhancement or blocking effects on cholinergic, alpha-adrenergic, or beta-adrenergic receptors and drugs with calcium channel effects might influence the lower urinary tract directly. A range of drugs can have a diuretic effect influencing urinary output.

If a patient is on a drug prescribed to them to influence lower urinary tract function, or on a drug with urinary side effects, then the investigator should interpret the subsequent urodynamic findings with this in mind. In certain circumstances, the clinician may prefer to withdraw the relevant drug a week in advance of urodynamic testing, or before completion of a bladder diary, if it is safe to do so.

Physical Examination

A general examination of the patient should always be undertaken. All patients must have a simple neurological examination. Consider whether any abnormality of speech, co-ordination, or walking may reflect a brain or spinal cord problem. Even when introducing yourself to the patient, you can note their gait, speech, co-ordination, and strength (Figure 4.15). A gross assessment of sensation, reflexes, and muscle function in the legs should be undertaken. The anal reflexes should be tested and documented. In patients found to have, or known to have, neurological abnormalities, a full neurological examination should be performed.

This section emphasises aspects of examination that are of special relevance to the lower urinary tract.

Abdominal Examination

Abdominal surgical scars should be noted. The lower abdomen should be palpated and percussed in an attempt to demonstrate the bladder. Only if it contains more than 300 ml is it likely to be palpable or percussed above the pubic symphysis. Often, the patient is unaware of their bladder distension. However, pressing on the suprapubic region, and asking if the patient feels a need to void, may suggest a full or enlarged bladder. Suprapubic examination also reveals the degree of sensitivity of the bladder in some cases where bladder pain is a symptom. The degree of obesity of the patient should be noted.

Pelvic Examination

Genital examination should be undertaken. In the female, abnormalities such as meatal stenosis or fusion of the labia are found occasionally. In male patients, phimosis should be excluded, and the foreskin retracted to reveal the external meatus, which should be examined for stenosis. The urethra should be felt for fibrous thickening, which may indicate inflammation or stricture.

Vaginal examination starts with the patient supine. Inspect the introitus, and check the position and appearance of the meatus. Consider whether the introital mucosa is well oestrogenised (pink, moist, and healthy) or whether there are signs of oestrogen deficiency (the mucosa appears thin, red, and atrophic). Inflammation and an offensive discharge suggest an infective vaginitis. Vaginal capacity and mobility can be very important, for example, deciding on choice of operation type. When the patient is asked to contract her pelvic floor, the perineum should be seen to elevate. The pelvic floor muscles should be palpated with two fingers (index and middle finger in the vagina) in the lateral vaginal walls and their strength assessed, for example, using the modified Oxford Grading classification:

- Grade 0 – no discernible contraction
- Grade 1 – very weak contraction ('flicker')
- Grade 2 – weak contraction (increase in tension without lift or squeeze)
- Grade 3 – moderate contraction with some degree of lift and squeeze
- Grade 4 – good contraction producing elevation with some resistance
- Grade 5 – strong contraction and strong resistance

Test for urine leaking by asking the patient to cough repeatedly and then to bear down (strain), observing the meatus.

When assessing for pelvic organ prolapse (POP), the most suitable assessment is the POP-quantification (POP-Q) developed by the ICS [11] (Table 4.2 and Figures 4.16–4.20). POP can most reliably be evaluated using a Sim's speculum with the woman asked to turn onto the left lateral position.

Staging of POP resulting from the POP-Q measurements is as follows:

- Stage 0: No prolapse is demonstrated (points Aa, Ba, C, D, Ap, and Bp are all $</ = -3\,cm$)
- Stage I: The most distal portion of the prolapse is more than 1 cm above the level of the hymen (points Aa, Ba, C, D, Ap, and Bp are all $<-1\,cm$)

Table 4.2 The measurements taken in pelvic organ prolapse-Quantification (POP-Q) evaluation (Figures 4.16 and 4.17).

POP-Q: Measurements

The locations of the six defined points when the prolapse is fully reduced.

Anterior vaginal wall

1. **Point Aa**: A point located in the midline of the anterior vaginal wall 3 cm proximal to the external urethral meatus.

The potential range of position of point Aa relative to the hymen is −3, indicating no anterior vaginal POP, to +3 cm which is full prolapse.

2. **Point Ba**: A point that represents the most distal (i.e. most dependent) position of any part of the upper anterior vaginal wall (between the vaginal cuff or anterior vaginal fornix and point Aa).

Point Ba coincides with point Aa (−3 cm) in a woman who has no anterior POP. In a woman with severe POP, Ba coincides with point C.

Upper vagina

3. **Point C**: A point on either the most distal (i.e. most dependent) edge of the cervix or the leading edge of the vaginal cuff (hysterectomy scar).

4. **Point D**: The posterior fornix in a woman who still has a cervix[a].

Posterior vaginal wall

5. **Point Ap**: A point located in the midline of the posterior vaginal wall 3 cm proximal to the hymen.

The potential range of position of point Ap relative to the hymen is −3 to +3 cm

6. **Point Bp**: A point that represents the most distal position of any part of the upper posterior vaginal wall (between the vaginal cuff or posterior vaginal fornix and point Ap).

Three further descriptive landmarks and measurements.

1) The **genital hiatus (GH)** is measured from the middle of the external urethral meatus to the posterior margin of the hymen.

2) The **total vaginal length (TVL)** is the length of the vagina (cm) from posterior fornix to hymen when point C or D is reduced to its full normal position.

3) The **perineal body (PB)** is measured from the posterior margin of the hymen to the midanal opening.

Source: Madhu et al. [12].
[a] *Point D is included as a point of measurement to differentiate suspensory failure of the uterosacral-cardinal ligament 'complex' from cervical elongation. When the location of point C is significantly more positive than the location of point D, this is indicative of cervical elongation which may be symmetrical or eccentric. Point D is omitted in the absence of the cervix.*

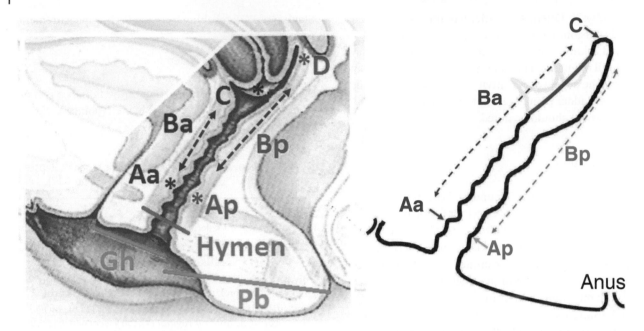

Figure 4.16 The six defined points used to quantify pelvic organ prolapse (POP) in women without (left) or with (right) a previous hysterectomy. Aa and Ap are 3 cm from the hymen when there is no POP, or any POP is fully reduced. POP-Q identifies where these points come to lie relative to the hymenal plane with the POP fully evident. Ba and Bp reflect the lowest point reached by a POP, relative to the hymenal plane. Any part of the vagina could potentially descend furthest, so Ba may lie anywhere from Aa-C, and Bp may lie anywhere on the posterior wall. Ba and Bp coincide with Aa and Ap in a woman who does not have POP. Three measurements complete the description; the genital hiatus (Gh), the perineal body (Pb), and the total vaginal length (not shown).

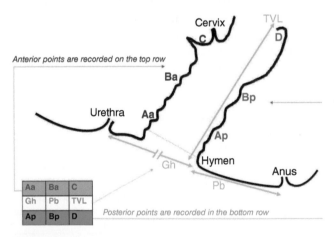

Figure 4.17 How the six defined points and three measurements relate to a 3 × 3 grid used for clinical documentation. Gh: genital hiatus; Pb: perineal body; TVL: total vaginal length.

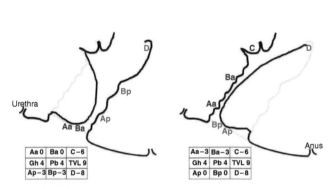

Figure 4.18 POP-Q staging of a second-stage anterior (left) and second-stage posterior (right) vaginal wall prolapse.

- Stage II (Figure 4.18): The most distal portion of the prolapse is situated between 1 cm above the hymen and 1 cm below the hymen (any of the points Aa, Ba, C, D, Ap, and Bp has a value between −1 cm and +1 cm)
- Stage III: The most distal portion of the prolapse is more than 1 cm beyond the plane of the hymen, but not completely everted, meaning no value is >/ = TVL −2 cm

(any of the points Aa, Ba, C, D, Ap, and Bp is >/ = +2 and </ = TVL −3 cm)
- Stage IV (Figure 4.19): Complete eversion or eversion to within 2 cm of the total vaginal length (TVL) of the lower genital tract is demonstrated (any of the points Ba, C, D, or Bp is >/ = to TVL −2 cm)

The POP-Q measurements and staging are summarised in Figure 4.20.

Figure 4.19 POP-Q staging of a stage IV pelvic organ prolapse (procidentia).

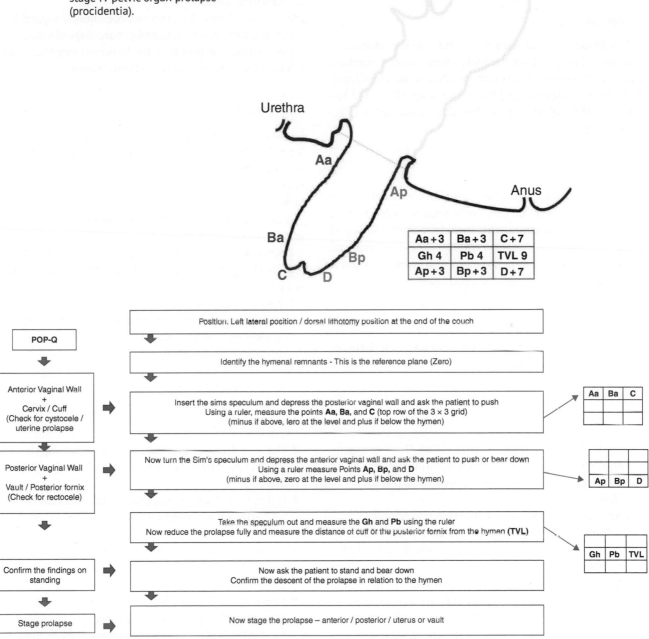

Aa +3	Ba +3	C +7
Gh 4	Pb 4	TVL 9
Ap +3	Bp +3	D +7

POP-Q

Position. Left lateral position / dorsal lithotomy position at the end of the couch

Identify the hymenal remnants - This is the reference plane (Zero)

Anterior Vaginal Wall + Cervix / Cuff (Check for cystocele / uterine prolapse)

Insert the sims speculum and depress the posterior vaginal wall and ask the patient to push
Using a ruler, measure the points **Aa, Ba,** and **C** (top row of the 3 × 3 grid)
(minus if above, lero at the level and plus if below the hymen)

Aa	Ba	C

Posterior Vaginal Wall + Vault / Posterior fornix (Check for rectocele)

Now turn the Sim's speculum and depress the anterior vaginal wall and ask the patient to push or bear down
Using a ruler measure Points **Ap, Bp,** and **D**
(minus if above, zero at the level and plus if below the hymen)

Ap	Bp	D

Take the speculum out and measure the **Gh** and **Pb** using the ruler
Now reduce the prolapse fully and measure the distance of cuff or the posterior fornix from the hymen **(TVL)**

Gh	Pb	TVL

Confirm the findings on standing

Now ask the patient to stand and bear down
Confirm the descent of the prolapse in relation to the hymen

Stage prolapse

Now stage the prolapse – anterior / posterior / uterus or vault

➤ *It is standard practice to assess the pelvic floor and perform a bimanual examination to complete the gynaecological examination*

Figure 4.20 Practical aspects of performing POP-Q.

Rectal examination should also be systematic. Does the anus appear normal? Does lateral traction cause the anus to begin to open? If the perineal skin is scratched, the anus should briefly tighten (anal reflex). As the examining finger passes into the anal canal, the tone of the anal sphincter can be assessed. In lesions such as meningomyelocele, anal tone may initially appear good, but after removal of the examining finger, the anus may remain open. Patients should be able to increase anal sphincter pressure by voluntarily contracting the levator ani. Any faecal impaction should be noted, as the subsequent urodynamics may be affected. In men, the prostate gland should be assessed for size, shape, consistency, and abnormal tenderness.

The pelvic examination is a chance to check preservation of the perineal skin sensation, which is the dermatome distribution of the S2–4 sacral spinal cord segments.

Other Investigations

Urinalysis

White blood cells and haematuria indicate the presence of inflammation, of which the most likely cause is infection, but other possible causes must always be considered. Urinalysis is a routine test for people with LUTS, and formal microbiological culture should be requested if infection is suspected.

Cytology

Since bladder malignancy can sometimes inadvertently be referred as LUTS, some cases may need a voided urinary cytology specimen check. This includes people with a past history of bladder cancer and smokers. Local and national guidelines will need to be followed as to when this test is requested.

Cystourethroscopy

Some people may need endoscopic evaluation if there are certain features, such as:

- inflammation on the urinalysis,
- a history of pain,
- a possible fistula (for example, continuous vaginal leakage in a woman who has had gynaecological surgery),
- possible mesh exposure in the lower urinary tract, and
- a flow pattern suggesting urethral stricture.

Radiology Department Tests

Ultrasound is a common evaluation, safely able to check for valuable information such as hydroureteronephrosis, post-void residual, and prostate size (either transabdominal or rectal). A translabial scan can look for relationships between surgical mesh and the LUT.

A micturating cystourethrogram can be used to check for vesicoureteric reflux.

Computerised Tomography scanning is a valuable tool for checking the structure of the LUT and adjacent organs.

Magnetic resonance imaging scanning is a more advanced structural examination, particularly useful for specific circumstances such as a suspected urethral diverticulum.

References

1. Ito, H., Young, G., Lewis, A. et al. (2020). Grading severity and bother using the IPSS and ICIQ-MLUTS scores in men seeking lower urinary tract symptoms therapy. *J. Urol.* 204 (5): 1003–1011.
2. Abrams, P. and Klevmark, B. (1996). Frequency volume charts: an indispensable part of lower urinary tract assessment. *Scand. J. Urol. Nephrol. Suppl.* 179: 47–53.
3. Abrams, P., Cardozo, L., Fall, M. et al. (2002). The standardisation of terminology of lower urinary tract function: report from the standardisation sub-committee of the international continence society. *Neurourol. Urodyn.* 21 (2): 167–178.
4. Bright, E., Drake, M.J., and Abrams, P. (2011). Urinary diaries: evidence for the development and validation of diary content, format, and duration. *Neurourol. Urodyn.* 30 (3): 348–352.
5. Bright, E., Cotterill, N., Drake, M., and Abrams, P. (2014). Developing and validating the international consultation on incontinence questionnaire bladder diary. *Eur. Urol.* 66 (2): 294–300.
6. Bright, E., Cotterill, N., Drake, M., and Abrams, P. (2012). Developing a validated urinary diary: phase 1. *Neurourol. Urodyn.* 31 (5): 625–633.
7. Drake, M.J. (2018). Fundamentals of terminology in lower urinary tract function. *Neurourol. Urodyn.* 37 (S6): S13–S19.
8. Gulur, D.M., Mevcha, A.M., and Drake, M.J. (2011). Nocturia as a manifestation of systemic disease. *BJU Int.* 107 (5): 702–713.
9. Drake, M.J. (2014). Do we need a new definition of the overactive bladder syndrome? ICI-RS 2013. *Neurourol. Urodyn.* 33 (5): 622–624.
10. Marshall, S.D., Raskolnikov, D., Blanker, M.H. et al. (2015). International consultations on urological D: Nocturia: current levels of evidence and recommendations from the international consultation on male lower urinary tract symptoms. *Urology* 85 (6): 1291–1299.
11. Haylen, B.T., Maher, C.F., Barber, M.D. et al. (2016). An international Urogynecological association (IUGA)/ international continence society (ICS) joint report on the terminology for female pelvic organ prolapse (POP): international urogynecological association (IUGA). *Neurourol. Urodyn.* 35 (2): 137–168.
12. Madhu, C., Swift, S., Moloney-Geany, S., and Drake, M.J. (2018). How to use the pelvic organ prolapse quantification (POP-Q) system? *Neurourol. Urodyn.* 37 (S6): S39–S43.

5

Treatments for Lower Urinary Tract Dysfunction

Sharon Yeo[1] and Hashim Hashim[2]

[1] *Department of Urology, Tan Tock Seng Hospital, Singapore, Singapore*
[2] *Bristol Urological Institute, Southmead Hospital, Bristol, UK*

CONTENTS

Following initial evaluation, a treatment plan can be formulated based on conservative therapies. Describing the nature of the condition, therapy options, and prognosis is important, ideally with written information and using easily understood language. Patients need to be given the chance to raise questions and must be given a meaningful response. A balance of nursing and medical contribution is appropriate to establish a good rapport, help two-way communication, and give adequate time. This helps identify factors patients find particularly problematic, notably:

- maintaining or recovering sexual function,
- cultural requirements, for example, post-micturition dribble (PMD) is particularly problematic for Moslems, while some groups cannot accept vaginal examination of an unmarried woman by a doctor,
- anxiety disorder, and
- psychological trauma, e.g. previous sexual assault.

Therapy selection must recognise that many patients are not 'ideal', meaning that not only do they have the issue under discussion, but also they may have a physical, medical, or psychological factor which could contribute to the mechanism of lower urinary tract dysfunction (LUTD), or which could influence outcome (Table 5.1). Furthermore, LUTD may well occur in conjunction with linked issues, such as bowel or gynaecological problems, which need to be managed alongside. Hence, there are many potential medical issues which might need to be considered:

- Pelvic organ prolapse (POP) in women
- Menopausal oestrogen deficiency in women
- Previous gynaecological surgery, notably vaginal mesh procedures (POP and stress incontinence operations)
- Urethral stricture/stenosis/tenderness
- Prior pelvic trauma
- Bowel problems, e.g. faecal incontinence, chronic constipation, irritable bowel syndrome (IBS), and inflammatory bowel disease
- Neurological disease
- Impaired cognition
- Mental health issues

Some of these may be amenable to supported conservative therapy. For example, healthy weight loss (>5%) in obese women may improve incontinence [1]. Topical oestrogen therapy may help women with atrophic vaginal epithelium. For older patients, possible causes of transient incontinence can be recalled using the mnemonic 'DIAPPERS' [2]; Delirium, Infection, Atrophic vaginitis,

---

Abrams' Urodynamics, Fourth Edition. Edited by Marcus Drake, Hashim Hashim, and Andrew Gammie.
© 2021 John Wiley & Sons Ltd. Published 2021 by John Wiley & Sons Ltd.

Table 5.1 Individual issues which potentially could influence patient attitudes to the condition and its treatment.

Regular commitments (e.g. journeys, meetings, and social events)

Personal or intimate (sexual) relationships

Cultural requirements (e.g. post-micturition dribble is a problem for a Moslem wishing to pray)

Prior pelvic surgery, especially in the presence of vaginal mesh

Pelvic trauma

Psychological trauma, e.g. sexual assault

Impaired cognition

Mental health issues

Anxiety disorder

Pharmaceuticals, Psychological, Excess urine output (diuretics, diabetes mellitus), Reduced mobility (hip fractures, deconditioning), and Stool impaction (opioid medication).

The managing team has to remain open-minded and alert to anticipate where to focus attention in assessment and therapy and ensure realistic expectations. Patients understandably think an operation will sort out all their symptoms, so the practitioner needs to be explicit about which ones actually will realistically improve. If someone has an incurable problem, it is important not to suggest a cure is possible (including when referring to someone else, even if they are an 'expert', since the patient may be given unrealistic expectations). Furthermore, if getting nowhere with treatment, it is best to step back and re-evaluate rather than persisting with futile treatments (Figure 5.1).

Follow-up is important to evaluate adequacy of response. If the patient reports insufficient improvement, the situation needs to be reviewed to ascertain the problem(s):

- Persistence of the symptoms (absent or insufficient response)
- New symptoms (e.g. disease progression)
- Adverse effects (the condition responded, but the treatment is poorly tolerated)
- Complication (e.g. the patient is now in chronic retention)
- Non-compliance with therapy
- Inadequate initial assessment
- Urinary tract infection

Once the problems are identified and investigated, therapy can be reviewed. It may be decided to alter the conservative approach, and again follow-up. Alternatively, the potential necessity to proceed with more interventional methods may mandate urodynamic evaluation, following which surgical approaches may be an option. Thus, management of LUTD is a stepwise and logical process of assessment, directed therapy, and follow-up, with escala-

2010	Oxybutynin 5 mg
2011	Tamsulosin 400 mcg
2011	Finasteride 5 mg (4 months)
2012	Indapamide 2.5 mg
2012	Desmopressin 200 mcg × 2
2013	Furosemide 20 mg
2013	Solifenacin 5 mg
2013	Fesoterodine 4 mg
2014	Furosemide 20 mg (again)
2014	Trospium Chloride 60 mg
2014	Mirabegron 50 mg

Figure 5.1 An example of why it is appropriate to review the situation if failing to improve with the current therapeutic strategy. Illustrated is a list produced by a patient showing medications he had been prescribed to try to reduce severe nocturia, each of which had proved ineffective. On direct questioning, he described heavy snoring and his wife described breathing interruptions when asleep. Screening for obstructive sleep apnoea proved positive, and nocturia resolved with continuous positive airway pressure treatment.

tion until adequate response is achieved (Figure 5.2). If the bladder serves adequately as a reservoir, intermittent self-catheterisation (ISC) may be a treatment in certain situations or may be used to open out additional options.

For some patients, it may be necessary to confine management to containment (e.g. incontinence pads and bed protection) [3, 4]. For men, collecting appliances (penile sheath or condom collecting devices) [5] are available. Ultimately, some individuals may proceed to indwelling catheterisation [6] to manage their incontinence.

This chapter is intended to provide basic principles involved in treatment and their relationship with urodynamic investigation at different levels. The books from the International Consultations on Incontinence (ICI), the sixth of which was published in 2017, provided detailed evaluation of the techniques used for the management of LUTD [7].

Storage Phase Problems

The relevant symptoms are most commonly:

- storage lower urinary tract symptoms (LUTS), which may principally present as overactive bladder (OAB) syndrome,
- nocturia, and
- incontinence.

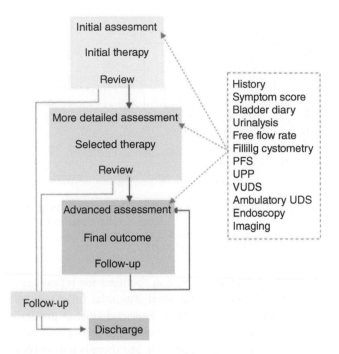

Figure 5.2 Managing benign lower urinary tract dysfunction can require successive iterations of assessment and therapy where outcome is unsatisfactory (red arrows), until satisfactory outcome is achieved (blue arrows). An increasing range of diagnostic tools may be needed as the assessments get more advanced. PFS: pressure flow studies; UPP: urethral pressure profilometry; VUDS: video urodynamics.

The urodynamic findings may be detrusor overactivity (DO), increased filling sensation, reduced detrusor compliance, or urethral sphincter incompetence causing urodynamic stress incontinence (USI).

OAB and/or DO

1) Conservative treatments consist of the following:
   a) Advice on fluid and food intake
      - Reduce intake if planning to go out. Advise patients about the likely time taken for a drink to result in urine production (a couple of hours).
      - Minimise intake before going to bed or during the night, e.g. 4 hours before going to bed.
      - Maintain an adequate urine output: 1–2 l.
      - Avoid fluids that contain caffeine, alcohol, or chemicals (e.g. artificial sweeteners). This improves symptoms of OAB but does not improve urinary incontinence [8, 9].
      - Some foods (fruit, salads, vegetables, rice, and pasta) can have enough liquid (300–500 ml) that the quantity and timing of intake should also be considered.
   b) Bladder training. The patient is encouraged to aim to control an urgency sensation when it commences,

either by resisting (pelvic floor/sphincter contraction) or relaxing (mental distraction, or conscious control). Initially, only small intervals should be aimed for (a matter of a few seconds), but larger intervals can be achieved over the ensuing weeks as the patient's skill and confidence grows.

   c) Pelvic floor muscle exercises (PFME). Increasing pelvic floor muscle contraction strength and durability may inhibit detrusor contraction in patients with OAB symptoms [10]. PFME may also help bladder training by aiding urethral closure until the involuntary contraction has passed. Strong consideration should be given to providing healthcare professional input in formal teaching of how to do these exercises, especially for female patients.

A bladder diary can be used to assess the success of these treatments.

2) Medical management

These should follow compliance with conservative measures and follow-up. The conservative measures are important since medications are not an antidote to inappropriate habits, such as excessive caffeine intake.

   a) Antimuscarinic medications reduce the effect of the low level of acetylcholine release seen during the storage phase. Oral preparations may be immediate or extended (sustained) release; the latter are considered more effective [11]. Antimuscarinics produce the common side effects of dry mouth, blurring of vision, constipation, and sometimes drowsiness. In addition, there is the possibility of central nervous system (CNS) effects, notably an effect on memory and cognition [12]; this is probably less likely if the specific drug has a quaternary amine structure (e.g. trospium chloride). Transdermal preparations of oxybutynin are available which may reduce the likelihood of systemic effects (due to an altered profile of generated metabolites) but carry a risk of local skin irritation. Flexible dosing of some antimuscarinics is an option to match the timing of intake to anticipated need (e.g. using an extended release preparation but only taking it on working days, or taking an immediate release preparation an hour before a journey, etc.) or to limit the adverse effects. Early review upon commencing an antimuscarinic should be done to monitor efficacy and side effects. Special attention is needed for vulnerable patients, such as the elderly, and those susceptible to CNS effects (e.g. early cognitive impairment). These medications are contraindicated in severe bowel disease, poorly controlled acute angle glaucoma, and myasthaenia gravis. Proper education is essential, since failure to convey exactly what to expect, or how to deal with issues, may contribute to the low proportions staying on an antimuscarinic long term [13].

b) Beta-3 agonist. Relaxation of the detrusor muscle during the storage phase occurs with the activation of sympathetic system via stimulation of ß₃-adrenoceptors [9]. Mirabegron is a ß₃-adrenoceptor agonist approved for use in several countries for treating OAB [14]. Side effects are infrequent and may be idiosyncratic; it is contraindicated in severe uncontrolled hypertension.

c) Drug combinations. Due to their differing mechanisms of action, it is appropriate to consider using antimuscarinics with mirabegron in patients not responding to either drug given separately. In the BESIDE study randomising more than 2,000 patients with persisting incontinence despite solifenacin 5 mg, the combination of mirabegron with solifenacin 5 mg was more effective than solifenacin 5 or 10 mg in terms of incontinence and frequency and was better tolerated than the higher strength antimuscarinic alone (Figure 5.3) [15].

3) Endoscopically administered OAB therapy

Onabotulinum toxin-A (BTX). *Clostridium botulinum* produces a neurotoxin which inhibits release of acetylcholine from nerve endings, resulting in paralysis. Medical formulations injected into the bladder wall have a range of effects which can reduce DO. There are different medical formulations (i.e. onabotulinum-A, abobotulinum-A, and incobotulinumtoxin-A); doses of the formulations are different and not interchangeable. Onabotulinum-A has received Food and Drug administration (FDA) approval for treatment of urgency incontinence in adults who have failed or could not tolerate anticholinergics; the dose for idiopathic DO is 100 units [16] and for neurogenic DO (multiple sclerosis or subcervical cord injury) 200 units [17]. After injection, response is seen within a couple of weeks, with

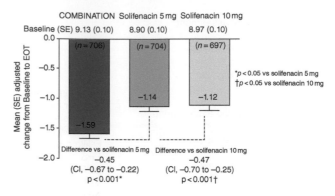

Figure 5.3 Combination of beta-3 agonist (mirabegron 50 mg) with antimuscarinic (solifenacin 5 mg) is more effective at reducing incontinence episodes than antimuscarinic monotherapy. *Source*: Drake et al. [15].

quite a varied duration and the need for repeat injections subsequently (at least 3 months later to avoid forming antibodies) [12]. Repeated dosing generally achieves a similar level of response to earlier treatments for an individual (Figure 5.4), but there is a drop-off in the number of people responding with ongoing repeated dosing. Urinary tract infection can be problematic after onabotulinum-A injections. All patients planned for this treatment need to learn ISC beforehand, because some people will develop voiding dysfunction. When the therapy was being developed, higher doses (200 and 300 U) were generally used, which resulted in a longer duration of effect but greater risk of needing to do ISC subsequently.

4) Nerve stimulation

a) Sacral nerve stimulation (SNS), also known as sacral neuromodulation (SNM), involves stimulation of the relevant sacral nerve root (usually S3 or S4) via an electrode connected to a pulse generator (Figure 5.5). In the initial/test phase (the percutaneous needle evaluation, or PNE), a temporary wire

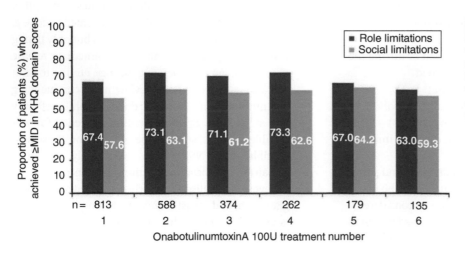

Figure 5.4 Mean improvement from baseline in the proportion of patients who achieved the minimally important difference (at least a 5-point decrease) in the Kings Health Questionnaire at week 12 over six treatment cycles using onabotulinum-A 100 units intravesical injection. *Source*: Ginsberg et al. [18].

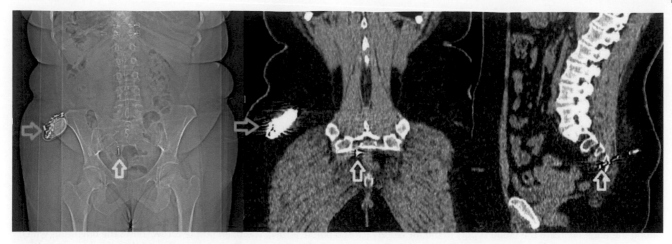

Figure 5.5 Computed tomography (CT) scan of a sacral nerve stimulator in position showing the battery pack (green arrow) and the electrode in the sacrum (yellow arrow). *Source*: Marcus Drake.

electrode is percutaneously inserted, and a temporary connection is made to an external stimulator. If this brings substantial improvement in symptoms, then the PNE electrode is removed for subsequent definitive therapy. The full SNS is fully subcutaneous, using a self-retaining 'tined' lead, and a stimulator with a battery. The patient is given a personal controller unit to enable them to alter the current delivery. SNS is currently recommended as treatment for urgency incontinence due to idiopathic DO after failed conservative therapy and non-obstructive urinary retention [19]. Complications may include pain and infection, which can necessitate implant removal. Lead displacement may result in loss of effect. Battery life is generally several years (5–7 years on average), but active follow-up for technical checks is needed to minimise battery depletion and hence prolong therapeutic response. As of 2020, the marketed devices by two companies are magnetic resonance imaging (MRI)-safe, and there is a rechargeable version which in theory could last for at least 15 years.

b) Tibial nerve stimulation. A percutaneous electrode placed near the tibial nerve at the ankle and used for short stimulations (typically 30 minutes at weekly intervals for 12 weeks) is an option for selected patients (Figure 5.6). It requires substantial input from healthcare professionals, and that may limit the number of patients able to benefit. Long-term outcome data is lacking [19]. Implantable tibial nerve stimulators are now also available.

5) Surgical management

Augmentation cystoplasty. The operation involves the bladder being cut almost fully in half ('bivalved'), right down to the bladder neck (Figure 5.7). The defect is bridged with a bowel patch, which has been isolated from the rest of the gut and opened along the edge away from its blood supply ('detubularised'). The augmentation increases the reservoir capacity and interrupts involuntary detrusor contractions from spreading to involve the entire organ. It also impairs voiding efficiency, so most patients will require ISC post-operatively. Early complications include infection, fistula, bowel obstruction, pulmonary embolism/deep vein thrombosis, patch necrosis, and death. In the long-term metabolic derangement, renal deterioration, urinary tract infection, bladder stones, perforation, and altered bowel habit have been described [20]. Malignancy is

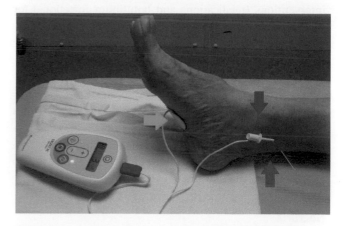

Figure 5.6 Applying treatment with a tibial nerve stimulator. The inserted electrode (red arrow) is placed posterior to the medial malleolus (blue arrow) and connected to the stimulator pack. This is also connected to a skin-patch electrode placed on the sole of the foot (green arrow). Current flows through the tissues to complete the circuit between the two electrodes; the tibial nerve lies in this region, and stimulating this has caused the toes to dorsiflex (point upwards). *Source*: Marcus Drake.

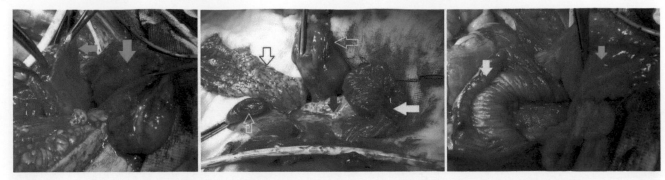

Figure 5.7 Three crucial steps in an augmentation cystoplasty. Left image: bivalving the bladder, i.e. fully cutting it in half down to the bladder neck; the blue arrow shows the back half, and the green shows the front half. Middle image: isolating and detubularising a bowel segment. The ileum has been divided at two points (open yellow arrows), and the part between (closed yellow arrow) cuts along the edge opposite the blood supply in the mesentery (closed purple arrow). The open purple arrow shows the omentum, which can be placed against the suture lines at the end of the operation to facilitate healing. Right image: the detubularised bowel (yellow arrow) has already been sutured to the posterior wall of the bladder (blue arrow) and is about to be closed to the front half (green arrow), aiming for watertight closure. *Source*: Marcus Drake.

rare, with a latency of 10 years or more, but means endoscopic surveillance may be needed [21]. Such radical surgery is an option in persistent debilitating symptoms but requires careful consideration in view of commonplace and potentially serious complications.

Increased Filling Sensation and Impaired Detrusor Compliance

OAB and DO have been the main research targets leading to the development of approved therapeutic interventions. In practice, these OAB interventions might be applied if people have increased filling sensation on urodynamics, but it is not clear whether the same response rates can be anticipated. Reduced detrusor compliance likewise relies on the same interventions (medications and botulinum injections) for attempting to reduce bladder pressures. However, the potential implication for renal dysfunction if response is poor means follow-up needs to be regularly and reliably done, and interventions may need to move quickly towards reconstructive options (augmentation cystoplasty).

Very rarely, reduced compliance may be treated with a sphincterotomy [22], i.e. deliberately damaging the sphincter by endoscopic incision. This aims at deliberately inducing leakage in order to avoid allowing the pressure to exceed an acceptable value for renal protection.

Nocturia

One of the key requirements in managing nocturia is to identify the underlying factors; it has many potential causes [23] derived from behavioural influences, medical conditions (notably cardiovascular, renal, or endocrine), sleep disorders (notably obstructive sleep apnoea [OSA]), or LUTD (Figure 5.8). These can be distinguished with the help of a properly completed bladder diary [25], thus enabling therapy to be directed at cause(s).

- A high proportion of people simply need advice on managing the fluid intake; the advice given to people with OAB is also relevant for people with nocturia. Since urine production reflects homeostatic needs to get rid of surplus water, salt, and toxins, these patients also need to reduce salt intake to avoid natriuresis.

- People need to consider suitable habits to encourage sleep as they head to bed, allowing time to relax before bedtime and ensuring a quiet and comfortable environment in the bedroom.

- Primary sleep disorders, such as restless legs syndrome might sometimes be present and would need specialist advice if considered likely.

- Some people have a medical condition which affects urine output, some of the key conditions being cardiac failure, chronic kidney disease, and diabetes (mellitus or insipidus). These patients may need their condition screened and optimised under the care of appropriate medical expertise [26]. If a specific medical cause is identified, therapy of the condition should be optimised. Sometimes, nocturia may indicate the need to review glycaemic control in diabetic patients [27]. In practice, the range of interventions is limited.

- LUTD is actually a relatively unusual contributor to nocturia. However, OAB syndrome or the presence of a significant post-void residual (PVR) may contribute, and specific therapy can be directed to these (see relevant section). Where bladder outlet obstruction (BOO) with associated PVR of urine has reduced functional capacity, then effective surgery could reduce nocturia. If there is a PVR without BOO (e.g. in detrusor underactivity [DUA]), ISC might be considered. Similarly, treatment of OAB/

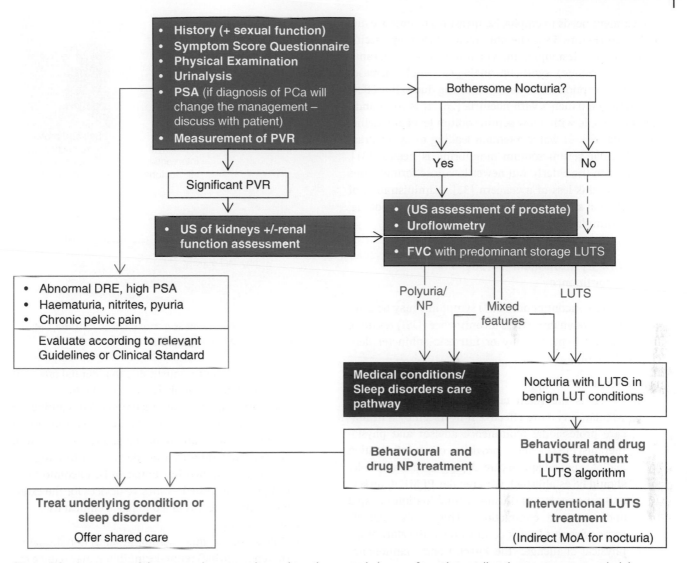

Figure 5.8 A summary of the approach to assessing and treating nocturia in men, focussing on directing treatment at underlying causative processes. DRE: digital rectal examination; FVC: frequency volume chart; LUTS: lower urinary tract symptoms; MoA: mechanism of action; NP: nocturnal polyuria; PCa: prostate cancer; PSA: prostate specific antigen; PVR: post-void residual; US: ultrasound. *Source*: Gratzke et al. [24].

DO can be considered, noting that the people most likely to respond are those who experience urgency overnight, not only in the daytime. If night-time voids are not driven by urgency, LUTD medications are not generally effective against nocturia [26].

STOP-Bang is a simple questionnaire in which the higher the STOP-Bang score, the greater is the probability of moderate-to-severe OSA [28]. A point is awarded for each question answered with 'yes':

- Snoring: Do you snore loudly (louder than talking or loud enough to be heard through closed doors)?
- Tired: Do you often feel tired, fatigued, or sleepy during daytime?

- Observed: Has anyone observed you stop breathing during your sleep?
- Pressure (Blood pressure): Do you have or are you being treated for high blood pressure?
- Body mass index (BMI): BMI more than $35\,\mathrm{kg\,m^{-2}}$?
- Age over 50 years old?
- Neck circumference greater than 40 cm (around 16 in., measured by staff)?
- Gender male?

There is an online tool which identifies the specific risk (http://www.stopbang.ca/osa/screening.php). This is a crucial consideration due to the possibility of a substantial reduction in nocturia using continuous positive airway pressure (CPAP) overnight [29].

Treatment needs to emphasise measures to improve diet and sleep (Figure 5.9). The only medical therapy specific for nocturia is desmopressin, which is a vasopressin (antidiuretic hormone) synthetic analogue which increases water reabsorption in the renal collecting ducts. It is effective for some patients with nocturia [26]. It is contraindicated in people with a low serum sodium level at baseline due to the risk of water retention leading to hyponatraemia. Regular serum sodium monitoring is needed [31], especially in the elderly, but newer low-dose formulations have made this less of a concern [32]. Administration of desmopressin should be about 90 minutes before bedtime. Several formulations are available.

Stress Urinary Incontinence/Urodynamic Stress Incontinence

Stress urinary incontinence (SUI) symptoms may be associated with urodynamic stress incontinence (USI) resulting from urethral hypermobility or intrinsic sphincter deficiency (ISD) or both:

1) Conservative therapy
   a) PFME is the main conservative intervention. In women, it is more effective if overseen by a healthcare professional (continence advisor and physiotherapist) [33] – mere provision of an information leaflet is not adequate care. A programme of activity should be established, with regular PFME done several times a day, and using a combination of rapid and sustained contractions. This helps establish responsiveness (quick contraction at the start of the physical challenge; 'the knack') and maintenance during prolonged activity. Pelvic floor muscle training (PFMT) can be augmented with biofeedback, weighted vaginal cones, and electrical or magnetic stimulation of pelvic floor muscle nerves. It is not full established how PFME works [34] – for example, it does not increase urethral closure pressure [35].
   b) For men, external compression can be applied to the penile shaft, and a range of such devices is available (Figures 5.10 and 5.11). Each individual may not find all options suitable [37]. These devices should

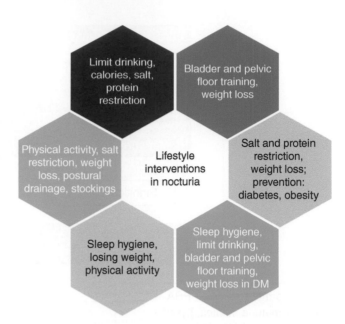

Figure 5.9 Conservative measures to manage nocturia. DM: Diabetes mellitus. *Source*: Everaert et al. [30].

not be worn continuously, due to potential effect on the penile blood supply [Figure 5.12] [36].

Currently, there is no recommended continence device for women. Intravaginal devices, supporting the bladder neck and reducing anterior vaginal wall descent, and intraurethral devices obstructing the outlet were trialled but found to be uncomfortable and poorly tolerated. Adhesive devices for the external urethral meatus failed to reach clinical use.

2) Medical therapy
   a) Duloxetine, a dual serotonin and noradrenaline (norepinephrine) reuptake inhibitor, may reduce the number of stress incontinence episodes [38]. It elicits an increase in resting tone and contraction strength of the urethral striated sphincter. It requires dose titration at initiation, as it can cause problematic side effects (sexual dysfunction, nausea, headache, dry mouth, somnolence, and dizziness). Two-week dose tapering has been recommended before discontinuation [39]. Duloxetine should not be offered to women or men who are seeking cure for their incontinence.

Figure 5.10 Some of the penile compression clamps available for managing male stress urinary incontinence. *Source*: Reproduced with permission from Lemmens et al. [36].

| Cunningham, Bard Medical | Wiesner, Wiesner Healthcare Innovation LLC | Dribblestop®, Rennich Industries Ltd. | Uriclak®, Vitalnovax Cb |

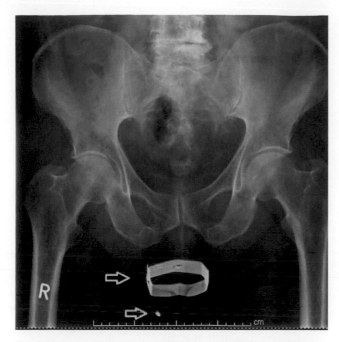

Figure 5.11 X-ray of a male with stress incontinence wearing a penile clamp (upper arrow). The lower arrow indicates the inactivation button of an artificial urinary sphincter which had failed, hence the need for the clamp. *Source*: Marcus Drake.

b) Vaginal oestrogen application may be considered as an adjunct in the management of common pelvic floor disorders in postmenopausal women [40, 41]. Practitioners need to be aware that systemic oestro-

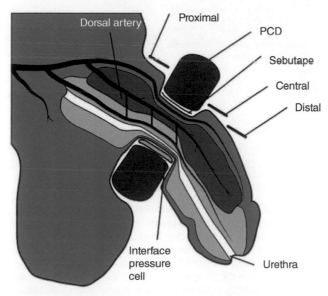

Figure 5.12 Penile compression device (PCD) and the penile blood supply. Diagram from a study measuring perfusion of the penis when a compression device is in place. This study indicated that application of a clamp for 1 hour with an equal clamp free time before reapplication is likely to be safe. *Source*: Lemmens et al. [36].

gen (as in oral hormone replacement therapy) apparently is associated with worsened symptoms of urinary incontinence [41].

3) Surgical treatment

For USI, this should be directed at the relevant mechanism.

Urethral hypermobility in women is treated with procedures to maintain urethral support and ensure the sphincter can function effectively:

a) Retropubic techniques. Burch colposuspension aims to approximate the inner aspect of the vaginal fornices retropubically to the pectineal ligament (a fascia condensation on the inner aspect of the pubis/ilium of the pelvis) with interrupted, non-absorbable, or absorbable sutures (Figure 5.13). The vagino-obturator shelf procedure, a modification with less elevation of the vaginal wall, uses sutures into the obturator fascia instead of the pectineal ligament. Long-term complete urinary continence rates are reported as 82% [42]. Colposuspension was the main procedure until the advent of midurethral tape procedures and is beginning to re-emerge [43] with the declining use of medical mesh in vaginal surgery. Laparoscopic and robotic Burch colposuspension is starting to gain ground.

b) Midurethral tapes were developed in the 1990s and steadily became the most used surgical intervention for women with SUI. They aim to support the midurethra with non-absorbable synthetic monofilament mesh and are placed tension-free. They lie paraurethrally and run either retropubically or through the obturator foramen (termed 'transvaginal' or 'transobturator', respectively).

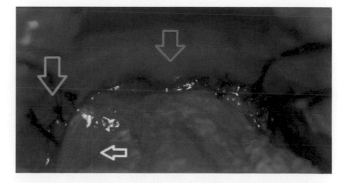

Figure 5.13 Colposuspension, viewed from the inside of the pelvis, with the pubic symphysis (grey arrow) at the top. Three sutures have been placed into the iliopectineal line (indicated on the left side with a green arrow) and used to elevate the vaginal fornix (blue arrow). The yellow arrow indicates the right lower edge of the bladder, which must not be caught by the sutures and is mobilised medially during the dissection. *Source*: Marcus Drake.

Midurethral tapes and colposuspension have broadly similar efficacy outcomes [44], but recovery time and risk of POP are a problem for colposuspension, while pain, voiding dysfunction, and bladder perforation can occur with tapes. Potential problems with medical mesh are increasingly being recognised [45, 46] leading to a clear decline in use in several countries.

Intrinsic urethral sphincter weakness in women is due to either neurogenic causes or trauma, for example, after repeated procedures for USI treatment. It may be treated by:

a) Urethral bulking injection. Injection of a bulking agent into the submucosal tissue of the urethra aims to increase the urethral resistance by improving the coaptation of the urethral lumen. They may be injected transurethrally or paraurethrally. There are a few substances marketed for urethral bulking, and no clear-cut conclusions could be drawn from trials comparing alternative agents [47]. Greater symptomatic improvement was observed with surgical treatments but set against likely higher risks [47]. Urethral bulking agent might be more cost-effective than surgery when used as an initial treatment in women without hypermobility or as a follow-up to surgery failure [47]. This approach is also sometimes used to treat hypermobility SUI, especially in countries where midurethral tapes are not available.

b) Sling procedures. Autologous fascial slings (rectus sheath or fascia lata) have also been available for years to support the mid and/or proximal urethra. Generally, a minimally invasive approach can be taken, referred to as a 'sling-on-a-string' [48], providing an approach which can be employed to manage primary stress incontinence without using medical mesh. Open autologous sling placement can also be used to treat ISD in a complex case (Figure 5.14), as well as serving as a treatment for urethral hypermobility. The autologous sling approaches are becoming an important option in current practice [48]. They provide urethral support and can be tensioned to provide urethral compression, which is needed in ISD. The compression may make it difficult to void, so patients generally need to be taught to do ISC before undergoing the operation.

c) Artificial urinary sphincter (AUS). The AUS is a rare operation in women, but it has a place in carefully selected patients, especially those with neurological disease [49]. The AUS system relies on a cuff placed around the urethra, connected to a pressurised reservoir which squeezes the urethra within the cuff (Figure 5.15). When wishing to pass urine, a third 'pump' component can be squeezed, which allows a couple of minutes to empty the bladder. In women, the pump for opening the cuff and allowing voiding is placed in a labium majorum. Implantation can be done by open surgery, laparoscopically [50], or robotically [51].

Intrinsic sphincter weakness in men. For men with post-prostatectomy incontinence (PPI), in contrast to women, formal healthcare professional pelvic floor training does not appear to give an additional advantage above an information leaflet [52]. Hence, operative intervention is often needed, with two main current options.

a) AUS. The AUS system in men has the cuff placed around the bulbar or proximal urethra, connected to an intra-abdominal pressurised reservoir. The pump component is placed in the scrotum (Figure 5.16). The AUS is an effective therapy for severe incontinence, though the evidence base is modest [53]. Patients with impaired dexterity or cognition, or previous pelvic radiotherapy may not be suitable for AUS. When the components are placed, scrupulous infection prevention measures are needed, because it is an implant and hence likely will need emergency removal if infection takes hold. Caution is needed for any subsequent operations or catheterisation. It may be possible to place an AUS after failure of a male sling [54].

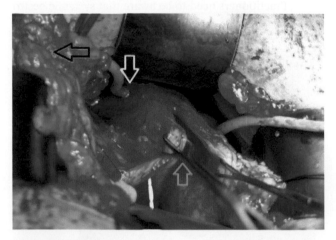

Figure 5.14 The anatomical location of an autologous sling. This figure illustrates open placement of an autologous sling in a patient with a complex background, including previous stress incontinence surgery. The inside of the pelvis is exposed, with the pubic symphysis hidden by a retractor at the top of the image. The route the sling will be placed along has been created and is held open by a rubber tube; the yellow arrow indicates the left hand end of the section behind the urethra itself. Pulling on the two ends of the tube will elevate and compress the urethra. The bladder has been opened (blue arrow) to be able to see into the urethra and check whether it has not been perforated. The omentum (black arrow) has also been mobilised to place along the track and provide some healthy tissue as protection. *Source*: Marcus Drake.

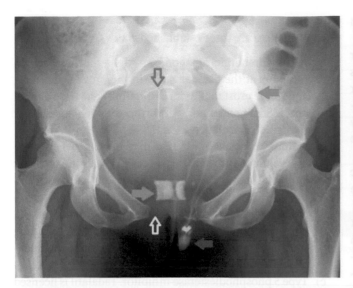
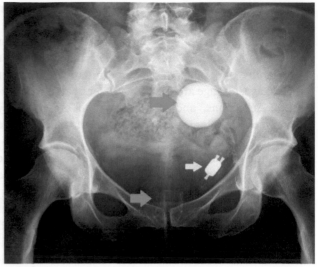

Figure 5.15 An X-ray of an artificial urinary sphincter (AUS) in two women. Above: the X-ray shows the cuff around the urethra (blue arrow), pressure reservoir filled with X-ray contrast (green arrow), and the pump component in the left labium majorum (red arrow). The AUS is visible because the components were filled with X-ray contrast when the device was inserted. There is also pubic diastasis (yellow arrow) and an intrauterine coil (orange arrow). Below: a different woman with an older model AUS, showing the reservoir (green arrow), cuff (blue arrow), and a connector (Picture on the right; yellow arrow). The labium is below the edge of the image, so the pump component is not visible. *Source*: Marcus Drake.

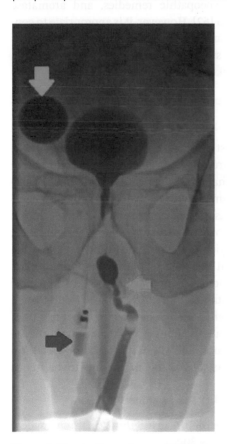

Figure 5.16 An X-ray of an artificial urinary sphincter in a man, showing the cuff around the urethra (just visible at the tip of the blue arrow), pressure reservoir filled with X-ray contrast (green arrow), and pump (red arrow). This has been compressed a couple of times to empty the cuff, and the man is passing urine. *Source*: Marcus Drake.

b) Male slings constructed from synthetic mesh. Restoration of continence in theory uses the concept of either urethral compression or repositioning of the bulb of the urethra [55]. Some male mesh-slings have adjustable tension but uncertain long-term outcomes and adverse events. There is no evidence that adjustability offers additional benefit over other types of sling [56].

A randomised trial has completed recruitment of male sling against AUS and results are awaited [57].

Intractable Incontinence

If age, physical status, mental state, or disease prevents the use of curative techniques, other methods of treatment may be needed. The proper management of incontinence depends on a nurse continence service which is properly integrated into care provision across the full scope of services where catheterised patients are encountered.

a) Pads. A wide range of products is available. All patients should be properly assessed as to their pad needs, with the appropriate size of pad being given, potentially with suitable incontinence pants to support the pad. All-in-one washable pants with fitted pads are preferred by many patients. Patients may require different protection at night from that used in the daytime. Bed protection, in the form of disposable or washable reusable protective sheets, should be considered. Often, absorbent pads are the first-line containment option

Table 5.2 Success rates of learning intermittent self-catheterisation in a well-supported service.

	Age < 65 years			Age > 65 years		
	Number of patients	Success rate (%)	Failure rate (%)	Number of patients	Success rate (%)	Failure rate (%)
Male	82	91	9	127	86	14
Female	69	80	20	31	68	32
Overall	151	86	14	158	82	18

Source: Parsons et al. [71].

b) ISC is used when possible, which is the case in the majority, provided the teaching is appropriately set up (Table 5.2), specifically considering requirements such as sending information about ISC in advance of a teaching appointment, additional information at the appointment, training under supervision, and access to follow-on support. [71]. ISC can generally be used by both sexes and all ages. If the patient is too young or too disabled, then intermittent catheterisation can be performed by the parent, relative, or carer.

c) Indwelling catheterisation is sometimes needed.

Medical Therapy

Medications are rarely successful. Use of alpha-blockers has been attempted in some functional obstruction situations, but evidence is of low quality.

Surgical Therapy

This was formerly the routine for functional obstructions, but the procedures are now undertaken infrequently due to the potential for ISC. If urethral ISC is impossible, for reasons of physical accessibility, outlet distortion, discomfort, or psychological aversion, then an extra-urethral

route may be created – a continent urinary diversion. In the Mitrofanoff procedure, the bladder is joined to the anterior abdominal wall by a small continent tube (appendix [72] or reconfigured small bowel segment [73]) as an alternative to the urethra for ISC (Figure 5.19). Complications and failure (at any stage) are common [74, 75]. Augmentation cystoplasty can be undertaken at the same time if bladder capacity is insufficient. If there is severe dysfunction of the bladder, a full reconstruction to fashion a storage reservoir ("neobladder") can be undertaken, which requires rather a large amount of ileum (Figure 5.20) or colon.

Detrusor Underactivity/Underactive Bladder

DUA [76] is a urodynamic observation which can occur as a primary problem or secondary to neurological disease. Recently, the International Continence Society (ICS) has introduced terminology for a symptom syndrome deriving from this form of LUTD; underactive bladder (UAB) syndrome is a clinical diagnosis characterised by a slow urinary stream, hesitancy, and straining to void, with or without a feeling of incomplete bladder emptying some-

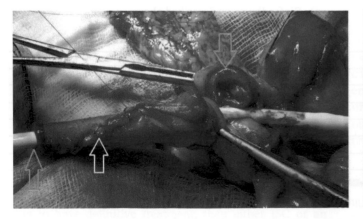
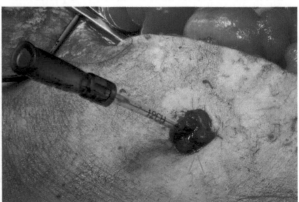

Figure 5.19 A Mitrofanoff extra-urethral channel to enable intermittent self-catheterisation of the bladder. A section of gut has been isolated from the ileum (green arrow) and reconfigured into a long thin tube (yellow arrow) using the Monti principle [73]. The outer end (blue arrow) is brought out to the abdominal surface, and the inner end is brought into the bladder with a valve configuration. *Source*: Marcus Drake.

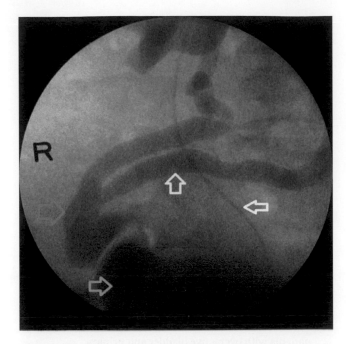

Figure 5.20 Video urodynamic study of a patient with a Mitrofanoff channel and a neobladder constructed by reconfiguring small intestine. The filling line inserted into the bladder along the Mitrofanoff channel is indicated by the white arrow. The point at which it enters the Mitrofanoff cannot be seen, and if knowledge of this location is needed (e.g. in patients being checked for incontinence along the channel), an external marker would have to be placed (see Figure 8.4). The green arrow indicates the reservoir, which has been constructed and reconfigured from detubularised bowel (usually small bowel, but sigmoid colon can also be used) to create a reservoir for storing urine as a replacement for the bladder ('neobladder'). In order to empty this, the patient self-catheterises along the Mitrofanoff. For this type of neobladder, the ureters are often joined side to side and attached to a non-detubularised bowel segment (orange arrow) which enters the neobladder ('Studer pouch'). Placing the ureters side to side is usually done by bringing the left ureter over to the right side of the abdomen (yellow arrow), passing it through the sigmoid mesentery in front of the spine. The ureters are fully visible because of grade IV/V vesicoureteric reflux. Patients can sometimes leak from the Mitrofanoff channel either (i) due to peristalsis in the neobladder, which would be reflected as overactive waves in p_{ves}, or (ii) due to weakness in the 'valve' mechanism at the join between the Mitrofanoff and the native bladder or neobladder. *Source*: Marcus Drake.

times with storage symptoms [77]. In men, the symptoms resemble those experienced by patients with BOO [78].

DUA management is challenging [79]:

- If symptoms or complications occur and there is significant PVR, then ISC may be required.
- Medical therapy aimed at increasing detrusor activity, for example, by cholinergic drugs or prostaglandin, is not evidently effective [80]. Alpha-adrenergic blockers to try

to improve sphincter relaxation likewise do not show consistent convincing results.

- There is little evidence that TURP will improve voiding function in men with DUA [81]. It is possible that bladder neck incision, prostatic incision, or TURP may improve voiding by allowing more effective straining.
- SNM can be helpful in women and worth trying in men.

Post-Micturition Symptoms

PMD is a common symptom in men and can be very bothersome. PMD is due to urine left in the bulbous and penile urethra, at the end of micturition (Figure 2.10). Rarely, it can occur in women, as a result of some voided urine entering the vagina (Figure 5.21). Since this urine is past the sphincter, it dribbles out and wets the underpants, and perhaps the trousers, after leaving the toilet. Treatment is by explaining the cause, advice on the need for unhurried conclusion of voiding, and advice about posture on the toilet (for women). Men should be taught how to manually express ("milk") the relevant part of the

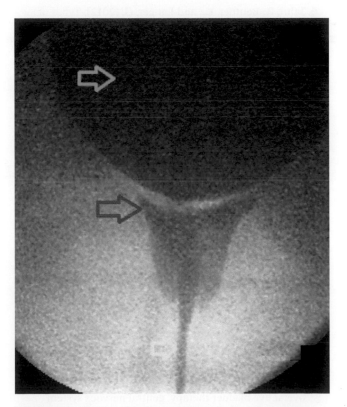

Figure 5.21 X-ray during pressure flow studies of a woman who reported post-micturition dribble as a frequent problem. While her bladder (green arrow) was emptying with a normal stream (yellow arrow), some contrast refluxed into the vagina and was seen pooling in the fornices (purple arrow). *Source*: Marcus Drake.

urethra by firm but not painful upward perineal pressure on the urethral bulb, slowly moving the pressure point along the urethra towards the penis, at which point the drops can readily be expelled (Figure 2.13). Sensation of incomplete emptying may benefit from ISC if a PVR is evident.

References

1. Hunskaar, S. (2008). A systematic review of overweight and obesity as risk factors and targets for clinical intervention for urinary incontinence in women. *Neurourol. Urodyn.* 27 (8): 749–757.

2. Resnick, N.M. (1987). Urinary incontinence. *Public Health Rep.* 102 (4 Suppl): 67–70.

3. Fader, M., Cottenden, A.M., and Getliffe, K. (2008). Absorbent products for moderate-heavy urinary and/or faecal incontinence in women and men. *Cochrane Database Syst. Rev.* 4: CD007408.

4. Fader, M. (2003). Review of current technologies for urinary incontinence: strengths and limitations. *Proc. Inst. Mech. Eng. H* 217 (4): 233–241.

5. Robinson, J. (2006). Continence: sizing and fitting a penile sheath. *Br. J. Community Nurs.* 11 (10): 420–427.

6. Jahn, P., Beutner, K., and Langer, G. (2012). Types of indwelling urinary catheters for long-term bladder drainage in adults. *Cochrane Database Syst. Rev.* 10: CD004997.

7. Abrams, P., Cardozo, L., Wagg, A. et al. Incontinence (2017). 6th International consultation on Incontinence, 6e. International Consultation on Urological Diseases/ International Continence Society.

8. Swithinbank, L., Hashim, H., and Abrams, P. (2005). The effect of fluid intake on urinary symptoms in women. *J. Urol.* 174 (1): 187–189.

9. Bryant, C.M., Dowell, C.J., and Fairbrother, G. (2002). Caffeine reduction education to improve urinary symptoms. *Br. J. Nurs.* 11 (8): 560–565.

10. Greer, J.A., Smith, A.L., and Arya, L.A. (2012). Pelvic floor muscle training for urgency urinary incontinence in women: a systematic review. *Int. Urogynecol. J.* 23 (6): 687–697.

11. Novara, G., Galfano, A., Secco, S. et al. (2008). A systematic review and meta-analysis of randomized controlled trials with antimuscarinic drugs for overactive bladder. *Eur. Urol.* 54 (4): 740–763.

12. Chancellor, M. and Boone, T. (2012). Anticholinergics for overactive bladder therapy: central nervous system effects. *CNS Neurosci. Ther.* 18 (2): 167–174.

13. Wagg, A., Compion, G., Fahey, A., and Siddiqui, E. (2012). Persistence with prescribed antimuscarinic therapy for overactive bladder: a UK experience. *BJU Int.* 110 (11): 1767–1774.

14. Warren, K., Burden, H., and Abrams, P. (2016). Mirabegron in overactive bladder patients: efficacy review and update on drug safety. *Ther. Adv. Drug Saf.* 7 (5): 204–216.

15. Drake, M.J., Chapple, C., Esen, A.A. et al. (2016). Efficacy and safety of mirabegron add-on therapy to solifenacin in incontinent overactive bladder patients with an inadequate response to initial 4-week solifenacin monotherapy: a randomised double-blind multicentre phase 3B study (BESIDE). *Eur. Urol.* 70 (1): 136–145.

16. Nitti, V.W., Dmochowski, R., Herschorn, S. et al. Group ES (2013). OnabotulinumtoxinA for the treatment of patients with overactive bladder and urinary incontinence: results of a phase 3, randomized, placebo controlled trial. *J. Urol.* 189 (6): 2186–2193.

17. Cruz, F., Herschorn, S., Aliotta, P. et al. (2011). Efficacy and safety of onabotulinumtoxinA in patients with urinary incontinence due to neurogenic detrusor overactivity: a randomised, double-blind, placebo-controlled trial. *Eur. Urol.* 60 (4): 742–750.

18. Ginsberg, D.A., Drake, M.J., Kaufmann, A. et al. (2017). Long-term treatment with onabotulinumtoxinA results in consistent, durable improvements in health related quality of life in patients with overactive bladder. *J. Urol.* 198 (4): 897–904.Investigators

19. Tutolo, M., Ammirati, E., Heesakkers, J. et al. (2018). Efficacy and safety of sacral and percutaneous tibial neuromodulation in non-neurogenic lower urinary tract dysfunction and chronic pelvic pain: a systematic review of the literature. *Eur. Urol.* 73 (3): 406–418.

20. Greenwell, T.J., Venn, S.N., and Mundy, A.R. (2001). Augmentation cystoplasty. *BJU Int.* 88 (6): 511–525.

21. Lane, T. and Shah, J. (2000). Carcinoma following augmentation ileocystoplasty. *Urol. Int.* 64 (1): 31–32.

22. Drake, M.J. (2015). Management and rehabilitation of neurologic patients with lower urinary tract dysfunction. *Handb. Clin. Neurol.* 130: 451–468.

23. Marshall, S.D., Raskolnikov, D., Blanker, M.H. et al. International Consultations on Urological D (2015). Nocturia: current levels of evidence and recommendations from the international consultation on male lower urinary tract symptoms. *Urology* 85 (6): 1291–1299.

24. Gratzke, C., Bachmann, A., Descazeaud, A. et al. (2015). EAU guidelines on the assessment of non-neurogenic

male lower urinary tract symptoms including benign prostatic obstruction. *Eur. Urol.* 67 (6): 1099–1109.

25. Cornu, J.N., Abrams, P., Chapple, C.R. et al. (2012). A contemporary assessment of nocturia: definition, epidemiology, pathophysiology, and management – a systematic review and meta-analysis. *Eur. Urol.* 62 (5): 877–890.

26. Sakalis, V.I., Karavitakis, M., Bedretdinova, D. et al. (2017). Medical treatment of nocturia in men with lower urinary tract symptoms: systematic review by the European association of urology guidelines panel for male lower urinary tract symptoms. *Eur. Urol.*

27. Chang, C.J., Pei, D., Wu, C.C. et al. (2017). Correlates of nocturia and relationships of nocturia with sleep quality and glycemic control in women with type 2 diabetes. *J. Nurs. Scholarsh.* 49 (4): 400–410.

28. Nagappa, M., Liao, P., Wong, J. et al. (2015). Validation of the STOP-Bang questionnaire as a screening tool for obstructive sleep apnea among different populations: a systematic review and meta-analysis. *PLoS One* 10 (12): e0143697.

29. Fitzgerald, M.P., Mulligan, M., and Parthasarathy, S. (2006). Nocturic frequency is related to severity of obstructive sleep apnea, improves with continuous positive airways treatment. *Am. J. Obstet. Gynecol.* 194 (5): 1399–1403.

30. Everaert, K., Herve, F., Bosch, R. et al. (2019). International continence society consensus on the diagnosis and treatment of nocturia. *Neurourol. Urodyn.* 38 (2): 478–498.

31. Chung, E. (2018). Desmopressin and nocturnal voiding dysfunction: clinical evidence and safety profile in the treatment of nocturia. *Expert. Opin. Pharmacother.* 19 (3): 291–298.

32. Juul, K.V., Malmberg, A., van der Meulen, E. et al. (2017). Low-dose desmopressin combined with serum sodium monitoring can prevent clinically significant hyponatraemia in patients treated for nocturia. *BJU Int.* 119 (5): 776–784.

33. Dumoulin, C., Hay-Smith, J., Habee-Seguin, G.M., and Mercier, J. (2015). Pelvic floor muscle training versus no treatment, or inactive control treatments, for urinary incontinence in women: a short version Cochrane systematic review with meta-analysis. *Neurourol. Urodyn.* 34 (4): 300–308.

34. Bo, K. (2004). Pelvic floor muscle training is effective in treatment of female stress urinary incontinence, but how does it work? *Int. Urogynecol. J. Pelvic Floor Dysfunct.* 15 (2): 76–84.

35. Zubieta, M., Carr, R.L., Drake, M.J., and Bo, K. (2016). Influence of voluntary pelvic floor muscle contraction and pelvic floor muscle training on urethral closure pressures: a systematic literature review. *Int. Urogynecol. J.* 27 (5): 687–696.

36. Lemmens, J.M., Broadbridge, J., Macaulay, M. et al. (2019). Tissue response to applied loading using different designs of penile compression clamps. *Med. Devices (Auckl)* 12: 235–243.

37. Macaulay, M., Broadbridge, J., Gage, H. et al. (2015). A trial of devices for urinary incontinence after treatment for prostate cancer. *BJU Int.* 116 (3): 432–442.

38. Li, J., Yang, L., Pu, C. et al. (2013). The role of duloxetine in stress urinary incontinence: a systematic review and meta-analysis. *Int. Urol. Nephrol.* 45 (3): 679–686.

39. Bitter, I., Filipovits, D., and Czobor, P. (2011). Adverse reactions to duloxetine in depression. *Expert Opin. Drug Saf.* 10 (6): 839–850.

40. Rahn, D.D., Ward, R.M., Sanses, T.V. et al. (2015). Vaginal estrogen use in postmenopausal women with pelvic floor disorders: systematic review and practice guidelines. *Int. Urogynecol. J.* 26 (1): 3–13.

41. Cody, J.D., Jacobs, M.L., Richardson, K. et al. (2012). Oestrogen therapy for urinary incontinence in post-menopausal women. *Cochrane Database Syst. Rev.* 10: CD001405.

42. Greenwell, T., Shah, P., Hamid, R. et al. (2015). The long-term outcome of the Turner-Warwick vaginal Obturator shelf urethral repositioning colposuspension procedure for Urodynamically proven stress urinary incontinence. *Urol. Int.* 95 (3): 352–356.

43. Lapitan, M.C.M., Cody, J.D., and Mashayekhi, A. (2017). Open retropubic colposuspension for urinary incontinence in women. *Cochrane Database Syst. Rev.* 7: CD002912.

44. Ward, K.L. and Hilton, P. (2008). Tension-free vaginal tape versus colposuspension for primary urodynamic stress incontinence: 5-year follow up. *BJOG* 115 (2): 226–233.

45. Chapple, C.R., Raz, S., Brubaker, L., and Zimmern, P.E. (2013). Mesh sling in an era of uncertainty: lessons learned and the way forward. *Eur. Urol.* 64 (4): 525–529.

46. Shah, H.N. and Badlani, G.H. (2012). Mesh complications in female pelvic floor reconstructive surgery and their management: a systematic review. *Indian J. Urol.* 28 (2): 129–153.

47. Kirchin, V., Page, T., Keegan, P.E. et al. (2017). Urethral injection therapy for urinary incontinence in women. *Cochrane Database Syst. Rev.* 7: CD003881.

48. Osman, N.I., Hillary, C.J., Mangera, A. et al. (2018). The midurethral Fascial "sling on a string": an alternative to midurethral synthetic tapes in the era of mesh complications. *Eur. Urol.* 74 (2): 191–196.

49. Phe, V., Leon, P., Granger, B. et al. (2017). Stress urinary incontinence in female neurological patients: long-term

Part III

Urodynamic Techniques

6

Uroflowmetry

Amit Mevcha[1] and Richard Napier-Hemy[2]

[1] *Urology Department, Royal Bournemouth Hospital, Bournemouth, UK*
[2] *Urology Department, Manchester Royal Infirmary, Manchester, UK*

CONTENTS

Uroflowmetry is relatively inexpensive and comparatively simple to undertake, serving as a useful screening study in a wide variety of patients of any age or either gender. It is a non-invasive evaluation (i.e. does not involve a catheter) [1] that measures the flow rate of the external urinary stream as volume per unit time in millilitres per second (ml/s) [2]. It is one of the basic tests included in the International Continence Society (ICS) standard assessment [1] and in guidelines for evaluation of lower urinary tract symptoms (LUTS) or urinary incontinence.

The generation of the urinary stream by the LUT requires sufficient propulsive forces (coming from contraction of the detrusor muscle and/or 'straining' to raise abdominal pressure) and an open bladder outlet (relaxation of the sphincter, along with the bladder neck in men and the pelvic floor in women). This requires coordination by the central nervous system (see Chapter 2). Slow and prolonged flow with incomplete emptying suggests impairment of one or more of these (Figure 6.1). It is not usually possible to be certain exactly which issue is present in a given individual purely from the uroflowmetry result, so additional evaluations are likely to be needed if an issue is identified. In this chapter, we describe how flow rates are measured and interpreted and also discuss how caution is necessary in some circumstances to avoid coming to false conclusions.

Principally, uroflowmetry is used in initial assessment. Flows should be measured before any procedure designed to modify the function of the bladder outlet, e.g. prostate or stricture surgery in men. This may also extend to situations where the outlet might be affected, for example, in women for whom surgery for stress urinary incontinence is being considered; when flow studies appear normal, it provides some reassurance about voiding being preserved after surgery. Slow flow rates on pre-operative testing indicates that risk of post-operative voiding problems may need to be considered. Uroflowmetry can also be used in follow-up for assessing treatment outcome and for detection of recurrence or progression, e.g. in urethral stricture disease. Flow rate testing is perhaps used less often in paediatric populations. Nonetheless, it can be used as a screening test [3, 4] and during follow-up after surgical intervention [5] in children and is sometimes combined with electromyogram studies to assess voiding dysfunction.

How to Do the Test

Bearing in mind that anxiety is problematic for uroflowmetry, it is good practice in advance of the appointment to send an information leaflet (the Bristol flow rate test

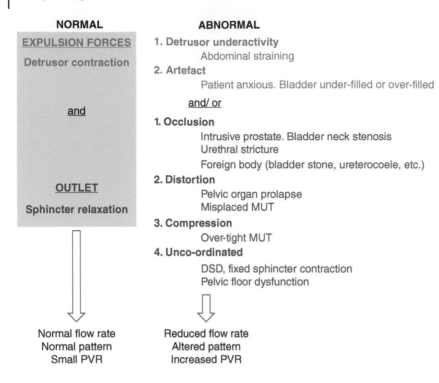

NORMAL

<u>EXPULSION FORCES</u>

Detrusor contraction

<u>and</u>

<u>OUTLET</u>

Sphincter relaxation

Normal flow rate
Normal pattern
Small PVR

ABNORMAL

1. **Detrusor underactivity**
   Abdominal straining
2. **Artefact**
   Patient anxious. Bladder under-filled or over-filled

   <u>and/ or</u>

1. **Occlusion**
   Intrusive prostate. Bladder neck stenosis
   Urethral stricture
   Foreign body (bladder stone, ureterocoele, etc.)
2. **Distortion**
   Pelvic organ prolapse
   Misplaced MUT
3. **Compression**
   Over-tight MUT
4. **Unco-ordinated**
   DSD, fixed sphincter contraction
   Pelvic floor dysfunction

Reduced flow rate
Altered pattern
Increased PVR

Figure 6.1 The factors that determine flow function are the bladder (detrusor) contraction and the state of the outlet. Several processes (listed on the right) may hamper free flow of urine. DSD: detrusor sphincter dyssynergia; MUT: midurethral tape; PVR: post-void residual.

patient information leaflet is included in Appendix C) and a 3-day bladder diary (Appendix A) to complete beforehand. Patients should be warned in advance that their clinic stay is likely to last 2–3 hours, since they may have to wait until they have a comfortably full bladder before performing the test each time (more than once). On arrival, the patient's bladder diary should be checked to see if the patient can be anticipated to achieve suitable voided volumes (VVs) (i.e. some voids in the diary are bigger than 150 ml). In children, older subjects, and someone with overactive bladder syndrome, the VV may never reach 150 ml. The test can still proceed, but the healthcare professional (HCP) responsible must not insist on the patient holding on to reach higher volumes; this may be unrealistic, unkind, and uninterpretable.

The patient may struggle with getting their hydration level appropriate. The ideal circumstance is a person with a normal or strong desire to void soon after they arrive for the appointment, to get the first flow rate measurement done promptly, but this is often not achieved. Nonetheless, it is vital that the HCP does not get the patient to consume large volumes of liquid quickly; this is ineffective at getting the bladder comfortably full and leads to an unrepresentative test result and difficulties with interpretation. Drinks are provided, but never advise a patient to 'drink this jug of water in five minutes'! Excessive rapid fluid intake combined with delay in being able to pass urine is likely to give a misleading result, by artificially reducing Q_{max} and increasing post-void residual (PVR), and is a surprisingly

common issue in flow rate clinics. In a paediatric population (and probably adults too), an excessive VV is associated with higher rate of abnormal uroflow pattern and/or elevated PVR [6].

Urine flow studies should be performed in a private undisturbed environment when the patient has a normal desire to void and is relaxed [7]. When a patient feels the need to pass urine, they should be given access to the flow equipment quickly and in privacy. Prompt access to the flowmeter is so vital that sometimes patients even report invasive urodynamic testing as easier and less uncomfortable than uroflowmetry because urodynamics does not involve having to wait with a full bladder [8]. The flowmeter is set up for the patient to pass urine in their usual position (sitting or standing), and instruction is given to pass urine naturally. For men, the stream should be aimed at the funnel, trying to maintain flow at a consistent point on the funnel. A full flowmetry test consists of the traces of two or three voids, which is necessary because the first void may not be representative (Figure 6.2). Soon after each void, a bladder scan is performed to assess PVR.

The bladder volume at the start of the void can easily be derived by adding the VV and PVR, known as 'total bladder capacity'. The aim is to obtain two or three flows, ideally done with a total bladder capacity of between 150 and 500 ml at the start of the void. The desired volume range is to make sure that the bladder is appropriately full so that it can perform the voiding contraction adequately. If the bladder has insufficient (<150 ml) or excessive (>500 ml) volume when start-

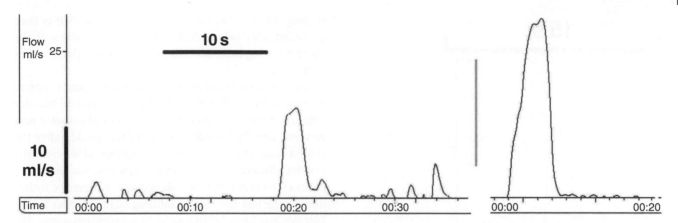

Figure 6.2 A visit to the flow clinic should be a chance to measure a few voids so that the effect of anxiety often encountered with the first void (left) can be excluded by focussing on voids where the patient was more relaxed and better prepared (right).

ing a void, generally it cannot work as well; consequently, if a slow stream is generated during that flow test, it could be the result of inappropriate filling volume, making interpretation more difficult. Obviously, a VV of 150 ml means they must have had at least sufficient total volume. If they do not generally pass 150 ml when voiding, considering the PVR as well helps decide whether the bladder was adequately full at the time they went to pass urine. Sometimes, a patient with overactive bladder always does small voids (as seen on their bladder diary) and has no PVR; it is not reasonable to force them to hang on in desperation before allowing them to void in the hope of getting to the 150 ml threshold. Such patients may well have a good flow rate even though the bladder volume was small, and this would be meaningful (Figure 6.3).

A dedicated urine flow clinic can be invaluable, as it provides a suitable environment for the patient to get their bladder comfortably full, giving the best chance to obtain a reliable flow pattern – something which might be impractical to obtain in the busy environment of the routine urological clinic. When the dedicated flow rate clinic was established in Bristol, there was a sharp drop in the number of small volume voids (the proportion of patients who failed to void 150 ml fell from 59% to 21%).

Reporting a Test Result

ICS Standardisations set out the definitions of the terms used in uroflowmetry [1, 7]. **Flow rate** is the volume of fluid expelled via the urethra per unit time and is expressed in ml/s. **Maximum flow rate (Q_{max})** is the maximum measured value of the flow rate *after correction for artefacts*. **VV** is the total volume expelled via the urethra (the area under the flow curve). In a clinical flowmetry report, data associated with each void is given, most importantly the VVs, the corrected maximum flow rates (Q_{max}), and the

PVRs. The corrected Q_{max} can be plotted on a flow rate nomogram, which relates maximum flow rate to VV, taking sex and age into account. Various authorities have produced such nomograms [9–15]. The traces are presented so that the pattern of flow can be interpreted, since certain patterns suggest particular situations, as described below. Thus, the four key parameters that should generally be presented are (Figure 6.4):

- Q_{max}, corrected for artefact. This is reported to the nearest ml/s (e.g. a reading of 12.6 ml/s is documented as 13 ml/s);
- VV. Reported to the nearest 10 ml (e.g. 418 ml is documented as 420 ml);
- PVR. Reported to the nearest 10 ml (e.g. 88 ml is documented as 90 ml); and
- The trace itself.

The ICS also described other parameters which provide further descriptive categorisation. Flow time (T_Q) is the time over which measurable flow occurs. Voiding time (T_{100}) is the total duration of micturition that also includes interruptions. Average flow rate (Q_{ave}) is VV divided by flow time. When calculating average flow rate, one should carefully review the flow pattern for terminal dribbling and interrupted pattern. Time to maximum flow ($T_{Q_{max}}$) is the elapsed time from the onset of flow to maximum flow.

Interpretation

The basic information necessary for interpreting the flow trace includes the environment in which the patient passed urine and the position, that is, sitting or standing (or even lying). It should also be stated whether the bladder filled naturally, or if diuresis was stimulated by fluid or diuretics, or whether the bladder was filled by a catheter.

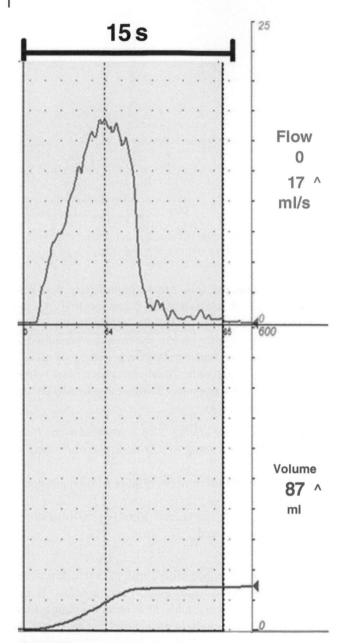

Figure 6.3 Example of a trace that provides useful information despite the voided volume being small because the maximum flow rate was good. In this case, the PVR was 30 ml, so the bladder volume at the start of voiding was 87 + 30 = 117 ml. It is principally when a slow flow is generated that the generally stated threshold of 150 ml becomes a consideration, as it brings doubt about adequacy of bladder filling. A volume of 117 ml is less than the desired 150 ml threshold often aimed at, so the case shows how the 150 ml is certainly not an indispensable requirement.

VV, PVR, and Bladder Voiding Efficiency

Knowing the VV is important; ideally, the flow test VV should be similar in volume to the largest voids on the patient's bladder diary. As a rule of thumb, a VV of at least 150 ml indicates the bladder was adequately full when voiding was started. For a smaller void, if a PVR is then identified, a VV below 150 ml could be compatible with the bladder having been adequately full, making the flow test meaningful.

Residual urine measurement is routinely done as soon as possible after uroflowmetry using an ultrasound bladder scanner. If none is available, then an in/out catheter may be used. The PVR needs to be recorded quickly after the void in order to gain a genuine impression of whether the bladder efficiently empties. Even a few minutes' delay in a patient who is in rapid diuresis because of excessive hydration for the test can lead to refilling of the bladder by the kidneys, erroneously suggesting incomplete emptying. For someone with vesicoureteric reflux (VUR), the bladder might empty fully but then have a significant volume restored as the refluxed urine drops back into the bladder within a few seconds (Figure 8.32).

The thinking behind measuring the PVR is to establish whether the bladder is fully emptied by voiding, as is expected for normal lower urinary tract function. Commonly, a small PVR (up to 30 ml) might be seen in someone with normal voiding under properly conducted test conditions. More than this may indicate voiding inefficiency, reflecting a possible underlying bladder outlet obstruction (BOO), and/or detrusor underactivity. This can be formalised by documenting the 'bladder voiding efficiency' (BVE), which is the VV as a proportion of the bladder volume (see below).

The bladder scanners generally used to measure PVR rely on ultrasound technology and aim to look for a fluid interface. Consequently, they may be confused if fluid-filled structures are present in the pelvis, which are not the bladder (Figure 6.5). This can lead to protracted problems if the clinical team mistakenly assumes the PVR is real and pursues a management pathway aimed at reducing it. Full radiology standard ultrasound equipment can also be used to obtain extra information, such as the presence of other structures which might be confusing the scanner (Figure 6.5) or a bladder diverticulum (Figure 6.6). It is important to recognise a diverticulum, if present, as these generally have very little detrusor muscle in the wall. Hence, they usually lead to a PVR, but this PVR tells us nothing about the detrusor activity generated by the rest of the bladder, or the state of the bladder outlet. If necessary, PVR can be calculated from a formal radiological ultrasound scan (Figure 6.7). The better-quality scans achieved in radiology departments can also be used for research parameters aiming at understanding lower urinary tract function, such as ultrasound-estimated bladder weight. However, more research is needed before these additional features can be used in routine clinical practice [16, 17].

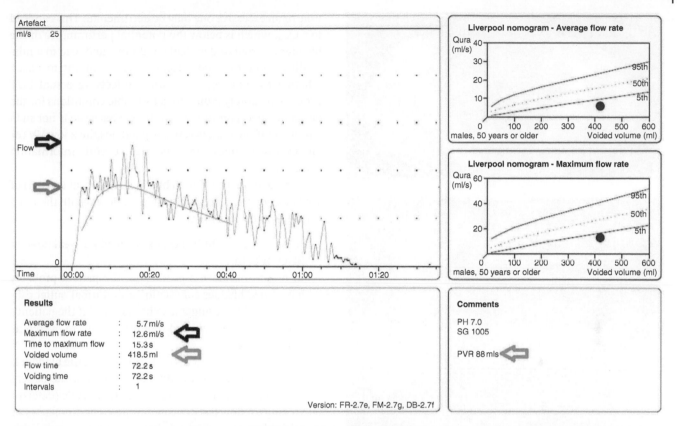

Figure 6.4 A standard reporting sheet for a free flow rate appointment. It displays the flow pattern with clarity, key parameters including the voided and post-void volumes (blue arrows), and nomograms. The trace given shows the limitation of modern equipment in recording peak flow rate without correcting for artefact (open black arrows), i.e. a spike in flow perhaps caused by a strain by the patient, or the stream not being aimed properly at the same spot in the funnel. The orange arrow is placed level with the top of the underlying smoothed curve of the flow removing the superimposed spikes, indicated by the orange line. Professional scrutiny of the trace hence yields the 'corrected Q_{max}' of approximately 8 ml/s, significantly lower than the misleading value given by the machine. This scrutiny is what the ICS recommends urodynamics units must do to make the flow data meaningful.

In summary, potential causes of a PVR are:

- bladder outlet obstruction,
- detrusor underactivity,
- the circumstances of the test (e.g. over-rapid excessive hydration, delay between onset of strong desire to void and getting access to the flowmeter, and prolonged interval between completing the void and getting the scan done),
- structural issues of the lower urinary tract (e.g. VUR or a bladder diverticulum), and
- scanner errors (either the machine or the operator).

There is currently no agreed threshold value where the PVR becomes 'clinically significant', in terms of implications for symptoms (sensation of incomplete emptying), diagnostics, or treatment. In practical terms, many people suggest 100 ml is the minimum volume where they would consider intermittent self-catheterisation (ISC) in someone who appears to be symptomatic from a PVR. A volume where ISC might be instigated in the hope of improving voiding efficiency is 300 ml [18].

Since VV and total bladder capacity at the start of the void (VV + PVR) are both needed to interpret a flowmetry result, combining the two into a single value could simplify interpretation. The BVE (or Void%) achieves this [19]. BVE is expressed as a percentage and is calculated by:

$$\text{BVE, or Void\%} = \left(\text{voided volume} \, / \, \text{total bladder capacity}\right) \times 100\%$$

As with PVR, there is no standardised consensus on threshold BVE values. As a practical guide, a BVE of 80% or more can be accepted as normal. For example, if VV was 400 and PVR was 100, then total bladder capacity was 500 ml. This would make the BVE calculation $(400/500) \times 100 = 80\%$.

Maximum Flow Rate

Detrusor muscle when suitably stretched achieves an optimal performance (like any other muscle), but if

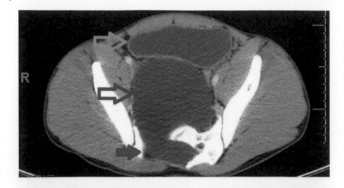

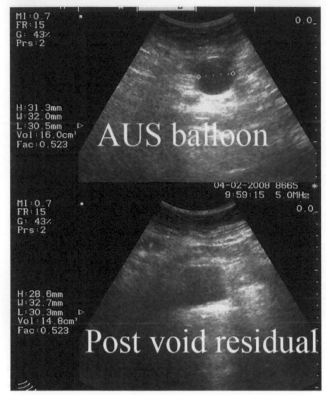

Figure 6.5 Some fluid-filled structures in the pelvis that a bladder scanner has erroneously reported as a PVR. Computed tomography (CT) scan of a myelomeningocoele; the bladder is indicated by a green arrow, and the myelomeningocoele is indicated by red arrows; the intrapelvic part was picked up as a PVR in a flow rate test. Ultrasound scan of the pressure reservoir of an artificial urinary sphincter (AUS) pressure balloon (reservoir). Because the radiologist was made aware of the presence of an AUS, they identified it appropriately. We have once experienced the disastrous situation of a needle aspiration of an AUS balloon being done, rendering the AUS non-functional, on the assumption that such a regular fluid-filled structure must be a cyst. *Source*: Marcus Drake.

stretched too far, it becomes inefficient and results in a poor flow rate. The total bladder capacity ideal for reviewing LUT performance is probably 200–400 ml for most adults, i.e. within the often-stated range of 150–500 ml. Since the Q_{max} achieved is influenced by the bladder volume when voiding was started, either an insufficient vol-

ume or an excessive one may be detrimental. This can lead to a Q_{max} which is below the potential performance of the bladder if tested under ideal conditions and lead to a misleadingly low flow rate. Here, it is important to check whether the low Q_{max} measured reflects an actual LUT problem or simply failure to get suitable conditions for the patient to give a representative flow. This issue is not such a problem if the Q_{max} is actually good despite a low VV (or an excessive one); this is still useful information (Figure 6.3).

With the influence of total bladder capacity at the start of void allowed for, when interpreting a flow result, the practitioner should recognise:

1) A slow Q_{max} might be because of bladder weakness, or BOO, or both.
2) In order to achieve a good Q_{max}, the patient probably has a good bladder contraction and normal outlet calibre. A good Q_{max} might also be achieved if the patient's bladder has strengthened (compensation) to overcome outlet resistance.
3) Temporary bladder weakness can occur if the bladder is insufficiently full at the time of voiding, or the patient had to resist a strong desire to void for a while (deferred voiding). A flow test done under these conditions can be misleading.
4) Q_{max} might be affected by factors other than bladder contraction and outlet relaxation:
   a) The patient coughed during the flow.
   b) An abrupt movement affecting the urethral meatus, e.g. a man who suddenly moves his penis manually, or a woman who shifts her weight.

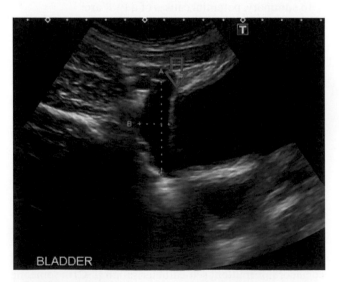

Figure 6.6 Ultrasound scan showing the septum (red arrow) between a bladder diverticulum (to the left) and the normal bladder (right). The presence of a diverticulum will often appear as a PVR on a bladder scanner. *Source*: Marcus Drake.

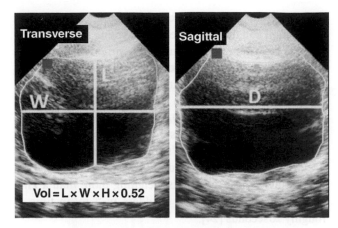

Figure 6.7 Calculating a PVR with an ultrasound uses the formula length × width × depth × 0.52, to give an approximate volume in ml. Length (L) is the distance in cm between the bladder neck and the fundus, and width (W) is the distance from side to side. Depth (D) is the distance from the anterior wall to the posterior wall. Some scanners will use a different factor (e.g. × 0.7), but the general principle is to derive an approximate volume mathematically. *Source*: Marcus Drake.

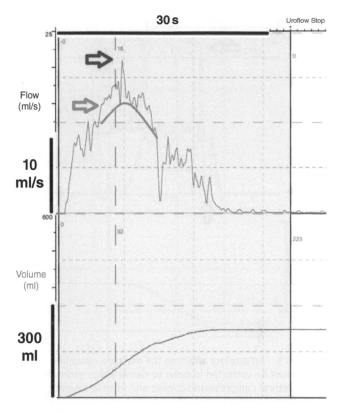

Figure 6.8 An artefact affecting the machine-measured Q_{max} which must be corrected to derive a true estimate of Q_{max}. This man did not consistently aim his stream at one spot in the funnel and moved it around such that the stream reached the flowmeter inconsistently. The machine will take the top spike to denote Q_{max} (red arrow; 18 ml/s), so the practitioner needs to apply a correction. In this case, the green line is more indicative of the underlying trend, so the green arrow (14 ml/s) is more appropriate. With this 'wandering stream/cruising' type of pattern, the flow rarely drops to zero, unless the stream is directed fully outside the funnel. If it does drop to zero, there will rarely be the abrupt spike afterwards that characterises the 'squeeze and release pattern' shown in Figure 6.9.

c) The urine stream not being aimed at the same consistent spot on the flowmeter funnel (Figure 6.8). This causes the flow to fall onto the measurement system in an unpredictable and inconsistent manner.

d) Flow being interrupted by manual urethral compression (Figure 6.9). Urethral compression 'squeeze and release' artefact reflects the fact that males hold the penis with a pinch grip, which can easily occlude flow temporarily, causing elastic energy to build up in the urethral tissue. Once released, this energy is released in a spike in the flow rate which is unrelated to normal voiding behaviour.

e) The flowmeter getting knocked or shaken, e.g. the patient's foot hit it or something dropped onto the funnel rim (e.g. the patient opened their bowels) or it was shaken (Figure 6.10). These often give rise to a transient negative flow rate, which is clearly a biological impossibility; hence, a clear warning sign an artefact is present.

5) Voluntary contractions of other muscles:
   a) Abdominal muscle contractions, i.e. 'straining' (Figure 6.10).
   b) Pelvic floor contractions, i.e. 'dysfunctional voiding' (Figure 6.11).

These issues give characteristic alterations in the flow pattern, and allowance must be made to correct the Q_{max} if any of these is identified. **Visual checking of the flow pattern and correcting the Q_{max} reported by the machine if an artefact is present is one of the most crucial aspects of running a flowmetry clinic.** Generally, a 'spike' is not a natural feature of the smooth muscle contraction by the detrusor or sphincter relaxation, so it should be excluded when deriving Q_{max}. Such spikes can arise from a range of artefacts as described above. The HCP must review the trace and check whether the value given by the machine truly reflects the patient's urinary function. Many departments fail to undertake this, and there are potentially serious implications for the patient as a result [20]. In a large study, more than 20 000 flow curves were reviewed and the machine readout compared with a manual assessment; there was a difference of more than 3 ml/s in 9% [21].

'Straining' signifies that the patient is using abdominal or diaphragmatic muscles in an attempt to initiate or increase the urinary flow, by providing an additional expulsion force alongside any detrusor contraction. An example is given in Figure 6.10, but straining affects the appearance in a very varied way, since the extent of detrusor contraction and BOO are both influential variables. The flow rate

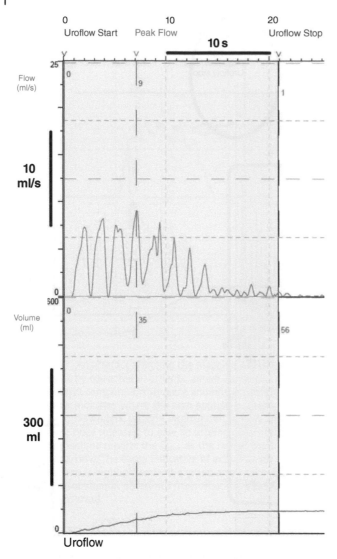

Figure 6.11 Behavioural muscle contractions can affect the flow pattern. The flow fluctuations seen here happen rapidly and in quick succession, with five such events seen in the first 10 seconds. This is much quicker than is generally seen with straining, where muscle recruitment is slower, though the appearance is otherwise similar. In a non-neuropathic patient, this is referred to as dysfunctional voiding.

accurate volume measurement. Density of the urine can affect the results, which should be considered when interpreting the reading. This method has a relatively slow response time and is prone to 'knocking' artefacts.

The **capacitance type of flowmeter** has two metallic strips in a set size container. The electrical capacitance between the strips changes as the height of the column of urine changes. This approach is not in common use. It has no mechanical parts and is relatively inexpensive. However, it is also prone to 'knocking' artefacts, and variable results are obtained depending upon the density and composition of the urine.

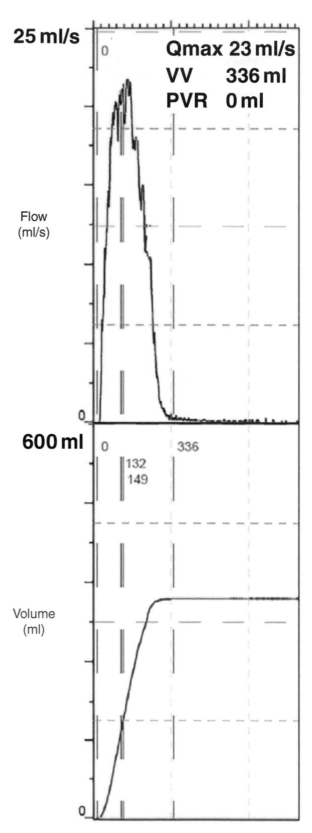

Figure 6.12 The normal flow curve characterised by a rapid upstroke, good Q_{max}, and a rapid drop back down to zero. *Source:* Drake [25].

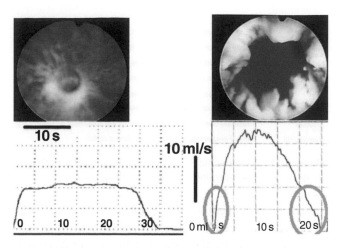

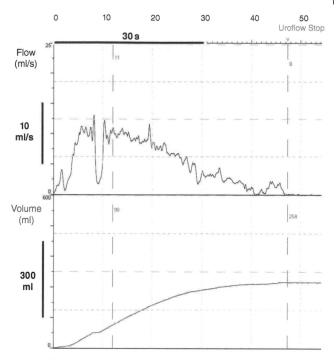

Figure 6.13 On the left is an endoscopic view and flow trace pattern for a significant urethral stricture. The upstroke is fast, and the downstroke is also fast (not quite as rapid as the upstroke), and there is a consistent restriction between, described as a 'plateau'. This pattern is sometimes referred to as 'constrictive' or 'box-like'. On the right is the endoscopic view and flow trace pattern once the stricturotomy had been done. Note how the beginning of upstroke and the conclusion of the downstroke (green ovals) are very similar to those before treatment, but the plateau effect between is fully resolved. Stricture recurrence appears likely in this case, based on the ragged appearance of the stricturotomy site, so he will be followed up with regular flow tests to see if the plateau pattern returns. PVR was not documented but some residual is fairly commonly seen in association with a plateau pattern.
Source: Marcus Drake.

Figure 6.14 A flow trace pattern characterised by a slow upstroke, low Q_{max}, and prolonged downstroke, commonly associated with a PVR. This is commonly seen in men with benign prostatic obstruction (this cannot be asserted for certain, since weak bladder contraction can produce a similar pattern). This pattern is sometimes referred to as 'compressive', though again this cannot be a reliable description without further data.

Most commercially available flowmeters have acceptable accuracy. However, the buyer should always seek independent information on the machine's performance [26] and, in particular, the accuracy (errors should be less than 5%), the linearity of response over the range 0 ml/s to 50 ml/s, the reliability of the apparatus, the compatibility with any existing equipment, the safety of the flowmeter, features of the software, and its ease of cleaning. It is wise to check the performance of the flowmeter at regular intervals, especially since a simple check of volume is very easy to do, by pouring in a known volume and checking whether the volume reported is accurate. The machine calculates the flow rate accurately if this volume figure is correct. Another simple test can give a less precise assessment of accuracy of volume and flow rate measurements and is straightforward (Figure 6.19).

The flow is recorded directly into the software, or using a chart recorder. The flowmeter package typically includes an automatic printout of descriptive measurements (notably VV and Q_{max}). However, since the software within these flowmeters does not distinguish physiological flow from flow changes produced by artefact, the traces must be examined and Q_{max} values corrected if necessary, as described above. Likewise, a proper description of the test needs to be documented at the time, since subsequent

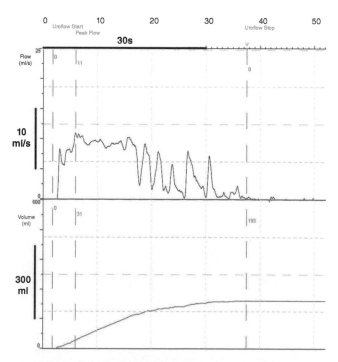

Figure 6.15 A fluctuating pattern, with several peaks and a prolonged voiding time. A PVR is commonly seen. The patient may well exert some straining during this type of flow. This pattern can signify contrasting mechanisms, such as an underactive bladder contraction or pelvic floor contractions during voiding.

3. Gupta, D.K., Sankhwar, S.N., and Goel, A. (2013). Uroflowmetry nomograms for healthy children 5 to 15 years old. *J. Urol.* 190 (3): 1008–1013.

4. MacNeily, A.E. (2012). The role of uroflowmetry in the diagnosis of lower urinary tract disorders in children. *J. Urol.* 187 (6): 1960–1961.

5. Capitanucci, M.L., Marciano, A., Zaccara, A. et al. (2012). Long-term bladder function follow-up in boys with posterior urethral valves: comparison of noninvasive vs invasive urodynamic studies. *J. Urol.* 188 (3): 953–957.

6. Chang, S.J., Yang, S.S., and Chiang, I.N. (2011). Large voided volume suggestive of abnormal uroflow pattern and elevated post-void residual urine. *Neurourol. Urodyn.* 30 (1): 58–61.

7. Gammie, A. and Drake, M.J. (2018). ICS: the fundamentals of Uroflowmetry practice, based on International Continence Society good urodynamic practices recommendations. *Neurourol. Urodyn.* 37 (S6): S44–S49.

8. Selman, L.E., Ochieng, C.A., Lewis, A.L. et al. (2019). Recommendations for conducting invasive urodynamics for men with lower urinary tract symptoms: qualitative interview findings from a large randomized controlled trial (UPSTREAM). *Neurourol. Urodyn.* 38 (1): 320–329.

9. Von Garrelts, B. (1958). Micturition in the normal male. *Acta Chir. Scand.* 114 (3): 197–210.

10. Backman, K.A. (1965). Urinary flow during micturition in normal women. *Acta Chir. Scand.* 130 (4): 357–370.

11. Backman, K.A., von Garrelts, B., and Sundblad, R. (1966). Micturition in normal women. Studies of pressure and flow. *Acta Chir. Scand.* 132 (4): 403–412.

12. Gierup, J. (1970). Micturition studies in infants and children. Normal urinary flow. *Scand. J. Urol. Nephrol.* 4 (3): 191–197.

13. Siroky, M.B., Olsson, C.A., and Krane, R.J. (1979). The flow rate nomogram: I. development. *J. Urol.* 122 (5): 665–668.

14. Haylen, B.T., Parys, B.T., Anyaegbunam, W.I. et al. (1990). Urine flow rates in male and female urodynamic patients compared with the Liverpool nomograms. *Br. J. Urol.* 65 (5): 483–487.

15. Haylen, B.T., Ashby, D., Sutherst, J.R. et al. (1989). Maximum and average urine flow rates in normal male and female populations – the Liverpool nomograms. *Br. J. Urol.* 64 (1): 30–38.

16. Malde, S., Nambiar, A.K., Umbach, R. et al. (2017). Systematic review of the performance of noninvasive tests in diagnosing bladder outlet obstruction in men with lower urinary tract symptoms. *Eur. Urol.* 71 (3): 391–402.

17. Bright, E., Pearcy, R., and Abrams, P. (2011). Ultrasound estimated bladder weight in men attending the uroflowmetry clinic. *Neurourol. Urodyn.* 30 (4): 583–586.

18. Bates, T.S., Sugiono, M., James, E.D. et al. (2003). Is the conservative management of chronic retention in men ever justified? *BJU Int.* 92 (6): 581–583.

19. Abrams, P. (1999). Bladder outlet obstruction index, bladder contractility index and bladder voiding efficiency: three simple indices to define bladder voiding function. *BJU Int.* 84 (1): 14–15.

20. Aiello, M., Jelski, J., Lewis, A. et al. (2020). Quality control of uroflowmetry and urodynamic data from two large multicenter studies of male lower urinary tract symptoms. *Neurourol. Urodyn.*

21. Grino, P.B., Bruskewitz, R., Blaivas, J.G. et al. (1993). Maximum urinary flow rate by uroflowmetry: automatic or visual interpretation. *J. Urol.* 149 (2): 339–341.

22. Reynard, J.M., Peters, T.J., Lamond, E., and Abrams, P. (1995). The significance of abdominal straining in men with lower urinary tract symptoms. *Br. J. Urol.* 75 (2): 148–153.

23. Wheeler, T.L. 2nd, Richter, H.E., Greer, W.J. et al. (2008). Predictors of success with postoperative voiding trials after a mid urethral sling procedure. *J. Urol.* 179 (2): 600–604.

24. Yang, P.J., Pham, J., Choo, J., and Hu, D.L. (2014). Duration of urination does not change with body size. *Proc. Natl. Acad. Sci. U. S. A.* 111 (33): 11932–11937.

25. Drake, M.J. (2018). Fundamentals of terminology in lower urinary tract function. *Neurourol. Urodyn.* 37 (S6): S13–S19.

26. Gammie, A., Clarkson, B., Constantinou, C. et al. (2014). International continence society guidelines on urodynamic equipment performance. *Neurourol. Urodyn.* 33 (4): 370–379.

27. Krhut, J., Gartner, M., Sykora, R. et al. (2015). Comparison between uroflowmetry and sonouroflowmetry in recording of urinary flow in healthy men. *Int. J. Urol.* 22 (8): 761–765.

28. Bray, A., Griffiths, C., Drinnan, M., and Pickard, R. (2012). Methods and value of home uroflowmetry in the assessment of men with lower urinary tract symptoms: a literature review. *Neurourol. Urodyn.* 31 (1): 7–12.

29. Heesakkers, J., Farag, F., Pantuck, A. et al. (2012). Applicability of a disposable home urinary flow measuring device as a diagnostic tool in the management of males with lower urinary tract symptoms. *Urol. Int.* 89 (2): 166–172.

30. Chan, C.K., Yip, S.K., Wu, I.P. et al. (2012). Evaluation of the clinical value of a simple flowmeter in the management of male lower urinary tract symptoms. *BJU Int.* 109 (11): 1690–1696.

7

Cystometry and Pressure-Flow Studies

Marcus Drake[1], Rachel Tindle[2], and Su-Min Lee[3]

[1] *Translational Health Sciences, Bristol Medical School, Southmead Hospital, Bristol, UK*
[2] *Urodynamics & Gastrointestinal Physiology, Southmead Hospital, Bristol, UK*
[3] *Department of Urology, Royal United Hospital, Bath, UK*

CONTENTS

The previous chapter on uroflowmetry examined the role of urine flow studies in defining bladder and urethral function. However, uroflowmetry cannot offer a precise diagnosis when flow rate is slow because it cannot distinguish between obstruction and detrusor underactivity. It also tells us little about the storage phase of micturition. Cystometry is used to study both the storage and the voiding phases of micturition to make urodynamic observations from which to derive diagnosis (in some patients, diagnoses). With specific diagnosis or diagnoses in mind, a rational treatment recommendation can be made, because the therapy can be aimed at the cause of the symptomatic problems, and potential risks for adverse outcome can be identified. Cystometry is the method by which the pressure–volume relationship of the bladder is measured. The indications for cystometry for given patient groups are dealt with in their respective chapters; below, we describe practical aspects and interpretation in terms of general principles.

When thinking about the diagnosis and treatment of lower urinary tract dysfunction, it is useful to consider both the bladder and the outlet during each phase (storage and voiding). For normal function, the bladder is relaxed and the outlet is contracted during the storage phase, whereas the reverse applies during voiding (Table 7.1). Abnormal function reflects failure of bladder and/or outlet during storage and/or voiding, and simple consideration can surmise what failure is responsible (Table 7.1).

'Underactive' and 'overactive' are relative to the expected behaviour. So, 'underactive' is never applied for the bladder during storage because, in normal function, it should be relaxed (how can you be less active than inactive?). Likewise, during voiding, the bladder cannot be described as overactive because its function is to contract with maximal efficiency to empty the bladder. Similarly, the outlet cannot be described as overactive during storage or as underactive during voiding because its function is to prevent any urine escape during storage and to permit full

---

Abrams' Urodynamics, Fourth Edition. Edited by Marcus Drake, Hashim Hashim, and Andrew Gammie.
© 2021 John Wiley & Sons Ltd. Published 2021 by John Wiley & Sons Ltd.

Table 7.1 Normal and abnormal observations in terms of bladder and urethral behaviour during urodynamics.

	Normal function		Abnormal function	
	Storage/filling	Voiding	Storage/filling	Voiding
Bladder	Relaxed	Contracted	Overactive	Underactive/acontractile
Outlet	Contracted	Relaxed	Incompetent with stress/effort or inappropriate relaxation	Partial obstruction (anatomical or functional)

Describing the observations for bladder during filling and voiding and for the outlet during filling and voiding thus constitute fundamental elements of the urodynamic report.

emptying when voiding. This leads to four considerations when evaluating a patient urodynamically:

- Is the bladder relaxed during storage?
- Is the outlet contracted during storage?
- Does the bladder contract adequately during voiding?
- Does the outlet open properly during voiding?

Although cystometry seems a simple technique, a number of areas present difficulties and limitations that must be appreciated. Crucially, the measurement of pressure is subject to numerous artefacts (see Chapter 18), so precise scientific method is vital in ensuring that valid data is obtained. Furthermore, there is increasing evidence that the approach the urodynamicist takes when running the test may well influence the results obtained. Both these points are discussed in full below.

Principles of Cystometry

Cystometry is used to study bladder and outlet function. To understand the storage phase, it is common practice to fill the bladder using a pump, so 'filling cystometry' is the main test used to evaluate storage properties. During voiding, both pressure and flow rate are measured, so 'pressure-flow study' (PFS) is the descriptive phrase applied to this stage of urodynamic tests.

What Pressures Are Used?

The bladder is an abdominal organ and so will be affected by changing abdominal pressure (in common with any other organ in the abdominal cavity). In the normal person, abdominal pressure directly influences the entire bladder and the proximal urethra lying above the pelvic floor. Intravesical pressure measurement thus reflects both detrusor activity and any changes in abdominal pressure since both of these affect pressure within the bladder lumen. Thus, throughout a urodynamic study, the pressure within the bladder (intravesical pressure, abbreviated to

p_{ves}) is measured, together with the pressure within the abdominal cavity (p_{abd}). The purpose of measuring p_{abd} simultaneously during bladder and urethral pressure recordings is to aid interpretation of the observed pressure changes. Without the facility to examine p_{abd}, a p_{ves} trace may be ambiguous, since the process causing the observed pressure changes could be impossible to identify. Hence, the synchronous measurement of bladder pressure with pressure in another abdominal organ allows the investigator to assess whether observed changes in p_{ves} are actually due to contraction of the bladder alone or whether they are due to the influence of abdominal pressure change.

The p_{abd} is generally estimated by measuring rectal pressure; vaginal pressure or other alternatives are sometimes used (see below). The abdominal pressure is principally affected by contraction of the diaphragmatic, abdominal wall, and pelvic floor muscles, which will happen if the patient speaks, coughs, lifts something, or is physically active. 'Straining' is sometimes used to denote physical exertion associated with lifting. Sometimes, straining is used in particular situations, such as physical effort used during defaecation. A cough or a Valsalva manoeuvre are controlled techniques commonly used in urodynamics (UDS) to reproduce the effect of abdominal straining on intravesical pressure and lower urinary tract function.

The pressures in the respective organs are picked up by catheters and are carried by connection tubing from the catheters to transducers, which convert the pressures for plotting as traces for p_{ves} and p_{abd} (Figure 7.1). The p_{ves} and

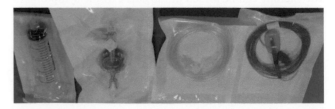

Figure 7.1 Disposable equipment used for measuring abdominal pressure; syringe used for flushing air out of the system (left), transducer (middle left), connection tubing (middle right), and rectal catheter (right). *Source*: Marcus Drake.

p_{abd} are called such, because those are the most important contributors to the pressure activity. However, it is important to recognise that the pressure recording uses a tube that runs between the patient and the transducer. The pressure measured can therefore be affected by additional influences on the tubing, not just the organ being recorded from. This could include a body structure, notably the anal and urethral sphincter, or an external influence, such as a heavy object coming to rest on the tube (Figure 7.2). It is also important to recognise that the physical relationship between the balloon and the abdominal catheter and the rectum can change; consequently, there can be a drop in the pressure if the balloon loses contact with the rectum, or an increase if the catheter moves into the anal canal, or further externally between the buttocks or fully out. For this reason, it is important to ensure the balloon of the catheter is fully in the rectum when the line is placed.

Intravesical pressure (p_{ves}) and rectal pressure (p_{abd}) are measured by transducers connected to the respective organ lumina with connecting tubes and catheters. By electronically subtracting abdominal pressure from intravesical pressure, the detrusor pressure (p_{det}) is derived by the urodynamic computer: $p_{det} = p_{ves} - p_{abd}$. The basic assumptions are as follows:

- If a pressure increase is seen in both p_{ves} and p_{abd} but not in p_{det}, then it is due to raised abdominal pressure.
- If a pressure increase is seen on p_{ves} and p_{det} but not on p_{abd}, then it is due to a detrusor contraction.
- If a pressure increase is seen on p_{ves}, p_{abd}, and p_{det}, then there is both a detrusor contraction and increased abdominal pressure.
- If a pressure change is seen on p_{abd} with no change in p_{ves} and a consequent fall in p_{det}, then this is due to a rectal contraction.

The appearance of a rectal contraction and a detrusor contraction is shown in Figure 7.3. These assumptions have to be made with constant alertness to be sure the catheters are recording properly, and there has not been any additional influence (such as one of the catheters shifting in relation to the relevant sphincter).

Since the bladder and rectal catheters have to cross the pelvic floor, it is important to appreciate that changes in pelvic floor function can affect the pressure in either catheter. Thus, a pelvic floor squeeze may cause a pressure change in p_{ves}, p_{abd}, or both. This squeeze can occur in response to a change in the pressure of one of the organs. For example, women often contract their pelvic floor just before a cough (a learned approach to reducing the leakage associated with stress incontinence) causing a rise on p_{abd} generated by pressure local to the rectal balloon but not affecting the bladder line. Likewise, pelvic floor relaxation often accompanies voiding for women, so p_{abd} can drop during voiding; the urodynamicist needs to be clear that this is due to pressure changes local to the rectal balloon only, which will manifest as an artefactual extra rise in p_{det} that needs to be corrected.

Whilst detrusor function can be assessed directly by observation of the pressure changes, outlet function is usually inferred indirectly from the pressure changes within the bladder, by measuring any urine leakage during filling, and by measuring urine flow during voiding.

Aims of Cystometry

The principal aim of UDS is to reproduce the patient's symptoms and to relate them to any synchronous urodynamic events. Some lower urinary tract symptoms (LUTS) are well suited to this aim and can readily be reproduced during testing as they occur spontaneously or in response to 'provocation'. Examples of provocation to observe urodynamic stress incontinence (USI) (Figure 7.4) include:

1) A single high-amplitude cough and a rapid series of high-amplitude coughs. A single cough often fails to elicit leakage as the patient will have a reflex contract

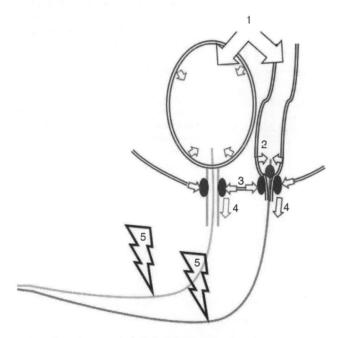

Figure 7.2 A rectal catheter measures abdominal pressure (1), but will also be affected by other influences; (2) a contraction of the rectum. (3) Anal pressure (squeeze or relaxation), which compresses the tube in the anus, (4) the balloon shifting into the anus and beyond if the catheter is displaced, and (5) something knocking or squashing the connection tube outside the patient. Equivalent influences also apply to the bladder catheter. Hence, each catheter shows pressure generated by the organ it is recording from, plus additional external influences.

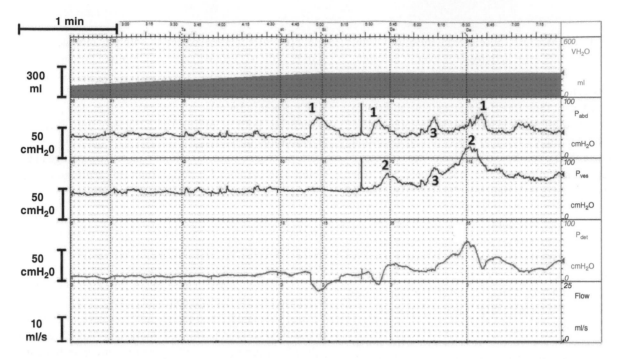

Figure 7.3 A filling cystometry showing rectal contractions (1) and detrusor overactivity (2). There is also a rise in abdominal pressure, which is picked up in both the rectum and bladder, so that is subtracted out on p_{det} (3).

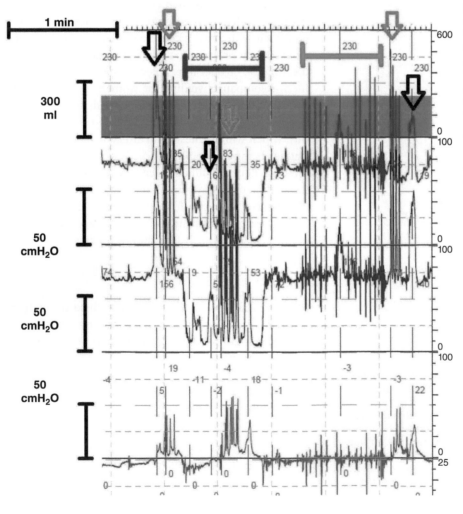

Figure 7.4 Attempting to provoke urodynamic stress incontinence. Valsalva manoeuvres are indicated by black arrows, and a powerful series of coughs is indicated by blue arrows. These can be done when squatting down (purple bar) to place the pelvic floor at a mechanical disadvantage. The green bar indicates running and jumping on the spot. Throughout, the urodynamicist has to look for leakage, since the patient is not above the flowmeter when doing this extensive testing. Note that the subtraction is not good (see main text).

their pelvic floor before the cough; it is very hard to do that with a series of rapid coughs.

2) A series of increasingly strong Valsalva manoeuvres.
3) Changing posture. USI is more easily provoked in women if they are asked to separate their legs widely, presumably because leg abduction weakens pelvic floor support to the sphincter mechanism.
4) High-level exertion.

A useful approach for detrusor overactivity (DO) is to generate the sound of trickling water (e.g. the noise generated by slowly running a water tap into a pool of water, e.g. into a sink with the plug in) (Figure 7.5). For some people, a cold stimulus can elicit DO, such as putting a hand in a bowl of cold water. Caution is needed with stress provocations, in case they actually provoke DO.

Provocation testing allows a symptom to be corresponded directly to a urodynamic observation. Other symptoms cannot be reproduced during standard UDS, such as nocturia, nocturnal enuresis, dysregulated voiding (see Chapter 16), and coital incontinence. The conclusions of a urodynamic test undertaken in a patient with symptoms that cannot be reproduced under standard testing conditions must be extremely cautious about linking any urodynamic observations to the symptom. If a symptom does not occur during testing, the underlying urodynamic mechanism is actually not known for sure, and the urodynamic report should state this.

Other aims of UDS are to define detrusor function and outlet function during both filling and voiding. This will give four elements about lower urinary tract function to describe in the report, as implied by Table 7.2. It is essential that the clinician relates these elements to the symptomatic complaints of the patient and any abnormal physical findings. These have to be presented alongside other important facets of the test as recommended by the International Continence Society (ICS) [1]. In this way, the relevance and reliability of the results can be assessed and, should the clinical problems not have been answered, further investigations can be planned.

Measuring Pressure Correctly

In standard practice, the pressure transducers for measuring p_{ves} and p_{abd} are placed at the same vertical height as the patient's pubis, and a mounting platform whose height can easily be adjusted is useful for this (Figure 7.6).

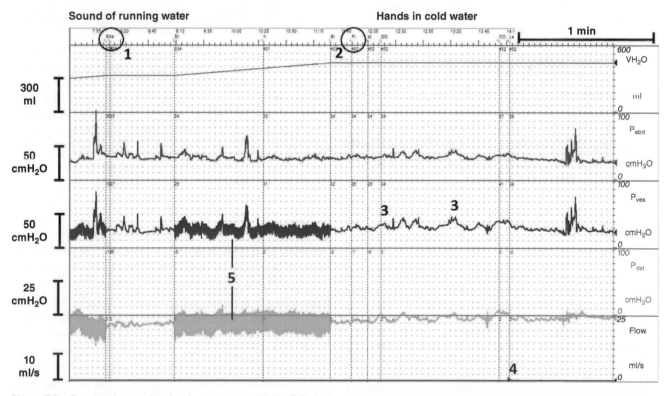

Figure 7.5 Provocation testing for detrusor overactivity (DO). At 1, the water taps were turned on gently to give a trickling sound. In this case, it had little effect, so the pump was restarted. It was stopped, and the patient was asked to put her hand in cold water at 2; this elicited low-amplitude DO (3) and consequent DO incontinence (4). The DO was more obvious in p_{ves} than in p_{det} because there was some pelvic floor contraction in response to the DO, giving an anal squeeze that slightly raised the pressure reported in p_{abd}, and hence reduced the amplitude of the p_{det} display of DO. This study used a double lumen catheter, leading to the pump artefact indicated by 5.

Table 7.2 The requirements that should be covered when compiling a urodynamics report, as recommended by the International Continence Society's Good Urodynamic Practices guidelines.

- Furthermore, the WG recommends reporting as follows:
- Overall judgement of the *technical quality* and the *clinical reliability* of the test to represent the lower urinary tract function 'as usual', to be evaluated by the person who performed the tests.
- Uroflowmetry: *Voiding position*, urge (before the test), and *representativeness*, as reported by the patient.
- Introduction of catheters: *sensation* (if occurring; pain), *muscular* (pelvic or adductor) *defence*, and – perceptibly unusual – *obstruction(s) during insertion*.
- *Position(s)* during cystometry and pressure-flow study.
- *Patient's ability to report* filling sensations and/or urgency and/ or urine loss.
- Method of urodynamic stress test (if applicable).
- Pressure-flow: position and representativeness, as reported by the patient.
- Accessory tests or measurements (if applicable – no further standard).
- Representativeness of the tests to reflect the 'usual LUT behaviour', as reported by the patient.
- Filling *sensation – diagnosis*.
- Cystometry (detrusor) pressure *pattern – diagnosis*.
- Pressure-flow – *diagnosis* (compared with uroflowmetry) includes:
  ○ Bladder outflow function or obstruction (and the method for assessment)
  ○ Detrusor *contraction* (and the method for assessment).

Source: Rosier et al. [1]. © 2017, John Wiley & Sons.

An arrangement is needed so that the transducers can efficiently be set up, record the pressure from the patient, and fix any problems as they happen. This basically means being able to switch between three configurations:

1) Recording atmospheric pressure, as this is needed for establishing the pressure reference 'zero' level – in line with the ICS Standard [1].
2) Recording from the catheter in the patient (with the pressure transducer placed at the same vertical height as the patient's pubis). This configuration is also used when calibrating the transducers.
3) Connecting to a saline-filled syringe that can flush air bubbles away from the transducer or catheter.

The arrangements for switching between configurations are illustrated in Figure 7.7.

For every urodynamic examination, setting zero and establishing the pressure reference level are needed for each patient.

Step 1: Setting zero: By convention, the reference pressure is the surrounding atmospheric pressure, which is taken as the zero pressure [1, 3]. Hence, once recordings are taken from the bladder and rectum, they are plotting how much higher the internal pressure is than atmospheric. Setting the zero is a simple process of opening the pressure transducer to the room and instructing the software to zero all pressures. The true 'resting pressures' within a patient are always higher than atmospheric, since the rectum and bladder are pelvic organs, so they are pressed on by all the abdominal and thoracic viscera. Similarly, changing from the supine position to seated greatly affects rectal pressure, since the heavy organs (notably liver and heart) are moved directly above the pelvis (Figure 7.8). A further change comes when moving to the standing position, as the support provided by a seat is gone, and the adipose can also now affect abdominal pressure (Figure 7.8). The zero should *not* be set when recording from the patient (yet this is a common mistake made in many units) (Figure 7.9). Zero to atmospheric pressure; do not zero to patient pressures.

Step 2: Establishing the reference level: The ICS has defined the reference height for external transducers and water-filled catheters (WFCs) as the top of the pubis. Most urodynamic equipment has the transducers mounted on a system which can be moved vertically, and all that is needed is to move the system to the same horizontal plane as the pubis using a button. If the patient's position is changed during a test (for example, going from seated position to standing), the transducers should be moved to the new height of the pubis. Effects of variations in the relationship between the heights of the patient and the transducers on measured pressures are shown in Figure 7.10. Catheter-tip transducers do not need a reference level in this way, but the p_{det} reading is affected by the change in relative position of the two catheter tips (see below).

Note that bladder filling can affect rectal pressure, without causing a general rise in abdominal pressure. This is because bladder expansion is constrained in front by the pubis forcing the dome backwards at higher volumes. This is unavoidable when the patient is supine and also can happen when the patient is upright (Figure 7.11). Consequently, the weight of the bladder increasingly compresses the rectum with filling. This is a direct compression of the rectum, so it does not mean a general rise in abdominal pressure. It is an explanation of why rectal pressure can change in a UDS test even if the only change has been to fill the bladder. This effect also applies if recording from the vagina, but not from a colostomy.

It is useful to include the setting up process when printing the trace (Figure 7.12).

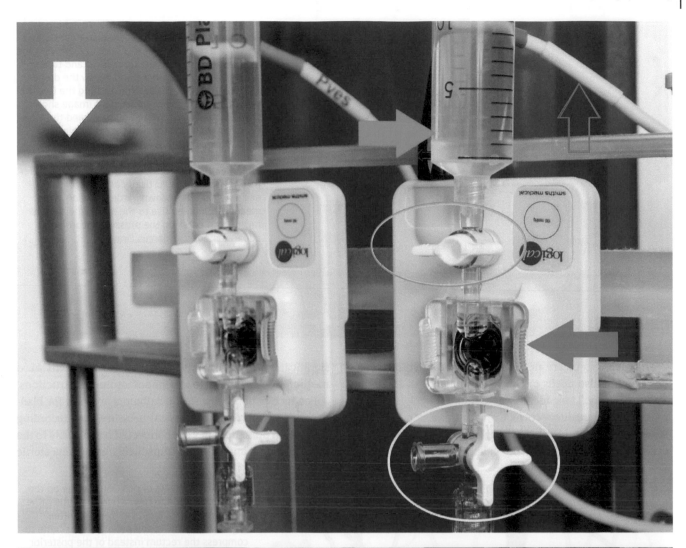

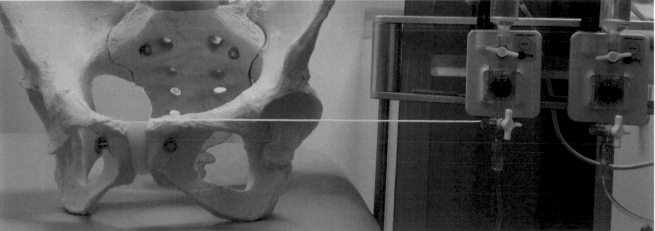

Figure 7.6 Top image: two pressure transducers are needed for standard urodynamics; one for p_{ves} and one for p_{abd} (closed orange arrow). A three-way tap below the transducer (yellow oval) allows the transducer to be connected to either atmosphere or the connection tubing to the catheter. An on-off switch (green oval), or another 3-way tap, allows the flushing syringe to be connected when needed. The open orange arrow indicates the electrical connection from the transducer to the computer. The transducers are mounted on a platform (white arrow), which can be moved up and down; when in position, the 3-way tap outlet used for atmospheric zero should be level with the top of the pubis (green line in the lower image). In practice, most units line the centre of the transducers level with the pubis, which is acceptable [2]. *Source*: Marcus Drake.

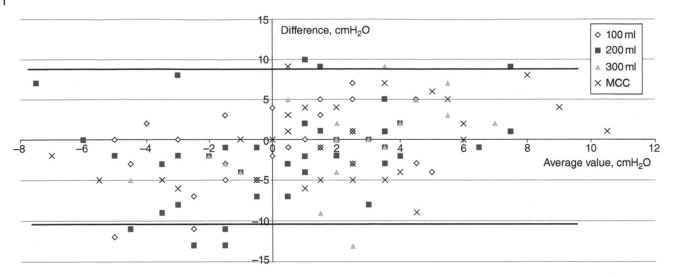

Figure 7.14 Bland–Altman graph comparing filling pressure values measured by air-filled catheters (AFCs) with those measured by water-filled catheters (WFC) after applying quality control checks. The graph plots the difference in values (AFC–WFC) against their average, with each mark representing a paired data point, taken at one of four bladder volumes; open diamond 100 ml, red square 200 ml, green triangle 300 ml, and cross maximum cystometric capacity (MCC). The 95% limits of agreement are −10.7 to +8.8 cmH$_2$O (mean = −0.9, SD 5.0), marked by solid lines. The difference in readings between the two systems is clearly appreciable. *Source:* Gammie et al. [5]. © 2016, John Wiley & Sons.

atmosphere and checking normal resting pressures should be maintained, though allowance should be made for slightly greater resting pressures than for water-filled systems, since the air-filled balloon is likely to be below the level of the symphysis pubis and thus register higher pressures. Since movement of the patient, and movement of the catheters within the patient, will change the relative positions of the catheter tips, such movement must be minimised and compensated for. Users of air-filled systems are advised to ensure they have a clear understanding of the mechanism of operation and the limitations of these systems in order to be able to interpret the results with appropriate caution.

What to Display

On screen, the urodynamic equipment plots events in real time. For cystometry, several parameters can suitably be displayed, most commonly, volume instilled, flowmeter

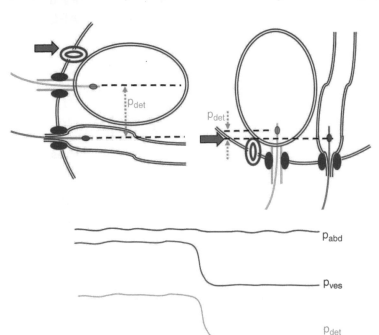

Figure 7.15 How position of the patient affects pressure for an *air-filled catheter*. The heights of the catheter tips (black dotted lines) change more for the vesical catheter than the rectal catheter when the patient moves from supine (left) to upright (right), affecting the vesical and detrusor pressure traces. The height of the pubis also changes (grey arrow), but this is not relevant for a catheter-tip transducer.

reading, p_{ves}, p_{abd}, and p_{det}. p_{ves} and p_{det} are most important, so they should be displayed further down on the screen (and paper printout if applicable) to ensure they are always fully visible when high values occur. The software allows for event markers to be placed at key moments, so specific aspects can be flagged up and recorded by the urodynamic practitioner. These annotations should be clear on both the screen and the printout, and it is helpful to set the software to print trace values at each marker.

Data sampling should be done at an adequate rate, and a minimum sampling rate of 10 data points per second (10 Hz) is necessary for a good-quality trace [4]. Sampling less often may mean the loss of important data during fast events (e.g. when the patient coughs). Sampling too often is unnecessary and may make the data file inconveniently large. The scale of each trace should be set so as to allow clear presentation of all features and should be standardised by the department. Pressure traces should all use the same scale. Variation in scales will cause confusion and possibly misinterpretation.

Technique of Filling Cystometry

To evaluate the storage phase of filling cystometry, some essential measurements must be made throughout filling:

- Intravesical pressure (p_{ves})
- Abdominal pressure (p_{abd})
- Detrusor pressure ($p_{det} = p_{ves} - p_{abd}$) – calculated electronically

In addition, the flowmeter can be used to detect any incontinence. In situations where the patient's perineum is not above the flowmeter (e.g. supine position filling cystometry), direct visual observation is needed to identify incontinence.

Other measurements recorded during cystometry can include volume instilled, electromyography (EMG), and urethral pressure measurement. Imaging is also done at suitable moments using video-urodynamics (see Chapter 8).

Dipstick urinalysis on the same day is valuable before filling cystometry, as it reduces the risk of the test being done with active urinary tract infection present (a risk factor for bacteraemia). Since free-flow rate testing is usually the first step in a UDS appointment, we evaluated whether doing the dipstick using a sample taken from the flowmeter collecting jug is a feasible option. We compared samples in the flowmeter with a sample taken from the same patient through the filling catheter. We found that nitrites were 100% consistent between flowmeter and catheterised specimens [7]. For some women, leukocytes were seen in the flowmeter specimen but not in the catheter specimen, suggesting that vaginal contamination may give a false positive result for leukocytes. It is thus our practice to use the flowmeter specimen for urinalysis, cleaning the jug carefully before the next patient's test.

Measurement of Bladder Pressure (p_{ves})

It is usual to measure p_{ves} with a urethral catheter. Once in place, it is joined to the external transducer with connection tubing; this tubing needs water-tight connections (e.g. Luer lock) at each end, and there should be no marked changes in calibre where the tubing joins the catheter or the transducer. The connection tubing needs to be flexible but kink resistant. It must not be elastic because the elasticity would affect the transmission of the pressure. The tubing should not be excessively long, narrow, or wide. The fluid in the tube is usually water.

It is advantageous to have two separate catheters in the bladder for filling and for measuring p_{ves}, i.e. the 'two catheter technique'. Firstly, the physical contact between two catheters is less than the contact between the two channels of a double lumen catheter, and this reduces pump artefact (see below). Secondly, once filling is complete at cystometric capacity (CC), the filling line can be removed. The filling catheter we use is 8 Fr size, and to measure p_{ves}, we use a 16-gauge catheter (similar to the type of tube used for epidural anaesthesia). The p_{ves} catheter is taped in place to stay present throughout filling cystometry and the PFS. In women, passing the tubes alongside each other simultaneously is quite straightforward. In men, the finer p_{ves} catheter would curl up in the urethra, so it needs to be 'piggy-backed' into the bladder on the filling catheter (Figure 7.16). In this technique, the tip of the p_{ves} catheter is introduced into one eyehole of the filling catheter. Both catheters are then passed into the bladder, until the urine drips from the filling catheter (indicating they are properly in the bladder). Both catheters are then withdrawn until the urine flow just stops (so the catheters will then be just below the bladder neck). Advancing by 1 cm (so urine drips again) means the catheters will now be lying only just inside the bladder. With one hand, the urodynamicist holds the filling catheter so it cannot move out again and slowly pulls the p_{ves} catheter gently until a subtle 'click' is felt, which indicates the tip has disengaged from the eyehole of the filling catheter. Both catheters can now be advanced together, so a good length of each is in the bladder. The 'click' is a valuable cue that the p_{ves} catheter has been freed from the filling catheter, i.e. 'disengagement'. If the p_{ves} catheter tip is still stuck in the filling catheter side hole (failure of disengagement), it will lead to unreliable p_{ves} recordings during filling cystometry and accidental removal of the p_{ves} catheter when the filling line is taken out for the PFS.

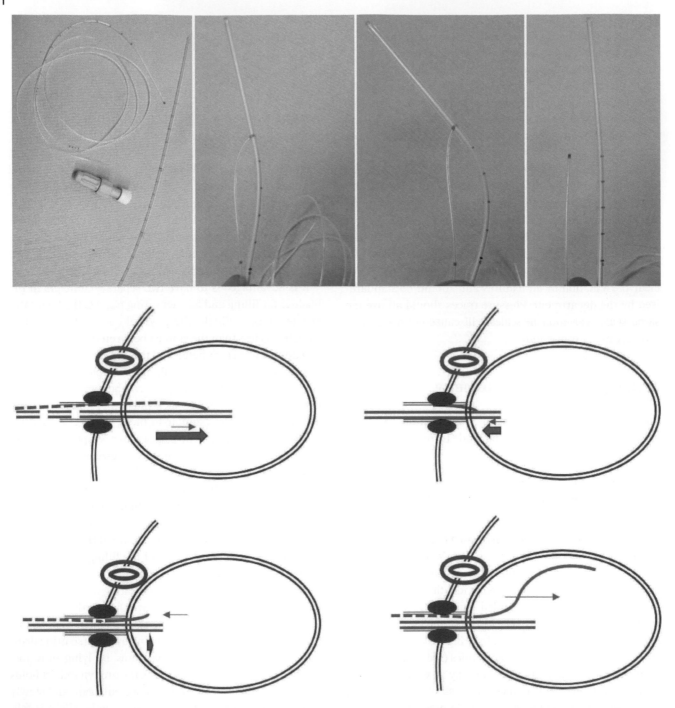

Figure 7.16 The two-catheter technique. Above: photographs of the catheters (top left), with the p_{ves} catheter piggy-backed into a side hole of the filling catheter (middle left), drawing back on the p_{ves} catheter to start disengagement (middle right), and disengaged (top right). Below the photographs are schematic diagrams of the process. The upper left diagram shows the piggy-backed catheters being advanced right into the bladder (urine will drop from the external end of the filling catheter when fully in). The upper right diagram shows them both being pulled slowly back to the bladder neck (if urine stops dripping, the filling catheter is in the prostatic urethra – advance the catheter back in by a few centimetres). Below left: disengaging by pulling the p_{ves} line slightly out, and slightly advancing the filling line. Feeling a 'click' sensation indicates full disengagement. Below right: advancing the p_{ves} catheter generously into the bladder to ensure it stays in properly for filling and pressure-flow study. It is important not to pull the 16G catheter into the prostatic urethra inadvertently, as it will not be possible to insert it into the bladder again without repeating the whole process. *Source*: Marcus Drake.

The two-catheter technique is inexpensive. It is also suitable for doing a urethral pressure profile to avoid the costs associated with triple-lumen catheters sometimes used for this. It also has some advantages for running urodynamic tests, due to the ability to remove the filling line at CC while leaving the p_{ves} line in place. Firstly, stress incontinence is easier to demonstrate (which can be difficult with a 6 or 8 Fr double lumen catheter, notably in post-prostatectomy incontinence). Secondly, the flow during PFS will be less impeded.

An alternative is to use a 'double lumen' catheter, which is a single catheter containing two channels, one for the measurement of p_{ves} and the other for bladder filling. A size 6 Fr double lumen catheter allows a filling speed of up to 50 ml/min and only rarely causes obstruction in adults (for example, if there is a urethral stricture). Larger catheters than 6 Fr should generally not be used.

When using a straight catheter in men, the natural curve of the urethral bulb and membranous urethra has to guide the catheter tip towards the bladder. Unfortunately, the bladder neck is often in the way, so a straight-ended catheter can snag, causing discomfort, and sometimes preventing catheterisation (Figure 7.17). A particularly valuable catheter to have available for men who are proving difficult to catheterise is the angle-ended 'Coudé' or 'Tiemann-tip' double lumen catheter, which can be used to help the catheter past the bladder neck very easily in a high proportion of cases, as illustrated in Figure 7.17.

The p_{ves} is kept separate from the filling tube, since the latter causes repetitive pressure variations – a result of the mechanism by which pumping is delivered (Figure 7.18). Unfortunately, this problem is often present with a double lumen catheter since the two lumina are so close together.

Accordingly, we prefer the two-catheter technique (see below) to give the best separation between the p_{ves} recording and the potential interference by the pump. If the pump seems to be interfering with the p_{ves} recording despite using two separate catheters, it is worth checking whether the connecting tubing of the pump is resting on the p_{ves} connection tubing outside the body, as they can easily be separated to resolve the problem.

For practical reasons, urethral catheters are used in most urodynamic tests. The percutaneous (suprapubic) route would be preferable in an ideal world to avoid impeding the outlet for doing the PFS. However, placing a suprapubic catheter can be uncomfortable and may be risky, particularly in obese patients and those who have had surgery in the lower part of the abdomen. In specific situations, they are valuable, for example, in some children, in adult patients with a psychological aversion to urethral access, in severe outlet structural abnormalities, and if there is a suprapubic catheter already in place. In a co-operative adult patient, blind puncture of the bladder with a special kit can be undertaken. This requires confident palpation of the bladder, which is only realistic in thin patients, and when the bladder volume is approximately 500 ml. Portable ultrasound machines allow a suprapubic catheter to be introduced with more confidence than for blind puncture.

Occasionally, a person with a long-term suprapubic Foley catheter comes for UDS. This can be used if the extent of urodynamic information needed is well defined. An example is UDS in a patient with neurological lower urinary tract dysfunction, where the main requirement is to establish the bladder compliance. In that case, the single lumen of the Foley catheter can be connected to the p_{ves} and filling connecting tubes using a 3-way tap. Having the

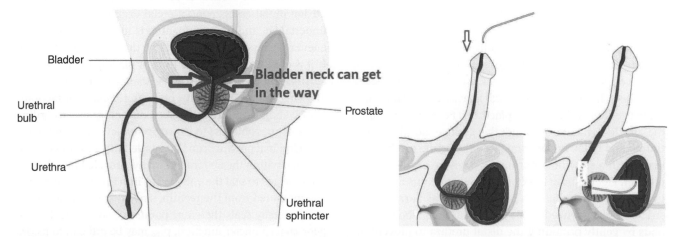

Figure 7.17 A straight catheter may be difficult to get past the bladder neck in men. A 'Coudé' or 'Tiemann-tip' double lumen catheter is an easy and safe way to avoid the bladder neck problem. It is placed like a normal catheter, but starting with the angle lined up to help the catheter find its way easily along the urethra. Hold the penis upwards and line the catheter so that the angled tip is pointing vertically downwards to the urethral meatus. The main length of the catheter should be above the patient's midline. As you advance the catheter from this starting point, the urethra will push it in the right direction.

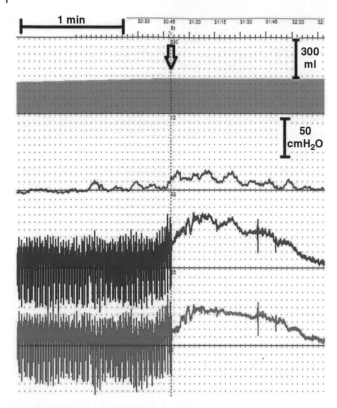

Figure 7.18 Pressure variations resulting from the filling pump mechanism, also known as 'pump artefact'. With the filling pump running, the flow is generated by a peristaltic pump, which gives a tiny surge several times per second. When the pump is stopped (black arrow), the artefact disappears.

tap switched to the filling pump for 100 ml, then changing to the p_{ves} line for a couple of minutes, allows intermittent recording of vesical pressure with good knowledge of bladder volume, so compliance can be calculated (Figure 7.19).

Anaesthesia for Urethral Catheterisation

In female patients, lubrication jelly is important for catheterisation. Local anaesthetic gel is probably unlikely to be effective, as it leaks out too quickly for the anaesthetic to take effect. In male patients, local anaesthetic gel may have some use. To get the gel into place, it is necessary to control the urethral meatus around the syringe nozzle with a thumb and index finger, straighten the penile urethra, and instil with a slow but continuous pressure on the syringe plunger. Gel pushing back out from the meatus as you are trying to get it in may indicate a urethral narrowing or stricture. The gel needs to be kept in place for about 60 seconds by gently occluding the distal urethra to prevent the gel escaping and gently easing the gel into the bulbar urethra with external compression, moving from distal to proximal. The patient may report an initial stinging sensation as the gel goes in because the product might contain an antiseptic; the easing of the stinging sensation is an

indicator that the anaesthetic effect has started. In most men, the anaesthetic jelly does not pass the sphincter into the prostatic urethra, meaning that the final part of catheter placement may be uncomfortable even with the anaesthetic gel.

Fixing the Catheter(s)

Careful attention to taping the catheters in place reduces the risk they could be displaced into the bladder outlet, or fall out altogether, during bladder filling or voiding. In the male patient, the p_{ves} catheter should be turned back over the shaft of the penis and held there with tape, ensuring that the tape does not compress the urethra (Figure 7.20). The filling catheter should be passed well into the bladder and secured with tape, leaving minimal gap between the external urinary meatus and the point at which the tape is placed on the catheter. The tape should be taken back over the dorsum of the penis, as shown in Figure 7.20. In the female patient, the two catheters should be held separately on the inside of the thigh using tape placed as close as possible to the external urethral meatus.

Measurement of Abdominal Pressure

The rectum generally should be empty, which means pressure recording usually works reliably. Constipation can be an issue for UDS, specifically if the rectum is loaded with faeces, as this might affect pressure recording for p_{abd}. It may also cause rectal contractions. Note that when claiming they have constipation, many patients are actually describing infrequent motions due to slow colon transit (colonic loading) rather than rectal loading, which is irrelevant for UDS. Hence, if someone reports constipation during initial assessment, a rectal examination should be undertaken, and if rectal loading is identified, a microlax enema can be self-administered on the morning of the test. If it is only identified at the time of placing the p_{abd} catheter, the test can still be run satisfactorily in many cases, allowing for the possibility of seeing rectal contractions. However, in a minority of tests, satisfactory p_{abd} recording proves impossible due to faecal occlusion of the catheter.

Abdominal pressure can be recorded from any organ with a lumen within the abdominal cavity, provided that there is some means to seal the entry point into the organ. It is usually measured from the rectum, since the anal sphincter at rest generally seals the entry point. For some people with poor anal sphincter function, p_{abd} may be difficult to record because the pressure differential from atmospheric pressure is obscured by the anal laxity and because it may be difficult to keep the tube in position. Sometimes, p_{abd} is measured from the vagina, placing the catheter high in the fornix so that some pressure seal is provided by the pelvic floor; this

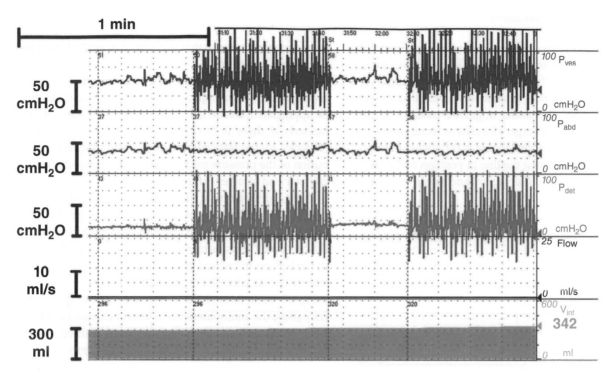

Figure 7.19 Single lumen bladder catheter for filling and p_ves measurement. A 3-way tap has been placed into the end of a suprapubic catheter to connect It to the filling pump and the bladder transducer. When the pump is not running, the transducer is measuring bladder pressure, but when it is running (which is obvious because of the pump artefact), the bladder transducer reading is dominated by the pump pressure. This is an approach to measuring bladder compliance, as it is possible to establish p_ves while controlling volume (see main text). This is an old trace; current practice is not to display the vesical pressure at the top.

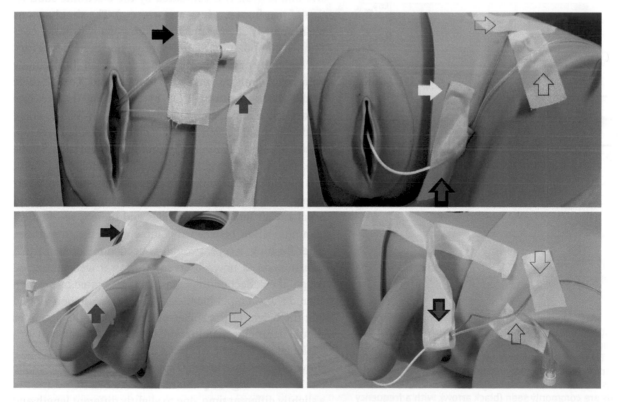

Figure 7.20 Two catheters (left side) and double lumen catheters (right) illustrating taping for women (above) and men (below). For women, the catheters are fixed to the perineum (solid arrows, black for filling catheter, purple for p_ves). An extra bit of tape on the thigh (open arrows) helps keep the weight off the perineal tape and separates the two lines to reduce transmission of pump artefact to p_ves. For men, the filling catheter or double lumen catheter uses two bits of tape; an anchor tape suprapubically, with a separate piece of tape securing the catheter to the anchor. In the two-catheter technique, the p_ves catheter, being more flexible, can be secured to the penis. Each piece of tape is placed with a little fold over at the end (yellow arrow) to facilitate removal. *Source*: Marcus Drake.

in p_{det} during a cough is fully acceptable, provided that the height above and below the baseline is similar. Reliable transmission of pressure can also be affected if one of the connectors works loose, leading to loss of pressure. This can lead to a steady drop in pressure on one of the lines (Figure 7.24). If this is seen, all connections should be checked, and the lines flushed.

Media Used for Bladder Filling

Water or physiological saline is the most commonly used filling medium in UDS, together with radiographic contrast medium if video urodynamics is being performed. We use fluid at room temperature. Formerly, we used to heat infusion fluid to body temperature (37°C), but there is no evi-

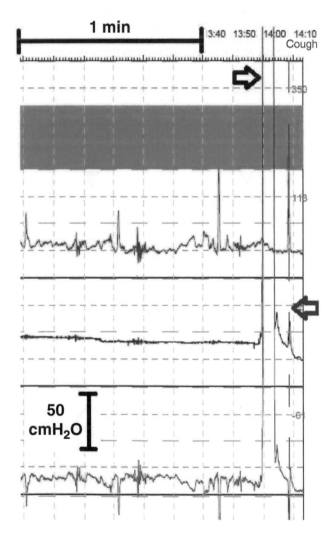

Figure 7.24 A steady declining pressure (here affecting p_{ves}, i.e. the blue line) indicates a significant problem; even after a flush-through of the bladder line (black arrow), the recording is still inadequate as shown by the poor pick of a cough in the p_{ves} line (blue arrow) compared with the big spike achieved at that moment in the p_{abd} line.

dence of any advantage for this [4]. The ICS recommends that temperature of filling medium is stated but does not instruct on which temperature should be in standard use [1], beyond warning that cold fluid (lower than 20°C) can influence detrusor activity at low bladder volumes [4]. This has been exploited as the 'ice water test' in some centres [9, 10].

Patient Position During Cystometry

The patient is catheterised when supine, but our practice is to undertake bladder filling with the patient upright, since most patients complain of bladder symptoms principally when they are active (upright), and making urodynamic observations while reproducing symptomatic complaints is the key reason for undertaking the test. Both DO and stress urinary incontinence (SUI) are generally more readily demonstrated when upright; this might be because the supine position does not reflect the everyday stresses to which the bladder is subjected. In order to make the transition from filling cystometry to PFS easier and quicker, we generally do the test seated (in the case of women) or standing (in the case of most male patients).

Some patients complain of symptoms when they change posture, for example, when rising from a sitting position. If the patient has symptoms related to change of posture, this should be tested during the urodynamic study. If the patient's position is changed, then the transducer height must be adjusted to remain level with the pubis and the new patient position recorded on the trace.

Supine bladder filling is a suitable consideration for some situations:

- If there is gross DO preventing proper filling when the patient is upright, it will be impossible to detect stress incontinence or sufficiently fill the bladder for voiding. In this case, stopping filling and transferring to the supine position, then recommencing filling at a slow rate can often help stabilise the bladder. This allows a proper examination for USI (Figure 7.25). This is far preferable to repeating the test after several weeks using overactive bladder (OAB) medications.
- Patients who are severely disabled by neurological disease may have to be investigated in the supine position. Flow rate measurement during PFS is problematic for this group, but a drainpipe run from the penis to the flowmeter can be used for male patients. This will mean a slight delay in recording the flow.
- Investigators who use video urodynamics sometimes use an X-ray tilt table, undertaking filling in the supine position and then tilting the X-ray table to fully upright for voiding. A disadvantage of this practice is the difficulty adequately reproducing the stresses on the bladder associated with upright posture during the storage phase.

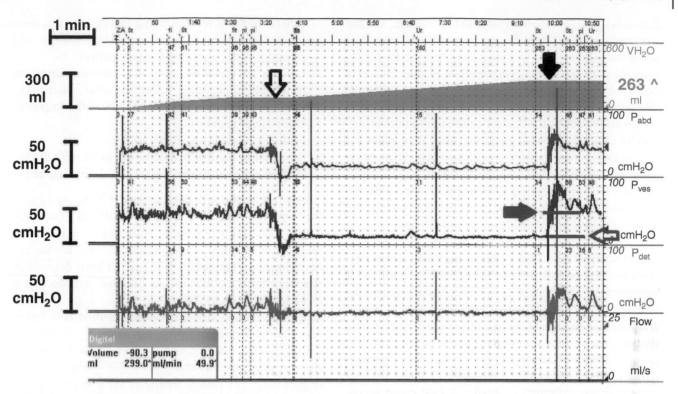

Figure 7.25 Filling cystometry, showing how position can affect detrusor overactivity. Right from the start of the study, there is considerable detrusor overactivity (DO). This limits the cystometry capacity, so this man was transferred from standing to supine (indicated by the open black arrow). As a result, the DO largely disappears, and filling can be restarted. The DO returned once he went back to the standing position (filled black arrow). The resting pressure in the p_{ves} and p_{abd} lines is lower when in the supine position (open purple arrow) than in the standing position (closed purple arrow).

Rate of Bladder Filling

Filling rate needs to be considered carefully for all patients. Once the test is complete, the filling protocol used needs to be stated clearly in the report for each test.

- For most patients, the bladder diary maximum voided volume (MVV) provides an indication of what the CC may turn out to be, though there is a high chance there will be a discrepancy. The ICS suggests dividing the MVV (in ml) by 10, to determine the filling rate (in ml/min) [1]. They also suggest stopping filling in case of urgency or if DO starts, waiting for them to settle before recommencing filling.
- If filling is started at the rate as described above, but the detrusor turns out to be poorly compliant (see below), the filling rate should be dropped to 10 ml/min, and the situation needs to be interpreted with care.
- For patients with neurological disease, filling rate is particularly influential on compliance [11]. Thus, slow-fill cystometry should be used to commence the test, meaning only 10 ml/min at most. The filling rate can be increased if bladder compliance proves to be normal.
- For children, the filling rate is derived as described in Chapter 12.

The ICS uses the term 'medium-fill cystometry' for speeds between 10 and 100 ml/min and fast-fill cystometry when the rate is greater than 100 ml/min. Fast-fill cystometry should not be used in routine practice, except for a very short time (for example, to try to provoke overactivity).

The rate of bladder filling has considerable influence on the resulting measurements. The faster the bladder is filled, the lower the apparent bladder compliance, which complicates interpretation. A series of cystometrograms repeated one after the other with a medium or rapid filling rate will show a gradually increasing capacity [12], and this can be avoided using the more restrained rates of filling described above. The slower filling rates lie closer to the maximum rate, the bladder might be expected to experience in life, i.e. the rate of urine production by the kidneys under maximum diuresis conditions [13]. The fastest physiological urine production for any individual can be estimated by dividing the body weight (in kg) by four (e.g. the maximum diuresis for a healthy 80 kg person is about 20 ml/min).

What to Do About Post-Void Residual Urine?

In general, before filling cystometry, the patient is asked to empty the bladder as fully as possible, usually into the flowmeter. They are then catheterised for the test, and the post-void residual (PVR) can be evacuated by aspiration along the catheter that will soon after be used for filling. How the patient normally empties their bladder currently needs to be factored in; if the patient usually uses intermittent self-catheterisation (ISC), then the patient is asked to do this and to empty the bladder before UDS commences.

More thought is needed regarding what to do about the PVR in situations where the specific urodynamic question needs consideration. For example, in a patient with neurological disease undergoing UDS solely to check that the lower urinary tract is compliant, then the issue is about the safety of their current approach to bladder emptying. If such a patient does not generally use ISC, then the PVR should not be emptied before beginning filling cystometry. Likewise, if a patient without neurological abnormalities has evidence of hydronephrosis, which could be secondary to elevated bladder pressure, the bladder should not be drained at the beginning of the filling phase of urodynamic studies. This is because removing the PVR and/or filling too quickly can fundamentally change the results, particularly in respect of bladder compliance, DO, and CC. For these patients, information about the PVR could be got with a bladder scanner or ultrasound before the test, or through a catheter after the PFS.

A practical point for video urodynamics is that filling with contrast without draining a urine residual may mean the contrast is too diluted to see properly. If so, it would be appropriate to remove some of the residual urine before filling with contrast.

What future treatment is being considered might also be relevant to deciding whether to empty a PVR. This is entirely dependent on individual situations, but we will generally plan to drain a PVR if a future surgical intervention plan includes a strategy for reliable bladder emptying, such as ISC or indwelling catheterisation.

Ensuring a High-Quality Recording

Once the catheters are in place and connected to the transducers, the tubing must be flushed to ensure that all bubbles are removed before starting recording. In addition, bubbles close to the transducer diaphragm must be removed by flushing (Figure 7.26). Failure to remove bubbles will lead to errors in measurement. All the connections between the catheters, tubing, and transducers should be air-tight; any leak will cause errors in the pressure measurement. Leaks, bubbles, or elastic-sided tubing will tend to lead to the recording of lower values of pressure.

Quality control must be scrupulously ensured by checking the following:

1) **Initial resting pressures** in the p_{ves} and p_{abd} traces are in the right range, with p_{det} close to zero.

2) **A 'live' signal** is seen, meaning that p_{ves} and p_{abd} show small fluctuations reflecting breathing, moving, and speaking, when recording from the patient.

3) **Coughs are present** at regular intervals during the investigation, including before and after voiding. The smaller cough response is at least 70% of the amplitude of the bigger response.

4) **Scales and labels** are clearly visible.

5) **Any quality control problems are dealt with during the test**, not once the test has concluded (see Chapter 18).

There are a range of feasible pressures for p_{ves} and p_{abd} in the supine, sitting, and standing positions (Table 7.3; Figure 7.27). Seeing that the pressure range is in the appropriate 'feasible' range is a good indicator that zeroing has been done appropriately, i.e. it has not been done while recording from the patient – a common mistake that is immediately obvious (Figure 7.9).

Before recording starts, the patient should be asked to raise their abdominal pressure, e.g. by doing a cough, and the p_{ves} and p_{abd} traces observed. There should be an equal rise in pressure on each when the patient coughs (Figure 7.22). The patient should be asked to give a cough that produces a clear deflection of approximately 50–100 cmH$_2$O. If the spikes are not identical, then the explanation may be that there are bubbles or leaks, that the catheters are malpositioned, or that there is interference with the measurement of p_{abd} e.g. due to faecal loading. These must be checked and corrected to get the cough response to the proper pattern. Sometimes, there may be

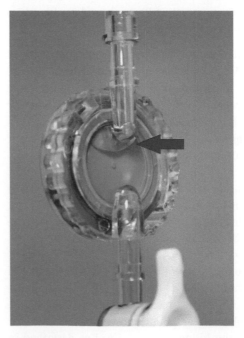

Figure 7.26 A bubble (red arrow) in a pressure transducer dome, which will dampen pressure changes and make accurate recording difficult. *Source*: Marcus Drake.

Table 7.3 Resting pressures [3].

	Supine	Seated	Standing
p_{ves}	5 to 20 cmH$_2$O	15 to 40 cmH$_2$O	30 to 50 cmH$_2$O
p_{abd}	5 to 20 cmH$_2$O	15 to 40 cmH$_2$O	30 to 50 cmH$_2$O
p_{det}[a]	−5 to 5 cmH$_2$O	−5 to 5 cmH$_2$O	−5 to 5 cmH$_2$O

[a] For the majority of prospectively evaluated patients [8]. Recorded p_{det} between 0 and 6 cmH$_2$O is acceptable in 80% of cases and in rare cases up to 10 cmH$_2$O [3].

difficulty recording p_{ves} if the bladder is empty (i.e. at the very start of the test); running the filling pump to infuse say 50 ml should quickly establish effective recording of p_{ves} if this is the case (Figure 7.28).

Once the initial cough gives a good-quality signal, bladder filling can commence. Throughout bladder filling, the fidelity of recording must be monitored, and a reliable way to do this is to ask the patient to cough regularly (e.g. at one-minute intervals). Good-quality signal is also indicated if both lines promptly and equally show the pressure changes associated with breathing and body movement. If at any stage the quality deteriorates in either of the measured pressure lines, then the investigation must be stopped, and the cause of the poor pressure transmission investigated. Once the fault is corrected, then the filling can recommence. Just before permission to void, and also after the PFS, the patient must cough again to ensure that the catheters have not moved during micturition. Failure to show an equal transmission of pressure after voiding means that the results of voiding cannot be confidently interpreted, and the investigation might need to be repeated if the voiding phase is vital for therapy decision-making.

Performing Filling Cystometry

Throughout cystometry, the principles of UDS must be considered, namely that 'The role of urodynamics is to reproduce the patient's symptoms' and 'The role of urodynamics is to provide a pathophysiological explanation for the patient's complaints'. This means there should be dialogue between the investigator and the patient *throughout* the investigation. It is particularly important when assessing the sensations the patient experience during cystometry. During bladder filling, the following should be assessed: bladder sensation, detrusor activity, bladder compliance, outlet function, and bladder capacity.

Bladder Sensation

Certain terms have been accepted relating to bladder sensation, though relating a precise bladder volume to any of them is subjective and is likely to vary considerably:

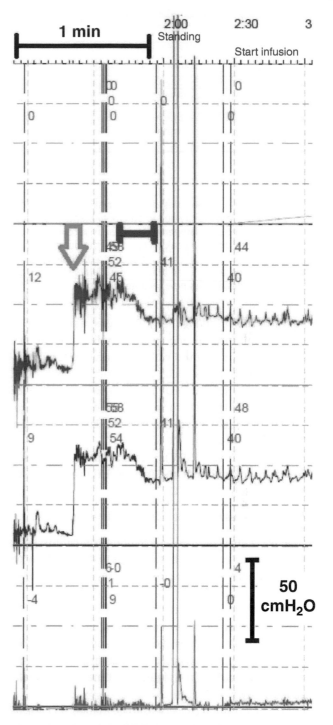

Figure 7.27 Resting pressures can change in response to both the position of the transducers and the position of the patient. When recording is restarted after a patient stands up (green arrow), a high pressure and noise from patient movement are evident. When the transducers are moved up to the level of the pubic bone (purple bar), the hydrostatic element of pressure gain is removed, but the raised resting pressure in the organs remains. With a change in position, the pressure in the organs does actually change. The transducers must be moved to the new height of the pubis during or after a position change (purple bar).

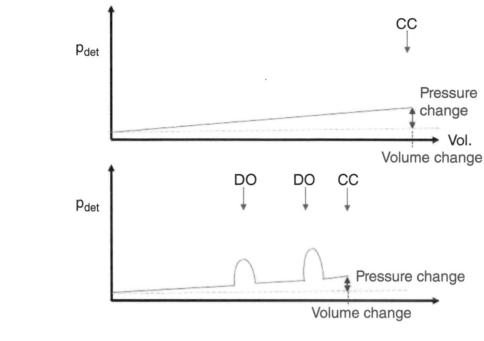

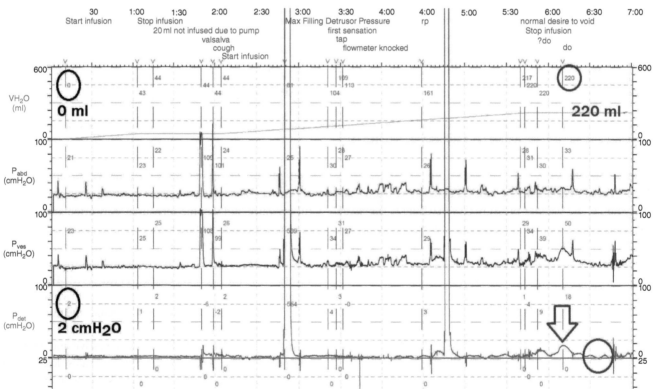

Figure 7.33 Calculating compliance requires pressure and volume values at two clear points; the top schematic diagram illustrates the measurements in an idealised trace. In practice, traces may have additional features that require adjustments identifying the two clear points. The lower schematic diagram shows how, if there is detrusor overactivity (DO), it is ignored in the calculation. The trace below shows this applied in practice. The volume change is 220−0 = 220 ml. The end pressure value (purple circle) needs to be taken once any DO (purple arrow) has settled down to baseline (purple circle). The exact value is not annotated, but the p_{det} appears to hit zero. This means pressure change would be −2 cmH$_2$O; in the event of a negative or zero pressure change, by convention, the value of 1 is used. Hence, in this example, the compliance is 220/1, i.e. 220 ml/cmH$_2$O. CC = cystometric capacity.

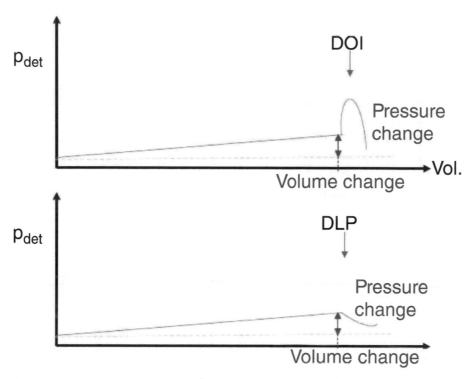

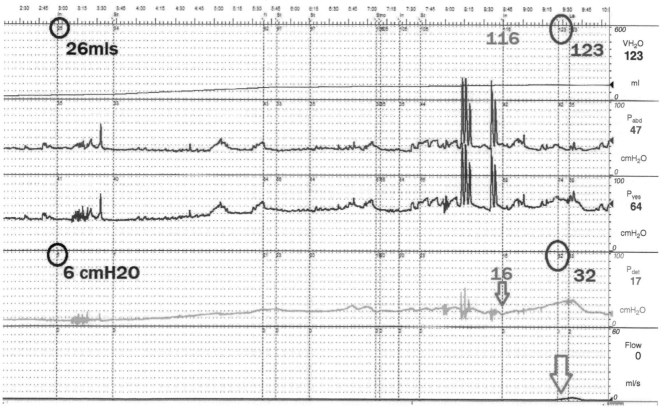

Figure 7.34 If leakage happens, the pressure change calculation should use the detrusor pressure fractionally before the leak. This may be a result of detrusor overactivity incontinence (DOI) or at a detrusor leak point (DLP). In the trace below, the volume change is $123 - 26 = 97$ ml, and the pressure change is $32 - 6 = 26\,cmH_2O$. Compliance is thus $97/26 = 3.7\,ml/cmH_2O$, which is abnormal, referred to as 'poorly compliant'. The end volume and pressure values (purple circles) were taken just before the leak (orange arrow). There is actually a subjective aspect to this trace, since the leak might actually be interpreted as resulting from DOI; in that case, the values indicated at the brown arrow can be taken for calculating compliance, which makes compliance $(116 - 26)/(16 - 6) = 9\,ml/cmH_2O$.

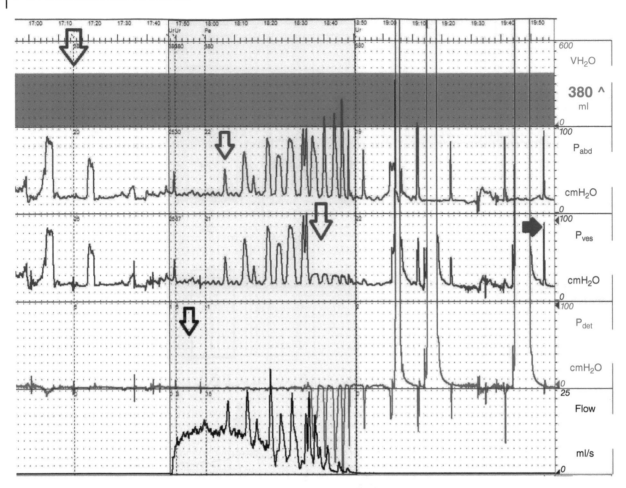

Figure 7.37 Urethral relaxation supplemented by straining. This figure illustrates the principle that bladder emptying in women may involve urethral relaxation rather than synchronous detrusor contraction and outlet relaxation. The illustration shows a pressure-flow study (permission to void is indicated by the purple arrow), with a good flow pattern associated with no detrusor pressure change at all (black arrow), i.e. voiding by urethral relaxation. In this PFS, the patient also used straining, and the first strain (after about 14 seconds of voiding by urethral relaxation) is indicated by the red arrow; with the urethra so relaxed, the straining is very effective at increasing flow rate. The vesical catheter blocked towards the end of voiding (open blue arrow), and three flushes were needed before the catheter was fully unblocked (closed blue arrow). Inappropriate urethral relaxation during storage is a rare mechanism of incontinence; being so unusual, we were not able to find an example to use for an illustration.

nence" is leakage due to urethral relaxation in the absence of raised abdominal pressure or a detrusor contraction. Urethral relaxation alone is an unusual cause of incontinence, and it is not clear whether or not it is a variant of a prematurely activated micturition reflex, in which the rise in detrusor pressure is of very low amplitude. The phenomenon is seen only in women.

Note that if incontinence occurs due to an involuntary detrusor contraction (DO incontinence), the urethral closure mechanism is not generally thought of as incompetent, even though leakage has occurred. However, there are some considerations in this situation:

1) Since urethral relaxation is a reflex action occurring as part of normal micturition, perhaps DO incontinence can be viewed as the premature activation of the micturition reflex. This is plausible where the amplitude of the DO exceeds the ability of the urethra to resist, or perhaps the outlet becomes fatigued as a DO contraction persists; this might then allow some urine to enter the proximal urethra, which can set off the reflex relaxation of the sphincter.

2) If outlet resistance is impaired, whether or not stress incontinence is present symptomatically, the entry of urine into the proximal urethra is more likely increasing the likelihood of DO incontinence. Urgency incontinence due to DO is seen more frequently in women because urethral and pelvic floor function are not as strong as in men, particularly after childbirth.

3) A reflex contraction of the pelvic floor is a natural reaction when DO starts (Figure 7.38). If the patient avoids leakage by maintaining voluntary pelvic floor contractions, the DO will in due course subside. Women with

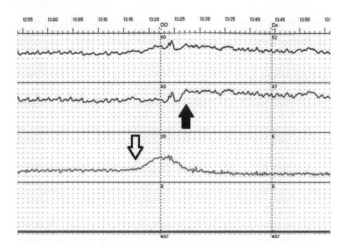

Figure 7.38 Pelvic floor contraction in response to detrusor overactivity (DO). A few seconds after the DO starts (open black arrow), there is a reflex pelvic floor contraction which includes an anal sphincter contraction. Even though a pelvic floor contraction does not increase abdominal pressure, this reflex shows up on the p_{abd} recording (closed black arrow). The illustrated order of traces is not consistent with modern standards (vesical pressure should not be at the top).

long-standing DO seem to have increased urethral closure pressures [19], suggesting that they have effectively done resistance training to strengthen their sphincter, and hence reduced their risk of DO incontinence.

4) Urine entering the proximal urethra generally does trigger a powerful sensation, but it does not inevitably lead to sphincter relaxation and leakage (Figure 2.19).

USI is the involuntary leakage of urine during increased abdominal pressure in the absence of a detrusor contraction. The provocation tests to elicit USI are shown in Figure 7.4, and a complete test evaluating someone with SUI symptoms is shown in Figure 7.39.

We sometimes find patients are reticent about engaging fully with provocation tests to elicit USI, due to the understandable embarrassment of leaking in public; they may therefore give rather weak coughs and hold their pelvic floor contracted. It takes a good rapport between the investigator and the patient to reassure them at this point and ask them not to 'hold on'. We encourage them to relax the pelvic floor since seeing the leak is really the point of doing the test. This is the reason to ask for a rapid

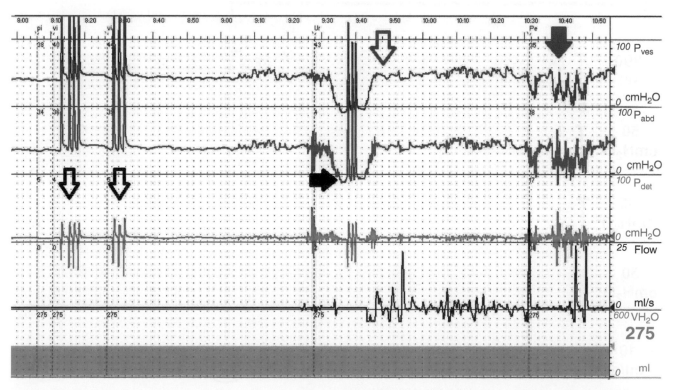

Figure 7.39 Evaluating a woman with stress urinary incontinence (SUI) symptoms. The bladder should be filled adequately (200 ml and cystometric capacity are commonly used). The patient is asked to do a rapid series of strong coughs (open black arrow). They are then asked to crouch, which makes it harder for them to contract their pelvic floor, and the cough series is repeated (closed black arrow). They can then be asked to jog on the spot (open purple arrow) or jump on the spot (closed purple arrow); this exertion can disturb the flowmeter, giving rise to the artefact shown (it is clearly an artefact, since it drops below zero). Throughout this, it is necessary to observe the urethral meatus to look for urodynamic stress incontinence. Additional options not illustrated include Valsalva manoeuvres and raising a leg (e.g. by resting a foot on a chair).

sequence of strong coughs, done with sufficient rapidity that the patient does not have a chance to recontract the pelvic floor before the next cough. We usually test for stress incontinence after 200 ml of filling; this is a suitable time, as the patient will generally not already have an SDV, as is likely to be the case at CC. If USI is not seen at 200 ml, we will repeat stress testing at CC. In the two urethral catheters technique, the filling line can be removed at this point. Removing the filling line facilitates seeing USI, particularly in men with post-prostatectomy incontinence (Figure 7.40), where 35% men may need catheter removal to show USI [20].

If standard UDS are used for a female patient and she is standing (i.e. not above the flowmeter to identify when the leak happens), then the external meatus must be viewed when the patient coughs in order to see the leak. Suitable lighting needs to be available to help see this reliably. An event marker must be applied to confirm incontinence has been seen and should be placed at the precise time it was observed. Women in particular may become embarrassed and must be reassured and put at their ease. With video

urodynamics, screening during the cough sequence is another chance to visualise a leak (Figure 8.44).

Bladder Capacity

In describing bladder capacity, there is a substantial influence of subjective judgement. A range of observations can be made which might be taken as some sort of measure of capacity.

- The MVV seen on the frequency-volume chart; this will be the everyday usable capacity in the patient's everyday life.
- CC is the bladder volume at the end of the filling cystometrogram, when the patient has an NDV and 'permission to void' has been given [14]. CC is volume voided plus any residual urine.
- Maximum cystometric capacity (MCC), in patients with normal sensation, is the volume at which the patient feels they can no longer delay micturition (has an SDV) [14].
- Maximum anaesthetic bladder capacity is the volume to which the bladder can be filled under either deep general or spinal anaesthetic and may often be very different

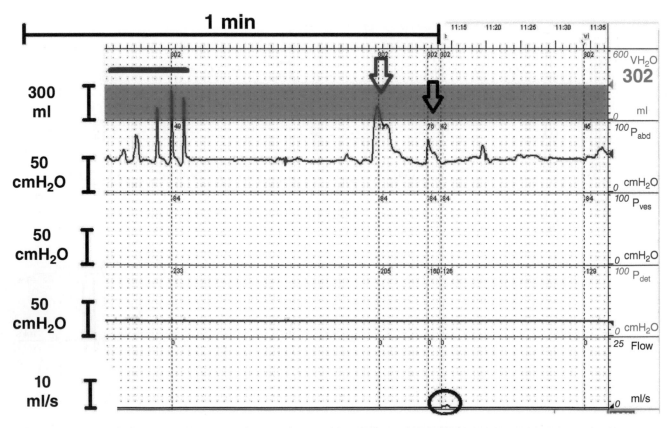

Figure 7.40 This man had stress urinary incontinence symptoms after radical prostatectomy. When catheterised for urodynamics, he was found to have a bladder neck stenosis (16 Fr calibre), so a double lumen Tiemann-tipped catheter was used for filling. No urodynamic stress incontinence (USI) was seen despite vigorous provocation manoeuvres (not shown). The double lumen catheter was then removed, and still no USI was seen despite good cough series (purple bar) and a high-amplitude Valsalva (purple arrow) – these are not seen on the p_{ves} line since the catheter was removed. Finally, he was told to relax his pelvic floor and not try to stop leakage; this enabled incontinence to be seen, elicited by a low-amplitude Valsalva (black arrow and oval).

from the MCC, particularly in conditions such as DO or bladder hypersensitivity.

For clinical management, consideration of PVR is important; if the patient were to be started on ISC, it could have the benefit of effectively increasing how much the bladder can usefully hold. As discussed in Chapter 6, caution is needed to check the PVR measured is genuinely representative of everyday life, or actually a consequence of the circumstances of testing. Hence, we often ask anyone started on ISC to keep a diary of some of their voided and catheter-obtained volumes so that we can decide about the actual contribution of PVR to everyday symptoms.

Artefacts During Cystometry

The urodynamicist is aware that UDS is not physiological, even with natural filling rates. This is due not only to the need for bladder filling and pressure measurement catheters but also because the patient is being observed. These limitations must be accepted and appreciated but not ignored. We have already discussed how technique must be adapted in the light of particular findings such as low compliance; further adaptations aimed at minimising artefacts are discussed in later chapters. The artefacts seen during cystometry can be divided into measurement and 'physiological' artefacts:

1) Measurement artefacts. This book tries to give sufficient practical detail to enable the urodynamicist to generate high quality traces and avoid measurement artefacts. Measurement artefacts are produced by problems in the equipment, somewhere between the tip of the catheters and the data recording. Setting up the equipment will uncover and deal with most of these problems. If there are problems with the transducers or the urodynamic equipment after proper calibration and transducer zeroing have been done, then the technical team, sales agent, or manufacturer will have to help. As filling cystometry is largely concerned with pressure measurement, this part of the test produces most pressure artefacts. Bubbles and leaks will alter the transmission of pressure from the patient to the transducer. The cough test is designed to identify this problem, so it can be dealt with and, hence, the importance of asking the patient to cough regularly. If there is unequal transmission of pressure on the p_{ves} and p_{abd} traces, then the catheters and lines should be flushed from the syringes attached to the transducer, especially for the line exhibiting the lower peak of cough amplitude (since that implies the cough impulse has not been fully picked up). The connections between catheter, tubing, and transducer should be checked for leaks. If unequal transmission of coughs continues, then catheter positions must be checked. Either catheter can slip down into the relevant sphincter region, causing a pressure transmission problem. This is rather more common with the rectal catheter, which can be difficult to keep in position in patients with poor anal function. A gradual emptying of the rectal catheter balloon can produce a confusing picture, with p_{abd} falling gradually (or else rising markedly if it enters the sphincter-active region), leading to an apparent increase in p_{det} (Figure 7.41). However, examination of the p_{ves} line shows that intravesical pressure is constant and focusses attention on p_{abd} as the cause of the artefact.

2) 'Physiological' artefacts. These are artefacts generated by patient activity. For example, rectal contractions are a cause of problems in interpretation and may lead to the misdiagnosis of DO. Rectal contractions are seen relatively frequently during urodynamic studies and may be single or multiple. If single, they should not create confusion, because there is then a single fall in p_{det} at the time of the rectal contraction. However, when they are repetitive, then the effect on the p_{det} trace can give the illusion of phasic DO.

Voiding Cystometry; Pressure-Flow Studies

Pressure-flow studies represent a natural progression from urine free-flow studies. Flow rate is dependent both on the outlet resistance and on the detrusor contraction, so a low flow rate may be associated with a high voiding pressure and outlet obstruction, or with a voiding pressure that is below normal. Similarly, the finding of a normal flow rate does not exclude bladder outlet obstruction (BOO), because normal flow may be maintained by a high voiding pressure in the presence of BOO. Thus, pressure measurement is needed to understand function fully.

We can be confident that when we see a genuine change in detrusor pressure, it indicates a bladder contraction is responsible. However, if the bladder outlet has a very wide calibre (as may be the case in women, especially those with USI), it can make pressure recording difficult. Also, when flow rates are high, the rate of volume expelled can be equal to the rate of contraction of bladder volume. Consequently, particularly in women, there may be minimal or no pressure change seen during voiding.

This may reflect two scenarios:

1) There is a normal bladder contraction, but pressure increase does not occur.

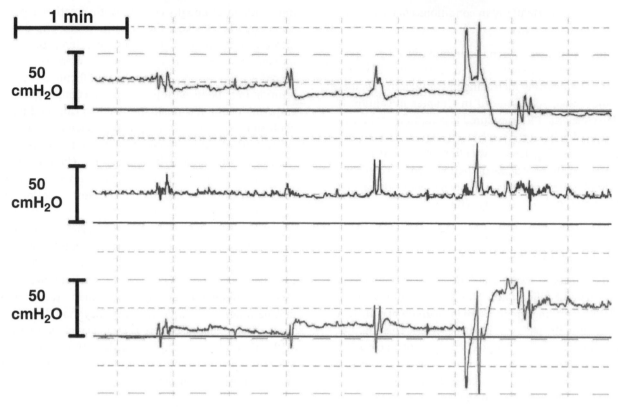

Figure 7.41 A problem with rectal recording in this filling cystometry causes p_{abd} to drop a few times. This has the effect of elevating the detrusor pressure in a manner that superficially looks like detrusor overactivity (DO). However, the lack of any similar activity in the vesical line indicates that this is not actually DO.

2) There is no bladder contraction, and voiding is principally a result of urethral relaxation (Figure 7.37).

Fundamentally, pressure generation is an indirect indicator of bladder contraction. Indeed, there is no technology currently able to measure the contraction in a living person directly in routine practice. This can be an important uncertainty, as normal bladder contraction (and the ability to increase the contraction strength to compensate if outlet resistance were to change) is needed if a woman intends to undergo surgery to treat USI. Consequently, it is worth considering some other aspects of voiding which might provide reassurance that micturition function is normal:

- Lack of voiding symptoms
- Prompt start of flow when given permission to void
- Normal duration of flow
- Absence of abdominal straining
- If using video urodynamics, a change in the bladder shape from 'floppy' to spherical in preparation for voiding
- A stop test might be considered if there is real uncertainty (see below)

The standardised ICS terminology applies the term *acontractile* if 'the detrusor cannot be observed to contract dur-

ing urodynamic studies resulting in prolonged bladder emptying and/or a failure to achieve complete bladder emptying within a normal time span' [21]. This definition is constrained by the fact that the only observation currently available in routine practice is pressure change, and the urodynamicist has to be alert to this limitation.

During PFS, detrusor pressure and flow rate are measured continuously, giving rise to some informative parameters (Figure 7.42). Each of these principally applies to p_{det} but can also be applied to p_{ves}:

- Premicturition pressure is the detrusor pressure recorded immediately before the initial isovolumetric contraction. It will be the same as the full resting pressure if the patient position has not been changed following the filling cystometrogram.
- Opening time is the time elapsed from the initial rise in detrusor pressure to the onset of flow. This is the initial isovolumetric contraction period of micturition.
- Opening pressure is the pressure recorded at the onset of measured flow. It should be remembered that there is a delay in the recording of flow because of the time taken for urine to reach the flowmeter. The delay is half a second to one second in duration and must be allowed for when interpreting the pressure-flow relationship. Such a

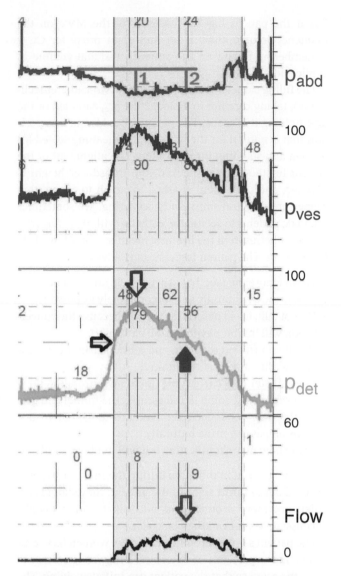

Figure 7.42 Pressure parameters during PFS in a male patient. The initial resting pressure at the start of the filling cystometry (not shown) was 5 cmH$_2$O; this should be subtracted from the voiding pressures to give the meaningful physiological change in detrusor pressure driving voiding. The brown line is placed to indicate that the apparent abdominal pressure has fallen during the void, which artefactually raises the apparent detrusor pressure. So, further correction of values is needed by subtracting the pressure drop at the applicable time. Maximum flow rate (Q$_{max}$) is indicated by the open purple arrow, 9 ml/s. Detrusor pressure at that time (p$_{detQmax}$; closed purple arrow) is particularly important. It starts out as 56 cmH$_2$O but is corrected for initial resting pressure (5 cmH$_2$O) and p$_{abd}$ drop (brown line 2, approx. 10 cmH$_2$O), giving a final value of 41 cmH$_2$O. Bladder outlet obstruction and bladder contractility indices are discussed in Chapter 14; in this case, their values are 23 and 86, respectively, meaning this man is equivocal for obstruction and he has detrusor underactivity. The blue arrow indicates the maximum detrusor pressure during the PFS (p$_{det.max}$), which should not be confused with p$_{detQmax}$. The black arrow indicates the 'opening pressure'.

delay is normally incorporated into urodynamic machine recording software.

- Maximum voiding pressure is the maximum value of the p$_{det}$ during voiding.
- Pressure at maximum flow (p$_{detQmax}$) is the pressure recorded at the time of maximum flow rate (Q$_{max}$). Again, allow for any delay in the recording of flow rate and for artefacts in the flow recording.
- Contraction pressure at maximum flow is the difference between the pressure at maximum flow and the premicturition pressure.
- After-contraction describes the common findings of a pressure increase after flow ceases at the end of micturition (Figure 7.43). The significance of this event is uncertain.

Outlet Resistance

A crucial issue is to identify the severity of the obstruction by measuring pressure and flow when the obstruction is the flow-limiting feature; an important thing to be clear about is the fact that people can actively increase outlet resistance. Clearly, this is a natural action during storage or filling cystometry when trying to resist physical forces and remain continent. However, if it occurs during a PFS, the assessment of BOO may well be completely erroneous. This particularly applies if a man has DO incontinence at the end of a filling cystometry; he will naturally respond by contracting the sphincter, which will lead to high pressure/ slow flow due to the voluntary sphincter action (Figure 7.44). It is only when a clear permission to void is given that the sphincter will be relaxed, meaning that the extent of prostatic obstruction can start to be understood. The BOO index must not be calculated unless preceded by permission to void. For this reason, it is good practice to avoid giving permission to void if terminal DO is present until the DO has settled. If it fails to settle, a clear 'permission to void' is needed to minimise the risk that the voluntary sphincter contraction is contributing to the outlet resistance.

The bladder and its outlet have independent functional properties which together determine the pressure–flow relationships of micturition. By knowing both factors, and relating them to the normal values of each, it is possible to ascertain whether voiding function itself is normal, more accurately than can be achieved from either measurement alone. To formalise the relationship of pressure and flow, various urethral resistance factors have been elaborated. Simple hydrodynamics of laminar flow through rigid straight tubes is not a good model, since the urethra is neither rigid nor straight and flow is often turbulent. The ICS recommends that pressure-flow data should be presented graphically, plotting one quantity against the other in a

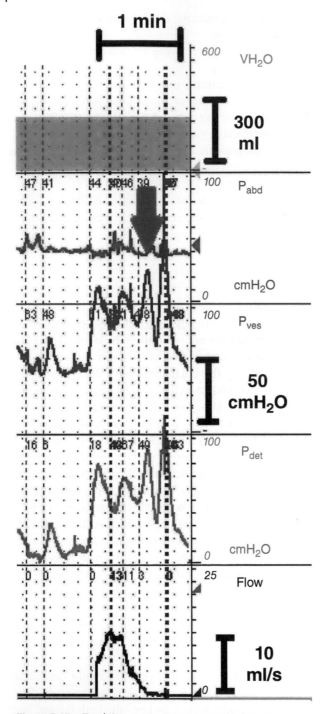

Figure 7.43 Two 'after contractions', meaning detrusor contractions following cessation of flow, the first of which is indicated by the purple arrow.

UDS report [1, 3], and it is this that gave rise to the nomograms used in the diagnosis of BOO.

Performing Voiding Cystometry

In most patients, it is quite clear when bladder filling should be stopped, since they experience strong sensations.

But if the patient has little sensation, the MVV on the frequency-volume chart is an important proxy for CC – remembering to add on the patient's residual volume as applicable.

The filling catheter is removed (in the two-catheter technique), taking care not to dislodge the p_{ves} catheter, or the tape holding it in place. The patient should void in a position that is natural for them, generally meaning seated for women and standing for most men. The alignment of the patient for the flow is checked, the transducer height is checked, and the patient is asked to cough to ensure that proper pressure transmission is occurring. We sometimes ask male patients to secure the catheter with their fingers a few centimetres from the urethral meatus, so it is less likely to come out. The patient is given some advice:

- Try to ignore the fact that other people are present.
- Pass urine as naturally and as completely as possible.
- Do not talk; avoid describing things (because the conversation will inhibit passing urine naturally).
- The liquid (filling medium and a bit of urine) will flow around the catheter, not within it.
- The catheter may carry some liquid away from the flowmeter funnel. If some liquid escapes the funnel and gets on the floor (or indeed the patient's foot), ignore it – focus on passing urine naturally.
- Urine flow may slightly sting but will not be painful.

Anyone present in the room during the PFS is instructed to stand out of direct sight of the patient; they should stay quiet, not move around, and not talk to other people. Permission to void can then be given.

The patient's privacy is important. Few women have ever voided in the presence of others, so it may be necessary to leave the room so that the patient can initiate voiding. The sound of gently trickling water (from slow running taps) may facilitate the initiation of voiding.

Interpretation of Voiding Cystometry

Detrusor activity and outlet function should be reviewed separately, whilst remembering that outlet characteristics will define the precise voiding pressure (Figure 7.45).

Detrusor Activity
This can be classified as follows (Figure 7.46):

- Normal, when the detrusor contracts to empty the bladder with a normal flow rate.
- Underactive, when either the detrusor contraction is unable to empty the bladder due to low pressure or the bladder empties at a lower than normal speed.
- Acontractile, when no measured detrusor contraction occurs during voiding.

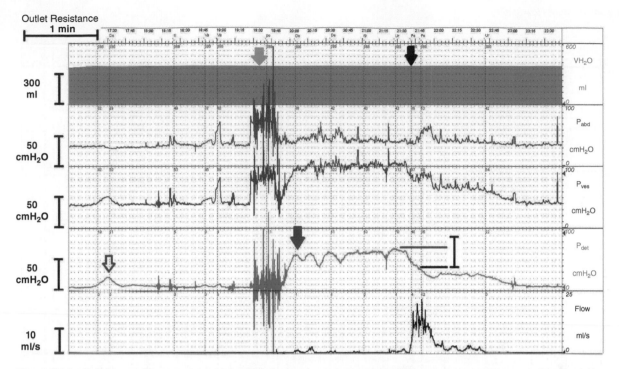

Figure 7.44 In this man, detrusor overactivity (DO) is seen towards the end of filling cystometry (open purple arrow). He stands and does some vigorous exercise as a stress test (closed light blue arrow), and this sets off high-amplitude DO (closed purple arrow), with incontinence. Some time is spent waiting for this to settle, but it does not do so. Accordingly, permission to void is given (closed black arrow); this defines the start of the pressure-flow study, and the detrusor pressure drops by about $30\,cmH_2O$ (scale bar = $50\,cmH_2O$). Calculating the bladder outlet obstruction index is only appropriate after permission to void, as the flow-limiting zone then is the prostate – in this case, not obstructed. Calculating it before permission to void is not acceptable, as the sphincter is the flow-limiting zone (as he tries to resist leaking). In cases such as this, if the pressure does not drop after permission to void, doubt remains as to the cause of the obstruction.

Figure 7.45 In this man, detrusor overactivity (DO) with some incontinence is seen towards the end of filling cystometry, and video urodynamic screening shows the contrast has been forced by the detrusor contraction into the prostatic urethra where it is held up by the urethral sphincter (closed orange arrow). He holds on resolutely until given permission to void (open black arrow), at which point he opens his sphincter fully and there is a precipitous drop in p_{ves}, as the flow-limiting zone shifts from the sphincter to the prostate. In this case, there is no prostatic obstruction. *Source*: Marcus Drake.

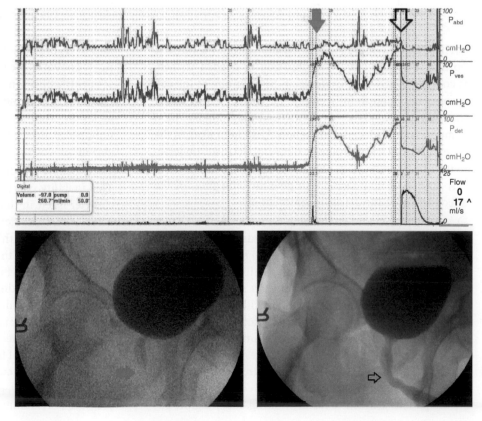

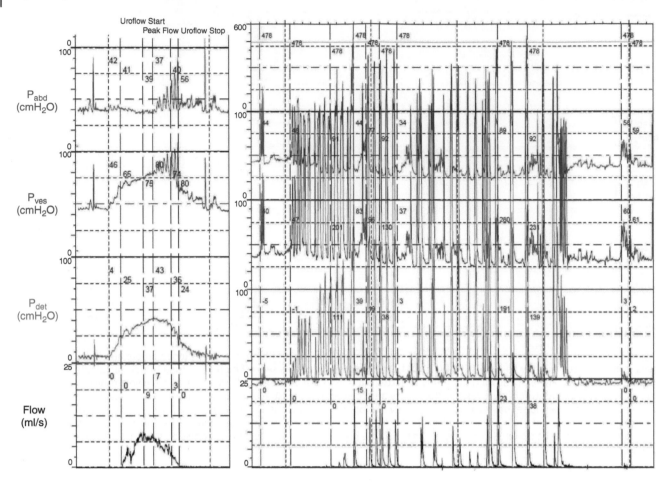

Figure 7.46 Detrusor activity during voiding may be normal, underactive (left, male patient), or acontractile (right, female patient).

These categories are fairly straightforward if the outlet is normal, but additional interpretation is needed if there is coexisting BOO. For example, in BPO, failure of the detrusor contraction to fully empty the bladder could reflect the obstruction alone, or there may additionally be a component of reduced contraction. UDS help discern the difference, since symptoms of BPO and detrusor underactivity are so similar [22]. This is discussed in Chapter 14.

A couple of approaches can give an indication of the effectiveness of the detrusor contraction:

1) An old way was to do the 'stop test' (Figure 7.47). Once the patient is voiding and when it judged that Q_{max} has been reached, the patient is asked to interrupt voiding. The patient achieves this by contracting the pelvic floor muscles. Pelvic floor contraction is usually achieved quickly, meaning that the bladder will still be contracting when flow stops. As the contraction is now against a closed outlet, it becomes an isovolumetric contraction (i.e. a contraction during which the volume does not change), and the intravesical pressure should increase sharply to a new maximum. After a couple of seconds, the patient is asked to restart voiding, meaning the p_{ves}

falls to its previous level. The height of the increase in p_{det} is known as the $p_{det.iso}$ and gives some idea of detrusor contractility. This test can be performed only if the patient is able to interrupt flow instantaneously and can mean the need for a second filling in order to see an unimpeded flow pattern. Stop tests are rarely done in current practice.

2) Many people are unable to interrupt their urine flow. This inability can be circumvented if a Foley balloon catheter is left in situ during voiding and when Q_{max} is achieved the catheter is pulled down so that the bladder outlet is blocked; this variant of the stop test is very rarely used (hence the absence of an illustration).

3) The t_{20-80} method (Figure 7.48) is used to calculate the 'Detrusor Contractility Parameter' (DCP). The DCP is an index of bladder contractility proposed by Fry et al. [23]. The DCP is derived from the maximum velocity of muscle element shortening (v_{CE}) during the isovolumetric phase of bladder contraction, i.e. before flow is initiated. As the calculation of v_{CE} is complex, surrogate markers for v_{CE} were assessed. The time for the pressure to rise from 20% to 80% of its maximum value

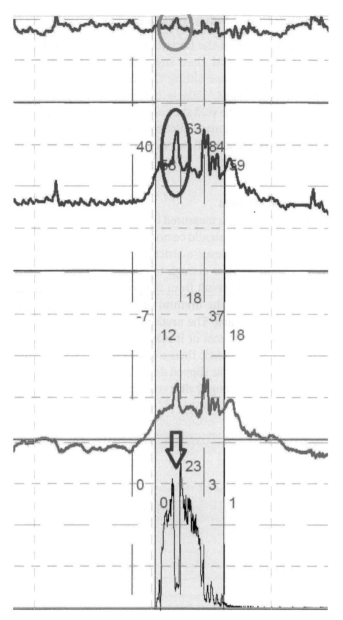

Figure 7.47 A 'stop test' to assess detrusor contractility (see main text). The patient attempted to interrupt flow (purple arrow), and this caused a sharp increase in vesical pressure (purple oval). The green oval shows the pelvic floor contraction needed to interrupt flow.

(a)

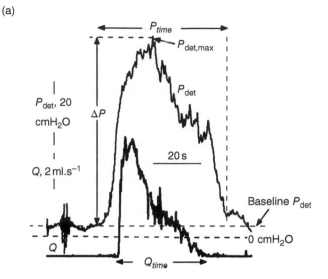

(b)

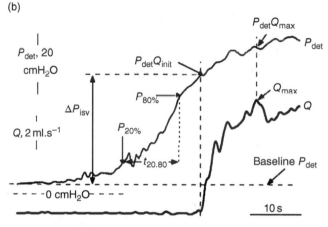

Figure 7.48 The t_{20-80} approach to estimating detrusor contractility; urodynamic recordings of detrusor pressure (p_{det}) and flow (Q), from which variables were measured. (A) Recordings over the timeframe of an entire bladder contraction defining values of the isovolumetric pressure change and flow time. (B) Faster time scale of the rise of p_{det}, showing the pressure values for 20% and 80% of the isovolumetric pressure change, from which the 20–80% isovolumetric pressure time is calculated. *Source*: Fry et al. [23]. © 2016, John Wiley & Sons.

during the isovolumetric phase of detrusor contraction (t_{20-80}) was found to correlate with v_{CE}. This alternative indicator of true detrusor contractility was termed DCP. DCP is calculated directly from pressure-flow traces. DCP is defined as the time interval between p_{det} rising from 20% to 80% of the difference in pressures between start of pressure rise and when flow starts. The detrusor pressure (cmH$_2$O) at the start of detrusor contraction (0% pressure) and at the start of flow (100% pressure) are recorded. From this, the pressures at 20% and 80% of the maximum pressure rise from baseline are calculated. The t_{20} and t_{80}, i.e. times at 20% and 80% of maximum pressure, respectively, are recorded. DCP was calculated as t_{20} subtracted from t_{80}. More research is ongoing in this area to define normative and urodynamic values.

Outlet Function During Voiding

During voiding, the urethra may be either normal or obstructive. A normal urethra is relaxed throughout voiding. An obstructive picture is most commonly a result mechanical obstruction. This can be due to issues such as extrinsic compression, a stricture, or an enlarged prostate. In such situations, sphincter relaxation is likely to be

be made of pressure-measuring quality, then unequal transmission will be seen, with the spike in p_{abd} being greater than in p_{ves}. If, on the other hand, the rectal catheter falls out, then the p_{abd} cough spike will be absent and the resting pressure reduced, or if it slips into the anal sphincter area, the cough spike will be reduced and the resting pressure raised. If the urethral catheter is voided at the beginning of voiding, the test will have to be repeated (unless the PFS is deemed a subordinate part of the examination). However, if the catheter moves after the maximum flow rate is achieved, a repeat test is perhaps not necessary (Figure 7.51). If problems occur with the rectal catheter, careful inspection of the p_{ves} trace is needed to assess whether a repeat test is required (Figure 7.52). If the cough spike on the p_{ves} trace after voiding is similar to that preceding voiding, then it is likely that p_{ves} has been accurately measured. However, if the p_{abd} recording is unreliable, it will not be possible to exclude straining as a significant part of the expulsive force used by that individual patient to void. Indeed, if the rectal catheter

has slipped down or come out, this could well be due (in part, at least) to the patient straining: hence, it may be necessary to repeat the PFS.

'Physiological' Artefacts

Voiding in the urodynamic setting is likely to be affected by a variety of factors:

- The environment may mean a patient who generally voids without problems could find it very difficult to void in the test situation. This is hardly surprising, as they are surrounded by complex equipment and have catheters in position, whilst being observed.
- Technique used may also be important. Overfilling of the bladder generally makes normal voiding difficult. The effect of relatively fast filling may also be detrimental.
- Voiding when the patient is experiencing terminal DO must be interpreted appropriately. They may have a very high premicturition p_{ves} and p_{det} (because they firmly hold their sphincter firmly shut to resist the powerful contraction). Once they are given clear and definite permission to void, intending that they should fully relax their sphincter, the pressures will drop, and the voiding can be interpreted (Figure 7.44).

'Straining' is a term used to denote an observation that the patient uses their abdominal muscles or a Valsalva manoeuvre in relation to the PFS. It can be used in various ways by patients who have at least some detrusor contraction (Figure 7.53):

1) To initiate voiding. Straining before a void might help to trigger a detrusor contraction directly, or indirectly by getting some urine in to the urethra, where the urethral afferents then facilitate the detrusor contraction.
2) To accelerate voiding. Increasing the rate of flow.
3) To perpetuate voiding. For people whose bladder contraction wanes, some straining may help with prolonging and increasing effectiveness of emptying.
4) To complete emptying. A few strains at the end is a common feature in people doing their best consciously to empty as best they can.

For those with an acontractile detrusor, straining serves to replace the detrusor contraction [25]. An alternative to abdominal straining is manual suprapubic pressure, pressing on the dome of the bladder above the pubis to help initiate voiding. This can accelerate voiding but is unlikely to perpetuate it, as the bladder becomes inaccessible behind the pubis when it decreases to a modest volume. It is also unlikely to be helpful in obese people or those with strong rectus muscles. Some people who use the seated position for voiding may lean forward a bit to apply some suprapubic pressure to the bladder dome.

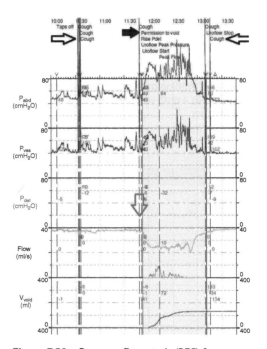

Figure 7.52 Pressure-flow study (PFS) for a woman. The cough before and after the void (open black arrows) are picked up well in both p_{ves} and p_{abd}. Permission to void is indicated by the closed black arrow. At this point, detrusor pressure drops considerably (orange arrow), the explanation being that the p_{abd} pressure has risen disproportionately. The reason is probably that there is some straining which is displacing the rectal catheter balloon into the anal canal so that it is no longer p_{abd} being measured but anal pressure. Consequently, p_{det} drops to negative, which is biologically impossible. Once straining stops, the balloon returns to the rectum. The p_{ves} recording seems reasonable, and so it makes sense to derive interpretation of this PFS more from p_{ves} than p_{det}; it appears that there is some small detrusor contraction to begin with (up to the vertical red dotted line) but a significant contribution by straining thereafter.

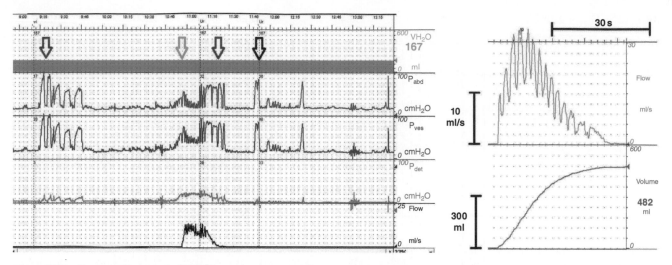

Figure 7.53 Pressure-flow study (left) illustrating how straining may be done to initiate voiding (purple arrow), increase the rate of flow (green arrow), perpetuate voiding (blue arrow), or in an attempt to complete emptying (black arrow). As with any urodynamic observation, it is important to check how this relates to other observations about the patient. In this case, the presence of straining to increase and perpetuate flow appeared to be present in her prior free-flow rate test (right), a trace which illustrates how the presence of both phasic detrusor contraction and superimposed straining can be surmised from examining flow rate pattern.

Abdominal straining during voiding may be either a habit or a necessity for the patient. The effect of straining on the voiding trace needs to be understood. The patient should always be asked to void normally and in as relaxed a way as possible. If the patient has an acontractile detrusor, then voiding can only be achieved by straining. If the detrusor contracts during voiding, but the patient also strains, then the trace can be difficult to interpret. It is also hard to know precisely what effect straining has on urine flow: in patients without obstruction, straining generally should increase flow rate during the Valsalva, but it usually does not in patients with partial BOO (Figure 7.54).

Electromyography

There are two approaches to EMG recording used in UDS – surface and needle. Many centres around the world have stopped using surface EMG, as it is difficult to get the pads to stay stuck to the body, and this approach measures pelvic floor activity rather than urethral function specifically. It may be helpful in children when combined with free uroflowmetry in diagnosing dysfunctional voiding.

Needle electrodes can be placed into the pelvic floor muscles for direct recording. Clearly, this would be a painful process for someone with normal sensation, so it is most often used where there is reduced sensory nerve function. This method is commonly used in spinal cord injury units, and it is a simple and effective method in this context, since pelvic floor behaviour generally seems to reflect sphincter function. Use of local anaesthesia might be con-

sidered in other contexts, but the potential effect on the electrical activity may make the injected anaesthetics unhelpful for reaching a confident diagnosis.

Sphincter EMG recording gives the most direct measurement of function. This is a technique of use in women with possible Fowler's syndrome [26–28] (Figure 7.55). Fowler's syndrome is a rare chronic problem, often initiated by an apparently unconnected precipitating event, such as a minor surgical procedure. It affects young women in the menarche, 40% of whom have polycystic ovary syndrome. They develop high-volume urinary retention (at least a litre in volume) which is remarkably painless. All investigations appear normal, including neurological evaluations. Excessive opiate use can also cause low-pain retention, so this must be excluded during evaluation. Women with Fowler's syndrome can usually pass some urine but with considerable difficulty (Figure 7.55). The striking urodynamic feature is a markedly raised maximum urethral closure pressure (Figure 7.55), and radiological imaging (ultrasound or magnetic resonance imaging (MRI)) can identify increased sphincter volume [29]. Given the remarkable strength of the sphincter, they are prone to sphincter spasm. Unfortunately, this makes treatment difficult; ISC would be ideal, but they experience severe sphincter spasm soon after catheter insertion, which is not only painful, it makes catheter removal extremely difficult. For these patients, sphincter EMG may be considered. However, it is a time-consuming technique, which requires considerable experience. It requires a urologist with the aptitude to identify the female urethral sphincter with a needle, based on an anatomical knowledge that the sphinc-

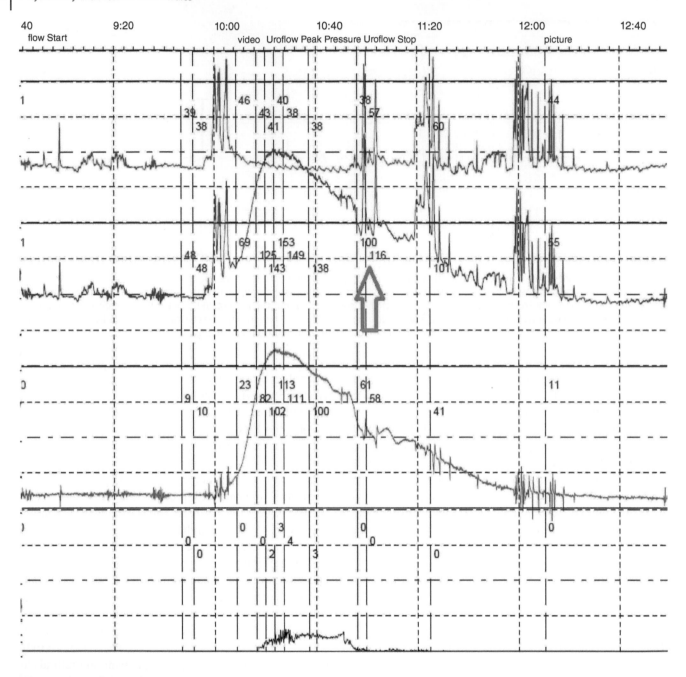

Figure 7.54 Attempts to increase flow rate do not have any effect if bladder outlet obstruction (BOO) is present. In this male pressure-flow study, there is obvious BOO, indicated by the flow rate despite high detrusor pressure. The orange arrow indicates two strains, with no associated effect on flow rate, perhaps even stopping it.

ter lies dorsally over the midurethra (Figure 2.1). Hence, the needle has to be inserted into the anterior vaginal wall a centimetre behind the external urethral meatus and a centimetre lateral to the midline, advancing horizontally to lie level with the dorsum of the urethra before deviating medially to probe for the muscle. This is done in conjunction with a neurophysiologist with expertise in EMG, able to interpret the waveforms picked up by the needle, and the

sounds coming from the EMG apparatus. This is a painful process for the patient. It may add prognostic value for sacral nerve stimulator (SNS) treatment [30]. Arguably, however, a percutaneous nerve evaluation for SNS can be undertaken anyway, since some women with retention may respond even without the characteristic features of Fowler's syndrome. Onabotulinum-A injections have also been evaluated [31].

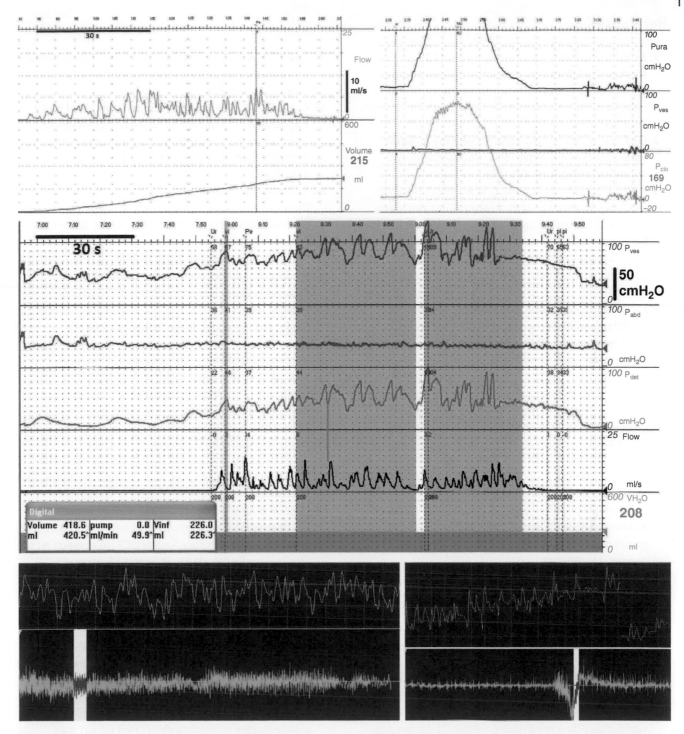

Figure 7.55 A woman with Fowler's syndrome. Free-flow rate testing (top left) showed prolonged, slow, and interrupted voiding. Urethral pressure profilometry (top right) showed very high maximum urethral closure pressure. Pressure-flow study (middle) showed the same flow pattern as free-flow testing and a detrusor pressure that dropped with each peak of flow (orange line, noting that there is a slight delay for the flowmeter to register the flow). This picture resembles that pattern of detrusor sphincter dyssynergia (see Figures 16.1 and 16.2), but it is not caused by lack of control by the pontine micturition centre. The bottom two figures are direct sphincter electromyography recordings, supporting the diagnosis of Fowler's syndrome. On the left, the trace was associated with a sound resembling whale song (the underwater singing often heard on nature documentaries). On the right, a cough led to a sound resembling the blades of a helicopter in flight. *Source*: DasGupta and Fowler [26]; Hoeritzauer et al. [27]; Osman and Chapple [28].

References

1. Rosier, P., Schaefer, W., Lose, G. et al. (2017). International Continence Society Good Urodynamic Practices and Terms 2016: urodynamics, uroflowmetry, cystometry, and pressure-flow study. *Neurourol. Urodyn.* 36: 1243–1260.

2. Gammie, A. (2018). The accuracy of static pressure measurement with water-filled urodynamic systems. *Neurourol. Urodyn.* 37: 626–633.

3. Schafer, W., Abrams, P., Liao, L. et al. (2002). Good urodynamic practices: uroflowmetry, filling cystometry, and pressure-flow studies. *Neurourol. Urodyn.* 21: 261–274.

4. Gammie, A., Clarkson, B., Constantinou, C. et al. (2014). International Continence Society guidelines on urodynamic equipment performance. *Neurourol. Urodyn.* 33: 370–379.

5. Gammie, A., Abrams, P., Bevan, W. et al. (2016). Simultaneous in vivo; comparison of water-filled and air-filled pressure measurement catheters: implications for good urodynamic practice. *Neurourol. Urodyn.* 35: 926–933.

6. Digesu, G.A., Derpapas, A., Robshaw, P. et al. (2014). Are the measurements of water-filled and air-charged catheters the same in urodynamics? *Int. Urogynecol. J.* 25: 123–130.

7. Hashim, H. and Abrams, P. (2006). Flow meter urine testing: a practical proposition in patients attending for urodynamics? *BJU Int.* 97: 1027–1029.

8. Sullivan, J.G., Swithinbank, L., and Abrams, P. (2012). Defining achievable standards in urodynamics-a prospective study of initial resting pressures. *Neurourol. Urodyn.* 31: 535–540.

9. Al-Hayek, S. and Abrams, P. (2010). The 50-year history of the ice water test in urology. *J. Urol.* 183: 1686–1692.

10. Deffontaines Rufin, S., Jousse, M., Verollet, D. et al. (2010). Cold perception of the bladder during ice water test. Study on 120 patients. *Ann. Phys. Rehabil. Med.* 53: 559–567.

11. Thomas, D. (1979). Clinical urodynamics in neurogenic bladder dysfunction. *Urol. Clin. North Am.* 6: 237–253.

12. Klevmark, B. (1974). Motility of the urinary bladder in cats during filling at physiological rates. I. Intravesical pressure patterns studied by a new method of cystometry. *Acta Physiol. Scand.* 90: 565–577.

13. Klevmark, B. (1999). Natural pressure-volume curves and conventional cystometry. *Scand. J. Urol. Nephrol. Suppl* (201): 1–4.

14. Abrams, P., Cardozo, L., Fall, M. et al. (2002). The standardisation of terminology of lower urinary tract function: report from the Standardisation Sub-committee of the International Continence Society. *Neurourol. Urodyn.* 21: 167–178.

15. Gajewski, J.B., Schurch, B., Hamid, R. et al. (2017). An International Continence Society (ICS) report on the terminology for adult neurogenic lower urinary tract dysfunction (ANLUTD). *Neurourol. Urodyn.* 37: 1152–1161.

16. Gajewski, J.B., Gammie, A., Speich, J. et al. (2019). Are there different patterns of detrusor overactivity which are clinically relevant? ICI-RS 2018. *Neurourol. Urodyn.* 38 (Suppl 5): S40–S45.

17. Wyndaele, J.J., Gammie, A., Bruschini, H. et al. (2011). Bladder compliance what does it represent: can we measure it, and is it clinically relevant? *Neurourol. Urodyn.* 30: 714–722.

18. Drake, M.J., Hedlund, P., Mills, I.W. et al. (2000). Structural and functional denervation of human detrusor after spinal cord injury. *Lab. Invest.* 80: 1491–1499.

19. Kapoor, D.S., Housami, F., White, P. et al. (2012). Maximum urethral closure pressure in women: normative data and evaluation as a diagnostic test. *Int. Urogynecol. J.* 23: 1613–1618.

20. Huckabay, C., Twiss, C., Berger, A., and Nitti, V.W. (2005). A urodynamics protocol to optimally assess men with post-prostatectomy incontinence. *Neurourol. Urodyn.* 24: 622–626.

21. Haylen, B.T., de Ridder, D., Freeman, R.M. et al. (2010). An International Urogynecological Association (IUGA)/ International Continence Society (ICS) joint report on the terminology for female pelvic floor dysfunction. *Neurourol. Urodyn.* 29: 4–20.

22. Uren, A.D., Cotterill, N., Harding, C. et al. (2017). Qualitative exploration of the patient experience of underactive bladder. *Eur. Urol.* 72: 402–407.

23. Fry, C.H., Gammie, A., Drake, M.J. et al. (2017). Estimation of bladder contractility from intravesical pressure–volume measurements. *Neurourol. Urodyn.* 36 (4): 1009–1014.

24. Austin, P.F., Bauer, S.B., Bower, W. et al. (2014). The standardization of terminology of lower urinary tract function in children and adolescents: update report from the Standardization Committee of the International Children's Continence Society. *J. Urol.* 191: 1863–1865, e1813.

25. Rachaneni, S. and Latthe, P. (2015). Does preoperative urodynamics improve outcomes for women undergoing surgery for stress urinary incontinence? A systematic review and meta-analysis. *BJOG* 122: 8–16.

26. DasGupta, R. and Fowler, C.J. (2003). The management of female voiding dysfunction: Fowler's syndrome – a contemporary update. *Curr. Opin. Urol.* 13: 293–299.

27. Hoeritzauer, I., Stone, J., Fowler, C. et al. (2015). Fowler's syndrome of urinary retention: a retrospective study of co-morbidity. *Neurourol. Urodyn.* 35: 601–603.

28. Osman, N.I. and Chapple, C.R. (2014). Fowler's syndrome-a cause of unexplained urinary retention in young women? Nature reviews. *Urology* 11: 87–98.

29. Wiseman, O.J., Swinn, M.J., Brady, C.M., and Fowler, C.J. (2002). Maximum urethral closure pressure and sphincter volume in women with urinary retention. *J. Urol.* 167: 1348–1351; discussion 1351–1342.

30. De Ridder, D., Ost, D., and Bruyninckx, F. (2007). The presence of Fowler's syndrome predicts successful long-term outcome of sacral nerve stimulation in women with urinary retention. *Eur. Urol.* 51: 229–233; discussion 233–224.

31. Panicker, J.N., Seth, J.H., Khan, S. et al. (2016). Open-label study evaluating outpatient urethral sphincter injections of onabotulinumtoxinA to treat women with urinary retention due to a primary disorder of sphincter relaxation (Fowler's syndrome). *BJU Int.* 117: 809–813.

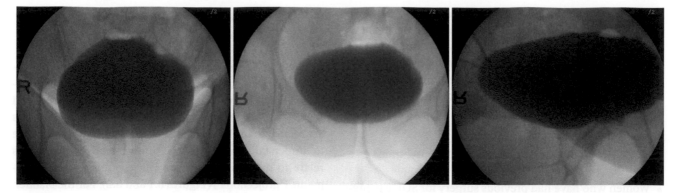

Figure 8.2 Images from three different viewpoints taken during video urodynamics for a woman undergoing filling cystometry. She is in the standing position and has 200 ml in her bladder. The left-hand image is antero-posterior, the middle image is postero-anterior, and the right-hand image is 45° oblique. The bladder looks quite small in the middle image, because the image intensifier is closer to it, meaning there is less magnification. *Source*: Marcus Drake.

3) Occasionally, oblique projections in the vertical plane are taken (Figure 8.4)

Identification of vesicoureteric reflux (VUR), i.e. passage of contrast going against the expected direction of urine transport, is an important advantage of VUDS. This problem can be clinically relevant for urinary tract infections and for chronic kidney disease. The severity of VUR is graded according to the level reached by contrast and structural changes in the upper urinary tract:

- Grade I: the urine flows back into one or both of the ureters but does not reach the kidney;
- Grade II: urine flows back up to the kidney but does not cause dilation of the renal pelvis;
- Grade III: there is mild to moderate dilation of the ureter and the renal pelvis;

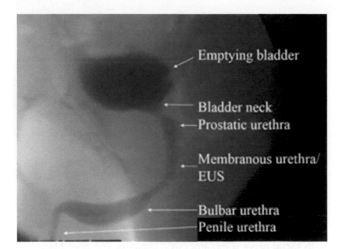

Emptying bladder

Bladder neck
Prostatic urethra

Membranous urethra/
EUS

Bulbar urethra
Penile urethra

Figure 8.3 45° horizontal oblique view of the male outlet during voiding. The exact location of the external urethral sphincter (EUS) is not obvious because, as expected, it is fully open for voiding. *Source*: Marcus Drake.

- Grade IV: the ureter, the renal pelvis, and calyces are dilated; and
- Grade V: there is severe dilation of the ureters, renal pelvis, and calyces, and tortuosity of the ureter.

The location of the ureteric orifice, also known as the vesicoureteric junction (VUJ), is worth noting. If it is in the normal position, then any VUR observed might reflect trauma to the VUJ, such as can happen during endoscopic surgery in the ureter. Alternatively, high pressures in the bladder may be responsible for VUR. If the VUJ is in a higher position than normal, then VUR may reflect a congenital problem preventing the normal valve function.

During VUDS, in order to view the ureters, and hence identify the presence of VUR and its severity, the centre point of the image is moved superiorly, keeping in the A-P plane. At the top end of the ureter, the top of the renal pelvis is usually level with the L1 vertebra (Figure 8.5). Tilting the C-arm in the vertical plane may be needed to view the renal collecting system fully.

A mobile C-arm, which includes an X-ray source and an image intensifier to visualise the X-rays, is the most convenient way to achieve these projections in a VUDS test. It can be rotated around the patient for horizontal oblique views, tilted for vertical obliques, flipped to switch between A-P and P-A, and elevated/depressed to the right anatomical level (Figure 8.6). It is also manageable to run the urodynamics test with the patient in supine, seating, and standing position as needed to make the essential observations of filling cystometry and PFS, including changes of position during the test. Sometimes, a standing patient is too tall to show the L1 level in the horizontal plane of a C-arm at maximum elevation; in that case, an oblique angulation in the vertical plane can be used to gain a little bit more height to view this level (Figure 8.6).

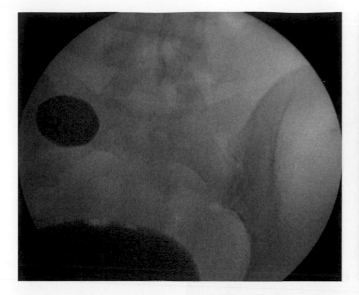 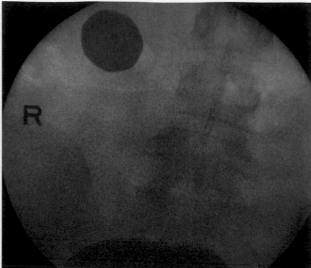

Figure 8.4 Vertical oblique centred above the bladder. This projection was used to look for contrast that might track along a Mitrofanoff channel (see Chapter 5, Figures 5.19 and 5.20) in a patient complaining of urine escaping from the channel onto her abdominal surface. A heptagonal coin was placed in the umbilicus to demarcate the external meatus of the Mitrofanoff to ensure the likely route of the channel was apparent. Shots from two different vertical oblique angles are illustrated showing how this increases the apparent separation of the marker from the bladder (an imaging property known as parallax). *Source*: Marcus Drake.

It is important to be aware that X-ray contrast is dense and so descends to the bottom of the bladder or other reservoir, e.g. a diverticulum. If there is any urine or saline present, it floats to the top, so the contrast will form a horizontal level with a slight upward curve at the edges ('meniscus'). The urine made by the kidneys between the start of the test (when the PVR was drained) and the time the X-ray image is taken will lead to this effect. Any air introduced from the catheters rises to the very top, curving to configure with the bladder dome, and appearing bright. Several of the images in this chapter show this feature.

As well as the contrast, bones and foreign objects are radio-opaque, while adipose tissue can impede X-rays sufficient to degrade image quality significantly (Figure 8.7).

The imaging can be used for:

1) Evaluating pelvic floor support
   a) In women, the base of the bladder normally lies at or just below the midpoint of the pubis (Figure 8.8). Screening during a cough or Valsalva will identify whether there is excessive descent of the pelvic floor, and any associated USI would be visible.
   b) In men with neurological disease or a background of major pelvic surgery, excessive movement of the pelvic floor with cough or Valsalva most likely indicates denervation of these muscles (Figure 8.9).
2) Evaluating sphincter function in filling cystometry and identifying incontinence

   a) In women, USI seen with minimal pelvic floor descent identifies intrinsic sphincter deficiency (ISD) (Figure 8.10).
   b) In men, leakage into the proximal urethral bulb indicates sphincter deficiency (Figure 8.11).
3) Identifying structural abnormalities of the bladder
   a) Configuration of the bladder neck, which should be closed during the filling phase. If open, it may be a result of neurological disease affecting the sympathetic nervous system in the thoracolumbar spinal cord (Figure 8.12). In adult men, this appearance can be a result of surgery, such as transurethral resection of the prostate (TURP). Some men who underwent radical retroperitoneal lymph node surgery as a treatment of testis cancer may also get this due to damage to the sympathetic chain. Many of these men will report retrograde ejaculation ('dry orgasm') if their sexual function is preserved.
   b) Trabeculation (large detrusor muscles strands sticking into the bladder lumen) and diverticulation (pockets of urothelium pushed outwards) are classic features of some neurological diseases (Figure 8.12). This appearance suggests it is likely to be a poorly compliant bladder.
   c) A bladder diverticulum (Figure 8.13), i.e. a small pocket joined to the bladder lumen, which is likely to have a thin wall and very little detrusor muscle (so it may well not empty during a PFS).

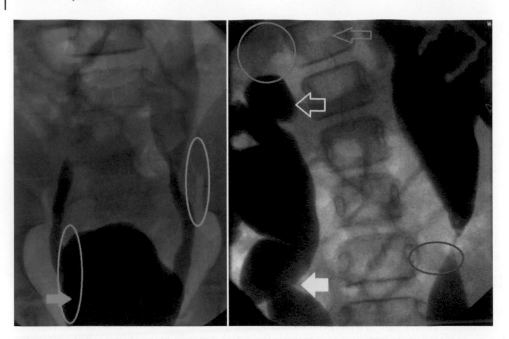

Figure 8.5 Severe bilateral vesicoureteric reflux; this is grade V, due to loss of angles ('clubbing') in the renal collecting system (open yellow arrow), marked dilation of the renal pelvis, and markedly dilated and tortuous ureters (closed yellow arrow). At the lower end, the vesicoureteric junction (closed blue arrow) can lie anywhere in the blue oval; a higher than normal location means the valve function of the junction is impaired – in this case, it is a bit higher than normal. The ureter crosses the pelvic brim near the sacroiliac joint (green oval). It ascends in front of the tips of the transverse processes of the lumbar vertebrae (red oval) to the renal pelvis. The top of the renal pelvis is level with the first lumbar vertebra. This can be identified as it is the one below the 12th thoracic vertebra (orange arrow), which has the lowest rib (orange circle). These anatomical landmarks are an approximate guide, as there is a lot of variability in the upper urinary tract. See also Figure 8.17. *Source*: Marcus Drake.

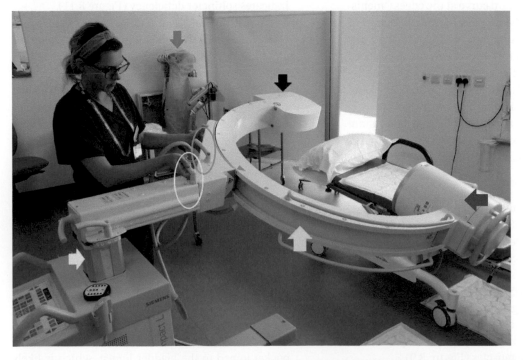

Figure 8.6 The mobile X-ray C-arm showing the X-ray source (black arrow), image intensifier (purple arrow), mounted on a C-arm (blue arrow). The C-arm can be moved into different planes with a release handle for horizontal (blue oval) and axial rotation (yellow). The illustration shows the arm being shifted to the position needed for vertical oblique projection in a standing person. The height of the column holding the C-arm (yellow arrow) can be varied. The orange arrow in the background illustrates how the protective lead aprons should be stored hung up carefully, with no creases to damage the lead. *Source*: Marcus Drake.

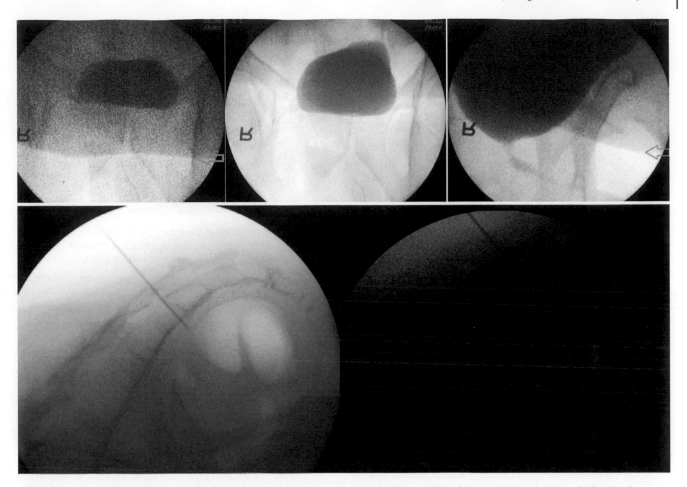

Figure 8.7 An obese patient can represent a challenge for X-ray imaging. In the top three images, the green arrow indicates the lower edge of an adipose apron in posteroanterior (left image) and oblique (right) projection in a male patient. In the middle image, he has been asked to lift the apron manually out of the shot, and the image is considerably clearer. The two lower images are of different patients undergoing the percutaneous nerve evaluation test phase for sacral neuromodulation, with the needle in one of the sacral foramina. This is easily seen in the slim patient on the left. On the right, the buttocks were sufficiently large to place a considerable amount of fat in line with the X-ray beam, causing severe degrading of the image quality. The needle can be seen, but the sacrum is hard to make out. *Source*: Marcus Drake.

d) Bladder 'distortion', e.g. part of the bladder entering a sliding hernia or being tethered by a misplaced stitch (Figures 8.14 and 8.15).

e) A ureterocoele, which is a thin-walled swelling of the lower ureter, expanding it and sometimes pushing it into the bladder lumen (Figure 8.16). Given that the VUJ is low down in the bladder, a ureterocoele can sometimes flop into the bladder neck and cause BOO.

4) Seeing escape of contrast from the bladder via non-urethral routes
a) VUR (Figures 8.5 and 8.17).
b) A vesico-vaginal fistula.

5) Identifying structural abnormalities of the bladder outlet
a) Defining the site of BOO in men. Potential sites of hold-up are: bladder neck (Figure 8.18), prostate (Figure 8.19), external urinary sphincter (Figure 8.20), urethral stricture (Figures 8.20–8.22), external urethral meatus (Figure 8.21), and preputial meatus (i.e. a tight foreskin entrance, known as a 'phimosis').

b) In women, VUDS may help identify BOO, for example, by demonstrating distortion, compression (Figure 8.23), or stricture (Figure 8.24).

c) A urethral false passage (Figure 8.25), which is where the urethral epithelium has been breached and a track created in the surrounding tissue which has persisted as it has become epithelialised. This is most often due to damage during catheterisation, and so commonly lies in line with the upward curve of the male urethra at the bulb.

d) A urethral fistula (Figure 8.26).

e) Intraprostatic reflux (Figure 8.27).

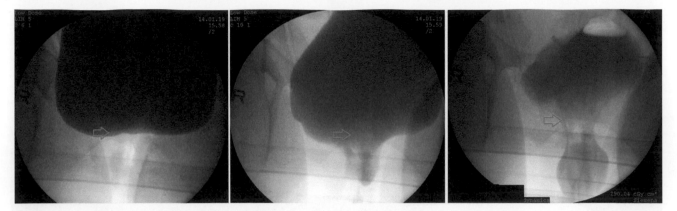

Figure 8.8 Female pelvic floor support. In the left image, the base of the bladder is located, as expected, level with the bottom of the pubic bones, indicated by the orange arrow. This lady used a lot of straining in order to pass urine, and this had the effect of prolapsing her bladder base, the middle and right images showing the progressive severity of the prolapse with one attempted void. *Source*: Marcus Drake.

f) Seminal vesicle reflux (Figure 8.28).

g) Posterior urethral valves (PUV) (Figures 8.29 and 8.30). This is a development abnormality of the prostatic urethra, in which tissue flaps block the proximal urethra, with profound effects on bladder development, and high risk for renal failure.

6) Checking post-voiding features

a) PVR (Figure 8.31), meaning that the bladder has not emptied fully once the person has completed voiding.

b) Pseudoresidual (Figure 8.32), which differs from a PVR in that the bladder actually has emptied fully on completion of voiding, but rapid entry of more urine into the bladder (within a few seconds) means that the bladder seems not to have emptied. This happens in people with severe VUR, where the void pushes urine (and contrast during VUDS) into the upper urinary tract as well as along the urethra. Refluxed urine simply drops back into the bladder once the detrusor contraction stops and vesical pressure returns to baseline.

c) Causes of post-micturition dribble (PMD); pooling of contrast in the male urethral bulb, or the vagina (Figure 8.33). A urethral diverticulum can also cause PMD if its entry point to the urethra is below the sphincter (Figure 8.34).

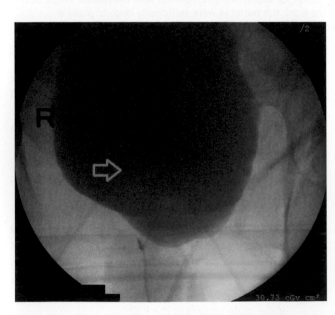

Figure 8.9 Male pelvic floor support. Denervation of the pelvic floor in a man allows the bladder to drop well below the bottom of the pubic bones (orange arrow). *Source*: Marcus Drake.

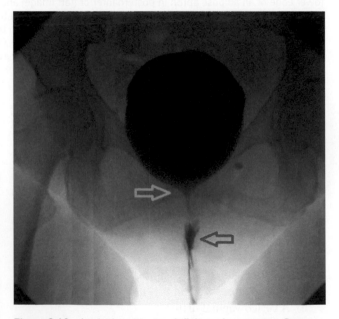

Figure 8.10 Intrinsic sphincter deficiency in a woman. Stress incontinence caused by a cough is indicated by the red arrow. The blue arrow indicates the base of the bladder, which lies close to the normal position (i.e. there was minimal urethral hypermobility). *Source*: Marcus Drake.

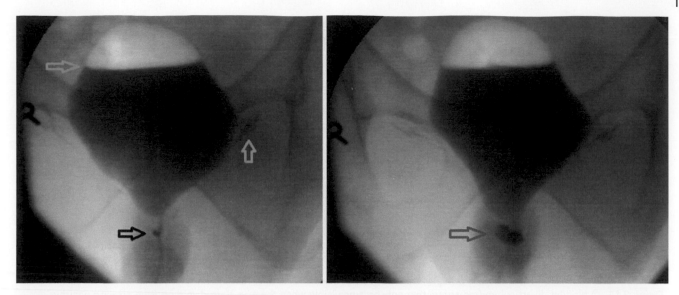

Figure 8.11 Intrinsic sphincter deficiency in a man after radical prostatectomy. On the left, the bladder holds contrast which has sunk to the lower part due to its density, leaving a fluid level (blue arrow), above which is either urine or air. The black arrow points to a kink in the filling line. The green arrow points to some clips used for haemostasis during the prostatectomy. On the right, following a cough, there has been clear contrast leak into the bulbar urethra (red arrow). *Source*: Marcus Drake.

Several features can show up on an X-ray image whose appearance is worth knowing about if seen in a particular patient during VUDS. These include internal foreign bodies, implants, external foreign bodies, and extrinsic compression (Figures 8.35–8.43).

a sensation of leakage but with no incontinence seen. In these men, it is worth screening the bladder neck region to see if the emergence of this complaint coincides with contrast entering the proximal urethra (Figure 8.46). If this is seen, it suggests the symptom may be driven by stimulation of the urethral receptors.

Roles of VUDS in Men

For men with post-prostatectomy incontinence, following radical prostatectomy or TURP, presentation with SUI symptoms prompts consideration of surgical interventions such as artificial urinary sphincter (AUS) or male sling. Here, it is necessary to observe the incontinence, and imaging helps confirm the exact moment of leakage to be sure of its mechanism. While the leakage is generally identified easily, the catheter can sometimes restrict the urethra, so it becomes difficult to demonstrate the leakage coming from the urethral meatus. In that case, VUDS screening below the sphincter location will readily identify contrast escaping into the urethral bulb, thus confirming USI (Figure 8.44).

VUDS can also be helpful for evaluating an AUS which is no longer functional, providing the device was charged with contrast when it was first placed (Figure 8.45). Here, it will be possible to evaluate whether the reservoir is still fluid filled and to observe the state of the cuff, along with its ability to resist a cough series or Valsalva. The assessment of USI in these patients is further discussed in Chapter 14.

Some men complain of urgency but are found not to have detrusor overactivity, and others may strongly complain of

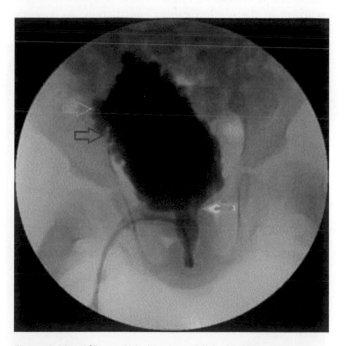

Figure 8.12 A 'fir tree' bladder in a child with neurological disease illustrated during filling cystometry. The bladder neck (green arrow) is open during the storage phase. There is trabeculation (red arrow) and diverticulation (blue arrow). *Source*: Marcus Drake.

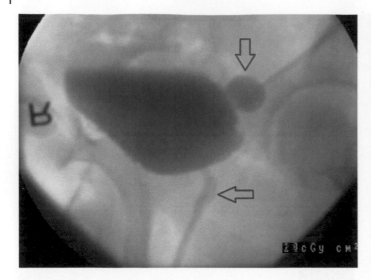
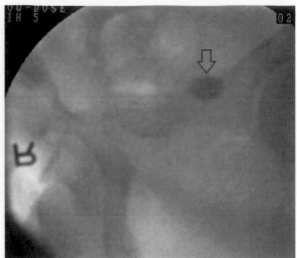

Figure 8.13 A bladder diverticulum (red arrow) that only became visible when the man started voiding. Blue arrow: a healthy-looking male outlet with no prostatic intrusion. Right: the diverticulum still had a small amount of contrast after voiding was completed. *Source*: Marcus Drake.

For young men with voiding symptoms, the aim of urodynamics is to distinguish the potential contributions of detrusor underactivity (DUA) and/or BOO, and the role of VUDS is in identifying the locus of any BOO identified, as described above.

The male bladder outlet is at risk of scarring related to previous surgery, trauma, or infection. Scars notoriously are prone to shortening, and since it is a tubular organ, scarring in the urethra causes constriction. As a result,

stricture or stenosis can develop. This can be anticipated in the following circumstances:

1) The patient who has a classic 'stricture pattern' on their flow rate.
2) Past history of urethral strictures.
3) History of previous stricture surgery, i.e. dilation, self-catheterisation for strictures, urethroplasty, or urethrotomy [5].

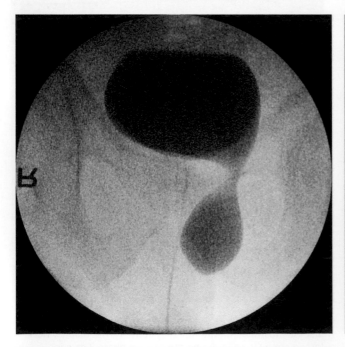
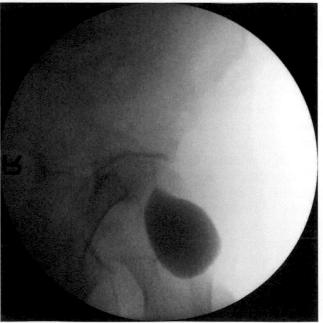

Figure 8.14 The appearance of a sliding hernia in a man undergoing video urodynamics. Left image: the bladder is in its normal anatomical location, but part of it is entering a large sliding left inguinal hernia. After voiding, the hernia still contained contrast (right image). *Source*: Marcus Drake.

4) Previous instrumentation of the lower urinary tract, e.g. cystoscopy, TURP, foreign body removal.

5) Clinical findings of extensive lichen sclerosis, with possible meatal stenosis [6].

6) Major surgery or radiotherapy, notably radical prostatectomy can cause bladder neck stenosis where the bladder is anastomosed to the urethra.

7) Previous sexually transmitted disease causing urethritis.

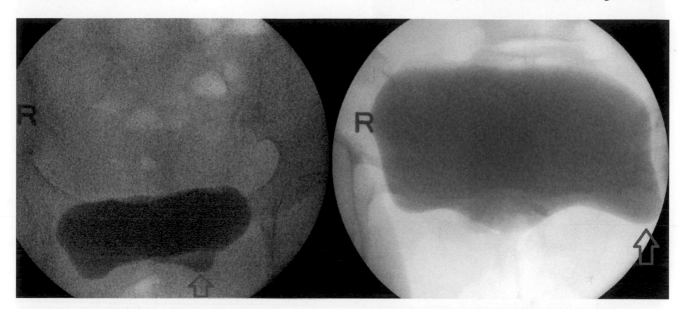

Figure 8.15 Two images which identified that part of the bladder had been caught in the closure stitch for a previous caesarean section scar; her obstetric history was placenta praevia and accreta, complicated by haemorrhage needing subtotal hysterectomy. Video urodynamics was undertaken to investigate storage and voiding lower urinary tract symptoms. *Source*: Marcus Drake.

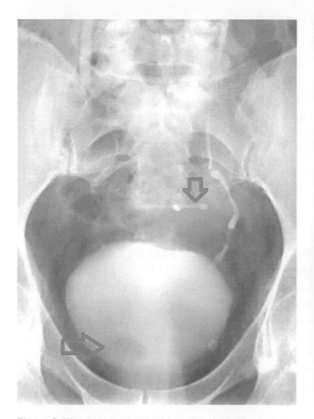
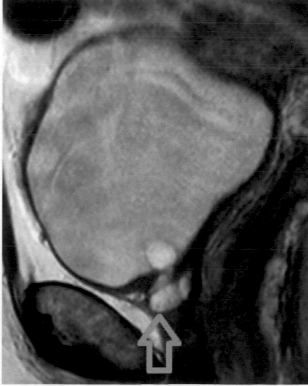

Figure 8.16 A ureterocoele (blue arrow), visible as it does not contain contrast on the intravenous urogram image (left). It lies close to the internal urethral meatus, so it could cause bladder outlet obstruction. The green arrow indicates an intrauterine contraceptive device. The magnetic resonance imaging scan on the right shows the lower ureter is dilated and tortuous. *Source*: Marcus Drake.

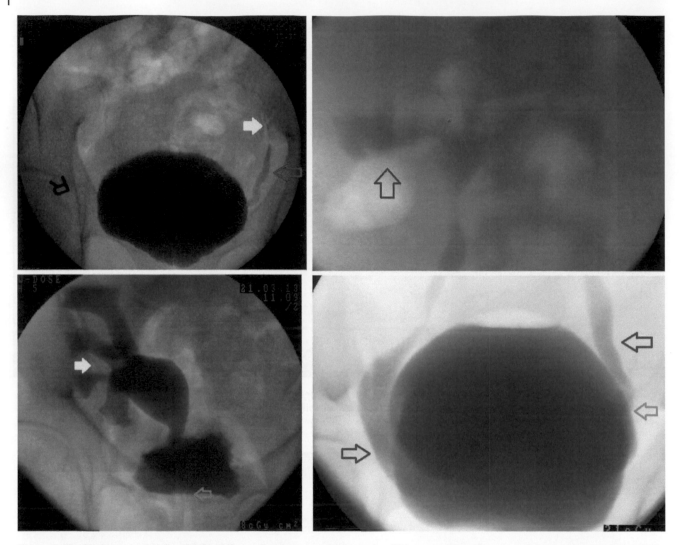

Figure 8.17 Vesicoureteric reflux (VUR). VUR can first become visible during filling or voiding. The top left image shows grade I VUR (red arrow). The yellow arrow indicates the sacroiliac (S-I) joint. At this severity, VUR can be treated with ureteric 'STING' injections. The two images on the right show grade III–IV reflux. This case showed bilateral VUR (red arrows) which reached the kidney on one side (blue arrow). The green arrow illustrates how a refluxing vesicoureteric junction is often anatomically in a higher location in the bladder than normal. Bottom left: VUR into a renal transplant. Transplanted kidneys tend to be placed with a refluxing anastomosis to the bladder and have a low-lying location as their blood supply is taken from the iliac vessels; hence, this transplanted kidney lies in front of the right S-I joint (yellow arrow) rather than the usual lumbar location. Orange arrow: base of bladder and pubic symphysis. *Source*: Marcus Drake.

This has important implications:

1) Voiding and post-voiding LUTS;
2) Difficulty with urodynamics, as the catheter can be hard to get fully to the bladder; and
3) More complex treatment decisions, since scars indicate impaired healing response that will mean further surgery carries additional implications (see Chapter 15).

Catheterisation can be difficult in this group of patients and can cause avoidable trauma, pain, and bleeding. The following are some measures to reduce this risk when catheterising a patient for VUDS with a potential urethral stricture:

1) Be liberal with the use of lubricant;
2) Use a small gauge catheter (6 French gauge at most) [7];
3) Catheterise gently – if resistance is encountered, stop and reassess;
4) Use an angle-ended (Coudé catheter) to help steer the catheter tip around any distortions which are causing a hold-up when trying to catheterise with a straight catheter; and
5) If catheterisation is unsuccessful and a lot of resistance is met, a guidewire can be used to see if the stricture is traversable, then a small gauge catheter can be railroaded over the wire to assess the density of the stricture.

Flexible cystoscopy can be used to see where to place the guidewire.

If catherisation is not possible, a urethrogram can be performed distally to assess the location and length of the stricture for operative planning. This is known as a retrograde urethrogram, or 'an upogram'. The upogram provides the full information about the extent of stricturing which is lacking if only conventional voiding studies are done as per VUDS (which would be classed as a 'downogram' in urethrogram terms). This is because the proximal part of the stricture slows down the contrast flow generated by the bladder contraction (hence is indicated by a proximal bulging of the urethra) so that everything beyond looks like a trickle. With an upogram, contrast is pushed against the distal end of the stricture, so the two types of study allow identification of the full stricture extent. In order to perform a retrograde urethrogram (upogram), the patient is positioned on a horizontal X-ray compatible table with the left hip raised (a towel can be used) and the right knee bent with the ankle nestled behind the opposite knee. This is done to angle the pelvis at 45° to best visualise the bulbar urethra. The penis is then placed on stretch in order to straighten the bend of the urethra at the penoscrotal junction [8]. A catheter tip is inserted into the meatus, and a penile clamp can be applied to ensure that contrast does not flow out of the urethra. Alternatively, the catheter balloon can be inflated in the distal penis with 5 ml of fluid to stop the catheter falling out and to occlude the lumen, as

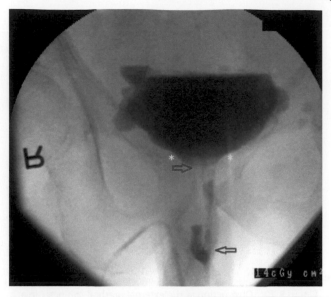

Figure 8.18 Obstruction at the bladder neck in a man undergoing pressure-flow studies (PFS). The contrast is held up at the bladder neck (red arrow); the bladder neck has been forced between the lobes of the prostate (yellow asterisks). Some contrast has got below the bladder neck, indicating this is not complete obstruction. Pooling in the bulbar urethra (blue arrow) is a risk factor for post-micturition dribble. *Source*: Marcus Drake.

shown in Figure 8.47. Contrast is then injected into the catheter under radiographic screening (Figures 8.47 and 8.48).

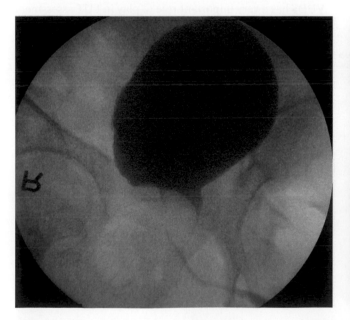
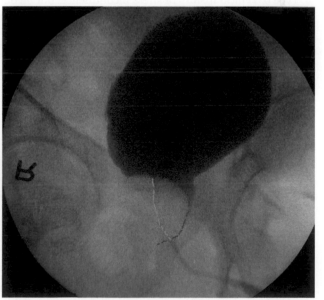

Figure 8.19 Obstruction at the prostate in a man undergoing pressure-flow studies. The prostate was not a particularly large gland in this case, showing up as rather radiotranslucent; on the right, the outline of the gland is marked in red (where it can be made out) and the course of the prostatic urethra in blue. *Source*: Marcus Drake.

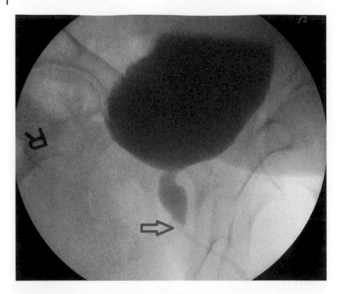

Figure 8.20 Obstruction at the external urethral sphincter in a man undergoing pressure-flow studies. Stenosis is present at the level of the sphincter (red arrow), with obvious dilation proximally, and minimal flow beyond the hold-up. *Source*: Marcus Drake.

Roles of VUDS in Women

Women reporting recurrent or persistent urinary incontinence may have either ISD or persisting hypermobility. These are readily distinguished with VUDS, as can be seen by comparing Figures 8.10 and 8.49.

VUDS can be used to classify the nature of the underlying mechanism, as described by Blaivas [9]:

- Type 0. Typical history of stress incontinence, but incontinence is not reproduced during the examination. The vesical neck and urethra descend during cough or strain and the urethra opens, but there is no leakage. Maximum urethral closure pressure is normal. In this type of incontinence, the patient is probably able to prevent leakage by momentarily contracting the external urethral sphincter.
- Type 1. Minimal descent of the vesical neck and urethra during stress with visible urinary leakage. No cystocoele. Normal maximum urethral closure pressure.
- Type 2. Obvious cystourethrocoele present with visible urinary leakage during stress. Normal maximum urethral closure pressure.
- Type 3. Vesical neck open during bladder filling without concomitant detrusor contraction. Visible urinary leakage with no or minimal stress. Variable vesical neck and urethral descent (often none at all). Maximal urethral closure pressure very low. This condition is usually due to failed previous surgery or a neurologic lesion involving the thoracolumbar and sacral spinal cord or peripheral nerves.

Women describing voiding difficulties following stress incontinence surgery may have DUA and/or BOO, and VUDS is helpful for pinpointing the location of BOO (Figure 8.23).

VUDS in People with Neurological Disease and Children

VUDS has a very important role to play in LUT assessment of neurological disease.

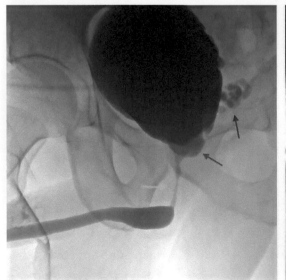

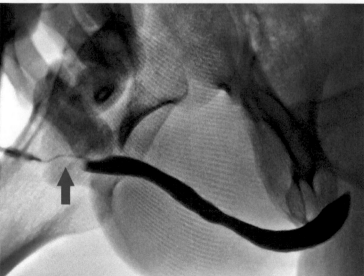

Figure 8.21 Male urethral strictures. Left image: a stricture affecting the proximal urethra and the proximal urethral bulb (blue arrow). The red arrow is dilation above the stricture, and the purple arrow indicates contrast in the seminal vesicle. Right image: a stricture of the navicular fossa, virtually at the external urethral meatus in a man (blue arrow). *Source*: Marcus Drake.

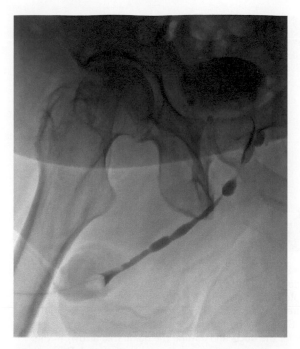

Figure 8.22 Urethrogram of a stricture affecting virtually the entire urethra, known as a 'panurethral' stricture. This is a radiology department urethrogram rather than a video urodynamics image. *Source*: Marcus Drake.

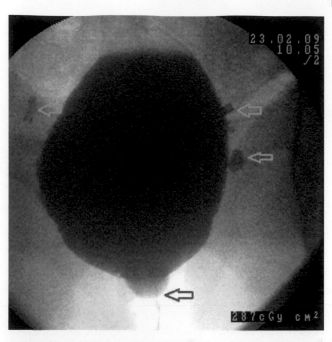

Figure 8.23 Bladder outlet obstruction in a woman where her previous midurethral tape is compressing the urethra. She had very clear obstruction (red arrow), indicated by ballooning of the proximal urethra. This was associated with an interrupted flow and high pressures with low maximum flow rate. She also had two laparoscopic sterilisation clips (blue arrows) and a small bladder diverticulum (green arrow). *Source*: Marcus Drake.

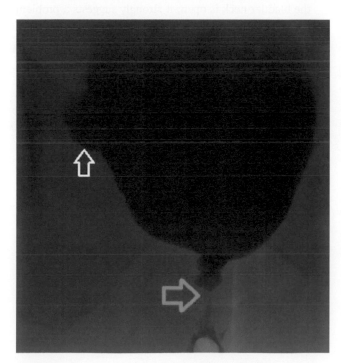

Figure 8.24 A urethral stricture in a woman (green arrow). There is also a small diverticulum on the right (white arrow). *Source*: Marcus Drake.

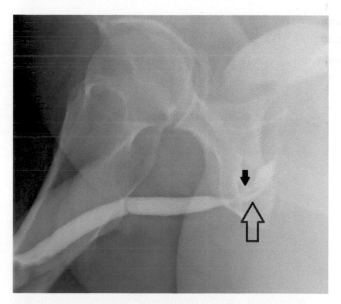

Figure 8.25 A urethral false passage in a man. At this point, two tracks can be seen; the higher is the normal upwards curve of the urethra at the bulb (filled black arrow). The lower is the false passage (open black arrow), where a previous attempt to place a catheter has failed to follow the line of the curve and instead pushed straight on into the tissues. This has healed and become an established structure, which can cause great problems for any subsequent attempts to catheterise. *Source*: Marcus Drake.

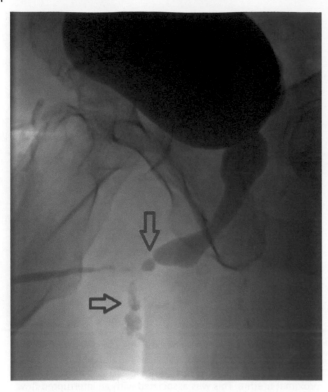

Figure 8.26 A urethral fistula in a man going to the perineum (blue arrow). There is also a urethral stricture (red arrow). *Source*: Marcus Drake.

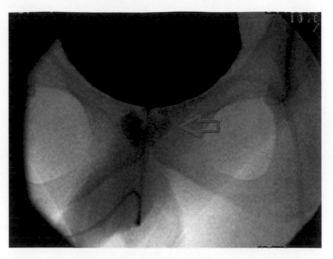

Figure 8.27 Reflux into the prostatic ducts in a man with neurological disease. The prostate is a secretory gland with multiple small ducts entering the prostatic urethra. Normally, they are not visible, but if a high pressure is generated in the prostatic urethra during pressure-flow studies, some contrast will enter the ducts and outline the gland (red arrow). In this young man, the prostate is small and heart-shaped. This observation suggests sphincter resistance and high voiding pressures, suggesting either detrusor sphincter dyssynergia or fixed sphincter obstruction (see Chapter 16). *Source*: Marcus Drake.

1) Imaging can pick up several factors which could be relevant for risk of developing or progressing renal failure:
   a) A bladder distorted by extensive diverticulation and trabeculation (the 'fir tree' bladder, Figure 8.12), combined with poor compliance on filling cystometry;
   b) VUR (Figure 8.5). It is important to record the pressure rise and the volume at which VUR starts, and the grading of the VUR;
   c) Sphincter dysfunction responsible for high pressure during voiding, such as detrusor sphincter dyssynergia (DSD) or fixed sphincter obstruction. These can be identified directly by observing the sphincter during X-ray screening, or they can be surmised if the resulting high pressures in the prostatic urethra cause contrast to enter the prostate ducts (Figure 8.27).
2) Site of neurological deficit. The location of a neurological deficit is not always confidently identified by a patient's neurologist, and the urodynamic assessment can help by cataloguing the LUT dysfunction and mapping it on to the problems expected for a given neurological deficit. One valuable observation by VUDS in this context is an open bladder neck in a man with no history of surgery of the prostate (which may have cut the bladder neck) or retroperitoneum (where the sympathetic chain can be damaged, for example, during lymphadenectomy for tes-

ticular cancer). If there is no such previous surgery, yet the bladder neck is open, it strongly suggests a problem in the thoracolumbar spinal cord, as this is the location of the sympathetic nucleus.
3) Understanding the mechanisms of symptoms; since history is rather unreliable in people with impaired nerve function, it is valuable to have the facility to spot the range of issues described in this chapter, since many of them can potentially exist in neurological disease.

In many cases, it is impossible to interpret the situation without the additional information that imaging offers (Figure 8.50).

The contribution of VUDS for children is rather akin to its use in neurological disease and is described in detail in Chapter 12. An important situation to be aware of is a specific type of BOO caused by congenital PUV (Figures 8.29 and 8.30).

Renal Failure and Transplant Patients

In patients awaiting transplant who have oliguria or bladder dysfunction, urodynamics can often reveal significant pathology. These patients may need to be screened for lower urinary tract dysfunction before joining the trans-

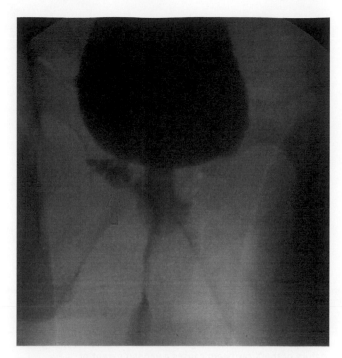

Figure 8.28 Reflux of contrast into a seminal vesicle (red arrow). This is a fairly common observation and does not necessarily imply high prostatic urethral pressures during pressure-flow studies. *Source*: Marcus Drake.

plant waiting list [10]. Appropriate treatment of these abnormalities aims at ensuring graft survival. A specific challenge is reflected in the urodynamic assessment of anuric patients, i.e. those with no urine production at all

as a result of severe kidney disease or dialysis. For these people, the absence of urine production means that the bladder gets no filling and voiding cycle, and this affects its properties, including a marked reduction in cystometric capacity and impairment of compliance. More prolonged anuria leads to more severe change [11]. This can provide a considerable dilemma, as the apparent severity of the urodynamic changes might seem to contraindicate placement of a transplant. We have encountered cases where a transplant was done in very severe reduction in cystometric capacity. In one case, capacity was as small as 30 ml, with highly symptomatic voiding frequency initially; this had markedly improved to 300 ml at 2 months after transplant. Consequently, the urodynamic assessment of an anuric patient does not necessarily give prognostic information for symptomatic and safety outcome once urine production is restored by transplantation. This subject has not been systematically studied, but anuria, even of long duration, does not prevent transplant, provided that the bladder was originally normal and is not infected [12]. Urodynamics is not routinely undertaken in this setting.

Urodynamics may be indicated to assess someone who has received a transplant which is not functioning as expected, and where hydronephrosis is worsening (Figures 8.51–8.54). Renal transplantation requires placement of the transplant ureter into the bladder. The organ takes its blood supply from the iliac vessels, so it is usually located low in the abdomen. The length of ureter is very

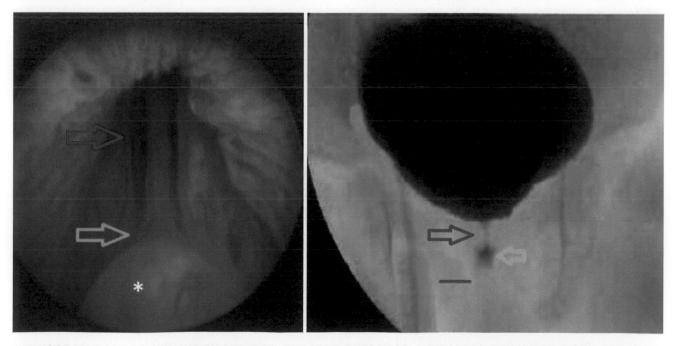

Figure 8.29 Posterior urethral valves (PUV) seen endoscopically (left) and during pressure-flow studies (right). Very fine tissue flaps are present (blue arrows). The green arrow is the prostatic urethra below the valve. The asterisk is on the verumontanum, an anatomical structure just proximal to the level of the sphincter (purple line). This is a very mild case of PUV. *Source*: Marcus Drake.

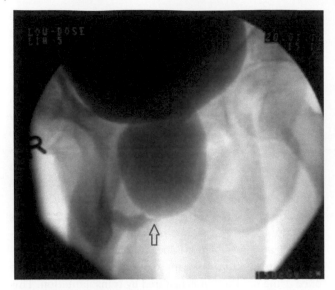

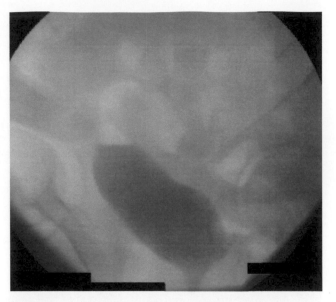

Figure 8.30 Severe PUV, indicated by a red arrow. There is enormous swelling of the outlet above the valves, a grossly swollen bladder, and severe hydronephrosis (not shown). *Source*: Marcus Drake.

Figure 8.31 After pressure-flow study, the presence of a post-void residual (PVR) is easily observed. It is unreliable to attempt to estimate how big the PVR is, since the diverging nature of the X-ray beam causes a varying extent of magnification of the final image, and because the image is two-dimensional, lacking the third dimension which is needed to derive volume (see Figure 6.7). *Source*: Marcus Drake.

short (due to the low location of the organ, and the better chance of avoiding ischaemia by minimising the length). Thus, bladder pressures can be transmitted very easily to the organ (Figure 8.51), so there can be a need for VUDS in some transplant patients. Many renal transplant patients have urodynamic abnormalities such as decreased bladder capacity and compliance.

Whitaker Testing

Occasionally, VUDS units may be asked to assess ureteric obstruction. The principle of the Whitaker test is to perfuse

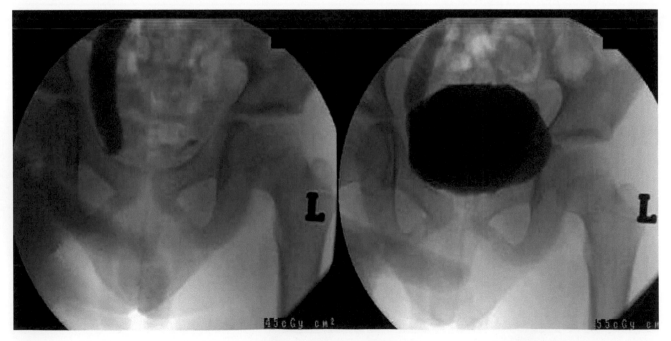

Figure 8.32 Pseudoresidual. Images taken at the end of voiding in a boy with vesicoureteric reflux [4]. Voiding has pushed contrast into the upper urinary tract. The left-hand image was timed nicely at the end of the voiding to confirm complete bladder emptying. The right-hand image was taken just 30 seconds later, by which time contrast had largely refilled the bladder, giving an appearance like a post-void residual. *Source*: Marcus Drake.

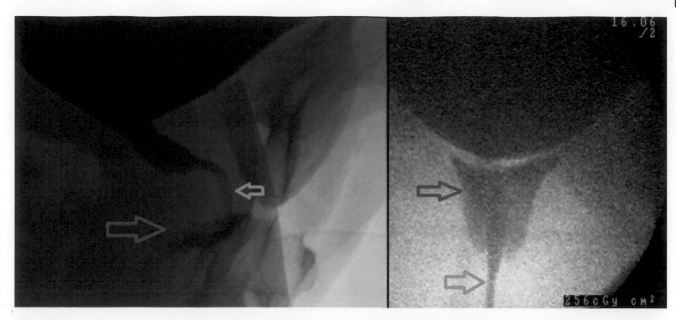

Figure 8.33 Intravaginal reflux. Two cases where a woman passing urine has experienced some urine entering the vagina. On the left, a woman with mild pelvic organ prolapse which affected the path of the stream, so it partly hit the perineal body. On the right, a nulliparous woman where the diversion may have been caused by the labia. In both cases, the main urinary stream is indicated by a green arrow, and the vaginal pooling is indicated by a red arrow. The urine captured by the vagina would escape soon after when the woman mobilised, giving the symptom of post micturition dribble. *Source*: Marcus Drake.

the upper urinary tract at a constant flow rate with saline or contrast medium from above downwards, through a nephrostomy tube, while recording the pressure in the renal pelvis [13, 14] (Figure 8.55). This pressure, when in steady state, is the pressure necessary to drive the fluid through the system at a fixed flow rate. The higher the pressure, the more likely that an obstruction is present (Figure 8.56), such as a ureteric stricture, or a pelvi-ureteric junction obstruction. With advances in renography, this test is rarely undertaken nowadays.

Using VUDS to Understand Limitations of Pressure Recording

The phrase 'filling cystometry' implies that the bladder is being filled to understand lower urinary tract function. Problems occur if the bladder has a structural deficit which causes the filling medium to fill other structures in addition, as this means it is not only the bladder being filled. Consequently, the term 'vesical pressure' may be misleading, since the reality is that the pressure properties reflect the combined structures being filled. This has enormous implications, as the bladder may be able to decompress into a low-pressure system to which it is attached. Indeed, it may be that harmful high pressures in the bladder were the initiating mechanism by which the abnormal communication has emerged. Two notable possibilities are severe

VUR (Figures 8.5 and 8.17) or a large diverticulum (Figure 8.57), both of which might be a consequence of chronic excessive vesical pressure. Both structures (upper urinary tract or diverticulum) are thin-walled and low pressure, and hence could obscure the properties of the bladder itself. As a result, it becomes difficult to identify either DO or impaired bladder compliance using only pressure recording. VUDS is the most reliable way to identify

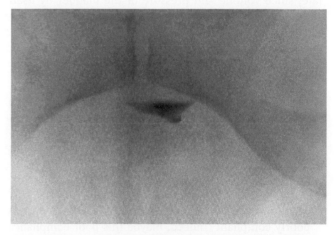

Figure 8.34 A urethral diverticulum in a woman can cause post-micturition dribble if its entry point to the urethra is below the sphincter. This image was taken after conclusion of voiding, showing contrast in a urethral diverticulum. This had not been visible before voiding, suggesting that its entry point probably is below the sphincter. *Source*: Marcus Drake.

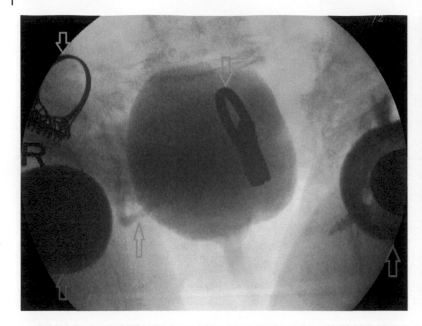
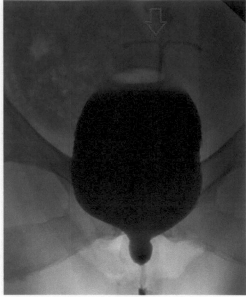

Figure 8.35 Internal and external foreign bodies seen on video urodynamics; any metallic objects will be seen on imaging. Here, this lady had two different types of hip replacement (red arrows), fixings and jewellery (blue arrows). She was also seen to have vesicoureteric reflux (green arrow). On the right, a uterine coil (purple arrow). *Source*: Marcus Drake.

the situation; it establishes that the bladder is not the only structure being filled, and hence provides a warning that the p_{ves} trace will potentially be unreliable for making diagnosis.

Identification of such communications necessitates caution when interpreting the vesical pressure. Since the p_{ves} recorded is not true bladder pressure, but a combination of the bladder with the extra storage space, it means that pressures are probably going to be lower than they would have been if only the bladder was filled. As a result, bladder compliance becomes extremely difficult to calculate, since volume and pressure of the bladder by itself cannot reliably be established. In this situation, the healthcare professional must be clear that any compliance calculation using p_{ves} actually reflects the whole system being filled and not just the bladder; if the bladder could be isolated, it might prove to be poorly compliant. An extreme example is illustrated in Figure 8.50, where a lot of contrast has been instilled but only a tiny proportion is in the bladder.

Uncertainty about true value of bladder compliance is very important when making major decisions:

- Is it safe to reimplant the ureters in a person with VUR? The answer would be 'definitely not' if the bladder is poorly compliant (indeed, maybe this poor compliance was what led to the VUR in the first place).
- Whether to place a renal transplant in a patient with severe VUR to the native kidneys. Again, the answer is 'no' if the bladder is poorly compliant. This response is

less clear-cut than the previous example, since it can be argued that the transplant might be protected by the pressure relief of VUR into the native kidneys. However, the protective nature of that situation may be uncertain, and consideration of the possibility that at some point in the future, one or both native kidneys may need removal (e.g. if a renal carcinoma develops or if the person starts to experience severe recurrent urinary tract infections).

There is no easy resolution to the issue of isolating the bladder in order to measure its compliance specifically. Conceivably, it can be possible to occlude the communication to the other structure with a balloon catheter if it is

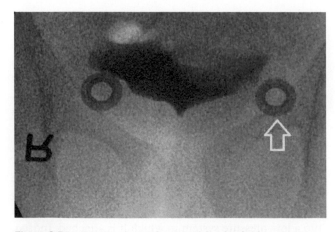

Figure 8.36 Another form of external foreign body seen on video urodynamics; eyelets used to secure the waist cord in a pair of trousers. *Source*: Marcus Drake.

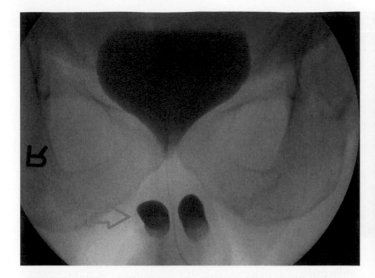
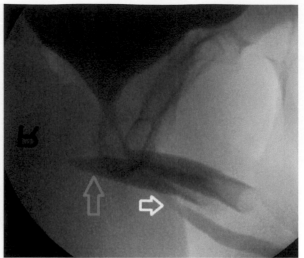

Figure 8.37 A two chamber penile implant seen during video urodynamics, the right chamber being indicated by an orange arrow. The left image is a postero-anterior projection during filling cystometry. The right image is an oblique view during pressure-flow studies, showing the relationship of the implant to the urethra. The white arrow indicates the urethral bulb. *Source*: Marcus Drake.

narrow, and then fill the bladder [15]. An attempt to do this in a case of severe VUR is described in Figure 8.58.

The issue of difficulty observing DO has less serious implications for the patient than failure to identify impaired compliance. Nonetheless, the test needs to make attempts to diagnose function fully. In the event that DO is suspected but not seen on the pressure trace, VUDS can be used to examine bladder shape. When the bladder contracts, its shape often changes, and this can be observed (Figure 8.59). This change could be used to decide on whether bladder contraction has occurred in the absence of measured pressure change. It is also a means of deciding whether the bladder is acontractile during voiding in women with a wide calibre urethra.

Equipment Needed

The equipment for filling the bladder, the capture of images, and how they are linked to the synchronous pressure data need to be considered. In order to achieve imaging of the urinary tract, contrast medium is instilled rather than saline. This means the filling pump should be able to handle contrast, and the different density of the contrast medium needs to be entered into the software (see below). The density of contrast medium means it settles in the base of the bladder, below any urine the patient makes (see Figure 8.11).

The image capture is most efficiently done with a C-arm, which includes an X-ray source and an image intensifier. An image intensifier within the urodynamic department, in a room set up for radiological procedures, allows the

unit to be independent of the Radiology department, making planning of VUDS investigations more flexible and straightforward. Taking the patient away from the busy Radiology department also means it is possible to create a better environment in which to perform the investigation. However, there is a significant cost to the department in purchasing and maintaining equipment. The C-arm should be used with an X-ray translucent urodynamics couch to avoid impeding the passage of X-rays.

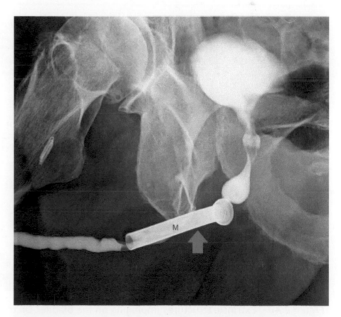

Figure 8.38 Another implant in a man, a Memokath intraurethral stent (orange arrow, "M"), used to treat a urethral stricture. This image was taken during a urethrogram. *Source*: Marcus Drake.

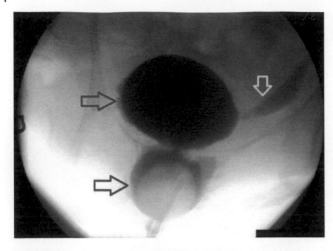

Figure 8.39 A man undergoing filling cystometry to assess bladder compliance, using single lumen filling and pressure measurement via a urethral Foley catheter (blue arrow). The retaining balloon is clearly sited in the prostatic urethra rather than the intended location of the bladder (red arrow). Vesico-ureteric reflux is seen (yellow arrow). *Source*: Marcus Drake.

An alternative is to do the urodynamic test in the X-ray department, employing a fixed X-ray unit, combined with a tilt table. These produce higher resolution images than the C-arm. However, using a tilt table can restrict the flexibility of how the test is run, as filling will generally mean the patient is supine. Furthermore, voiding will mean the table is transferred to the vertical position, which is unnatural for passing urine (women) and awkward for frail or neurologically impaired patients with balance problems. It can

also be difficult to get the oblique view needed to see the bladder outlet and urethra fully in men.

One further consideration is the urodynamic computer software, as this needs to be able to adjust for the contrast medium density when measuring urine flow and also has to be able to record the video images synchronously with the pressure-flow tracings in real time.

Considerations when Using X-rays

Radiation Safety

It is important to minimise radiation exposure as far as possible, considering the patient, the staff, and other bystanders. VUDS is a radiological investigation, and the unit needs to be constructed accordingly. Suitable materials must be used in the walls and windows (typically lead and/or barium) to prevent X-ray passage, and warning signs must be in position, with warning lights available which are illuminated while the test is running (Figure 8.60).

Protective clothing, such as lead aprons and thyroid shields, is vital. This applies not just for staff, but for any friends or relatives who are present in the room during the investigation. This shielding must be suitably cared for (Figure 8.61) and checked regularly. The lead is at risk of cracking when folded, and this will allow X-rays through, with accumulating inadequacy if careless use persists. Thus, the lead aprons should always be hung on a specific

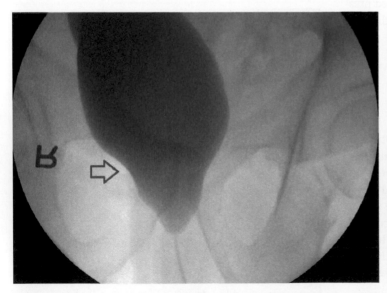
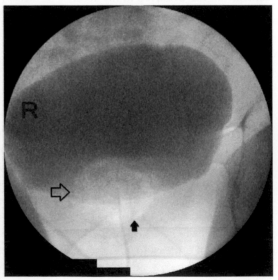

Figure 8.40 Extrinsic structures impinging on the bladder. On the left, compression by an intrapelvic fluid collection (red arrow). In this case, the fluid was a lymphocoele caused by pelvic surgery more than a year previously. On the right, a faecal mass, showing up as a paler structure (right margin indicated with open black arrow). It is clearly not a filling defect within the bladder, as its lower margin (filled black arrow) is below the lowest extent of the bladder. *Source*: Marcus Drake.

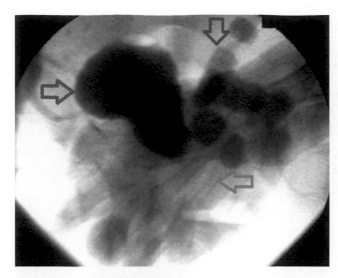

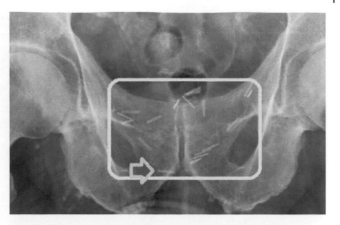

Figure 8.41 Oblique view of a man using his hand (orange arrow) to direct his penis when about to do a pressure-flow study. He was asked to move his hand out of the way before being giving permission to void. The purple arrow is colonic contents, as he had had a small bowel contrast study a few days previously. The red arrow indicates his bladder. *Source*: Marcus Drake.

Figure 8.42 Plain X-ray of a man who had previously undergone radical prostatectomy. Multiple clips used to stem bleeding ('haemostatic clips') are visible in the operative field (yellow rectangle). The lowest of these (arrowed) appears to lie very close to the expected location of the sphincter. *Source*: Marcus Drake.

hanger and never dumped thoughtlessly. Staff undertaking this test should wear dosimeters under their lead aprons. These are X-ray sensitive radiation exposure badges containing photographic films to detect accumulating exposure over time.

Staff training requires that all people responsible for this type of test are compliant with the applicable regulatory expectations. In the UK, these are the Ionising Radiation (Medical Exposure) Regulations, known as IR(ME)R. The

regulations stipulate the importance of minimising unintended, excessive, or incorrect medical exposures, ensuring the benefits outweigh the risks of each exposure (justification), and keeping doses 'as low as reasonably achievable' for their intended use (optimisation). Patient dose monitoring is thus essential [16]. Accordingly, while the number of images taken must be tailored to the complexity of the urodynamic question, it has to be balanced with minimising the number of images.

Due to the risk of radiation to the developing foetus, it is important to rule out pregnancy before performing X-rays on women of childbearing age. If there is any doubt, a

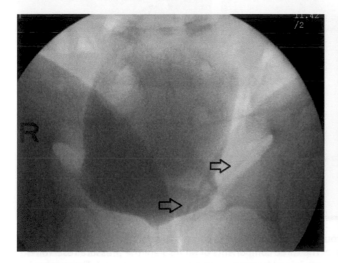

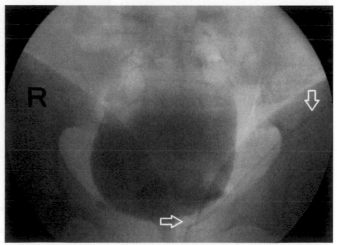

Figure 8.43 The left image was interpreted as showing vesicoureteric reflux (black arrows) due to a line of contrast near the bladder base heading towards the sacroiliac joint. However, a subsequent image (right) showed a different position (white arrows), away from the bladder base and running on the inside of the patient's thigh. At this stage, it was identified the structure was actually the contrast-containing filling line. *Source*: Marcus Drake.

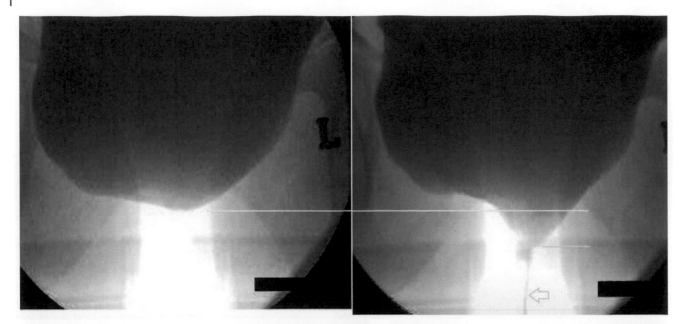

Figure 8.49 Urodynamic stress incontinence caused by urethral hypermobility. Left image: the bladder base prior to a cough. Right image: during the cough, the bladder base descends (hypermobility) and leakage occurs (arrow). *Source*: Marcus Drake.

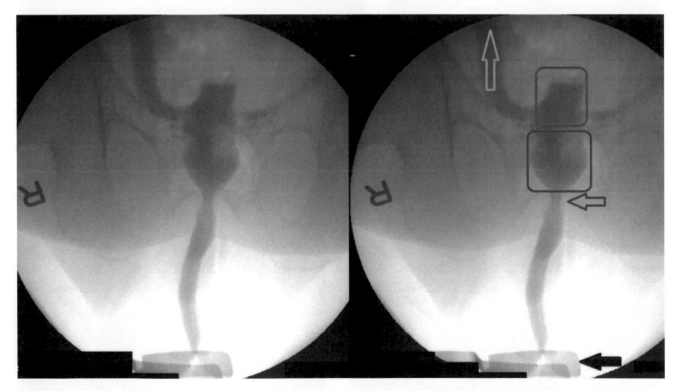

Figure 8.50 Filling cystometry of extreme neurogenic lower urinary tract dysfunction. In this case, the bladder (red square) was exceptionally small in volume and actually smaller than the prostatic urethra (purple square). The bladder neck was open (where the red and purple squares meet) and the sphincter (blue arrow) incompetent so that a penile clamp had to be applied (black arrow) in order to enable bladder filling. There was substantial right-sided vesicoureteric reflux (green arrow). *Source*: Marcus Drake.

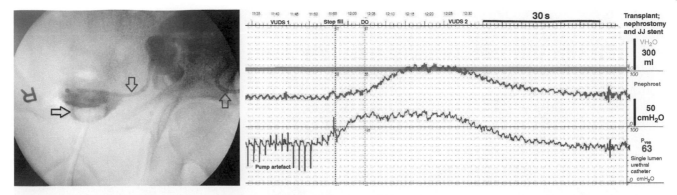

Figure 8.51 A transplant patient with a Foley catheter (black arrow), a ureteric stent (purple arrow), and a nephrostomy (blue arrow) in place due to renal dysfunction of the transplant graft. He underwent filling cystometry (right image) using the Foley catheter for bladder filling and vesical pressure recording (blue trace, p_{ves}). The red line is the pressure trace recorded from the nephrostomy. High-amplitude DO occurred in the bladder, and this was shortly afterwards readily visible in the nephrostomy pressure. *Source*: Marcus Drake.

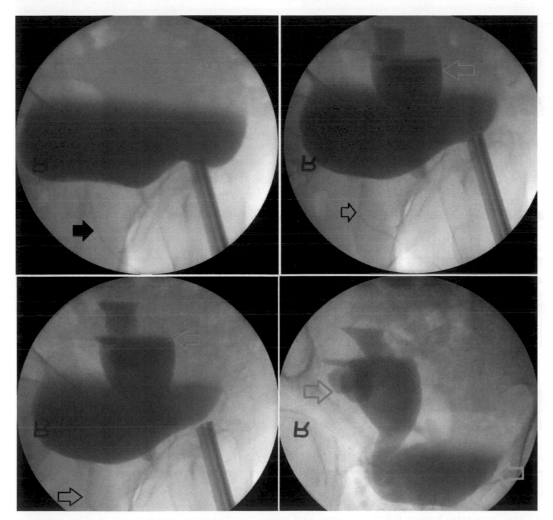

Figure 8.52 Pressure-flow studies in a transplant patient. Top left: before permission to void – the closed black arrow shows the course of the contrast-filled filling catheter. Top right and bottom left: after permission to void, showing a small extent of flow along the urethra (open black arrow), and more voluminous filling of the transplant renal pelvis. Bottom right: after voiding has concluded, the renal pelvis is full of contrast, and there is a lot of contrast in the bladder (green arrow). Careful screening enabled confirmation this was a true post-void residual, not a pseudo-residual. This patient was managed with intermittent self-catheterisation to prevent the need for voiding, which stabilised his transplant function. *Source*: Marcus Drake.

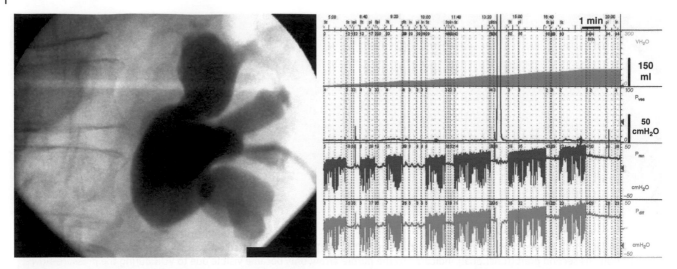

Figure 8.56 A Whitaker test showing the contrast perfusion (left) and pressure recording (right). The climbing pressure and visible dilation indicate that upper urinary tract obstruction was present. *Source*: Marcus Drake.

check the volume in the flowmeter jug at the end of the test and adjust the machine measurements accordingly.

Performing the Test

The patient's identity should be checked to ensure the right person is undergoing the investigation. The indications should be reviewed to make sure the test can be justified and to anticipate the key points at which images might be captured. Pregnancy should be excluded. The door should be locked, and the radiological warning lights illuminated. The catheters are placed as for conventional urodynamic testing.

Positioning of the Patient

Men should be stood next to the funnel (if that is their normal voiding position). During filling, the X-rays run in a P-A direction, i.e. the X-ray source is placed behind the patient and the image intensifier that captures them is in front (Figure 8.63). The intensifier is kept close to the abdominal wall suprapubically to minimise dose and misleading estimates of bladder size. During voiding, the axis is turned to a 45° oblique projection. This gives optimum view of the whole male bladder outlet and avoids the incomplete visualisation of the bulbar urethra resulting if the P-A projection is retained. It is important to have the male urethra fully in the field of view before giving permission for the patient to void. A mobile C-arm has benefits in

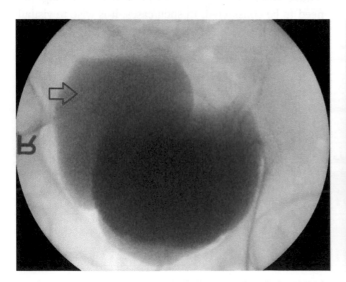

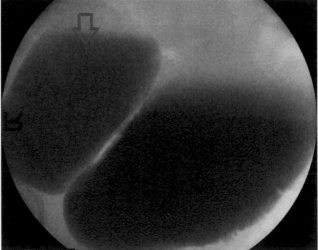

Figure 8.57 Filling cystometry showing a large bladder diverticulum (red arrow) viewed in postero-anterior (left) and oblique (right) projections. *Source*: Marcus Drake.

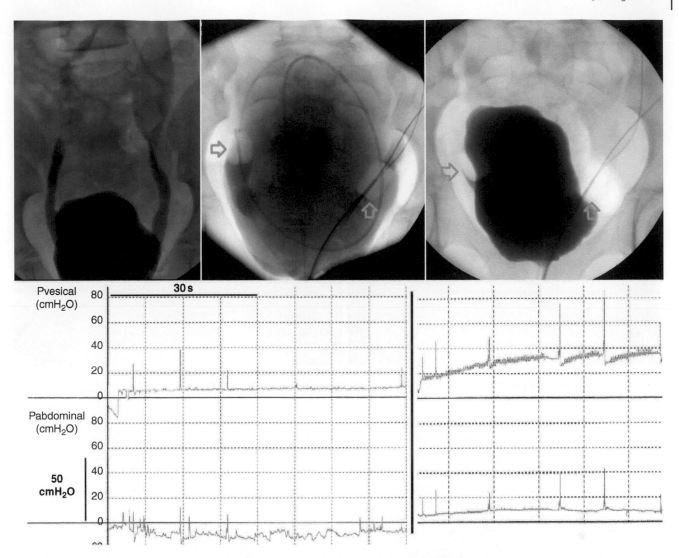

Figure 8.58 A case of severe vesicoureteric reflux is shown in the top left X-ray, with placement of bilateral ureteric occlusion catheters (green arrows) shown in the middle X-ray. As shown in the right X-ray, the catheters largely stopped the reflux. Vesical and abdominal pressure recordings during filling are shown below, before (left) and after (right) the occlusion catheters were placed. An obvious change in compliance is seen. *Source*: Marcus Drake.

this respect as its position can be adjusted without having to move the patient several times before permission to void can be given.

For women, who tend to be seated for filling cystometry and PFS, the bulk of the image intensifier makes the P-A projection uncomfortable, as the thighs get in the way. Thus, an A-P projection is generally used (Figure 8.64). This applies both during filling and voiding, as it generally achieves good views during both phases.

For patients with limited mobility, notably those with neurological disease, specialist equipment must be available. A hoist may be needed to get them into position, and grab rails and cushioned supports help maintain their position while running the test. Extra time should be allowed for the appointment so that positioning can be done safely.

Taking the Images

The C-arm needs to be lined up with the relevant organ (bladder, urethra, or ureter), and a pilot shot can be taken to confirm the beam includes the relevant structure with an unimpeded line of sight.

At the start of the test, the bladder is the centre of interest.

- An early image can be taken (after a few ml have been instilled) if there is doubt about the filling line having made it to the bladder – for example, if the catheter may have stuck in the urethra in a man, or slipped out of the urethra into the vagina in a woman.
- Generally, an image is taken at 200 ml. A stress test (rapid series of strong coughs) can be done, the C-arm being activated as the patient breathes in to do the first cough.

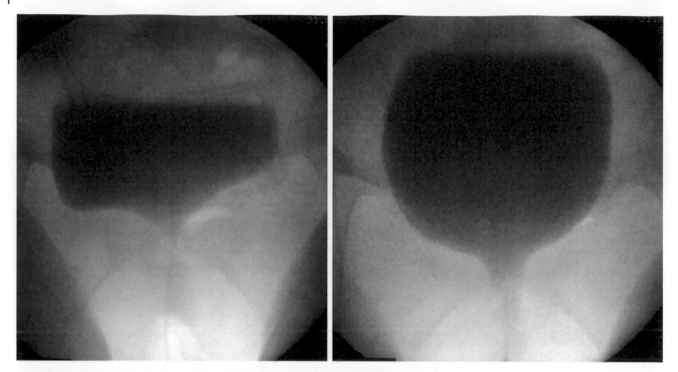

Figure 8.59 Visible shape change associated with bladder contraction. Source: Marcus Drake.

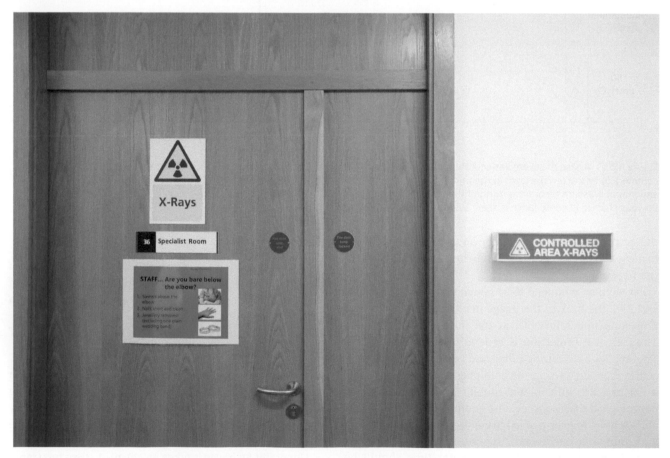

Figure 8.60 As a radiological test, the study room needs to have warning notices and warning signs that can be illuminated when X-rays are in use. *Source*: Marcus Drake.

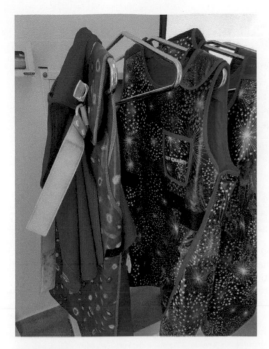

Figure 8.61 Good practice caring for lead aprons is vital to ensure they maintain safe protection for the wearer. Lead cracks if folded, so the apron can become X-ray permeable. Thus, these aprons should be hung up carefully on a strong rack designed for the purpose. Most of the aprons in the illustration are suitably hung, but the red apron has been thrown carelessly on to the rack, and lead cracking may result. *Source*: Marcus Drake.

- When looking for VUR, the C-arm is moved upwards to look at the line of the ureters bilaterally, up as far as the kidneys.
- An image can be taken if urgency is described by the patient, which can identify whether there is opening of the bladder neck and stimulation of the proximal urethra.
- Imaging during provocation tests can be repeated at cystometric capacity.

Before permission to void, the C-arm is moved for the oblique projection in men. The outlet is now the centre of interest, so the C-arm may need to be lowered. Flexibility to move the C-arm upwards to evaluate VUR is also appropriate.

- An image can be taken when detrusor pressure starts to rise.
- An image or video is taken when it is estimated flow rate is at its peak.
- A post-void image can be taken to look for a PVR. This must be taken promptly in patients with VUR to avoid misinterpreting a pseudoresidual (Figure 8.32) as a PVR.

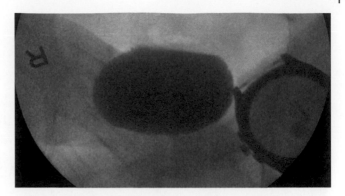

Figure 8.62 The distorting effect on relative size due to different distances from the image intensifier. In this case, a small wrist watch ends up looking larger than a bladder containing over 100 ml of contrast. *Source*: Marcus Drake.

Advantages and Disadvantages of VUDS

Advantages

VUDS provides the additional anatomical information that can make a vital difference to understanding an individual patient's urinary tract dysfunction, of greatest value where pathophysiological mechanisms are varied and potentially complex.

Disadvantages

The most significant disadvantage of VUDS is exposure to radiation for both the patient (Table 8.1) and the staff performing the investigation. Dose for the staff must be minimised by use of protective barriers, lead aprons, minimising screening time, and standing back from the patient to avoid 'scatter' radiation. VUDS also carries additional costs, since

Table 8.1 Comparative doses of ionising radiation for different situations encountered by patients.

Event	Radiation dose (mSv)
Chest X-ray	0.014
Transatlantic flight	0.08
Video urodynamics	0.34
UK resident (average annual background radiation)	2.7
CT scan of the chest	6.6
Annual limit for nuclear industry employees	20

CT: computed tomography. *Source*: www.gov.uk.

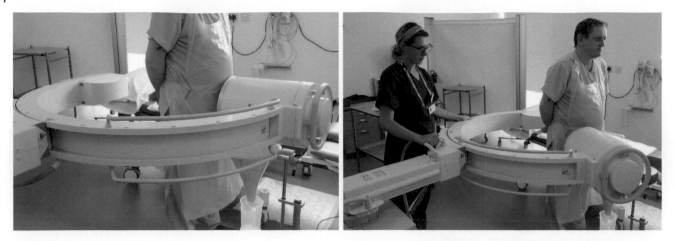

Figure 8.63 C-arm position for men during filling cystometry (left) and transitioning to a horizontal oblique view for pressure-flow study (right). These pictures are purely illustrative; for taking images during a video urodynamics (VUDS) test, hands should be kept out of the way of the X-ray beam, i.e. resting by the patient's sides, on their thighs, or <u>gently</u> resting on the C-arm. *Source*: Marcus Drake.

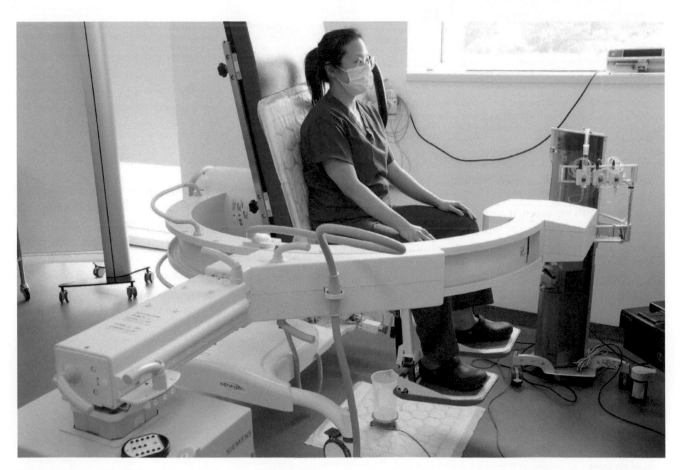

Figure 8.64 C-arm position for women during filling cystometry and pressure-flow study. The subject is seated on a radiolucent chair, which is specifically designed for urodynamics; height and angles can be varied, it can be placed into a horizontal couch configuration for catheterising, and the legs are separately supported, with a holder for the flowmeter funnel. *Source*: Marcus Drake.

the room has to be specially constructed, the equipment is expensive to purchase and maintain, there is additional staff training, and contrast media are more expensive than saline.

In order to take images during voiding, the staff operating the equipment generally need to be in the room. This can increase the chance of the patient being unable to void.

Alternatives to VUDS

Micturating Cystourethrogram

If VUDS is not available locally, micturating cystourethrogram (MCUG) is a test done by radiologists to evaluate the structure of the bladder and outlet. It involves catheterisation and instillation of a defined volume of contrast into the bladder. P-A films are taken at rest and with the patient coughing or straining, and during voiding for women.

Oblique lateral films are taken during voiding for men. No pressure data is obtained during the test, so it is purely an anatomical evaluation. While it can provide additional information, it is not aligned with the real-time progression during filling and voiding that makes VUDS so informative.

Ultrasound

Ultrasound is used in some units instead of fluoroscopy. This avoids radiation exposure. Some investigators report excellent imaging of the bladder outlet in women. It is possible to estimate parameters such as bladder wall thickness and weight; while these have been evaluated as potential diagnostic parameters [17], they remain experimental [18]. It is not practical to obtain images of the whole of the male urethra with ultrasound on a routine basis. It is also challenging to visualise the upper tracts and the bladder synchronously.

References

1. Wyndaele, M. and Rosier, P. (2018). Basics of videourodynamics for adult patients with lower urinary tract dysfunction. *Neurourol. Urodyn.* 37: S61–S66.

2. Drake, M.J., Apostolidis, A., Cocci, A. et al. (2016). Neurogenic lower urinary tract dysfunction: clinical management recommendations of the neurologic incontinence committee of the fifth international consultation on incontinence 2013. *Neurourol. Urodyn.* 35: 657–665.

3. Stohrer, M., Blok, B., Castro-Diaz, D. et al. (2009). EAU guidelines on neurogenic lower urinary tract dysfunction. *Eur. Urol.* 56: 81–88.

4. Drake, M.J. and Abrams, P. (2018). A commentary on expectations of healthcare professionals when applying the international continence society standards to basic assessment of lower urinary tract function. *Neurourol. Urodyn.* 37: S7–S12.

5. Spilotros, M., Sihra, N., Malde, S. et al. (2017). Buccal mucosal graft urethroplasty in men-risk factors for recurrence and complications: a third referral Centre experience in anterior urethroplasty using buccal mucosal graft. *Transl. Androl. Urol.* 6: 510–516.

6. Bhargava, S. and Chapple, C.R. (2004). Buccal mucosal urethroplasty: is it the new gold standard? *BJU Int.* 93: 1191–1193.

7. Agrawalla, S., Pearce, R., and Goodman, T.R. (2004). How to perform the perfect voiding cystourethrogram. *Pediatr. Radiol.* 34: 114–119.

8. Breyer, B.N., Cooperberg, M.R., McAninch, J.W., and Master, V.A. (2009). Improper retrograde urethrogram technique leads to incorrect diagnosis. *J. Urol.* 182: 716–717.

9. Blaivas, J.G. (1983). Classification of stress urinary incontinence. *Neurourol. Urodyn.* 2: 103–104.

10. Rude, T., Nassiri, N., Naser-Tavakolian, A., and Ginsberg, D. (2019). The role of Urodynamics in the pre-transplant evaluation of renal transplant. *Curr. Urol. Rep.* 20: 26.

11. Chen, J.L., Lee, M.C., and Kuo, H.C. (2012). Reduction of cystometric bladder capacity and bladder compliance with time in patients with end-stage renal disease. *J. Formos. Med. Assoc.* 111: 209–213.

12. Frantz, P., Guerrieri, M., Leo, J.P. et al. (1987). Restoration of urinary tract continuity in a non-functioning bladder after renal transplantation. *Ann. Urol.* 21: 130–134.

13. Farrugia, M.K. and Whitaker, R.H. (2019). The search for the definition, etiology, and effective diagnosis of upper urinary tract obstruction: the Whitaker test then and now. *J. Pediatr. Urol.* 15: 18–26.

14. Whitaker, R.H. (1973). Methods of assessing obstruction in dilated ureters. *Br. J. Urol.* 45: 15–22.

15. Bomalaski, M.D. and Bloom, D.A. (1997). Urodynamics and massive vesicoureteral reflux. *J. Urol.* 158: 1236–1238.

16. Rosier, P., Schaefer, W., Lose, G. et al. (2017). International continence society good urodynamic practices and terms 2016: Urodynamics, uroflowmetry,

cystometry, and pressure-flow study. *Neurourol. Urodyn.* 36: 1243–1260.

17. Bright, E., Oelke, M., Tubaro, A., and Abrams, P. (2010). Ultrasound estimated bladder weight and measurement of bladder wall thickness--useful noninvasive methods for assessing the lower urinary tract? *J. Urol.* 184: 1847–1854.

18. Malde, S., Nambiar, A.K., Umbach, R. et al. and European Association of Urology Non-neurogenic Male, L. G. P. (2017). Systematic review of the performance of noninvasive tests in diagnosing bladder outlet obstruction in men with lower urinary tract symptoms. *Eur. Urol.* 71: 391–402.

9

Ambulatory Urodynamics

Julie Ellis-Jones[1] and Wendy Bevan[2]

[1] *Department of Adult Nursing, University of the West of England, Bristol, UK*
[2] *Urodynamics Department, Bristol Urological Institute, North Bristol NHS Trust, Southmead Hospital, Bristol, UK*

CONTENTS

Ambulatory urodynamics (AUDS) is a useful tool in the armamentarium of the urodynamicist, primarily in the investigation of those patients where conventional urodynamic tests have failed to provide an explanation for their symptoms, yet a definite diagnosis is needed to inform management. In half to two-thirds of such cases, AUDS can deliver a meaningful diagnosis [1, 2].

The philosophy behind AUDS, as in conventional urodynamics, is to evaluate filling and voiding function and to use provocation tests to elicit important urodynamic observations, such as stress urinary incontinence (SUI) or detrusor overactivity (DO). In AUDS, p_{ves} and p_{abd} are measured to enable calculation of p_{det}, but relying on the natural urine output from the kidneys (rather than artificial filling by a pump through a second lumen into the bladder). The p_{ves} and p_{abd} catheters are connected to a lightweight recording device worn by the patient, which allows pressure recording without any onwards connection to fixed apparatus (Figure 9.1).

This arrangement allows real freedom of movement, to the extent that the patient can undertake many more activities than can be done in a conventional urodynamics setting. Furthermore, much more time (a few hours) potentially becomes available. The freedom of movement and time makes the provocation testing more effective. Accordingly, the chances of reproducing symptoms are improved due to a better chance of modelling the situations that the patient reports as generally precipitating the symptoms.

In undertaking the test, the patient should record their activities in an activity log so that leakage episodes can be correlated with sensations or physical activities. Thus, the test provides a sensitive approach for observing DO (Figure 9.2) and for allowing realistic provocation testing for urodynamic stress incontinence.

Modern-day equipment allows wireless communication with the equipment so data can be reviewed in real time, which enables the urodynamicist to intervene when needed to troubleshoot pressure recording issues. Generally, this is done each time the patient returns to void – before and after the void. Following the test, the healthcare professional can download from the recording box, for analysing the findings and generating the report.

Indications for AUDS

The International Continence Society (ICS) Urodynamics Committee recommends the use of AUDS as a second-line diagnostic tool when office laboratory urodynamics have failed to achieve a diagnosis [4, 5]. The ICS principally views the roles of AUDS as being [5]:

- To confirm the patient's history of incontinence where conventional UDS has been normal;
  To determine whether DO or sphincter weakness is the main cause of incontinence if the patient desires further treatment; and

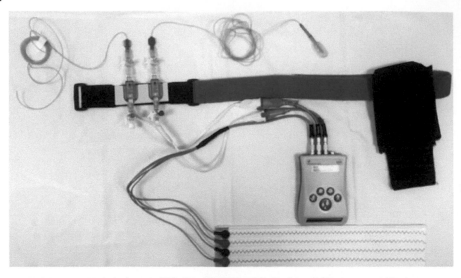
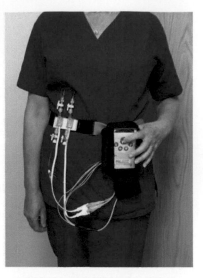

Figure 9.1 Equipment for ambulatory urodynamics, set up and in use. The equipment comprises p_{ves} (blue) and p_{abd} (red) catheters connected to transducers mounted on a belt. These go to a small recording device, which can go into a pocket on the belt. The recording device is also connected by four electrodes to a pad which can detect leakage. The arrangement is shown in use on the right, with the recording device in the belt pocket. The event markers (blue buttons on the recording device) are indicated. *Source*: Reproduced with permission from Cantu et al. [3].

- In situations in which conventional urodynamics may be unsuitable.

AUDS provides the chance to observe over a more prolonged period, and this improves the chance of observing unusual events, such as inappropriate urethral relaxation incontinence (Figure 13.16).

In addition, AUDS can be used to provide additional insight into mechanism and outcomes, of value in the context of research and clinical trials [6].

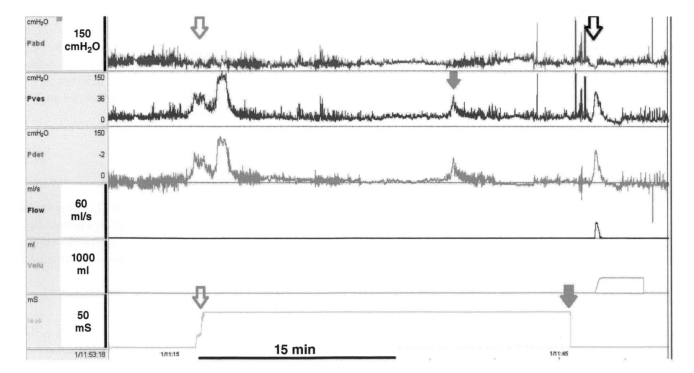

Figure 9.2 Ambulatory trace for a woman, who experienced detrusor overactivity (DO: open green arrow), which was associated with a leak (open blue arrow), i.e. DO incontinence. A lower amplitude episode of DO without leakage was seen a bit later (closed green arrow). The pad was removed, meaning that the leak detector reset to baseline (closed blue arrow), just before voiding (black arrow). The volume trace refers to voided volume.

Technique of AUDS

Patients undertake urinary flow rate, post-void residual, and urinalysis before proceeding to the test, as with conventional urodynamics. Specific gravity can be a useful indicator of hydration before starting as well. The patient is given clear explanation of how to use the device and activity log to record events and asked to maintain a good fluid intake. After the catheters are inserted, between one to three filling and voiding cycles are completed, but the duration is ultimately determined by clinical context and reproduction of urinary symptoms. The patient initially rests at the start of the first cycle to allow recording without movement artefacts. The patient is then encouraged to move actively around the hospital. They are encouraged to drink to maintain their urine output. At the end of each cycle, when the patient feels that their bladder is full, an exercise regime is performed. This should include any specific incontinence-provoking measures the patient has identified. For example, they may report leakage with walking downstairs, exertion (such as running), or other physical activity. Prior to voiding, the patient is asked to do a series of strong coughs when their bladder is full to screen for SUI (Figure 9.3). It is important that regular quality checks are performed during the test to ensure that the lines have not slipped during movement or voiding. This is now possible as AUDS traces can be viewed 'live' while the patient is a short distance away from the host computer using wireless technology.

Because one of the prime indications for AUDS is the detection of incontinence, it is important that the episode of leakage is recorded synchronously with the pressure data (Figure 9.4). Methods to measure this have included a pad following similar principles to a bedwetting mat alarm. The more common approach involves the patient wearing a pad in which there is a series of parallel wires (Figure 9.1). A small electrical potential is applied from the recording device, but electrical current only passes if the circuit is completed by the presence of urine (leakage), which conducts electricity due to the large number of ions present. By measuring the resistance between the wires, the severity of leakage can be estimated (though this is not necessarily very accurate). As an additional measure, the pad is also weighed pre- and post-test, and the pad may need to be changed at the end of each filling and voiding cycle. Another method utilises a temperature-sensitive device, able to detect the temperature change caused by leakage.

To pass urine, the patient uses a flowmeter in the usual way. The flowmeter has a wireless connection with the AUDS recording box so that urine flow rate is recorded synchronously with intravesical and abdominal pressure. Therefore, it is important that the patient uses the relevant

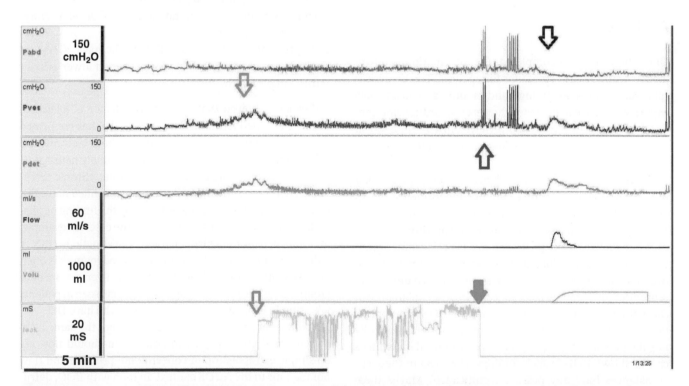

Figure 9.3 A short series of coughs (red arrow), followed by a longer cough series as a provocation stress for urodynamic stress incontinence, which was negative. Just before this, she had experienced DO (green arrow) with incontinence (open blue arrow), so the leak monitor had to be reset (closed blue arrow) before the stress testing. The test concluded with a pressure-flow study.

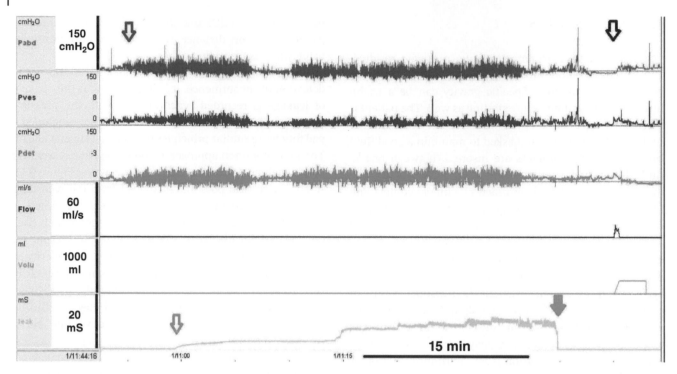

Figure 9.4 A study which identified urodynamic stress incontinence. The provocation was a long run (starting at the red arrow). Leakage started at the open blue arrow, with cumulative increase of leakage throughout the run. The leak monitor was reset (closed blue arrow) before the pressure-flow study (black arrow).

event marker on the recorder to record the start of voiding.

Analysis

Once the full test is completed, the information is downloaded onto the host computer for analysis. The analysis is relatively time-consuming and requires considerable expertise. There can be up to 6 hours of recording, and generally the test is expanded and reviewed in 4-minute screen shots to provide a detailed review, analysis, and interpretation of the test.

As well as providing the evidence for the presence and underlying mechanism of a patient's incontinence, much additional interesting information is generated by AUDS [7]. AUDS on normal individuals can show a significant prevalence of DO [8, 9]. Yet, this is of doubtful significance to the individual in the absence of urgency and urgency incontinence. Since the aim of urodynamics is 'to reproduce and provide a pathophysiological explanation of the patient's symptoms', the finding of DO here appears not to be significant in an asymptomatic neurologically normal person, particularly if a third of normal individuals can be shown to have such findings. Does DO in these circumstances have any positive significance? Maybe these findings could suggest:

- All people might have DO if studied long enough.
- DO is an artefact of investigation that results from the presence of an intravesical catheter.
- Thirty percent of normal individuals will develop symptoms in future years.
- People with asymptomatic DO might have a risk of adverse outcomes if they have some sort of lower urinary tract surgery in the future.

Klevmark showed that bladder compliance is related to the speed of bladder filling [10], and AUDS has confirmed this fact. In two groups of patients in whom conventional UDS frequently shows low compliance (namely neurogenic patients and older men with 'high-pressure chronic retention'), AUDS has shown that if the bladder is filled naturally, then low compliance may be replaced by the finding of phasic DO [7]. However, this is not always the case, for example, in women without bladder outlet obstruction (BOO), reduced compliance with conventional urodynamics is often not associated with DO on AUDS [11]. Even so, in both groups, there are higher filling pressures than seen in patients with simple BOO or neurogenic patients who have DO.

Voiding parameters during AUDS are not the same as in conventional UDS [12], so interpretation should not rely on simple extrapolation of conventional pressure and flow nomograms to the AUDS context. In men with BOO, detrusor contractility is higher and obstruction grade lower on

AUDS compared with conventional testing [13]. It appears that the maximum flow rate depends significantly on the voided volume, but the associated detrusor pressure does not [14]. Differing equipment and context may explain the lower pressures recorded [12]. On the other hand, physiological factors must also be considered. For example, comparatively fast filling (as used in conventional cystometry) may prevent the detrusor from generating its full contractile force, either because fast fill interferes with the mechanical reorganisation of the muscle or because the biochemical environment of the detrusor is altered. A similar phenomenon can be experienced by any of us if we allow our bladder to overfill, with the result that we have hesitancy and poor flow.

By its very nature of being a more active test, AUDS traces tend to have more artefacts than conventional urodynamic traces. Nonetheless, during urgency episodes, patients tend to move less to assist the holding reflex, so the increased incidence of artefacts does not necessarily impede diagnosis at that key time. In addition to standard UDS reporting, the subsequent report (and interpretation of traces) should include comments on all the filling/voiding cycles completed throughout the test:

- Detrusor activity during the filling phase – did this correspond with the patient recorded urinary event markers (or activity log during the test), and were any of these events associated with any urgency or leakage (DO incontinence)?
- Urinary leakage – was this recorded as an event? If so, was the leakage with or without sensation, and with or without a detrusor contraction?
- Provocation – what manoeuvres/exercises were undertaken and recorded (e.g. coughing, Valsalva, running, and squatting), and what was the outcome of stress pad testing at full bladder capacity?
- Reproducibility of the patient's symptoms – were all symptoms reproduced or partially reproduced?
- Conclude with a final comment on the overall quality of the AUDS trace – was it a reliable test throughout? It is important to comment on any technical difficulties or artefacts that may have occurred and made subsequent analysis difficult.

A summary of the Bristol experience with AUDS has been published, derived from a retrospective review of the database (Figure 9.5) [3]. This showed a strong female preponderance in the patients undergoing the test (92%). Standard UDS had failed to explain the patients' symptoms satisfactorily in all cases, and 1 in 10 of the patients previously had more than one standard or video UDS. All examinations were interpreted with the aid of event markers and activity

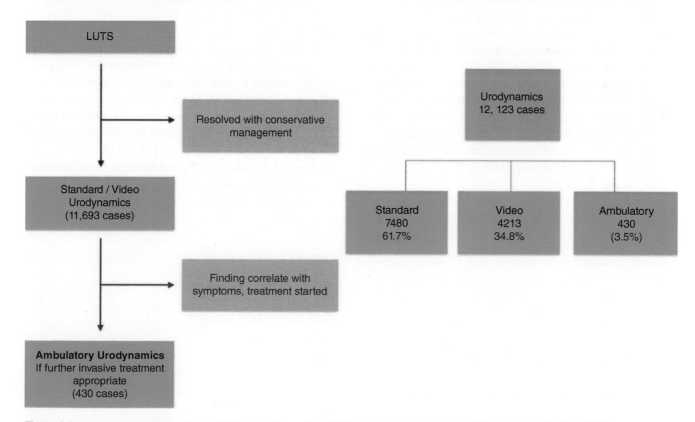

Figure 9.5 Bristol experience with ambulatory urodynamics. LUTS: lower urinary tract symptoms. *Source*: Cantu et al. [3].

logs during the test. AUDS lasted between 60 and 300 minutes. Patients' symptoms were reproduced in 74% of cases, with symptoms partially reproduced in 11% and not reproduced in 15%. In 17% of the studies, the findings were normal, 29% revealed DO (with or without DO incontinence), 25% had urodynamic stress incontinence, 17% had mixed urinary incontinence, and 12% had voiding dysfunction. Overall, additional urodynamic findings which correlated with symptoms were made in 69% of the patients.

In summary, AUDS is a valuable method of investigating the lower urinary tract in cases where diagnosis has been difficult, and it is generally used in the context of failure to reproduce any significant symptoms with conventional testing. The tests require considerable urodynamic expertise and interpretative skills, which are both costly (in terms of staff and resources) and time-consuming. AUDS is therefore best used only in the larger units with extensive experience of basic UDS.

References

1. Swithinbank, L.V., James, M., Shepherd, A., and Abrams, P. (1999). Role of ambulatory urodynamic monitoring in clinical urological practice. *Neurourol. Urodyn.* 18: 215–222.

2. van Koeveringe, G.A., Rahnama'i, M.S., and Berghmans, B.C. (2010). The additional value of ambulatory urodynamic measurements compared with conventional urodynamic measurements. *BJU Int.* 105: 508–513.

3. Cantu, H., Sharaf, A., Bevan, W. et al. (2019). Ambulatory urodynamics in clinical practice: a single Centre experience. *Neurourol. Urodyn.* 38: 2077–2082.

4. Digesu, G.A., Gargasole, C., Hendricken, C. et al. (2017). ICS teaching module: ambulatory urodynamic monitoring. *Neurourol. Urodyn.* 36: 364–367.

5. van Waalwijk van Doorn, E., Anders, K., Khullar, V. et al. (2000). Standardisation of ambulatory urodynamic monitoring: report of the Standardisation Sub-Committee of the International Continence Society for Ambulatory Urodynamic Studies. *Neurourol. Urodyn.* 19: 113–125.

6. Rosario, D.J., Smith, D.J., Radley, S.C., and Chapple, C.R. (1999). Pharmacodynamics of anticholinergic agents measured by ambulatory urodynamic monitoring: a study of methodology. *Neurourol. Urodyn.* 18: 223–233; discussion 223–224.

7. Bristow, S.E. and Neal, D.E. (1996). Ambulatory urodynamics. *Br. J. Urol.* 77: 333–338.

8. Schmidt, F., Jorgensen, T.M., and Djurhuus, J.C. (2004). Twenty-four-hour ambulatory urodynamics in healthy young men. *Scand. J. Urol. Nephrol. Suppl.* 38 (215): 75–83.

9. Robertson, A.S. (1999). Behaviour of the human bladder during natural filling: the Newcastle experience of ambulatory monitoring and conventional artificial filling cystometry. *Scand. J. Urol. Nephrol. Suppl.* 201: 19–24.

10. Klevmark, B. (1999). Natural pressure-volume curves and conventional cystometry. *Scand. J. Urol. Nephrol. Suppl.* 201: 1–4.

11. Harding, C., Dorkin, T.J., and Thorpe, A.C. (2009). Is low bladder compliance predictive of detrusor overactivity? *Neurourol. Urodyn.* 28: 74–77.

12. Valdevenito, J.P., Leonard, A., Griffiths, C.J. et al. (2014). Differences in urodynamic voiding variables recorded by conventional cystometry and ambulatory monitoring in symptomatic women. *Int. Braz. J. Urol.* 40: 666–675.

13. Rosario, D.J., MacDiarmid, S.A., Radley, S.C., and Chapple, C.R. (1999). A comparison of ambulatory and conventional urodynamic studies in men with borderline outlet obstruction. *BJU Int.* 83: 400–409.

14. Groen, J., van Mastrigt, R., and Bosch, R. (2000). Factors causing differences in voiding parameters between conventional and ambulatory urodynamics. *Urol. Res.* 28: 128–131.

10

Studies Assessing Urethral Pressures

Dharmesh Kapoor[1] and Marcus Drake[2]

[1] *Gynaecology Department, Global Hospital, Mumbai, India*
[2] *Translational Health Sciences, Bristol Medical School, Southmead Hospital, Bristol, UK*

CONTENTS

Lower urinary tract (LUT) function reflects activity of both the bladder and its outlet (bladder neck, external urethral sphincter, pelvic floor, and urethra). To an extent, effects of bladder dysfunction can be counterbalanced by the bladder outlet. For example, urgency and detrusor overactivity (DO) is a bladder issue which would be expected to give rise to incontinence, but in many people, the bladder outlet steps up resistance in order to stop the leakage actually happening (Figure 10.1). Indeed, the sphincter appears to become stronger over the years in people who experience long-standing DO without incontinence – a sort of muscle training for the sphincter [1]. Conversely, normal bladder storage function does not prevent leakage if the bladder outlet is impaired; this is the basis of stress urinary incontinence (SUI). Thus, an appreciation of bladder outlet function is essential in order to interpret any urodynamic observations related to the bladder, and the urodynamic practitioner needs to consider both elements when evaluating the situation in a specific patient.

The key role of the outlet during storage is continence. This must mean that there are forces achieving urethral closure which exceed the forces in the bladder lumen at all times. In real life, there is constant closure in the resting state, and supplementary reinforcement (both reflex and volitional) is also available to cope with any dynamic high-amplitude stresses that might otherwise overcome the urethral closure. Studies looking at the resting and dynamic pressures generated in the urethra accordingly can elaborate the deficiencies in a symptomatic individual; they are looking to identify 'closure pressures', the extent to which the urethral pressure (p_{ura}) exceeds the pressure in the bladder (p_{ves}), and whether this is sufficient to protect against leakage. In contrast, during voiding, the outlet needs to be able to relax and thereby open out to a good calibre channel, avoiding impeding the flow of urine. Sometimes, dysfunction of an outlet component (sphincter or bladder neck) or enlargement of the prostate might prevent normal outlet relaxation.

To an extent, urethral function can be inferred from the findings during filling and voiding. Absence of leakage during filling cystometry suggests that urethral function during storage is satisfactory, provided that adequate physical provocation testing is done to provide a genuine challenge to the outlet. Likewise, observation that voiding is unobstructed during the pressure-flow study indicates that full urethral relaxation must have taken place. Nonetheless, greater confidence in the assumptions can be achieved if additional assessments are undertaken to evaluate the

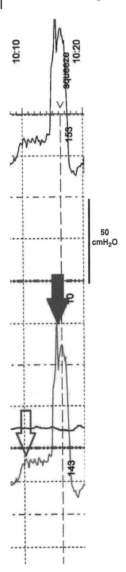

Figure 10.5 A urethral pressure recording taken from the maximum closure pressure point for 10 seconds, demonstrating the resting closure (approx. 90 cmH₂O; open red arrow) and the additional active component when she was asked to 'squeeze'. This generated an extra 50 cmH₂O closure (closed red arrow).

due to prostatic tissue. The pre-sphincteric pressure area blends with the pressure zone attributed to the distal urethral sphincter mechanism, which should be more or less symmetrical. The normal female UPP is symmetrical in shape and reflects the urethral sphincter.

When planning a test in an individual patient, it is sensible to consider what features are likely to be obvious in order to keep a mental track of where in the urethra the catheter eyeholes may have reached. This is to ensure the catheter is not pulled too far, causing it to drop out of the external urethral meatus. The key landmark in women is the urinary sphincter, and it is prudent to stop removing the catheter when the

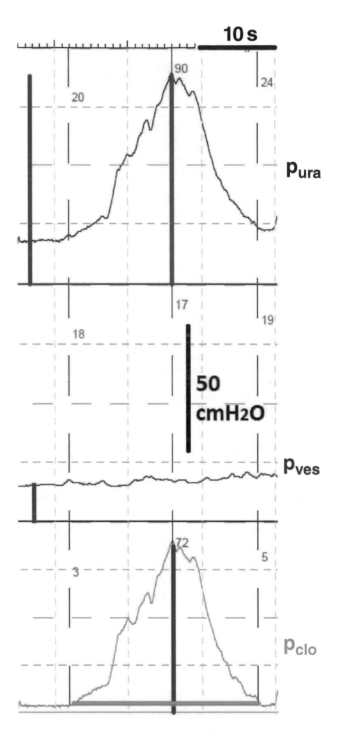

Figure 10.6 Urethral pressure profile nomenclature. Maximum urethral closure pressure (MUCP) (purple lines) is the surplus of the maximum urethral pressure (red line) above the intravesical pressure (blue line). The functional profile length (green bar) is the reserve the urethra has in women to prevent leakage for situations causing a rise in intravesical pressure. Note that the p_{ura} initial value is raised above the p_{ves} by 2 cmH₂O by the pump. This amount needs to be subtracted to obtain MUCP of 70 cmH₂O and MUP of 88 cmH₂O. *Source*: Based on Abrams et al. [4].

profile is showing the downslope at the distal end of the sphincter. For men, the bulbar urethra is often the point beyond which the catheter is not allowed to pass.

To keep note of progress when running a UPP test, distance from the bladder neck is not always reliable, since the start of the outlet may not be very obvious (in women, and men who previously had outlet surgery), and distances vary from person to person. Instead, the UPP features can be identified in sequence (see section on UPP shape below), being careful to ensure that the potential changes in the features are anticipated from the clinical history so that they can actually be recognised (Figure 10.7):

- In men, previous transurethral resection of the prostate means the bladder neck and prostatic plateau are hard to see.
- In men, previous radical prostatectomy means the bladder neck and prostatic plateau are absent.
- In people with SUI, the urinary sphincter profile may be of low amplitude.
- In people with neurological disease, the patient may not be able to contract the pelvic floor.
- In men with neurological disease affecting the sympathetic nervous system, the bladder neck may not be obvious.

Some events can also affect the bladder pressure (Figures 10.8 and 10.9):

1) Detrusor overactivity
2) A person who erroneously contracts abdominal and gluteal muscles when attempting to do a voluntary pelvic floor contraction
   Other factors affecting abdominal pressure
   a) Coughing
   b) Breathing can very occasionally be picked up in the vesical pressure.

Occasionally, the p_{ura} line can show pulsations (Figure 10.10). These might be caused by arterial pulsations, if p_{ura} is high, which is easily checked by feeling the patient's radial pulse. A neurological tremor might also be apparent in p_{ura}. If a peristaltic pump is used for the catheter perfusion, pump artefact might be visible. p_{ura} should not be higher than systolic blood pressure; if so, it is probably an artefact.

UPP Equipment

Figures 10.2, 10.3, and 10.11 illustrate the requirements for urethral closure pressure profile measurement.

A motorised syringe pump (or a very accurate peristaltic pump) is used for the constant-rate perfusion through the catheter. A perfusion rate of between 2 and 10 ml/min gives an accurate measurement. Below 2 ml/min, recording the true urethral pressure is unlikely, since changes in the urethral pressure will be faster than the flow of perfusion can

Figure 10.7 Features on a urethral pressure profile of a woman (left) and a man (right). Sphincter: dark brown arrow; bladder neck: red arrow; prostate: pale brown arrow.

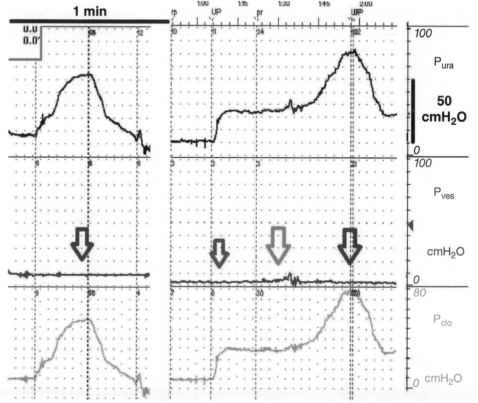

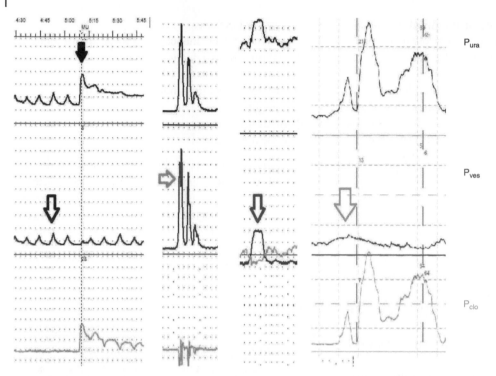

Figure 10.8 The p_{ves} line is usually comparatively featureless in a urethral pressure profilometry, and the principal reason for recording it is to establish resting pressure so that urethral closure pressures can be derived. However, occasionally, it is possible to see the effects of breathing; in the left-hand image, there are numerous small waves caused by breathing (black arrow) and coughing (middle left; orange arrow). As the p_{ura} catheter passes from the bladder into the urethra (closed black arrow) in this male patient, the visible respiratory activity is no longer seen. Coughing (middle left; orange arrow) is visible in the p_{ves} and p_{ura} lines. Likewise, a gluteal contraction caused by someone contracting their buttocks when attempting a sphincter contraction is visible in both the p_{ves} and p_{ura} lines (middle right; purple arrow). Detrusor overactivity (right image; green arrow) can also sometimes be seen.

react to. Above 10 ml/min, it is usually too fast for the perfused liquid to escape, leading to falsely high readings, and discomfort. A motorised 'puller' is most appropriate in order to withdraw the catheter mechanically at a constant speed. Puller speeds are usually 1 or 3 mm/s. Speeds below 7 mm/s are satisfactory when used with perfusion rates of 2–10 ml/min. A speed of 1 mm/s allows easier interpretation and calculation of length of urethra (where the reading is printed on graph paper). The puller needs to be able to disconnect so that the catheter position can be adjusted manually, e.g. for reinserting the catheter after the pull through. Transducers are used to measure the syringe driver pressure (which is used to indicate urethral pressure) and the vesical pressure. The vertical height reference point is the superior edge of the symphysis pubis (as in cystometry). When reporting a UPP clinically, it is necessary to specify the catheter type and size, the measurement technique, the rate of infusion, the rate of catheter withdrawal, the bladder volume, and the position of the patient.

Running a UPP Test

The patient is catheterised using the two-catheter technique described in Chapter 7 (Figure 7.16). Once the catheters have been passed fully into the bladder, the p_{ves} is fixed in position, and the puller mechanism (if used) is connected to the p_{ura} line. The perfusion pump is started and the p_{ura} catheter is pulled back, until the eyeholes start to register the beginning of the bladder outlet. It is then slowly withdrawn, ideally using a constant rate (1 mm/s), observing the expected anatomical features in sequence. The start and end point of each feature can usually be seen during the running of the test. If the withdrawal is done at a constant rate (with a mechanical puller), the distance from the bladder to the feature can be derived by measuring the relevant time points. Before the eyeholes reach the external urethral meatus, the puller is stopped and disconnected so that the catheter can be pushed smoothly back to the bladder by hand. The puller is then restarted to repeat the UPP measurement from start of outlet to beyond the sphincter in order to check the observations are consistent. The final step is to disconnect the puller and advance the catheter back to the sphincter by hand. When in position, the patient is asked to do a pelvic floor contraction, enabling assessment of the voluntary increment in sphincter pressure achieved (Figure 10.5). Thus, the study generally displays two complete in-to-out pull throughs, with an out-to-in

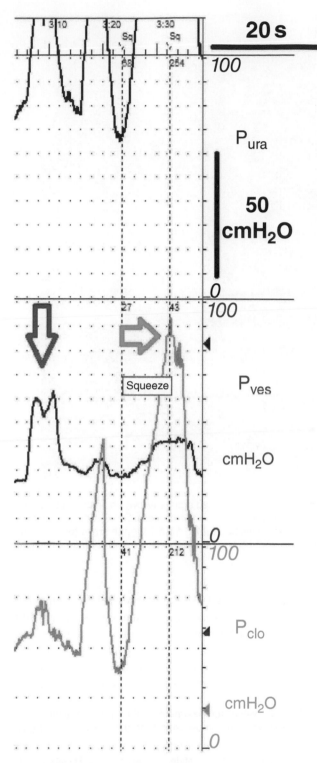

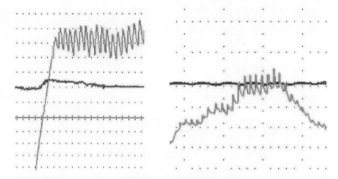

Figure 10.10 Pulsations in p_{ura} caused by the arterial pulse (left) and a tremor caused by cerebellar ataxia (right).

manual reinsertion between, and concludes with a partial reinsertion to the level of the sphincter. Having checked the voluntary sphincter contraction, the catheter is fully reinserted for the filling cystometry. Sometimes, three complete in-to-out pull throughs are conducted, and the MUCP would be calculated from the average of the measurements taken. The various steps can be seen on the full trace of a study (Figure 10.12).

It is easier to perform urethral profiles if the patient is supine, and most tests are performed in this position. The normal response to the assumption of a more upright posture is a small increase in the MUCP. In some patients with abnormal urethral function, this increase may not occur. Indeed, the absence of an increase in pressure on standing may be a diagnostic test for urodynamic stress incontinence [5]. In others, notably some people with neurological disease, the increase in pressure upon standing may be excessive (greater than 100%).

Reproducibility of the UPP

Provided that suitable attention has been paid to details of technique, the results are highly reproducible. There are certain 'normal' variations in the UPP:

1) Pressure variations may be seen, which are most commonly due to voluntary contraction of the urethral or periurethral musculature. If the patient is not relaxed during UPP measurement, the pelvic floor, which lies in close proximity to the urethra, may by its contraction produce a pressure increment along the urethra.

2) If the urethra is sensitive, it is not uncommon for the first urethral profiles to be of a higher pressure because of the failure of the patient to relax. If reproducible profiles cannot be obtained in any particular case, then this is an indication for the performance of a profile which records the maximum urethral pressure with a stationary catheter over a longer period of time.

Figure 10.9 The difference between gluteal and sphincter contraction is seen in this patient attempting sphincter contraction three times, getting better at each attempt. The first attempt (red arrow) is almost entirely due to buttock contraction, the last one is a very strong sphincter contraction (green arrow) with minimal gluteal contribution. Accordingly, careful description of what is being requested and a chance to try more than once are necessary to evaluate voluntary sphincter contraction.

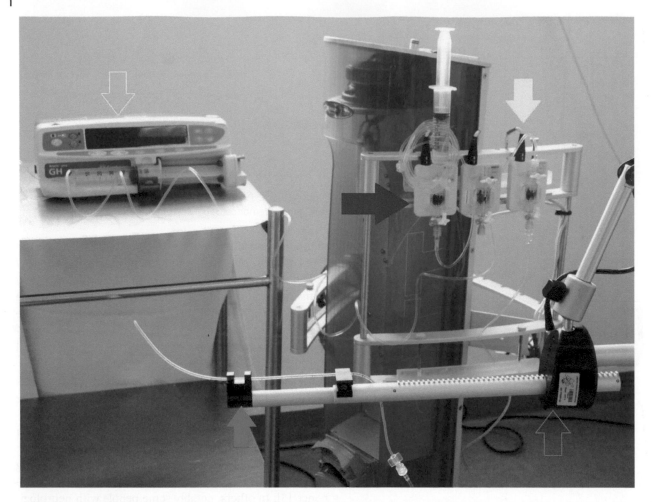

Figure 10.11 Photograph of a urethral pressure profile setup. The catheter is mounted (closed orange arrow) on an arm with a puller mechanism (open orange arrow) which can move the catheter forwards and backwards at controlled speeds. Connection tubing joins the catheter to the p_{ura} pressure transducer (solid yellow arrow), which receives connection tubing from a syringe driver (open yellow arrow). Along with p_{ura}, p_{ves} is measured; the purple arrow indicates the connection tubing, transducer and flushing syringe placed in readiness. *Source*: Marcus Drake.

Interpreting the UPP

MUCP

The figures for normal urethral pressures in the available literature are all taken from very small series. Table 10.1 reports values taken from a large number of our patients who have been assessed and considered to be both clinically and urodynamically normal, recorded in a supine position with the bladder empty. Adequate information on normal pressures in other postures and for other bladder volumes is not available. This does limit the value of UPP measurement because it is the urethral response to bladder filling and postural change which may be most important in diagnosis. Others have described a normal MUCP in women as a simple calculation, subtracting the patient's age from 92 [6].

More recent review of the urodynamic database in Bristol evaluating only women identified a clear decline in MUCP with ageing [1] (Table 10.2), notably after the menopause. The very low values in older women are also described in other centres [7]. In the female, the functional urethral length also tends to decrease with ageing. It is evident that there is a wide overlap between the range for normal

Table 10.1 Values for maximum urethral pressure (cmH$_2$O) in patients in whom no urodynamic abnormality was been found.

	Male		Female	
Age (years)	Mean	Range	Mean	Range
<25	75	37–126	90	55–103
25–44	79	35–113	82	31–115
45–64	75	40–123	74	40–100
>64	71	35–105	65	35–75

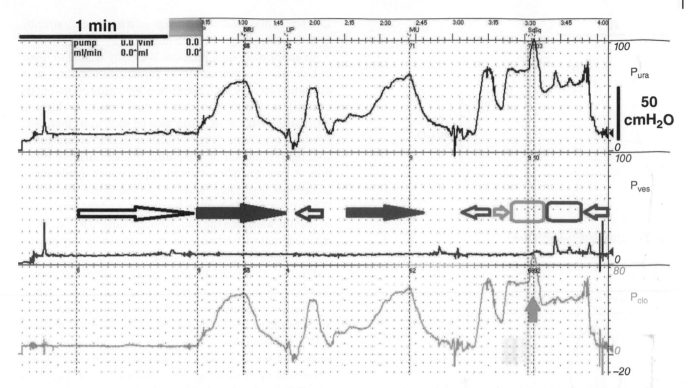

Figure 10.12 The trace from a complete urethral pressure profilometry in a woman. Right-facing arrows represent in-to-out pulls of the p_{ura} catheter, and left-facing are out-to-in movements. The black arrow shows the p_{ura} catheter in the bladder being pulled outwards. The brown closed arrow is the first full-profile recording. The open brown arrow is the manual reinsertion preparatory for the second full-profile recording (closed purple arrow). The open purple arrow is a manual reinsertion, and the open green arrow is bringing the p_{ura} catheter to the level of the external urethral sphincter. It is held at the sphincter (green rectangle) to allow the test of voluntary sphincter contraction (closed green arrow), which concludes the profilometry. The red rectangle is when the puller is being disconnected from the p_{ura} catheter, and the red arrow is manual reinsertion. The end of the trace shows p_{ura} catheter measuring vesical pressure, and the catheters are in position ready to transition to filling cystometry.

urethral parameters and for abnormal situations, e.g. stress incontinence. This means that MUCP on its own is not a suitable technique to constitute a diagnostic test (at least in women [1]). In the male, the maximum urethral pressure

Table 10.2 Mean and 95% confidence interval values for maximum urethral closure pressure (cmH_2O) in continent and incontinent women.

Age (years)	USI	USI+DOI	DOI	Continent
20–29	70 (64–77)	68 (59–78)	91 (88–94)	92 (88–97)
30–39	61 (59–64)	65 (62–68)	84 (82–86)	81 (78–84)
40–49	54 (53–56)	57 (55–59)	74 (72–75)	73 (70–75)
50–59	48 (47–50)	51 (49–53)	63 (62–65)	61 (59–63)
60–69	39 (38–41)	43 (41–45)	53 (51–55)	54 (51–57)
70–79	33 (31–35)	34 (31–37)	43 (40–45)	47 (36–45)
80+	27 (22–32)	35 (29–41)	40 (35–45)	40 (30–50)

Source: Kapoor et al. [1].
USI: urodynamic stress incontinence; DOI: detrusor overactivity incontinence.

does not decline significantly with age. In the male, the prostatic length tends to increase with age.

UPP Shape

Abnormalities may be classified according to the part of the urethra affected and the sex of the patient. Pre-sphincteric abnormalities in male patients are usually seen with bladder neck or prostatic problems. A peak in the midprostatic region may be related to the meeting of the lateral lobes caused by prostate enlargement due to benign prostatic hyperplasia. Commonly, the prostatic plateau may be elevated or elongated (Figure 10.13). This plateau may be flat, or there may be a prostatic peak between the bladder neck and the distal urethral sphincter mechanism. The significance of this peak is uncertain. If it is at the region of the bladder neck, then it is sometimes due to bladder neck hypertrophy. A bladder neck peak may also occur on penile erection. Pre-sphincteric abnormalities in the female are usually produced by a past history of surgery, where an elongation is related to operations to treat SUI (Figure 10.14).

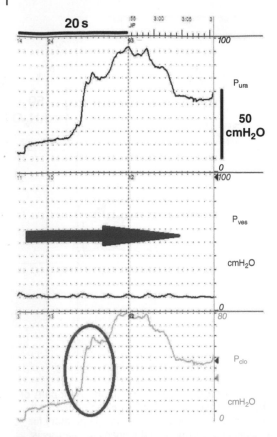

Figure 10.13 An enlarged prostate can show up during urethral pressure profile as elevation of the 'prostatic plateau'. In this case, it was a residual unresected part of the prostate after previous transurethral resection of the prostate, here highlighted in red. The brown arrow indicates in-to-out movement of the catheter.

Sphincteric abnormalities are evident in the area of the main urethral pressure peak, which is at the midurethra in the female and just near the prostatic apex in the male.

Low pressure is related to damage (often surgical), atrophy, or denervation (Figures 10.15 and 10.16).

An abnormally high pressure is usually related to involuntary sphincter overactivity or pelvic floor contraction. In the latter case, the high pressure is seen only on voluntary contraction when the pressure may reach as high as 300 cmH$_2$O. High MUCP can also be seen in women with Fowler's syndrome (Figure 10.17), which is idiopathic voiding dysfunction or idiopathic painless urinary retention in younger adult women [8]. Fowler's syndrome is sometimes associated with polycystic ovary syndrome. While the urinary retention is painless, catheterisation can be painful, and often the pain is elicited after a few seconds, meaning that withdrawing the catheter can be very painful even if placing it was not. MUCP in these cases is over 100 cmH$_2$O. Conventional urodynamic testing is characterised by a reduced sensation on filling, but otherwise normal bladder pressures, and no observed voiding contraction. Since women with SUI may also have pelvic organ prolapse (POP), it is sometimes necessary to undertake urodynamic evaluation with a pessary in place to reduce the POP and ensure full understanding of sphincter function. The effect on sphincter function before and after pessary placement can be evaluated during UPP assessment (Figure 10.18). Occasionally, a urethro-vaginal fistula may be detected on a UPP, visible as a drop in pressure between two peaks, since the perfused saline is easily able to escape through the fistula. Figure 10.19 illustrates a UPP with a very small urethro-vaginal fistula; a large fistula will generally make the UPP undetectable, since the perfused saline simply escapes through the defect.

In men after radical prostatectomy, the complete removal of the prostate requires anastomosis of the bladder base to the

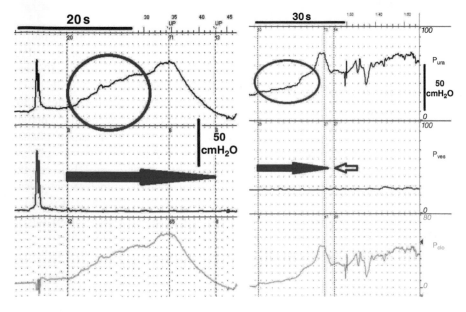

Figure 10.14 Urethral pressure profiles for two women who previously underwent stress urinary incontinence surgery. The closed brown arrows indicate in-to-out movement of the catheter, and the open brown arrow out-to-in movement. On the left: colposuspension, illustrating an elongation of the pre-sphincteric component of the functional profile (brown oval). On the right: a woman who had an autologous fascial sling, showing an elongation of the functional urethral length, and a step-up at the site of the sling (brown oval), just proximal to the sphincter. This lady could not achieve a voluntary sphincter contraction.

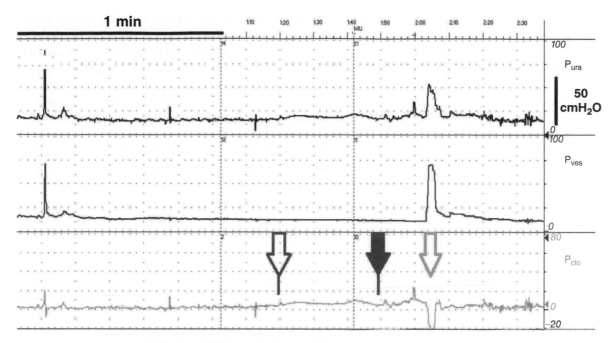

Figure 10.15 A urethral pressure profile for a man who had TURP where prostate cancer was identified, and who, therefore, underwent radical radiotherapy. He had severe stress urinary incontinence, and this corresponded with almost total absence of resting urethral contraction; the extent of the functional profile is indicated by the purple arrows (open arrow at the start, closed at the end). The green arrow indicates a gluteal contraction when he was asked to contract his sphincter.

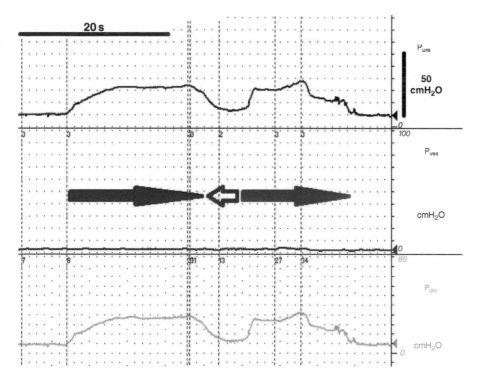

Figure 10.16 A urethral pressure profile for a 37-year-old woman with severe stress urinary incontinence following a complicated obstetric history. Two profiles are shown, each having a severe reduction in maximum urethral closure pressure. The closed brown arrow indicates in-to-out movement of the catheter, and the open brown arrow out-to-in movement; the difference in length between these arrows is because different speeds were used while doing the study- the catheter was pulled out slowly, and pushed back in quickly. The slower the puller speed, the longer the profile length. Hence, it is important to specify the puller speed to allow accurate measurement of the functional profile length.

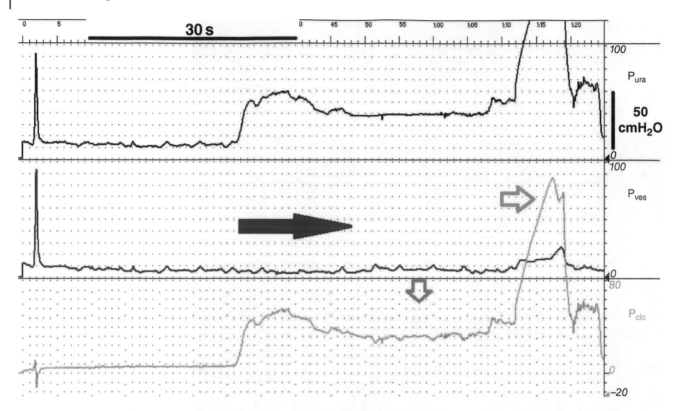

Figure 10.21 A severely incontinent man with previous radical prostatectomy. The functional profile is shown by the closed brown arrow, illustrating markedly reduced maximum urethral closure pressure. The orange arrow indicates pressure in the bulbar urethra. The green arrow shows that he had excellent voluntary sphincter/pelvic floor contraction.

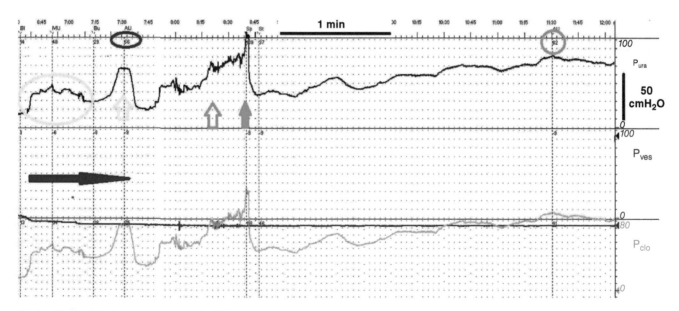

Figure 10.22 Urethral pressure profile (UPP) in a man with stress urinary incontinence after previous radical prostatectomy, treated with a subsequent artificial urinary sphincter (AUS). The brown arrow indicates a UPP made up of a plateau caused by a rather tight vesico-urethral anastomosis (yellow oval) and the AUS in its inactivated state. The P_{ura} catheter was then held at the location of the AUS (open green arrow), and the AUS was activated; this requires a sharp squeeze on the pump AUS component, which causes a short pressure spike (closed green arrow). As a result of activation, the pressure reservoir AUS component is able to fill the cuff, a slow process, indicated by the steadily rising pressure in the following three minutes. Before activation, the urethral pressure was 66 cm H_2O (yellow arrow), and it peaked at 82 afterwards (green circle). Thus, the additional active contribution provided by the pressure reservoir was a rather low 16 cmH_2O.

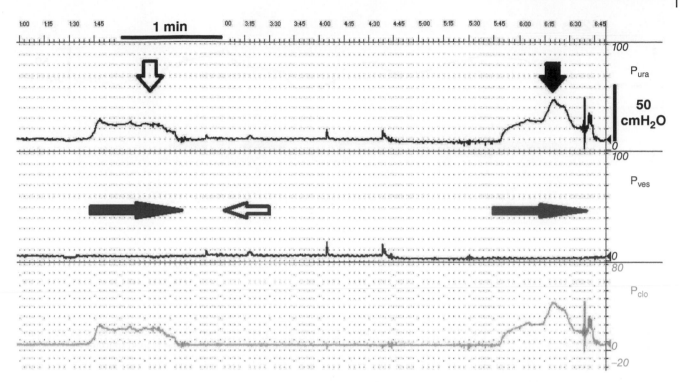

Figure 10.23 Urethral pressure profiles in another man with stress urinary incontinence after previous radical prostatectomy, treated with a subsequent artificial urinary sphincter (AUS), before (brown arrow), and after (purple arrow) AUS activation. The open (inactivated) and closed (activated) black arrows indicate the AUS location. Again, the additional active contribution was rather low at around 20 cmH$_2$O.

Urethral Leak Point Pressure Measurement

Abdominal Leak Point Pressure

This technique seeks to define overall urethral function in terms of the intravesical pressure at which urine starts to leak from the urethra. The abdominal leak point pressure can be divided into a cough leak point pressure (CLPP) and Valsalva leak point pressure (VLPP). It is defined as the intravesical pressure at which urine leakage occurs due to increased abdominal pressure in the absence of a detrusor contraction. The Valsalva manoeuvre (expiration against the closed glottis) is the easiest and most controlled way of achieving a graded increase in intravesical pressure. If the concept of a Valsalva is difficult to communicate to the patient, we sometimes ask them to seal their lips around the end of a syringe and exhale, as if trying to blow the plunger out (akin to blowing up a party balloon) or blowing against the back of their hand. Assessing VLPP requires some assumptions; firstly that the urethral catheter does not significantly alter the seal of the urethra, secondly that straining does not produce urethral distortion (falsely elevating the VLPP), and finally that there is no pelvic floor relaxation or contraction during the test. An example is illustrated in Figure 10.25.

VLPP measurement provides an assessment of dynamic pelvic floor function, in contrast to the static nature of UPP [10]. While the technique has not been examined as closely as UPP from the technical point of view, it is clear that there is an association between poor urethral function and a low VLPP. The VLPP has been used to identify those women with USI who have intrinsic sphincter deficiency (Table 10.3) rather than urethral hypermobility as the cause of their incontinence [11]. This can influence what type of operation may be chosen for treatment (e.g. autologous sling or AUS).

Table 10.3 Comparison of Valsalva leak point pressure (VLPP) and maximum urethral closure pressure (MUCP) in differentiating between intrinsic sphincter deficiency and urethral hypermobility in women.

	VLPP	MUCP
Urethral hypermobility	>90 cmH$_2$O	>20 cmH$_2$O
Equivocal	60–90 cmH$_2$O	
Intrinsic sphincter deficiency	<60 cmH$_2$O	≤20 cmH$_2$O

Source: Based on Park et al. [11].

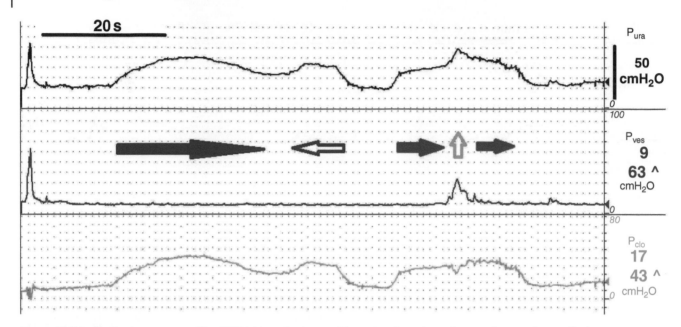

Figure 10.24 Urethral pressure profiles (UPPs) in another man with stress urinary incontinence after previous radical prostatectomy, treated with a subsequent male sling operation. Two UPPs were done, indicated by the solid arrows. The second (purple) was interrupted with a short pause to evaluate voluntary sphincter squeeze (green arrow); this showed only gluteal contraction.

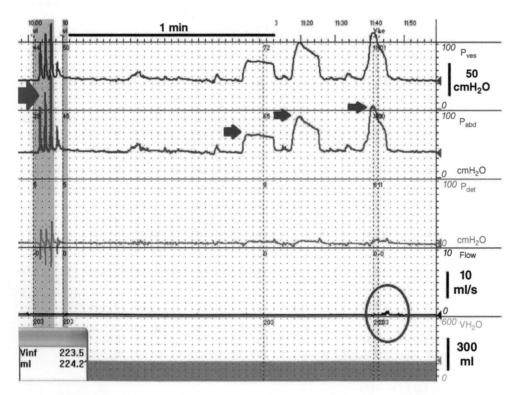

Figure 10.25 Demonstrated urodynamic stress incontinence in a man where a series of high-amplitude coughs (red arrow) has failed to show incontinence. A series of Valsalva manoeuvres of increasing amplitude (purple arrows) was undertaken, the biggest of which caused a leak (purple oval). Accordingly, the abdominal leak point pressure was between the amplitudes of the two bigger Valsalvas (the exact value is uncertain, since the precise moment of leakage is hard to ascertain when pressure change is swift). This trace does not comply with current International Continence Society expectations that p_{ves} and p_{det} should be displayed lower down on the display.

Detrusor Leak Point Pressure

The detrusor leak point pressure (DLPP) is defined as the lowest detrusor pressure at which leakage occurs in the absence of either a detrusor contraction or increased abdominal pressure. An example is illustrated in Figure 10.26. DLPP assessment is a factor in deciding risk of damage to renal function in patients with a poorly compliant detrusor. A threshold of $40\,cmH_2O$ is commonly used, based in the seminal work of McGuire evaluating patients with myelodysplasia [12, 13]. However, there is not much information across the full spectrum of patients, and thresholds for risk have not been standardised [14].

Indications for Urethral Function Testing

The measurement of static UPP has several uses:

- In postprostatectomy incontinence, there is a close association between sphincter damage and reduction in MUCP. UPP can also be used in assessment of an AUS that is failing to control leakage despite a device that appears to be functioning from the point of view of fluid transfer in the device pump.

- In women with USI, there is some evidence that a preoperative MUCP of less than $20\,cmH_2O$ is associated with poor outcome of SUI surgery. This suggests that UPP assessment may define a group of women who require a degree of obstruction to be introduced in order to become continent when surgery is undertaken. In so doing, they may then be at risk of voiding dysfunction, and hence could require training in intermittent self-catheterisation pre-operatively.

- In women with unexplained incontinence, measurement of MUCP for a period of minutes may suggest inappropriate urethral relaxation incontinence. This might be a feature in people with incontinence after neobladder formation.

- In patients being considered for undiversion (a rare procedure in current practice), the MUCP gives a good indication as to whether implantation of an artificial sphincter or bladder neck suspension is necessary. If the MUCP is greater than $50\,cmH_2O$, then the patient will probably be continent if a good volume, low-pressure reservoir is created.

- In women with voiding dysfunction/Fowler's syndrome, where the MUCP may be over $100\ cmH_2O$, perhaps indicating that sacral neuromodulation may be helpful.

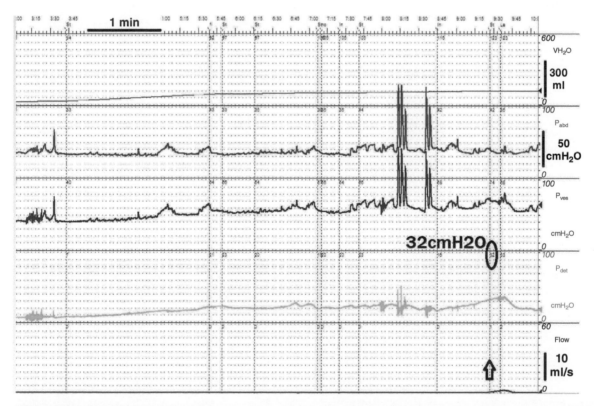

Figure 10.26 Detrusor leak point pressure in a man with a poorly compliant detrusor. The start of the leak is indicated by the black arrow, and at that moment, detrusor pressure was $32\ cmH_2O$; hence, this is the DLPP. This point arguably could coincide with detrusor overactivity, in which case the phrase 'detrusor overactivity leak point' could be applied (see Chapter 16 for further discussion about leak points); either way, the presence of leakage at such a low p_{det} is clearly abnormal.

References

1. Kapoor, D.S. et al. (2012). *Maximum urethral closure pressure in women: normative data and evaluation as a diagnostic test. Int. Urogynecol. J.* 23 (11): 1613–1618.

2. Griffiths, D. (1985). *The pressure within a collapsed tube, with special reference to urethral pressure. Phys. Med. Biol.* 30 (9): 951–963.

3. Brown, M. and Wickham, J.E.A. (1969). *The urethral pressure profile. Br. J. Urol.* 41: 211–217.

4. Abrams, P. et al. (2002). *The standardisation of terminology of lower urinary tract function: report from the standardisation sub-committee of the international continence society. Neurourol. Urodyn.* 21 (2): 167–178.

5. Tanagho, E.A. (1979). *Urodynamics of female urinary incontinence with emphasis on stress incontinence. J. Urol.* 122 (2): 200–204.

6. Edwards, L. and Malvern, J. (1974). *The urethral pressure profile: theoretical considerations and clinical application. Br. J. Urol.* 46 (3): 325–335.

7. Edwards, L.E. (1973). *The investigation and management of incontinence of urine in women. Ann. R. Coll. Surg. Engl.* 52 (2): 69–85.

8. DasGupta, R. and Fowler, C.J. (2004). *Urodynamic study of women in urinary retention treated with sacral neuromodulation. J. Urol.* 171 (3): 1161–1164.

9. Ulmsten, U., Asmussen, M., and Lindstrom, K. (1977). *A new technique for simultaneous urethrocystometry including measurements of the urethral pressure profile. Urol. Int.* 32 (2–3): 127–136.

10. Martan, A. et al. (2007). *Weak VLPP and MUCP correlation and their relationship with objective and subjective measures of severity of urinary incontinence. Int. Urogynecol. J. Pelvic Floor Dysfunct.* 18 (3): 267–271.

11. Park, K.K. et al. (2017). *A study of clinical predictors associated with intrinsic sphincter deficiency in women with stress urinary incontinence. Int. Neurourol. J.* 21 (2): 139–142.

12. McGuire, E.J. et al. (1981). *Prognostic value of urodynamic testing in myelodysplastic patients. J. Urol.* 126 (2): 205–209.

13. McGuire, E.J. et al. (1981). *Prognostic value of urodynamic testing in myelodysplastic patients. J. Urol.*, 2002. 167 (2 Pt 2): 1049–1053; discussion 1054.

14. Tarcan, T. et al. (2017). *Is 40 cm H2 O detrusor leak point pressure cut-off reliable for upper urinary tract protection in children with myelodysplasia? Neurourol. Urodyn.* 36 (3): 759–763.

11

Non-invasive Urodynamics

Alison Bray[1], Christopher Blake[2], and Christopher Harding[3]

[1] *Northern Medical Physics and Clinical Engineering Department, The Newcastle upon Tyne Hospitals NHS Foundation Trust, Royal Victoria Infirmary, Newcastle upon Tyne, UK*
[2] *Urology Department, Royal Cornwall Hospital, Truro, Cornwall, UK*
[3] *Urology Department, Freeman Hospital, Newcastle upon Tyne Hospitals NHS Foundation Trust, Newcastle upon Tyne, UK*

CONTENTS

Introduction

Standard urodynamics testing involves catheterisation and is comparatively expensive. Consequently, various groups have explored the possibilities of less invasive techniques to support clinical assessment and diagnosis, to aid clinical discussion with patients, and to better predict outcomes from treatment. The main aim of the majority of these non invasive techniques has been to look at novel ways of diagnosing bladder outlet obstruction (BOO) in men. The novel techniques that have been studied broadly fall into two categories [1]:

- Measures of established urodynamic parameters, typically an assessment of isovolumetric bladder pressure during voiding, which can be combined with a flow rate to give pressure-flow information.
- Other variables that may be related to BOO.

Some of these are already done routinely in some settings, such as free flow rate testing (discussed in Chapter 6), but many are still experimental. The first half of this chapter describes and summarises the evidence surrounding the following eight non-invasive urodynamic techniques: Doppler ultrasound, near-infrared spectroscopy (NIRS), bladder wall thickness (BWT), intravesical prostatic protrusion, penile cuff test, condom catheter, urethral connector, and penile compression-release (PCR). For these, the current evidence base allows estimation of test performance (Table 11.1). However, this evidence is rather patchy due to heterogeneity of definitions and thresholds for index tests and reference standards [2]. The second half of the chapter provides practical information and examples for the penile cuff test, which is a commercially available non-invasive urodynamic system (UroCuff® Test, https://www.srsmedical.com/the-urocuff-test, SRS Medical Systems, Inc. North Billerica, MA 01862 US) in use in many centres.

Non-invasive Urodynamic Techniques

Doppler Ultrasound

Doppler ultrasound works by projecting high-frequency sound waves and detecting reflections from moving elements, which in the flowmetry context are microbubbles in the flowing urine. By using transperineal ultrasound to measure flow velocity in the prostatic urethra, its cross-sec-

Table 11.1 Summary of performance of non-invasive urodynamic tests derived from systematic review of published literature.

Test	Studies (n)	Pts (n)	Sensitivity Median (IQR)	Sensitivity Range	Specificity Median (IQR)	Specificity Range	Positive predictive value Median (IQR)	Positive predictive value Range	Negative predictive value Median (IQR)	Negative predictive value Range
Penile cuff test	7	546	88.89 (76.5–95.3)	64–100	70.2 (64.5–78.3)	55.6–84	69 (67.9–72.5)	66.7–92	93 (89.2–100)	78–100
Uroflowmetry	16	2580	72 (58.4–89.9)	16–100	64 (38.5–81)	25–100	70 (57.5–79)	32.5–100	70 (57.7–85.2)	46.5–100
DWT	8	848	69 (64–82.8)	43–100	88 (72–93.8)	15–100	89.5 (82.7–93.1)	64–100	75.5 (63.8–85.7)	50–100
Bladder weight	2	258	73.6	61.9–85.3	73.45	59.8–87.1	60.85	33.8–87.9	83.5	82.6–84.4
ECC	1	56	90.9		92.3		96.7		80	
IPP	10	1013	75.5 (60.9–80)	46–95	78.5 (69.2–81.3)	50–92	73.8 (72.4–85)	69.6–100	69.6 (69–85)	46–85.1
Doppler US	2	51	No data	No data	No data	No data	97.5 (96.2–98.7)	95–100	57	No data
Prostate volume	3	245	72 (61.5–79.5)	51–87	38 (33.8–49.5)	29.6–61	65 (58.1–74.5)	51.3–84	44 (43–58.3)	42–72.7
NIRS	5	282	85.71 (68.3–86)	61.1–100	87.5 (62.5–87.5)	40–87.5	88.89 (82.7–892)	78.6–93.8	84 (42.9–85.71)	22.2–100

Pts: patients; IQR: interquartile range; DWT: detrusor wall thickness; ECC: external condom catheter; IPP: intravesical prostatic protrusion; US: ultrasound; NIRS: near-infrared spectroscopy.
Source: Malde et al. [2].

tional area can be estimated [3]. A small study by the developers showed good correlation between 'velocity ratio' (the ratio of distal to proximal urethral flow velocity) at maximum flow rate (Q_{max}) and BOO index ($p_{detQmax}-2Q_{max}$), with Spearman's rho of 0.73 and $p < 0.001$ [4]. All men with a ratio above 1.6 were obstructed, and all below 1.0 were equivocal or unobstructed. Further research is needed both to further validate this technique and to confirm the proposed thresholds when larger numbers of men are tested.

Near-Infrared Spectroscopy

NIRS is a way to study changes in bladder perfusion and oxygenation, which can show significant reduction as a result of voiding in the presence of BOO [5]. The imaging modality uses an infrared-emitting and -detecting abdominal patch and can detect the oxygenated and deoxygenated haemoglobin in bladder tissue quantitatively. From this, it is possible to derive blood flow. BOO in conventional urodynamics relies on high pressure associated with slow flow; this high pressure should decrease blood flow more substantially, so, in theory, it is an indirect measure of pressure. However, a study evaluating 87 men with lower urinary tract symptoms (LUTS) found the accuracy of an NIRS-derived measure combined with Q_{max} and post-void residual to diagnose BOO to be relatively poor (67%) [6]. Again, this technique is not appropriate for widespread uptake based on current knowledge.

Anatomical Techniques

Anatomical measurements to determine whether BOO is present rely on an indirect assumption that the structural change is a direct cause or consequence of the physiological change. It necessitates an assumption that other influences play a modest role in the structural changes.

Bladder Wall Thickness

Anatomical measurements of BWT assume that the work required for the bladder to empty past substantial resistance leads to detrusor hypertrophy. On the face of it, this makes sense, but additional factors might also be relevant; for example, a background of detrusor overactivity might also cause hypertrophy potentially unrelated to BOO. The hypertrophy is potentially reversible following relief of the obstruction. Quantification of BWT by transabdominal ultrasound has thus been proposed to evaluate BOO. Modern technology can enable measurement of detrusor wall thickness (DWT) (Figure 11.1), which might be important as hypertrophy of the urothelium can also be caused by mechanisms independent of BOO, such as urinary tract infections. Unfortunately, BWT and DWT might be affected by bladder

volume. This is because a more distended bladder must have the wall stretched out to a greater extent. An attempt to address this has been made by estimating bladder weight [7].

These are relatively new approaches which lack standardisation of technique and diagnostic thresholds. This has led to conflicting evidence of utility [8], with one study reporting DWT ≥2 mm to diagnose BOO with 89% accuracy in 160 men with LUTS [9], whilst another failed to measure any difference between symptomatic and asymptomatic populations [10].

Intravesical Prostatic Protrusion

The extent to which the prostate protrudes into the base of the bladder can be estimated using either transabdominal or transrectal routes. Here, the anatomical measurement assumes that the structural change (prostate enlargement) is a direct cause of the physiological change (BOO). This is not clear-cut, since the enlargement of the prostate is not necessarily proportionate to the effect on the prostatic urethra. Specifically, a relatively small enlargement may cause BOO if it is principally sited nearby the urethra. Conversely, considerable enlargement may have minimal obstructing effect if it is outward-directed. Sensitivity and specificity of 67% and 81% in diagnosing BOO have been reported for the threshold 5.5 mm [11], rising to 75% and 83%, respectively, for 8.5 mm [12]. Clearly, the thresholds (and underlying assumptions) are crucial, and the techniques have to be easily communicated for replication in other centres, so this approach is not routine practice currently.

Isovolumetric Techniques

Non-invasive isovolumetric measurements estimate bladder pressure under conditions which restrict flow ($p_{ves.isv}$). These are appealing because they aim to avoid the dependence of pressure on flow. This gives a theoretical maximum pressure that the bladder can generate, as detrusor pressure rises in response to the outlet closing. On a practical level, these techniques tend to require several centimetres of penile shaft and so are not suitable for all men. Further, the pressure measurements are related to intravesical rather than detrusor pressure, so these are of less value and can be compromised by abdominal straining.

Condom Catheter

Patients are asked to void into a modified incontinence sheath, which is a semi-rigid plastic 'condom' sealed to the penis and connected to a system of tubing (Figure 11.2). This allows both the flow of urine and pressurisation. The outlet is then closed, meaning that, as the condom fills with urine, the pressure will rise until it equalises with that in the bladder, and flow will cease. This technique allows a direct meas-

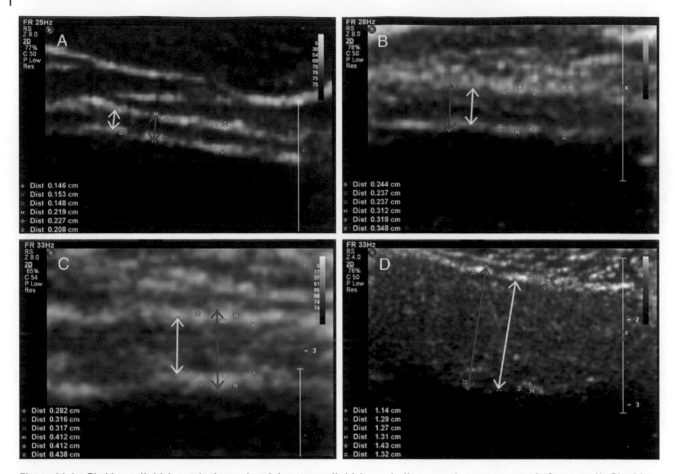

Figure 11.1 Bladder wall thickness (red arrow) and detrusor wall thickness (yellow arrow) measurements in four men (A–D) with urinary symptoms, at bladder filling volume of 250 ml. Patient A had symptoms but no obstruction. Patients B to D had LUTS and increasing severity of BOO. A–C, reduced from ×8. D, reduced from ×4. *Source*: Marcus Drake.

urement of $p_{ves.isv}$. The design of the condom catheter has had to overcome problems with leaking and prolonged duration of pressure equalisation, which can lead to inhibition of the voiding contraction. Accuracy is worse at low flow rates, which clearly is a disadvantage when dealing with BOO assessment. More recent studies used a condom catheter in which the outflow resistance can be varied in order to

extrapolate $p_{ves.isv}$ mathematically. It gives greater confidence that the pressure in the condom more accurately reflects the pressure in the bladder. This method will accurately diagnose BOO in around 70% of patients, but test failure for technical reasons is an important problem. Diagnostic performance may be no better than uroflowmetry [13].

Urethral Connector

The urethral connector device involves the patient employing a 'digital manoeuvre' to interrupt flow during voiding [14]. It is somewhat invasive as it requires insertion of a portion of tubing into the distal urethra and measurement of abdominal pressure by a rectal manometry catheter. The developers of the technique reported sensitivity and specificity to diagnose BOO of 67% and 79% [14]. At present, this investigation requires considerable further research before it can be considered diagnostically useful.

Penile Compression-Release

Essentially a manual equivalent of the tests above, the patient occludes their urethra after the onset of flow by

— **Condom catheter**

— **Pressure transducer**

— **Outlet closed manually during voiding**

Figure 11.2 Schematic diagram of the condom catheter method. *Source*: Blake and Abrams [1].

compressing the penile shaft. Once compression is released, a characteristic flow pattern results, with a surge of flow (Q_{surge}) as urine is expelled from the distended urethra. This then settles to a more normal steady state flow (Q_s). Analysis of these flow patterns suggests that the magnitude of change in flow rate between Q_{surge} and Q_s is determined by the magnitude of $p_{ves.isv}$. Patients with BOO tend to have a high Q_{surge} and low Q_s, whereas those with detrusor underactivity (DUA) during voiding have both a low Q_{surge} and low Q_s. These patterns are reliable as long as the flow controlling zone is proximal to the urethral compression, e.g. prostatic obstruction, but no surge is seen if the flow controlling zone is distal, e.g. meatal stenosis. The PCR index was defined as the surge increase as a proportion of steady flow: $(Q_{surge}-Q_s)/Q_s$. An index of 1 (a surge doubling steady flow) had sensitivity and specificity 91% and 70%, the index being higher in patients with BOO [15].

The Penile Cuff Test

Penile Cuff Test

Using a technique analogous with non-invasive sphygmomanometry (blood pressure measurement), this test estimates isovolumetric bladder pressure by interrupting urine flow with an automated pneumatic penile cuff (Figure 11.3). The resulting maximum cuff interruption pressure ($P_{cuff.int}$) is combined with Q_{max} from the same test in order to diagnose BOO using a bespoke nomogram [16]. In the automated setting, PCR index of 1.6 was shown to have sensitivity of 78% and specificity of 84% for diagnosing BOO [17]. $P_{cuff.int}$ has shown relatively poor agreement with simultaneously measured intravesical pressure, with

standard deviation of 28 cmH$_2$O [18]. However, a recent review presented median sensitivity and specificity to diagnose BOO of 88% and 75%, respectively, [2], indicating good diagnostic performance.

In addition to diagnostic accuracy, the ability of the penile cuff test to predict outcome from endoscopic prostatectomy was investigated in a consecutive cohort of 208 men. Good outcome from surgery was defined as a 50% or greater reduction in International Prostate Symptom Score. Men categorised by the penile cuff test as obstructed had an 87% chance of a good outcome from surgery, whilst those deemed not obstructed had a 56% chance (both had $p < 0.01$ when compared to the whole group, 77% of whom experienced good outcome) [19].

Practicalities of the Penile Cuff Test

The cuff test should be performed when the patient feels the normal desire to pass urine following natural bladder filling.

Explaining the Test

The principle of the cuff test can be explained to the patient using the analogy of non-invasive sphygmomanometry. The penile cuff inflates to stop urine flow in order to measure bladder pressure, instead of stopping flow in the blood vessels of the arm to measure blood pressure.

Once the cuff is fitted, the patient passes urine into the flowmeter. Once flow is detected, the cuff inflates until flow stops (or cuff pressure reaches its limit). The cuff then deflates to allow flow to resume, and this cycle repeats, usually several times, until there is no resumption of flow.

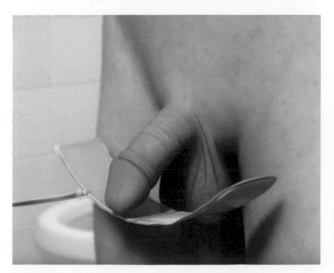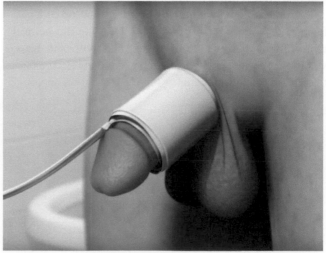

Figure 11.3 Illustration of the setup for the penile cuff test. The cuff should be fitted as close to the body as possible, ideally with the glans visible at the end. *Source*: Marcus Drake.

Stress to the patient the importance of not straining their abdominal muscles during the test. The sensation of flow slowing and then stopping artificially may cause a strong desire to do so, but straining compromises the measurement. Inflation of the cuff around the penis is an unusual sensation, which may sting, but is generally well tolerated. Around 2% of men notice a small amount of blood in their urine after the test [19].

Fitting the Cuff and Conducting the Test

The cuff should be fitted as close to the body as possible, ideally with the glans visible at the end (Figure 11.3). It may help to fit the cuff whilst the patient lies on his back and to push gently against his lower abdomen to lengthen the shaft. Placing tape around the cuff circumference can prevent the Velcro, or its adhesive, becoming unstuck during the test. It is possible to fit a penile cuff for most men but might not be feasible for those with a short penile length. The longest cuff that it is possible to fit should be used [20]. Once the cuff is in place, it can be connected to the pneumatic port on the machine, the test can be started, and the patient given permission to void. It is useful to remind the patient again at this point not to strain.

Interpreting the Test

Example cuff test time series data are shown in Figure 11.4. Flow rate, shown in black, decreases to zero as cuff pressure, shown in orange, increases. When the flowmeter detects the absence of flow, the cuff deflates. This causes a surge in flow due to the release of urine stored in the proximal urethra and the increase in bladder pressure under isovolumetric conditions. Flow then returns to a steady state, and this cycle repeats.

The measurements required for interpretation of a cuff test are Q_{max} and maximum $P_{cuff.int}$. Q_{max} should be read ignoring the post-deflation surges, and with the usual smoothing-by-eye of high-frequency changes that applies to conventional uroflowmetry. Figure 11.4 shows an example of Q_{max} marked in blue. $P_{cuff.int}$ is read from pressure versus flow plots for each inflation and then the maximum value chosen. Before doing so, invalid inflations must be excluded. An inflation cycle is invalid if:

- Flow does not surge after cuff deflation (for example, the last two inflations on Figure 11.4; there is no clear flow surge following each inflation as there is after the first two), implying that the cuff was not restricting flow.
- The flow trace is erratic, making cuff interruption pressure difficult to determine from the pressure-flow plot (Figure 11.5). This may be due to the patient straining their abdominal muscles or knocking the flowmeter.

On occasion, flow is not interrupted, i.e. the flow rate is not reduced to zero despite the cuff pressure reaching its limit (Figure 11.6). This means that the pressure required to interrupt flow is an unknown value above $200\,cmH_2O$. The inflation is still usable (unless the cuff has come off) by equating $P_{cuff.int}$ to $200\,cmH_2O$, as a value above this would not change the interpretation.

$P_{cuff.int}$, the cuff pressure required to stop flow, should be measured for all valid inflations. This is done by examining the point at which flow drops to zero on a graph of pressure versus flow and fitting a line to the approximately straight portion of the plot up to this point. $P_{cuff.int}$ is the point at which this straight line intersects the horizontal axis. Figure 11.7 shows three examples, where $P_{cuff.int}$ is 115, 133, and $127\,cmH_2O$, respectively. Small portions of very low flow at the highest pressure (indicated by the arrow on Figure 11.7, inflation 1) can be ignored; this is due to flow from urine in the distal urethra after the cuff has closed the urethra more proximally.

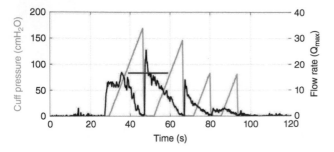

Figure 11.4 Example cuff test time series data. Cuff pressure is shown in orange, flow rate in black, and Q_{max} is marked in blue.

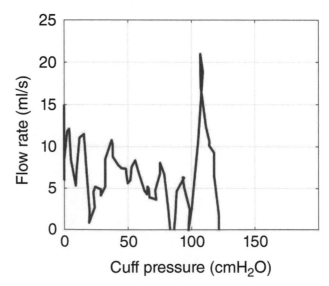

Figure 11.5 Example pressure-flow plot from an inflation where erratic flow prevents determination of cuff interruption pressure.

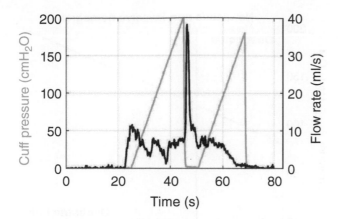

Figure 11.6 Example cuff test where the first inflation reaches the pressure limit of 200 cmH$_2$O without interrupting flow. (The second inflation is invalid as there is no flow surge.)

The marking of $P_{cuff.int}$ is not always obvious; inflations where the correct pressure is unclear should be excluded.

Newcastle Non-invasive Nomogram

Once Q_{max} and maximum $P_{cuff.int}$ have been determined, they are plotted and interpreted using the Newcastle non-invasive nomogram [16]. This nomogram was created by starting with the line separating the obstructed and equivocal regions on the International Continence Society (ICS) nomogram (Figure 11.8). The line was modified to account for the differences between the penile cuff test and invasive urodynamics. Firstly, the line was raised by 40 cmH$_2$O, an assumed correction factor to account for the abdominal pressure for all patients, based on a study by McIntosh et al. [21], given that cuff pressure represents intravesical rather than detrusor pressure. This is why it is important for patients not to strain during the test; abdominal pressure would be unpredictable and likely much higher than this. Based on studies examining the behaviour of the blad-

der in response to interrupted flow [22], the steepness of the line was doubled to account for the increase in bladder pressure under isovolumetric instead of flow conditions (taking its gradient from 2 to 4 cmH$_2$O per ml/s). Finally, a line was added at $Q_{max} = 10$ ml/s to separate the obstructed and unobstructed categories (Figure 11.9).

Example Penile Cuff Test Studies

Below are examples of cuff test time series, pressure-flow, and nomogram plots for three different diagnoses: BOO, DUA, and unobstructed. BOO is indicated by high cuff interruption pressure with low maximum flow rate (Figure 11.10). A low pressure-low flow cuff test result suggests a diagnosis of DUA (Figure 11.11). In Figure 11.12, moderate cuff interruption pressure with a normal maximum flow rate places this patient in the unobstructed area of the nomogram.

Current Standing

The penile cuff test and BWT-related measures, evaluated prospectively, are promising non-invasive tools for the evaluation of LUTS. However, the evidence is generally of low quality, with many reports confounding technique development and evaluation, often led by interested parties, and with unblinded analyses. This has led to an unclear message about the value of non-invasive urodynamics. Issues with invasive urodynamics, the inevitable comparator, such as the effect of catheterisation on flow rate, interdependence of pressure and flow, and uncertainty surrounding reproducibility, may also have contributed. We recommend that future studies evaluating non-invasive urodynamics are performed and reported robustly, according to methodological standards such as

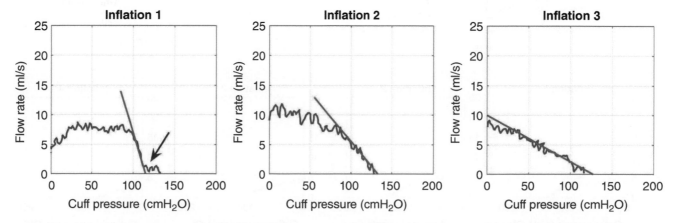

Figure 11.7 Examples of marking cuff interruption pressure for three inflations. $P_{cuff.int}$ is 115, 133, and 127 cmH$_2$O for inflations 1–3, respectively.

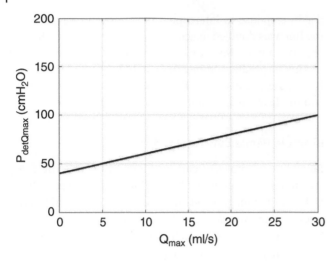

Figure 11.8 The line separating the obstructed and equivocal regions in the International Continence Society nomogram.

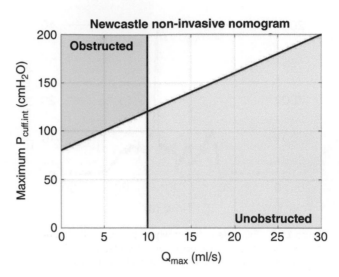

Figure 11.9 The Newcastle non-invasive nomogram. *Source*: Based on Griffiths et al. [16].

those described by the EQUATOR Network [23], with careful consideration of the most appropriate comparators and/or outcome measures. Current non-invasive tests are unlikely to ever replace conventional urodynamics but may be usefully positioned in clinical pathways as screening tests which could be applied to significant numbers of men with LUTS. They may also be useful when invasive urody-

namics cannot replicate the patient's symptoms. An International Consultation on Incontinence – Research Society paper provided a series of research priorities around development and assessment of non-invasive techniques [24]. Meanwhile, the pressure-flow study remains the standard test in determining BOO [2].

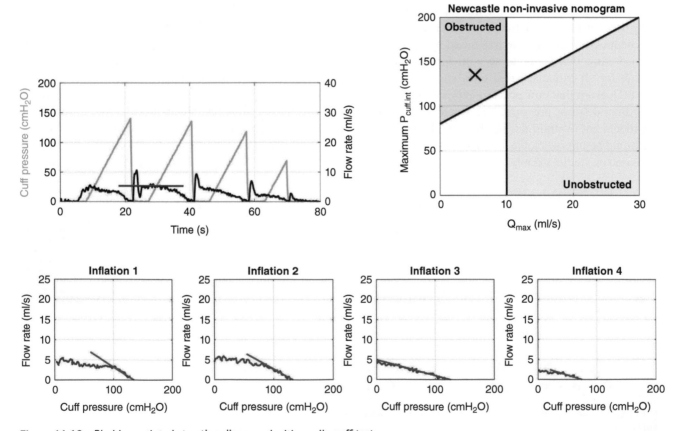

Figure 11.10 Bladder outlet obstruction diagnosed with penile cuff test.

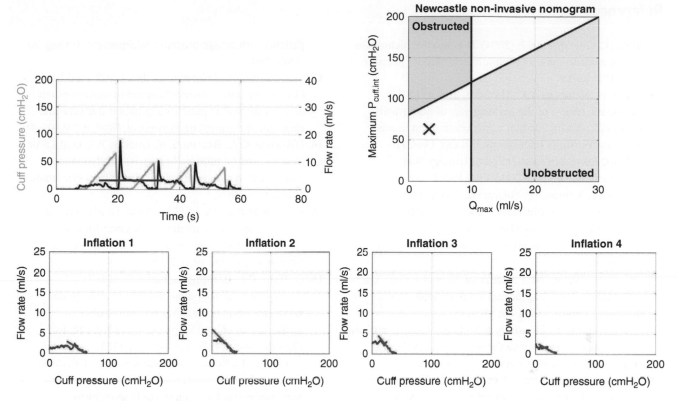

Figure 11.11 Detrusor underactivity diagnosed with penile cuff test.

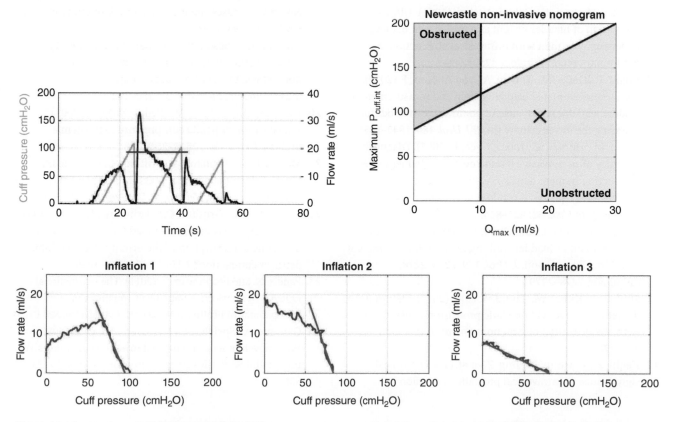

Figure 11.12 Unobstructed finding for penile cuff test.

References

1. Blake, C. and Abrams, P. (2004). Noninvasive techniques for the measurement of isovolumetric bladder pressure. *J. Urol.* 171: 12–19.

2. Malde, S., Nambiar, A.K., Umbach, R. et al. (2017). Systematic review of the performance of noninvasive tests in diagnosing bladder outlet obstruction in men with lower urinary tract symptoms. *Eur. Urol.* 71: 391–402.European Association of Urology Non-neurogenic Male LUTS Guidelines Panel

3. Ozawa, H., Kumon, H., Yokoyama, T. et al. (1998). Development of noninvasive velocity flow video urodynamics using Doppler sonography. Part II: clinical application in bladder outlet obstruction. *J. Urol.* 160: 1792–1796.

4. Ozawa, H., Watanabe, T., Uematsu, K. et al. (2009). Use of Doppler ultrasound for non-invasive urodynamic diagnosis. *Indian J. Urol.* 25: 110–115.

5. Greenland, J.E. and Brading, A.F. (1996). Urinary bladder blood flow changes during the micturition cycle in a conscious pig model. *J. Urol.* 156: 1858–1861.

6. Zhang, P., Yang, Y., Wu, Z.J. et al. (2013). Diagnosis of bladder outlet obstruction in men using a near-infrared spectroscopy instrument as the noninvasive monitor for bladder function. *Urology* 82: 1098–1102.

7. Kojima, M., Inui, E., Ochiai, A. et al. (1996). Ultrasonic estimation of bladder weight as a measure of bladder hypertrophy in men with infravesical obstruction: a preliminary report. *Urology* 47: 942–947.

8. Bright, E., Oelke, M., Tubaro, A., and Abrams, P. (2010). Ultrasound estimated bladder weight and measurement of bladder wall thickness – useful noninvasive methods for assessing the lower urinary tract? *J. Urol.* 184: 1847–1854.

9. Oelke, M., Hofner, K., Jonas, U. et al. (2007). Diagnostic accuracy of noninvasive tests to evaluate bladder outlet obstruction in men: detrusor wall thickness, uroflowmetry, postvoid residual urine, and prostate volume. *Eur. Urol.* 52: 827–834.

10. Blatt, A.H., Titus, J., and Chan, L. (2008). Ultrasound measurement of bladder wall thickness in the assessment of voiding dysfunction. *J. Urol.* 179: 2275–2278; discussion 2278–2279.

11. Shin, S.H., Kim, J.W., Kim, J.W. et al. (2013). Defining the degree of intravesical prostatic protrusion in association with bladder outlet obstruction. *Korean J. Urol.* 54: 369–372.

12. Keqin, Z., Zhishun, X., Jing, Z. et al. (2007). Clinical significance of intravesical prostatic protrusion in patients with benign prostatic enlargement. *Urology* 70: 1096–1099.

13. van Mastrigt, R., de Zeeuw, S., Boeve, E.R., and Groen, J. (2014). Diagnostic power of the noninvasive condom catheter method in patients eligible for transurethral resection of the prostate. *Neurourol. Urodyn.* 33: 408–413.

14. D'Ancona, C.A., Bassani, J.W., Querne, F.A. et al. (2008). New method for minimally invasive urodynamic assessment in men with lower urinary tract symptoms. *Urology* 71: 75–78.

15. Sullivan, M.P. and Yalla, S.V. (2000). Penile urethral compression-release maneuver as a non-invasive screening test for diagnosing prostatic obstruction. *Neurourol. Urodyn.* 19: 657–669.

16. Griffiths, C.J., Harding, C., Blake, C. et al. (2005). A nomogram to classify men with lower urinary tract symptoms using urine flow and noninvasive measurement of bladder pressure. *J. Urol.* 174: 1323–1326; discussion 1326; author reply 1326.

17. Harding, C.K., Robson, W., Drinnan, M.J. et al. (2004). An automated penile compression release maneuver as a noninvasive test for diagnosis of bladder outlet obstruction. *J. Urol.* 172: 2312–2315.

18. McIntosh, S.L., Drinnan, M.J., Griffiths, C.J. et al. (2004). Noninvasive assessment of bladder contractility in men. *J. Urol.* 172: 1394–1398.

19. Harding, C., Robson, W., Drinnan, M. et al. (2007). Predicting the outcome of prostatectomy using noninvasive bladder pressure and urine flow measurements. *Eur. Urol.* 52: 186–192.

20. Drinnan, M.J., Robson, W., Reddy, M. et al. (2001). Transmission of penile cuff pressure to the penile urethra. *J. Urol.* 166: 2545–2549.

21. McIntosh, S., Drinnan, M., Griffiths, C. et al. (2003). Relationship of abdominal pressure and body mass index in men with LUTS. *Neurourol. Urodyn.* 22: 602–605.

22. McIntosh, S.L., Griffiths, C.J., Drinnan, M.J. et al. (2003). Noninvasive measurement of bladder pressure. Does mechanical interruption of the urinary stream inhibit detrusor contraction? *J. Urol.* 169: 1003–1006.

23. Pandis, N. and Fedorowicz, Z. (2011). The international EQUATOR network: enhancing the quality and transparency of health care research. *J. Appl. Oral Sci.* 19 (5).

24. Gammie, A., Speich, J.E., Damaser, M.S. et al. (2020). What developments are needed to achieve less-invasive urodynamics? ICI-RS 2019. *Neurourol. Urodyn.* 39 (3): S36–S42.

Part IV

Urodynamics in Clinical Practice

12

Urodynamics in Children

Jonathan S. Ellison[1], Guy Nicholls[2], and Mark Woodward[2]

[1]*Urology Department, Children's Hospital of Wisconsin & Medical College of Wisconsin, Milwaukee, WI, USA*
[2]*Bristol Royal Hospital for Children, Bristol, UK*

CONTENTS

Urodynamics is an essential tool for evaluating bladder function in selected children. In broad terms, three different situations may necessitate urodynamic evaluation for children:

- Specific neurological disorders known to affect vesicourethral function;
- Non-neurological disorders known to affect vesicourethral function; and
- Lower urinary tract symptoms (LUTS) suggestive of vesicourethral dysfunction but with no known underlying disorder.

The same general principles as for adults hold true for children. However, several factors add complexity to paediatric urodynamics, notably the range of potential body sizes, temperament and cooperation, and sensitivity to radiation exposure. This chapter will thus focus not only on indications and findings of urodynamic studies but also on specific technical considerations for the paediatric population.

As with adults, it is important to use standardised terminology, as defined in the paediatric population by the International Children's Continence Society (ICCS) [1]. Additionally, the ICCS has also published specific guidance on urodynamic studies [2].

Children with Neurological Disorders

Any disorder that interrupts normal bladder innervation can result in abnormal bladder function, including sacral agenesis, spinal cord injury, or iatrogenic denervation. Most common are spinal cord dysraphism, which range in severity from spina bifida occulta to myelomeningocele – the latter commonly resulting in vesicourethral dysfunction. The goals of urodynamics in these patients are to evaluate whether the bladder can store urine at safe pressures and to identify the cause(s) of incontinence, if present.

Urodynamics are utilised by the majority of paediatric urologists in both initial evaluation and follow-up of patients with myelomeningocele [3]. However, the timing of such studies is debated. Early investigations (under one year of life) may be technically challenging, but focussed management based on these studies can spare need for augmentation in the future [4, 5]. Furthermore, patients with delayed presentation of neurogenic bladder in the form of occult dysraphism appear to risk irreversible dysfunction, suggesting that investigation early in life is appropriate where possible [6]. Other authors argue for a more conservative approach, with ultrasound screening initially proceeding to urodynamics only on the basis of an abnormal ultrasound or clinical factors suggestive of bladder dysfunction (notably urinary tract infections [UTIs] or symptoms). This approach may initially spare 66% of children from urodynamics, though ultimately the majority of children managed with this approach eventually require a formal urodynamic investigation [7].

Acquired spinal cord lesions present first with an areflexic bladder regardless of the level of the lesion, a situation known as spinal shock. Thus, initial urodynamics studies are best deferred to allow the neurological changes in the bladder to manifest themselves, for example, allowing an interval of three months following the injury. Management of other, less common, neurological disorders can be managed similar to adults. The level of the actual spinal lesion is generally predictive of lower urinary tract function. Lesions above the brainstem cause detrusor overactivity (or rarely acontractile bladder) with coordinated sphincter function.

Lesions between the brainstem and the sacral spinal cord are associated with detrusor overactivity and loss of coordinated sphincter control. These patients generally have poor compliance and high detrusor leak point pressures, which have the potential to cause upper tract deterioration if the bladder is not managed appropriately. Lesions of the sacral spinal cord or peripheral innervation often result in an areflexic bladder; however, depending on the lesion, they may also cause a fixed bladder neck that can result in unsafe storage pressures.

Surveillance of the neurogenic bladder patient is important, as bladder function may evolve over time. Most paediatric urologists utilise urodynamics in the surveillance protocol [3]. At a minimum, these patients must be followed with routine symptom evaluations and upper tract imaging. New onset or worsening incontinence, UTIs, hydronephrosis, or urinary stone disease should prompt repeat urodynamics to assess bladder function.

Urodynamics and the Neurogenic Bladder

There are several aspects of urodynamics for the neurogenic bladder which are further complicated by the additional challenges of diagnostic testing in children. We illustrate this with an example case as follows:

Case 1

An 11-year-old male with spina bifida was referred with incontinence and poor adherence to catheterisation regimens and medication. He had a solitary kidney following a nephrectomy for Wilms's tumour. Fluoroscopic images and urodynamic tracings are shown in Figure 12.1. Standard rectal and urethral catheters were used to obtain pressure measurements, and only the filling phase is shown. The video urodynamic image in Figure 12.1b is taken during a cough. The situation needs to be interpreted in terms of storage parameters and any abnormalities on the fluoroscopic images, and thence consideration of the next steps in management.

Discussion

The patient has evidence of both poor storage capacity and stress urinary incontinence, classic findings in spina bifida resulting from a neurogenic bladder, a fixed open bladder neck, and weak sphincter. The detrusor pressure rose to 40 cmH$_2$O following 140 ml of filling during the study. The expected bladder capacity (Table 12.1) in a patient of this age would be at least 300 ml.

Table 12.1 Comparison of formulae to estimate bladder capacity in infants and children.

Author	Formula (ml)	Notes
Hjalmas et al. [8]	[age (yr) × 30] + 30	Based on data from unspecified number of children aged 0–16 years undergoing cystometry, and citing historical data from series of 203 non-enuretic children
Koff [9]	[age (yr) × 30] + 60	Validated in 35 children without bladder pathology, ages 0–14 years, using cystometry under anaesthesia
Kaefer et al. [10]	< 2 yr: 30 × [age (yr) × 2] ≥ 2 yr: 30 × [age (yr)/2 + 6]	Validated in 2066 children undergoing awake radionucleotide cystography
Fairhurst et al. [11]	7 × weight (kg)	For infants <12 months of age; validated in 125 infants undergoing voiding cystourethrography

Case 1   (Continued)

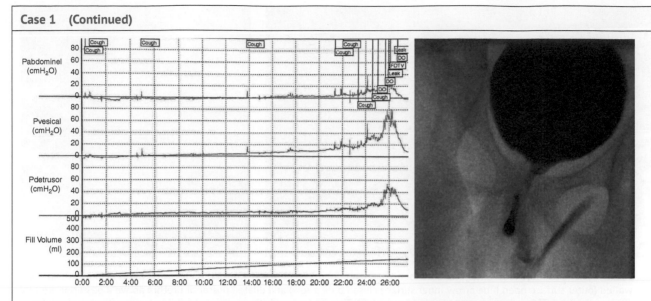

Figure 12.1   Video urodynamic filling cystometry of an 11-year-old boy with spina bifida. There was impaired detrusor compliance (steadily increasing p_{det} during filling) and detrusor overactivity. Note the lack of resting pressures at the start of the trace suggests the zeroing was done while recording from the patient, which is not International Continence Society recommended practice. The image on the right was taken during a cough and demonstrates stress incontinence. *Source*: Marcus Drake.

With regards to spinal dysraphism, urodynamic studies are especially important for two key reasons. First, there is poor correlation between the identified level of the spinal lesion and bladder function [12]. Second, as defined by McGuire, such evaluations are imperative for identifying bladders that maintain 'unsafe' storage pressures. Those patients with poor compliance or detrusor sphincter dyssynergia have a much higher risk of upper tract deterioration leading to renal failure and warrant decisive management and follow-up [13].

The patient is scheduled to undergo bladder augmentation, formation of a Mitrofanoff catheterisable channel, and a procedure to reinforce the bladder outlet (bladder neck artificial urinary sphincter), in order to improve compliance and treat the stress incontinence. It is important to note that undertaking an outlet procedure by itself would be contraindicated, as there would be a high risk of upper tract deterioration if the impaired bladder compliance were left untreated; in that case, the outlet procedure would be harmful in raising still further the storage pressures that the bladder could reach.

Children with Non-neurological Disorders

Posterior Urethral Valves

Posterior urethral valves (PUV) refers to a congenital abnormality in boys in which abnormal tissue leaflets are present below the bladder neck and cause blockage to urine flow. PUV is a rare condition that potentially has a lifelong impact on urologic function even if the initial obstruction is relieved relatively early in life with valve ablation [14, 15]. The use of prenatal sonography has increased early recognition and treatment of this disease. Classic prenatal findings include bilateral hydronephrosis, a thickened bladder wall, and a dilated posterior urethra, commonly referred to as a 'keyhole sign' (Figure 12.2).

Importantly, however, even in contemporary series, a large proportion of boys with PUV may present after birth [16, 17]. Bladder function evolves in a well-documented fashion, often progressing from an overactive bladder with poor storage parameters early in life to detrusor failure as the child enters adolescence (Figure 12.3) [14, 15, 18]. Long-term progression to end-stage renal disease and need for renal replacement therapy is high in these patients, despite aggressive and early bladder management, suggesting a degree of unalterable renal damage acquired during embryonic development. Accordingly, it is necessary to observe both renal function and bladder function during childhood [19]. Polyuria, especially nocturnal, from chronically damaged kidneys may contribute to bladder dysfunction, with poor bladder storage parameters and progressive upper tract deterioration as the outcome [20, 21].

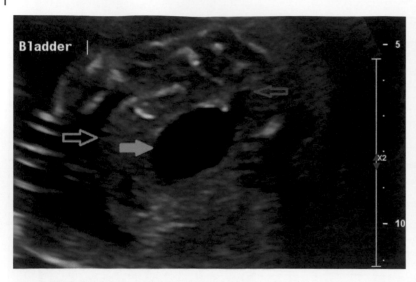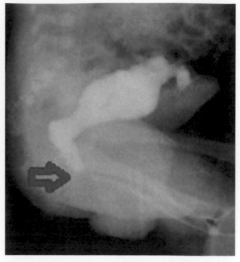

Figure 12.2   The left image is an antenatal ultrasound of a male foetus at 22 weeks of gestation showing a full bladder which is very thick-walled (outer surface open blue arrow, inner surface closed blue arrow) and dilated posterior urethra above a posterior urethral valve (PUV: red arrow). This is known as the 'keyhole sign' (left). The right image is the post-natal voiding cystourethrogram on day of life 3, revealing a dilated and elongated posterior urethra with notable obstruction at the level of the PUV. *Source*: Marcus Drake.

Lower Urinary Tract Symptoms

Assessment of neurologically normal children with LUTS comprises a large part of paediatric urology practice. These children may present with incontinence or urine infections as a result of detrusor overactivity or dysfunctional voiding, or a combination of both. Urodynamics are used selec-

tively in this population to fully define vesicourethral function if conservative treatment options fail in order to target symptom relief and to rule out occult bladder pathology.

Given the invasive nature of urodynamics, the use of such studies in this population is controversial. While studies have shown some benefit to invasive urodynamics in a

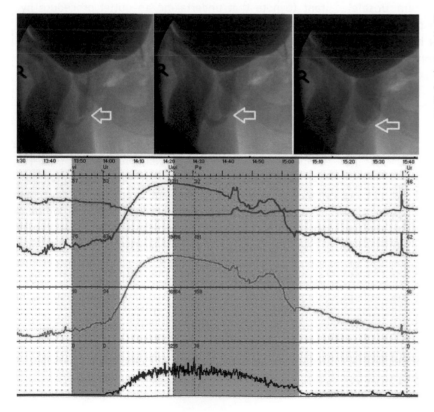

Figure 12.3   Video urodynamic pressure-flow study (PFS) of a teenager with PUV. The top images are X-rays during voiding, showing the PUV (yellow arrow), and steadily increasing filling of the proximal urethra above it. The PFS confirms a very high pressure and slow flow, i.e. bladder outlet obstruction. *Source*: Marcus Drake.

non-neurogenic paediatric population, interpretation of data is problematic in that a heterogeneous group of patients is often reported together [22].

Overactive Bladder Syndrome

Overactive bladder syndrome (OAB) is a common complaint, manifesting with urgency with or without increased daytime frequency and/or incontinence [1, 23]. Urodynamics have been proposed as an essential part of the treatment algorithm for this population [24]. However, in a prospective randomised trial comparing oxybutynin to placebo in children, only one-third of children with symptoms suggestive of OAB were found to have detrusor overactivity on urodynamic studies, whilst two-thirds of patients with detrusor overactivity following treatment were new onset. As no correlation was seen between pretreatment findings and treatment outcomes, the authors did not recommend routine urodynamic studies in management of OAB [25]. Others have shown a high likelihood of finding detrusor overactivity in these patients,

though a low proportion had additional findings, suggesting the diagnostic value of such studies is low [26]. Detrusor overactivity may underlie giggle incontinence (see Chapter 13, Figure 13.19).

Dysfunctional Voiding

The term 'dysfunctional voiding' is used by many to describe a wide variety of voiding complaints but should be viewed as the habitual inability to relax the external urethral sphincter and/or pelvic floor during voiding. Diagnosis relies on:

- Uroflowmetry identification of interrupted voiding pattern (Figure 12.4) and
- Pressure-flow studies (PFSs) revealing external sphincter contractions during the voiding phase (Figure 12.5).

In a study comparing children receiving standard treatment or pelvic floor physical therapy for dysfunctional voiding symptoms, a similar proportion of patients were found to have increased pelvic floor activity pre- and post-

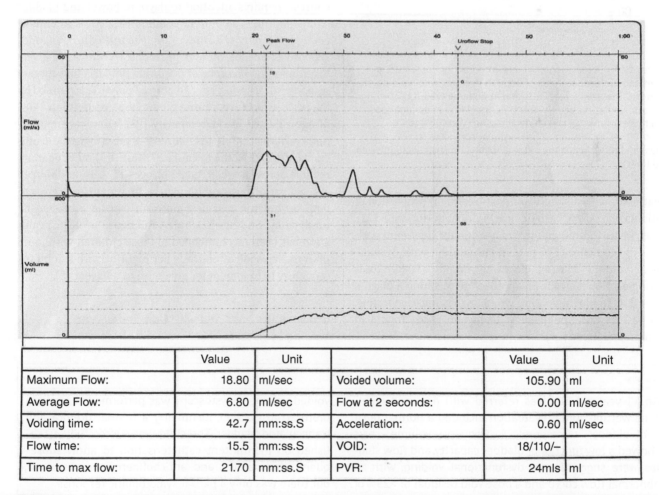

	Value	Unit		Value	Unit
Maximum Flow:	18.80	ml/sec	Voided volume:	105.90	ml
Average Flow:	6.80	ml/sec	Flow at 2 seconds:	0.00	ml/sec
Voiding time:	42.7	mm:ss.S	Acceleration:	0.60	ml/sec
Flow time:	15.5	mm:ss.S	VOID:	18/110/–	
Time to max flow:	21.70	mm:ss.S	PVR:	24mls	ml

Figure 12.4 A representative pre-intervention free flowmetry trace for a child with dysfunctional voiding showing the intermittent stream.

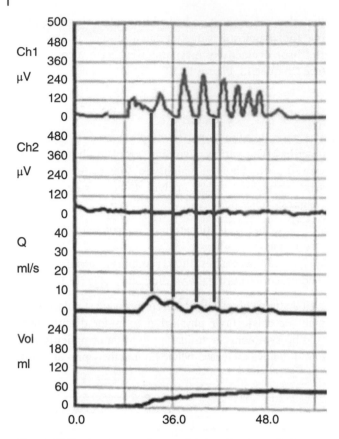

Figure 12.5 A representative pre-intervention trace during animated biofeedback on a child with dysfunctional voiding, with external sphincter (Ch 1) and abdominal wall (Ch 2) electromyographic activity (from perineal and abdominal pad electrodes), flow (Q), and voided volume (Vol). Flow is intermittent, increasing as the external sphincter relaxes (red lines) and reducing as the external sphincter contracts (between red lines).

treatment, with a significant post-treatment proportion of patients presenting with de novo voiding dysfunction [22]. Thus, invasive urodynamics may not alter treatment decisions in the majority of patients presenting with dysfunctional voiding. Placing electromyography (EMG) leads during uroflowmetry is an approach to reaching a diagnosis of dysfunctional voiding which avoids invasive testing. The ICCS has published diagnostic and treatment recommendations [27].

Enuresis

Enuresis is both a symptom and a condition of intermittent incontinence that occurs during periods of sleep [1]. Enuresis, typically defined as more than one night-time incontinence episode per month, is the preferred current terminology for night-time wetting and can be divided into two main groups: monosymptomatic (those with only night-time complaints) and non-monosymptomatic (those patients with daytime complaints including incontinence, OAB, or other LUTS) [23, 28]. These sub-groups are likely to represent two separate disease processes and differ in terms of urodynamic findings and treatment responses [29, 30]. Adolescents (average age 14.7 years) with anorexia nervosa have a prevalence of nocturnal enuresis of 17%, and patients generally did not mention it to the medical team without prompting [31]. Follow-up identified that this can resolve with weight gain.

Monosymptomatic enuresis is typically managed with a focus on healthy night-time bladder habits, alarm systems, and medications such as desmopressin to reduce nocturnal urine production [23]. Meanwhile, non-monosymptomatic enuresis requires attention to daytime bowel and bladder habits and other comorbid conditions such as attention-deficit hyperactivity disorder [28]. The role of urodynamics is poorly defined in these populations. Non-invasive investigation for the presence of nocturnal polyuria may predict response to desmopressin. Nocturnal polyuria is defined by the ICCS as nocturnal urine production greater than 130% of age-adjusted bladder capacity [23]. However, this formula is most accurate in children 7–8 years of age, and others have proposed the formula $20 \times (age + 9)$ ml to be more reliable across a wider range of ages [32]. In addition to assessment of nocturnal polyuria, treatment responses to both oxybutynin and desmopressin can be predicted by urodynamic findings [33, 34]. A full neuro-urologic evaluation has been recommended in those children with more than one episode of enuresis per night or with symptoms refractory to treatment for greater than one year [8].

Urodynamics in a Child with Non-neurogenic Voiding Symptoms

Case 2

An 11-year-old boy was referred with day- and night-time wetting. Initial evaluation included a normal renal and bladder ultrasound. A frequency-volume chart showed a low functional bladder capacity, and flow studies were suggestive of dysfunctional voiding, with an abnormal flow curve and a post-void residual of >25% of voided volume. A cystoscopy was performed to exclude urethral obstruction, identifying a normal urethra and trabeculated bladder. The child was successfully established on intermittent catheterisation to allow subsequent urodynamics, and anticholinergics commenced, but there was only a partial symptomatic response.

Case 2   (Continued)

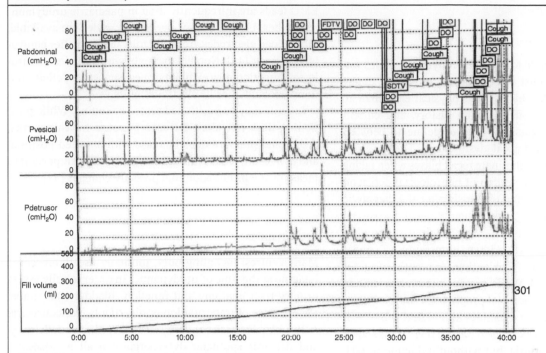

Figure 12.6   Video urodynamic filling cystometry of an 11-year-old boy with wetting and low functional bladder capacity on frequency-volume chart (FVC). The PFS reveals marked symptomatic detrusor overactivity from approximately 150 ml fill.

When electing to proceed with urodynamics, it is important to consider what primary questions need to be answered and how findings may guide the next steps in management. Indications, if any, for invasive urodynamics need to be clear-cut, and fluoroscopy to detect additional information may need to be considered.

The urodynamics are presented in Figure 12.6. Standard rectal and urethral catheters were used to obtain pressure measurements, and only the filling phase is shown. When interpreting this study, characterise the patient's compliance, functional bladder capacity, and any abnormalities that are noted. What is the diagnosis and what are the next management options?

Discussion

One approach to the identification of children likely to have abnormal urodynamic studies is with use of the following risk factors: history of UTI, small capacity bladder, symptoms refractory to treatment, dysfunctional pattern on uroflowmetry, and abnormal ultrasound findings. Only 6.2% of patients selected based on these factors actually have normal invasive urodynamic studies [35]. However, it is unclear whether such findings altered management decisions in these children. Thus, a reasonable approach could be an assessment with history, physical examination, voiding diary, non-invasive urodynamic techniques

and imaging, followed by a trial of pharmaceutical and/or behavioural therapies. Prior evaluation in this case included flow studies and a renal-bladder ultrasound, and further non-invasive studies were unlikely to yield additional information. Urodynamics were additionally indicated as the child's symptoms were refractory to medical management.

The main question to be answered by this study was the cause of the child's incontinence, which was clinically presumed to relate to detrusor overactivity. The expected bladder capacity of a child of this age would be 300–330 ml. During the study, symptomatic detrusor contractions were identified from 150 ml fill confirming a diagnosis of detrusor overactivity. The end-fill detrusor pressure was approximately 20 cmH$_2$O at a capacity of 330 ml, confirming a good capacity, reasonably compliant bladder, although the detrusor overactivity was marked. In this case, a magnetic resonance imaging (MRI) of the lumbosacral spine was undertaken to ensure there was no occult spinal dysraphism, and the child is scheduled to undergo a trial of intra-vesical botulinum toxin A injection, with counselling regarding the lack of licence for this indication in children. As seen above, those children with refractory symptoms or extenuating circumstances suggestive of an underlying neurological or anatomical abnormality would likely benefit most from invasive urodynamic studies [27].

Practical Aspects of Urodynamic Studies

Pre-test Considerations

Prior to subjecting a child to invasive urodynamics investigation, several factors must be considered. Important to any evaluation is a detailed history and physical examination. Duration of problem, toilet training history, and current bowel and bladder habits can help to delineate between behavioural and physiological dysfunction. The use of a voiding diary can help to eliminate recall biases when taking a voiding history. Any suggestion of neurological deficit on physical examination should obviously alter the diagnostic algorithm, as delayed diagnosis of neurological disease can have long-reaching effects [6]. Occult spinal dysraphism should be evaluated with either ultrasound (if under six months of age) or MRI (if older than six months of age) of the spinal cord [36, 37]. While pre-operative urine culture may help to guide antimicrobial prophylaxis, antibiotics are used routinely prior to urodynamics although this has been called into question. A Cochrane database review has shown reduced rates of bacteriuria, but without reduction in UTI, using pre-investigation prophylactic antibiotics [38]. Likewise, no deleterious effects were shown in performing urodynamic studies in children with asymptomatic bacteriuria without antibiotic prophylaxis [39]. Findings from previous imaging studies may be useful in preparing for urodynamic studies. Evidence of bladder wall thickening may suggest abnormal bladder function and anticipate treatment response [40]. Hydronephrosis may indicate the presence of high storage pressures or vesicoureteral reflux (VUR) and the need for video urodynamics.

Technique Modification in Children

Children differ from adults in both size and ability to co-operate with the examination, requiring some modification to standard urodynamic techniques. The paediatric urology nurse specialists generally meet the child and their family prior to the test to ensure they will be able to tolerate the procedure. Double-lumen 6 Fr urethral catheters and 4.5Fr rectal catheters are generally used. Volumes used to flush the catheters are small (usually 2–5 ml). Filling fluids ideally should be warmed close to body temperature, but at a minimum, they should be at room temperature. In cases where it is not possible to insert a urethral catheter, a suprapubic catheter kit is available. Usually, the child has the catheter inserted in the morning under sedation or anaesthesia and then has the urodynamics in the afternoon once the effects of the anaesthetic have worn off.

Other Considerations in Children

EMG leads are infrequently used in paediatric urodynamics studies. If used, pad or needle electrodes are available, though pad electrodes are better tolerated and offer equivalent efficacy [46]. Notably, patients with impaired neurological function may exhibit perineal sensation deficits and so may tolerate needle electrodes quite well.

Patients may be positioned seated or supine. While positioning does not alter detrusor pressure measurements, abdominal pressure does increase with a seated position, and as a result, rectal catheter use is especially important to measure any intra-abdominal pressure changes [47].

Radiation Exposure in Children: Video Urodynamics

Many centres, including ours, routinely use fluoroscopic imaging at the time of urodynamics in order to fully assess urinary tract anatomy and function. Bladder wall shape, the presence of trabeculation or diverticula, vesicoureteric reflux, bladder neck support, intrinsic sphincter deficiency, and detrusor sphincter dyssynergia can all be assessed. These observations inform the assessment of overall bladder function and can help define actual versus measured bladder capacity and compliance.

However, use of radiation is not without risks, especially in a susceptible population. Radiation exposure during fluoro- or video urodynamics varies widely among practitioners, though interpretation is limited given non-standardisation of reported parameters. Overall radiation exposure may be as high as 10 mGy [48]. In general, the effective radiation dose may be as low as that received during a chest X-ray, but sometimes it may be as high as a computed tomography scan of the abdomen and pelvis (roughly 500 chest X-ray equivalents). Increased bladder capacity and weight or body mass index may increase risk of radiation exposure during these studies [48, 49]. The ALARA ('As Low As Reasonably Achievable') principle suggests that modification of both equipment and techniques used during the study can decrease unnecessary radiation exposure to both the patient and practitioner. Thus, collaboration with a knowledgeable radiographer and careful consideration of radiography use is important to a safe and effective video urodynamic study. In addition, the practitioner should consider at the beginning of the study if fluoroscopy will add any additional information. If the answer is no, radiation use should be avoided.

Ureteral Occlusion in Severe Reflux

High-grade VUR can introduce additional complexity to urodynamic investigations. The following situation (Case 4) exhibits these challenges:

Case 3

The following example illustrates several of the challenges specific to performing invasive urodynamic studies in children. A four-year-old girl was referred with partial sacral agenesis and a resultant neuropathic bladder. During toilet training, she had been noted to pass small volumes of urine frequently and had evidence of incomplete bladder emptying on ultrasound. Urodynamics were planned to evaluate her bladder function. However, she was unable to tolerate urethral catheterisation and so suprapubic filling and vesical pressure lines were therefore placed under general anaesthesia the day prior to the procedure. During filling, she was noted to have significant urethral leakage. Fluoroscopic images are shown in Figure 12.7, along with urodynamics tracings.

Discussion

This child typifies the unique challenges seen in paediatric practice. First, she was young and unable to tolerate urethral catheterisation. Urethral catheterisation can be difficult for both the patient and the parents, and a thorough and informed discussion is required prior to proceeding with urodynamics. Catheter placement can be

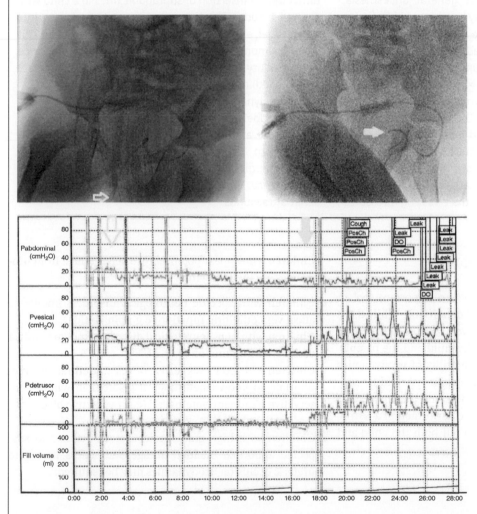

Figure 12.7 Video urodynamic filling cystometry on a four-year-old girl with partial sacral agenesis. The top images are X-rays during filling. On the left, the suprapubic catheter that had been placed 24 hours previously to record vesical pressure and for filling is seen to have migrated beyond the bladder down into the urethra (open yellow arrow). In this location, the catheter is unable to record p_{ves}. This is clear from the filling cystometry below, where p_{ves} shows a very different trace to p_{abd}, suggesting that it is not recording from the same body cavity. Once this problem was recognised, the catheter was repositioned into the bladder (right image, closed yellow arrow). In the cystometry trace, this repositioning was performed between 16 and 18 minutes (closed yellow arrow) and then proper recording of p_{ves} is seen. It is at this point that high-pressure neurogenic detrusor overactivity with associated leakage is observed. *Source*: Marcus Drake.

(Continued)

Case 3   (Continued)

viewed as one of the most psychologically traumatic experiences of the entire urodynamics process. If the child is able to tolerate urethral catheterisation, then a tour of the urodynamics facility with reassuring staff for both the child and parents may help to ease the anxiety [41]. Some patients may require sedation or even general anaesthetic for catheter placement, as in this case. Sedation does not appear to alter urodynamic findings in small series [42]. It may occasionally prove necessary to perform the filling cystometry under general anaesthesia; PFS is not possible in this circumstance. Most elements of the filling phase of urodynamics appear to be observable under general anaesthesia, though detrusor overactivity may be blunted [43].

Second, due to both her age and her partial sacral agenesis, she had a small bladder. Expected bladder capacity can be measured a number of different ways, utilising either age or weight. Many units use a range generated from the first two formulae in Table 12.1 [9–11]. A maximum filling rate of 10% of expected bladder capacity per minute is often used for children [41]; many units, including ours, actually start with lower filling rates of 5–10 ml/min. The rate of filling may influence detrusor pressure; one-third of patients will have filling pressures at least 10% higher than resting pressures during urodynamic studies [44]. As such, some groups have argued for natural-filling cystometry as a more accurate measure of bladder pressures while eliminating the need for a filling line [45]. This generally necessitates insertion of suprapubic vesical pressure recording line under general anaesthesia, resulting in a more invasive procedure with a higher risk of complications.

In this case, suprapubic lines were utilised to avoid urethral catheterisation. Initial filling resulted in urethral leakage within a few minutes, and visual inspection of the introitus revealed that the catheter had migrated through the urethra, demonstrating one of the potential difficulties of insertion of suprapubic lines in a child with a small bladder. The lines were repositioned back into the bladder, and a successful study was performed. This clearly demonstrates the importance of staff experience, as the ability to troubleshoot is particularly important during paediatric studies.

The urodynamics showed a small capacity, poorly compliant bladder, with high-pressure neurogenic detrusor overactivity and associated leakage. It was eventually possible to establish urethral catheterisation, and anticholinergics were commenced, with resolution of the incontinence. Her upper tracts have remained stable on serial ultrasounds.

Summary and Recommendations

Urodynamic studies in children are an important tool in management of multiple urological conditions. While these studies are generally safe, the invasive nature of the tests can cause significant anxiety for both the child and the parents. Thus, as with any investigation, the utility of urodynamics and any potential alternative investigations should be considered. Care should be taken to understand the anxieties of the children. Urodynamics should be performed in a setting with experienced personnel able to put both the child and parents at ease.

Children who appear potentially to benefit most from urodynamics are the following:

- Children with specific neurological disorders known to affect vesicourethral function (e.g. spina bifida);
- Children with non-neurological disorders known to affect vesicourethral function (e. g. PUV);
- Children with LUTS suggestive of vesicourethral dysfunction but no known neurological disorder in whom conservative treatment options fail (e.g. overactive bladder or dysfunctional voiding); and
- Children with high-grade vesicoureteric reflux and suspected abnormal bladder storage parameters in whom ureteric occlusion urodynamics may be required.

Case 4

A nine-year-old boy was referred for assessment with a background history of dysfunctional voiding, vesicoureteric reflux, and chronic kidney disease. He required bladder evaluation prior to renal transplantation. In addition, it was possible that bilateral nephrectomies might be necessary as he had both significant proteinuria and previous UTIs. With conventional urodynamics, high-grade VUR increases the apparent bladder capacity as upper tract storage occurs, and so bladder evaluation is unreliable. Any need for subsequent native nephrectomy could clearly affect storage parameters by removing this upper tract reservoir.

Case 4   (Continued)

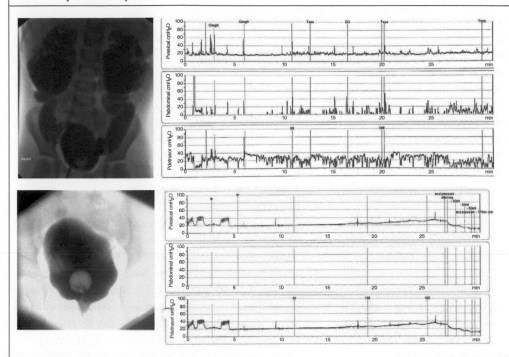

Figure 12.8   Top images: cystogram showing the severity of vesicoureteric reflux (VUR), and cystometry which apparently suggests a compliant detrusor (note technical issues with p$_{abd}$ recording). Lower images: cystogram showing that VUR has been prevented using balloon catheters placed in each ureteric orifice, and cystometry indicating the detrusor is poorly compliant (p$_{abd}$ not recorded). *Source*: Marcus Drake.

Fluoroscopic images and corresponding urodynamic studies under general anaesthesia are shown in Figure 12.8. In the top figure, severe reflux is present, and the filling cystometry shows little pressure change. Below, ureteric occlusion balloons have been placed bilaterally in the lower ureters, and elimination of vesicoureteric reflux is achieved by inflating the balloons. Repeat cystometry shows a pressure increase with filling, and hence impaired compliance of the isolated bladder.

Discussion

High-grade vesicoureteric reflux results in a 'pop-off' effect, in which both the bladder and the upper tracts hold urine during bladder filling. In this situation, measurement of 'bladder' capacity and compliance with routine urodynamics is misleading and potentially falsely reassuring, as the measurement is in reality the capacity and compliance of the whole urinary tract. In addition, without additional information, it is impossible to predict what effect removal of upper tract storage (with bilateral nephrectomy) might have on bladder pressure. Over the course of a young person's lifetime, nephrectomy may eventually be indicated; even if this is decades later, the consequence of impaired bladder compliance for remaining kidney function or a transplanted kidney may be very serious.

Techniques to improve assessment of bladder function in these cases have been described, wherein ureteric occlusion catheters are placed, often under anaesthetic [50, 51]. In a series of patients having paired studies, compliance measurements were up to 16% worse, and capacity was reduced by up to 33% when occlusion was in place [51]. Thus, occlusion of the ureters, by maintaining better retention of fluid within the bladder, facilitates assessment of the lower urinary tract.

In this case, pre-occlusion urodynamics did indeed provide a falsely reassuring assessment of compliance. Further evaluation with ureteric occlusion urodynamics demonstrated poor compliance, with a detrusor pressure rise of 21 cmH$_2$O for a 170 ml filled volume (expected bladder capacity 300 ml). Thus, elimination of the reflux, through either subsequent native nephrectomy or ureteric reimplantation, would result in a potentially unsafe situation for a transplanted kidney. Ultimately, nephrectomy was required, and a ureterocystoplasty was therefore performed at the same time as nephrectomy, using the dilated ureter and pelvis of one kidney, to ensure an adequate storage reservoir for an anticipated renal transplant. The patient subsequently underwent renal transplantation, and his renal function remains stable a year following his transplant.

References

1. Austin, P.F., Bauer, S.B., Bower, W. *et al.* (2016). The standardization of terminology of lower urinary tract function in children and adolescents: update report from the standardization committee of the International Children's Continence Society. *Neurourol. Urodyn.* 35 (4): 471–481.

2. Bauer, S.B., Nijman, R.J., Drzewiecki, B.A. et al., International Children's Continence Society Standardization Subcommitee (2015). International Children's Continence Society standardization report on urodynamic studies of the lower urinary tract in children. *Neurourol. Urodyn.* 34 (7): 640–647.

3. Elliott, S.P., Villar, R., and Duncan, B. (2005). Bacteriuria management and urological evaluation of patients with spina bifida and neurogenic bladder: a multicenter survey. *J. Urol.* 173 (1): 217–220.

4. Kaefer, M., Pabby, A., Kelly, M. et al. (1999). Improved bladder function after prophylactic treatment of the high risk neurogenic bladder in newborns with myelomentingocele. *J. Urol.* 162 (3 Pt 2): 1068–1071.

5. Wu, H.Y., Baskin, L.S., and Kogan, B.A. (1997). Neurogenic bladder dysfunction due to myelomeningocele: neonatal versus childhood treatment. *J. Urol.* 157 (6): 2295–2297.

6. Satar, N., Bauer, S.B., Shefner, J. et al. (1995). The effects of delayed diagnosis and treatment in patients with an occult spinal dysraphism. *J. Urol.* 154 (2 Pt 2): 754–758.

7. Hopps, C.V. and Kropp, K.A. (2003). Preservation of renal function in children with myelomeningocele managed with basic newborn evaluation and close follow-up. *J. Urol.* 169 (1): 305–308.

8. Hjalmas, K., Arnold, T., Bower, W. *et al.* (2004). Nocturnal enuresis: an international evidence based management strategy. *J. Urol.* 171 (6 Pt 2): 2545–2561.

9. Koff, S.A. (1983). Estimating bladder capacity in children. *Urology* 21 (3): 248.

10. Kaefer, M., Zurakowski, D., Bauer, S.B. et al. (1997). Estimating normal bladder capacity in children. *J. Urol.* 158 (6): 2261–2264.

11. Fairhurst, J.J., Rubin, C.M., Hyde, I. et al. (1991). Bladder capacity in infants. *J. Pediatr. Surg.* 26 (1): 55–57.

12. Blaivas, J.G., Labib, K.L., Bauer, S.B., and Retik, A.B. (1977). Changing concepts in the urodynamic evaluation of children. *J. Urol.* 117 (6): 778–781.

13. McGuire, E.J., Woodside, J.R., Borden, T.A., and Weiss, R.M. (1981). Prognostic value of urodynamic testing in myelodysplastic patients. *J. Urol.* 126 (2): 205–209.

14. De Gennaro, M., Capitanucci, M.L., Silveri, M. et al. (2001). Detrusor hypocontractility evolution in boys with posterior urethral valves detected by pressure flow analysis. *J. Urol.* 165 (6 Pt 2): 2248–2252.

15. Holmdahl, G. (1997). Bladder dysfunction in boys with posterior urethral valves. *Scand. J. Urol. Nephrol. Suppl.* 188: 1–36.

16. Vasconcelos, M., e Silva, A.S., Dias, C. et al. (2019). Posterior urethral valves: comparison of clinical outcomes between postnatal and antenatal cohorts. *J. Pediatr. Urol.* 15 (2): 167.e161–167.e168.

17. Brownlee, E., Wragg, R., Robb, A. et al., BAPS-CASS (2019). Current epidemiology and antenatal presentation of posterior urethral valves: outcome of BAPS CASS National Audit. *J. Pediatr. Surg.* 54 (2): 318–321.

18. Ghanem, M.A., Wolffenbuttel, K.P., De Vylder, A., and Nijman, R.J. (2004). Long-term bladder dysfunction and renal function in boys with posterior urethral valves based on urodynamic findings. *J. Urol.* 171 (6 Pt 1): 2409–2412.

19. Heikkila, J., Holmberg, C., Kyllonen, L. et al. (2011). Long-term risk of end stage renal disease in patients with posterior urethral valves. *J. Urol.* 186 (6): 2392–2396.

20. Dinneen, M.D., Duffy, P.G., Barratt, T.M., and Ransley, P.G. (1995). Persistent polyuria after posterior urethral valves. *Br. J. Urol.* 75 (2): 236–240.

21. Woodhouse, C.R. (2001). The fate of the abnormal bladder in adolescence. *J. Urol.* 166 (6): 2396–2400.

22. Kaufman, M.R., DeMarco, R.T., Pope, J.C. et al. (2006). High yield of urodynamics performed for refractory nonneurogenic dysfunctional voiding in the pediatric population. *J. Urol.* 176 (4 Pt 2): 1835–1837.

23. Neveus, T., Eggert, P., Evans, J. et al., International Children's Continence Society (2010). Evaluation of and treatment for monosymptomatic enuresis: a standardization document from the International Children's Continence Society. *J. Urol.* 183 (2): 441–447.

24. Curran, M.J., Kaefer, M., Peters, C. et al. (2000). The overactive bladder in childhood: long-term results with conservative management. *J. Urol.* 163 (2): 574–577.

25. Bael, A., Lax, H., de Jong, T.P. et al., European Bladder Dysfunction Study (2008). The relevance of urodynamic studies for Urge syndrome and dysfunctional voiding: a multicenter controlled trial in children. *J. Urol.* 180 (4): 1486–1493; discussion 1494–1485.

26. Soygur, T., Arikan, N., Tokatli, Z., and Karaboga, R. (2004). The role of video-urodynamic studies in managing non-neurogenic voiding dysfunction in children. *BJU Int.* 93 (6): 841–843.

27. Chase, J., Austin, P., Hoebeke, P., and McKenna, P., International Children's Continence Society (2010). The management of dysfunctional voiding in children: a report from the Standardisation Committee of the International Children's Continence Society. *J. Urol.* 183 (4): 1296–1302.

28. Franco, I., Von Gontard, A., and De Gennaro, M., International Children's Continence Society (2013). Evaluation and treatment of nonmonosymptomatic nocturnal enuresis: a standardization document from the International Children's Continence Society. *J. Pediatr. Urol.* 9 (2): 234–243.

29. Whiteside, C.G. and Arnold, E.P. (1975). Persistent primary enuresis: a urodynamic assessment. *Br. Med. J.* 1 (5954): 364–367.

30. Kajiwara, M., Kato, M., Mutaguchi, K., and Usui, T. (2008). Overactive bladder in children should be strictly differentiated from monosymptomatic nocturnal enuresis. *Urol. Int.* 80 (1): 57–61.

31. Kanbur, N., Pinhas, L., Lorenzo, A. et al. (2011). Nocturnal enuresis in adolescents with anorexia nervosa: prevalence, potential causes, and pathophysiology. *Int. J. Eat Disord.* 44 (4): 349–355.

32. Rittig, S., Kamperis, K., Siggaard, C. et al. (2010). Age related nocturnal urine volume and maximum voided volume in healthy children: reappraisal of International Children's Continence Society definitions. *J. Urol.* 183 (4): 1561–1567.

33. Rushton, H.G., Belman, A.B., Zaontz, M.R. et al. (1996). The influence of small functional bladder capacity and other predictors on the response to desmopressin in the management of monosymptomatic nocturnal enuresis. *J. Urol.* 156 (2 Pt 2): 651–655.

34. Radvanska, E., Kovacs, L., and Rittig, S. (2006). The role of bladder capacity in antidiuretic and anticholinergic treatment for nocturnal enuresis. *J. Urol.* 176 (2): 764–768; discussion 768–769.

35. Hoebeke, P., Van Laecke, E., Van Camp, C. et al. (2001). One thousand video-urodynamic studies in children with non-neurogenic bladder sphincter dysfunction. *BJU Int.* 87 (6): 575–580.

36. Guggisberg, D., Hadj-Rabia, S., Viney, C. et al. (2004). Skin markers of occult spinal dysraphism in children: a review of 54 cases. *Arch. Dermatol.* 140 (9): 1109–1115.

37. Korsvik, H.E. and Keller, M.S. (1992). Sonography of occult dysraphism in neonates and infants with MR imaging correlation. *Radiographics* 12 (2): 297–306; discussion 307–308.

38. Foon, R., Toozs-Hobson, P., and Latthe, P. (2012). Prophylactic antibiotics to reduce the risk of urinary tract infections after urodynamic studies. *Cochrane Database Syst. Rev.* (10) (Art. No.: CD008224). DOI: https://doi.org/10.1002/14651858.CD008224.pub2.

39. Shekarriz, B., Upadhyay, J., Freedman, A.L. et al. (1999). Lack of morbidity from urodynamic studies in children with asymptomatic bacteriuria. *Urology* 54 (2): 359–361; discussion 362.

40. Bright, E., Oelke, M., Tubaro, A., and Abrams, P. (2010). Ultrasound estimated bladder weight and measurement of bladder wall thickness--useful noninvasive methods for assessing the lower urinary tract? *J. Urol.* 184 (5): 1847–1854.

41. Drzewiecki, B.A. and Bauer, S.B. (2011). Urodynamic testing in children: indications, technique, interpretation and significance. *J. Urol.* 186 (4): 1190–1197.

42. Bozkurt, P., Kilic, N., Kaya, G. et al. (1996). The effects of intranasal midazolam on urodynamic studies in children. *Br. J. Urol.* 78 (2): 282–286.

43. Ameda, K., Kakizaki, H., Yamashita, T. et al. (1997). Feasibility of urodynamic study (combined cystometry and electromyography of the external urethral sphincter) under general anesthesia in children. *Int. J. Urol.* 4 (1): 32–39.

44. Kaefer, M., Rosen, A., Darbey, M. et al. (1997). Pressure at residual volume: a useful adjunct to standard fill cystometry. *J. Urol.* 158 (3 Pt 2): 1268–1271.

45. Yeung, C.K., Godley, M.L., Duffy, P.G., and Ransley, P.G. (1995). Natural filling cystometry in infants and children. *Br. J. Urol.* 75 (4): 531–537.

46. Maizels, M. and Firlit, C.F. (1979). Pediatric urodynamics: a clinical comparison of surface versus needle pelvic floor/external sphincter electromyography. *J. Urol.* 122 (4): 518–522.

47. Lorenzo, A.J., Wallis, M.C., Cook, A. et al. (2007). What is the variability in urodynamic parameters with position change in children? Analysis of a prospectively enrolled cohort. *J. Urol.* 178 (6): 2567–2570.

48. Ngo, T.C., Clark, C.J., Wynne, C., and Kennedy, W.A. 2nd (2011). Radiation exposure during pediatric videourodynamics. *J. Urol.* 186 (4 Suppl): 1672–1676.

49. Hsi, R.S., Dearn, J., Dean, M. et al. (2013). Effective and organ specific radiation doses from videourodynamics in children. *J. Urol.* 190 (4): 1364–1369.

50. Woodside, J.R. and Borden, T.A. (1982). Determination of true intravesical filling pressure in patients with vesicoureteral reflux by Fogarty catheter occlusion of ureters. *J. Urol.* 127 (6): 1149–1152.

51. Bomalaski, M.D. and Bloom, D.A. (1997). Urodynamics and massive vesicoureteral reflux. *J. Urol.* 158 (3 Pt 2): 1236–1238.

13

Urodynamics in Women

Wael Agur[1], Ruben Trochez[2], Antonin Prouza[3], George Kasyan[4], and Abdelmageed Abdelrahman[2]

[1] *Gynaecology Department, NHS Ayrshire & Arran University Hospital Crosshouse, Kilmarnock, UK*
[2] *Liverpool Women's Hospital NHS Foundation Trust, Liverpool, UK*
[3] *Bristol Urological Institute, Southmead Hospital, Bristol, UK*
[4] *Urology Department, Moscow State University of Medicine and Dentistry, Moscow, Russia*

CONTENTS

For women, urodynamics (UDS) is used to assess symptoms which continue to impair quality of life despite having complied with conservative therapy. The affected patient needs to be adequately healthy to undergo interventional therapy, and she needs to be willing to consider it. The dominant context for urodynamic evaluation of women generally is urinary incontinence. However, overactive bladder syndrome (OAB) without incontinence and voiding dysfunction are also important issues.

In this chapter, we discuss how a range of contexts influences the running of a UDS test and the interpretation of findings. The technical side is largely covered in the preceding chapters, in particular Chapter 7. It is worth noting that measurement of abdominal pressure can sometimes use vaginal recording, provided that the catheter is placed high in the posterior fornix (Figure 13.1). For this to work, the pelvic floor function needs to be reasonable for the pressures to record reliably and to hold the catheter in place without falling out.

About half of the women with incontinence suffer stress urinary incontinence (SUI), with 11% having urgency urinary incontinence (UUI), and 36% having mixed urinary incontinence (MUI) [1]. Key to the predisposition of women to incontinence is the anatomical vulnerability of the bladder outlet. The urethra is relatively short, and the sphincter is reliant on pelvic floor support, which is vulnerable to the demands of pregnancy and childbirth. Table 13.1 summarises the data from a large epidemiological study (over 15 000 women) evaluating urinary incontinence according to mode of delivery [2]. Ageing further compounds the risk of incontinence, due to increasing risk of OAB, and a tendency for the urethra to become less competent. The pattern of presentation varies with age, and the overall prevalence increases with age.

It is unrealistic and indeed unnecessary for all women developing incontinence to have urodynamic studies to confirm a diagnosis when they first present. Initial treatment should begin with conservative approaches:

- Formal pelvic floor muscle training (PFMT) for SUI;
- Bladder training, fluid advice, and prescribed medications (antimuscarinics or beta-3 agonist) for OAB; and

Abrams' Urodynamics, Fourth Edition. Edited by Marcus Drake, Hashim Hashim, and Andrew Gammie.
© 2021 John Wiley & Sons Ltd. Published 2021 by John Wiley & Sons Ltd.

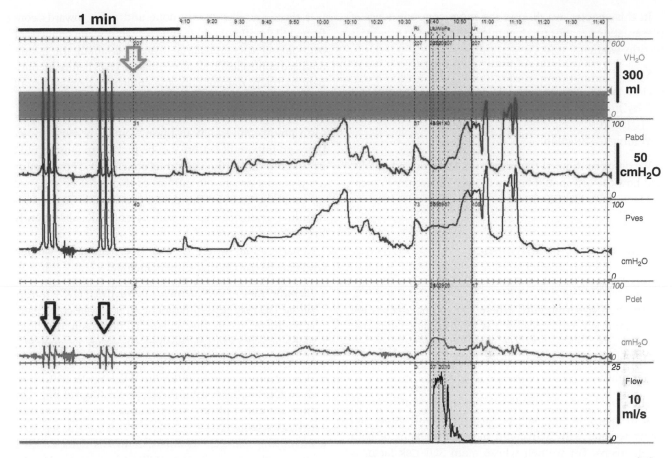

Figure 13.1 Recording from the posterior fornix of the vagina can provide a good approach to recording p_{abd}. This patient was nulliparous, and she had excellent pelvic floor function. The biphasic artefact in p_{det} for two successive cough sequences showed excellent subtraction (black arrows). After permission to void (blue arrow), there was straining visible both before and after flow, and this likewise was well subtracted in p_{det}. However, for many women, this route is not effective.

- Weight loss for body mass index (BMI) over 30.

UDS become relevant if a woman has complied with conservative treatment but remains symptomatic and is bothered by her symptoms. Sometimes, it is needed because conservative treatment is contraindicated (e.g. unable to tolerate OAB medications) or unrealistic (e.g. a woman who cannot voluntarily contract her pelvic floor), and before surgical treatment.

UDS has the role of defining the underlying vesico-urethral disorders when empirical treatment has failed so

that directed therapy to counteract the underlying cause can be derived. This can be an embarrassing situation for patients, and much effort must be made to put the woman at ease so that she will tolerate such intrusive examinations. Throughout, a considerate attitude towards the patient's embarrassment must be maintained. She should be asked to relax her pelvic floor and try to avoid resisting leakage if it is going to happen (this will be very much against her natural instincts). Women will need reassuring that a successful test is one that reproduces her symptoms in an environment where pressures and flows could be measured.

Table 13.1 Urinary incontinence categorised by mode of delivery [2].

Mode of delivery	Any incontinence (%)	Moderate/severe incontinence (%)	SUI (%)	UUI (%)	MUI (%)
Nulliparous	10.1	3.7	4.7	1.6	3.1
Caesarean section	15.9	6.2	6.9	2.2	5.3
Vaginal delivery	21	8.7	12.2	1.8	6.1

SUI: stress urinary incontinence; UUI: urgency urinary incontinence; MUI: mixed urinary incontinence. *Source*: Based on Rortveit et al. [2].

In this chapter, we discuss the more common types of presentation seen for urodynamic assessment in otherwise healthy women:

- SUI;
- OAB, which may be with UUI (OAB 'wet') or without it ('dry');
- MUI; and
- Voiding dysfunction.

We describe some of the associated features and pitfalls, and how the test should be run to help ensure the influential factors are identified.

Stress Urinary Incontinence

SUI is caused by:

1) Urethral hypermobility, where the sphincter does not function properly because it is inadequately supported and
2) Intrinsic sphincter deficiency (ISD), where the sphincter muscle has lost contractile strength.

These are often described as if they are separate entities, but, in fact, this may well be an oversimplification, and many women with SUI could have an element of both mechanisms. For women whose main SUI risk factor is previous childbirth, hypermobility is likely to be the main cause. Some women appear to be at risk of hypermobility without previous childbirth, and this is a notable feature of young women who participate in activity that generates longitudinal impact forces, such as gymnastics and competitive trampolining. This may well reflect the fact that many sporting activities generate abrupt and substantial intra-abdominal pressures [3], much of which will impact directly on the pelvic floor.

Is UDS 'Necessary' in Uncomplicated SUI?

Women with risk factors for ISD, such as neurological disease or previous relevant surgery (e.g. urethral diverticulum excision [4]), need urodynamic assessment to categorise the type of SUI. However, there is controversy on whether UDS are required prior to surgical treatment in women with pure SUI who do not have ISD risk factors. Good-quality assessment is essential:

1) History to exclude risk factors for ISD;
2) Examination to exclude risk factors for ISD and to confirm stress incontinence and urethral hypermobility;
3) Symptom score and bladder diary to exclude OAB; and
4) Free flow test and post-void residual (PVR) scan to exclude voiding dysfunction.

If these are all properly done and point towards confirmed SUI without additional risk factors, the chances of overlooking a complicating feature is small. In a randomised controlled trial, pre-operative UDS before incontinence surgery did not alter the clinical outcomes overall for uncomplicated patients [5]. Nonetheless, there is wide variation in clinical practice, and many surgeons still perform pre-operative UDS in these women, because sometimes an important feature can be picked up which could be very relevant to the individual concerned. These factors are potential prognostic influences that must be weighed up properly, both by the doctor responsible for recommending treatment and the patient who will subsequently live with the outcome.

Considerations where UDS can be helpful for women who may be considering surgery include:

- *Identification of any detrusor overactivity (DO) during filling.* DO may be asymptomatic, or it may be considered subordinate when the patient is first seen in clinic. Nonetheless, DO could become symptomatic after SUI surgery, or increase in severity.
- *Assessment of voiding function.* SUI surgery can introduce some outlet resistance, so pre-existing voiding dysfunction might place a woman at risk of post-operative urinary retention.
- *Identifying sphincter weakness.* If ISD is detected, SUI surgery that treats hypermobility may not resolve the problem.
- *Confirmation that incontinence is indeed present, its severity, and the mechanism.* A history may be unreliable for this. Careful physical examination can achieve a diagnosis of SUI in ideal circumstances if leakage is seen immediately with the first cough. This necessitates an easily seen urethra (so that the timing of leakage can be seen precisely), symptoms that occur in the supine position (since it is difficult to see the urethra in an upright woman while keeping the line of sight, i.e. the observer's face, out of the direction any leak will take), and knowledge of bladder filling state (an underfilled bladder is unlikely to leak). For many women, the physical aspects render the conclusions uncertain. For others, leakage occurs not with the first cough but a subsequent one in a series of coughs. In fact, this is often the case in SUI, because women hold their pelvic floor contracted for an individual cough, but this gets difficult with each repeated cough occurring in quick succession.

The ability to evaluate these aspects of a woman's lower urinary tract function means that some tests can yield results that mandate careful consideration by the surgeon and the patient. These include the following possibilities:

1) **Urodynamic stress incontinence (USI) not seen;**

2) **Low-severity USI;**

If either of these is the conclusion after comprehensive provocation testing (Figure 13.2), the woman needs careful and sympathetic counselling. Symptoms are hard to quantify, as women do not have a benchmark against which to compare their experiences. Thus, urodynamic assessment that finds that incontinence is absent or insubstantial is an important way to establish the possibility there might be only limited potential for improvement with surgery. There is a risk the patient may feel worse off if she has surgery, especially where there is a surgical complication. Roughly 10% of women presenting with SUI had normal UDS (i.e. USI not seen) in an audit at our unit [6]. We would recommend not to undergo surgery for those women due to the low chance of improvement. It is important to review the context, since some people can experience worsening SUI later in the day (presumably due to increasing pelvic floor fatigue). Hence, UDS done in the morning might miss a problem that only really gets bothersome later in the day. If the patient disagrees with a conservative treatment recommendation, then we may proceed to ambulatory urodynamics (AUDS), in order to have the chance of more representative and sustained provocation testing (see Chapter 9).

3) **Mechanism(s) found on UDS that contrasts with that anticipated from symptoms**. Fairly often, symptomatic presentation can suggest one mechanism, while the urodynamic observation establishes a different situation. There are two principal symptomatic/urodynamic discordances applicable:

a) A woman reporting symptoms of stress incontinence found on UDS to have stress-provoked DO incontinence (Figure 1.2). In this situation, the stress test (usually coughing) does not directly cause leakage, it does so indirectly; the urodynamic report must make it totally clear that the mechanism is DO incontinence, not USI. Sometimes, it can be very hard to tell what the mechanism is with certainty (Figure 13.3), in which case more provocation testing is essential in order to come to a reliable conclusion.

b) A woman reporting symptoms of urgency or UUI found to have USI. An important minority of patients living with SUI might describe their symptoms with words suggesting urgency. In this situation, the urgency is probably explained by the strong sensation elicited when urine stimulates urethral sensory nerves, i.e. when the SUI causes a leak which stimulates urethral afferents.

4) **Abnormal voiding.** Since surgery to treat any USI may place a woman at risk of urinary retention, the presence of voiding dysfunction increases potential concern about post-operative retention. For example, some women use straining to enhance a rather weak detrusor contraction and thereby achieve voiding (Figure 13.4). This works where there is no bladder outlet obstruction (BOO), but if SUI surgery leads to any BOO (see below), it would place her at risk of being unable to void.

5) **Multiple symptomatic and urodynamic problems.** MUI is very important to identify (Figure 13.5). Where incontinence is multifactorial, or risk factors such as voiding abnormalities are also present (Figure 13.6), it stands to reason that all identified causes need successful treatment in order to restore continence.

Hence, the confirmation of incontinence and the categorisation of its cause are highly desirable for individual cases, even if the evidence to use UDS routinely in all cases is lacking. USI means that leakage is directly brought on by the cough/raised p_{abd}; subsequent treatment for USI is appropriate. In stress-provoked DO incontinence (DOI), seen as leakage which happens after a short delay while DO becomes established, the subsequent treatment must target the DO. For MUI, in which both direct USI leakage and delayed DOI leakage are seen after coughs, curing incontinence will require successful treatment of both USI and DOI. If USI occurs in a woman who also has DO, but the DO does not cause leakage, treatment is aimed at the most bothersome symptom, with counselling about the risk of adverse outcome resulting from DO if the SUI is treated first. Some women with USI and asymptomatic DO diagnosed on pre-operative UDS could experience symptomatic progression of their DO after USI surgery. Certainly, if DO is found pre-operatively, counselling should include persistence of DO (whether symptomatic or not), and the possibility that UUI could become a post-operative problem, impairing the surgical outcome. This is probably a

---

Fill bladder to 200 ml
- Sequence of strong coughs
- Valsalva

Fill to cystometric capacity
- Remove filling line (2 catheter technique)
- Ask patient to relax her pelvic floor
- Sequence of strong coughs and Valsalvas
- Running on the spot
- Squatting position; coughs/Valsalvas
- Standing with one leg raised; coughs/Valsalvas

Figure 13.2 Maximising the chances of identifying Urodynamic stress incontinence.

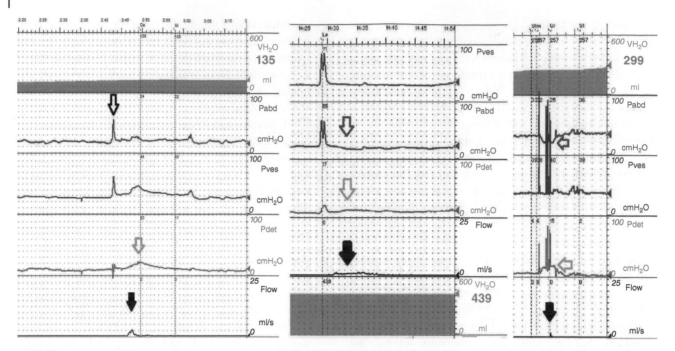

Figure 13.3 Urinary leaks may have uncertain mechanism during urodynamics. Left trace: A cough (open black arrow) is followed by a leak (closed black arrow) and detrusor overactivity (DO; green arrow). However, the leak is very soon after the cough and appears to precede the DO, so there is doubt as to the nature of the leak. In the middle trace, a cough is followed by a leak (black arrow), and at the same time, it looks like there is DO (green arrow). However, the apparent rise in p_{det} is actually caused by a drop in p_{abd} (red arrow), perhaps due to pelvic floor relaxation – there is no rise in p_{ves}. Accordingly, this is not DO incontinence, but secondary to a Valsalva and pelvic floor relaxation, hence related to stress incontinence. The right hand trace is similar to the middle one; again, there is a leak (black arrow), with an appearance to suggest DO (green arrow), but in reality, there is no bladder contraction – again a drop in p_{abd} (red arrow) is seen.

greater risk if DO occurs at low filling volumes, or reaches high amplitude. Similarly, if the detrusor is underactive or acontractile on voiding (even in the absence of voiding symptoms), then pre-operative counselling should include possible consequent voiding difficulties, including potential prolonged catheterisation or the need for intermittent self-catheterisation (ISC). Such urodynamic diagnosis would allow suitable selection of women to be offered an ISC teaching session before SUI surgery. Obtaining the full urodynamic picture allows the surgeon to counsel each woman on the likely outcome of surgery.

The Diagnosis of USI

USI is the involuntary leakage of urine during increased abdominal pressure in the absence of a detrusor contraction during filling cystometry. Thus, with a stable detrusor, the following stress tests can be used to reproduce the symptoms during the UDS test:

- A single cough; this may be all that is needed to confirm USI in some badly affected women.
- Series of coughs; several strong coughs in quick succession. The succession of coughs means that it is difficult for the woman to resist the leakage by holding the pelvic

floor contracted. The interval between coughs needs to be short to avoid her recontracting the pelvic floor after each one.

- Valsalva manoeuvre; this develops a sustained change in abdominal pressure, and again this may be needed to uncover SUI. If it is difficult to communicate what is required, the patient could be asked to blow into the end of a large syringe, as if trying to blow up a party balloon.
- Physical exertion challenge (in the standing position); e.g. running on the spot, jumping on the spot, or star jumps.
- Positional adjustment before cough series or Valsalva; adjusting the legs to make pelvic floor contraction more difficult, e.g. thigh abduction (seated position), or raising one leg on to a chair with a thigh abducted (standing).

Once any of these stress tests has identified a leak, the diagnosis of USI has been made (provided the detrusor stays stable). It is then unnecessary to undertake further stress testing; to do so would potentially be humiliating for the patient. The focus can shift instead to evaluating detrusor function.

A practical step-wise way to run the test for a woman seated on a commode for the filling phase could be:

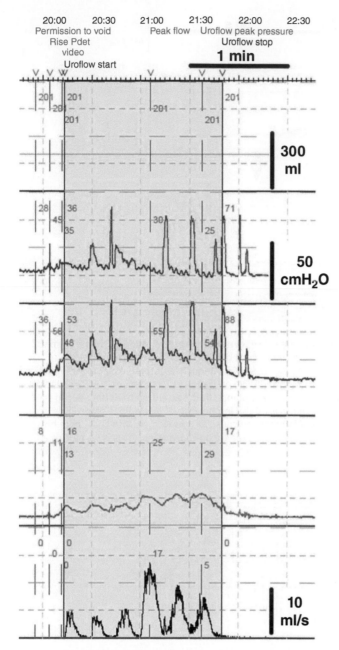

Figure 13.4 Pressure-flow study in a woman with stress incontinence (not shown), illustrating abnormal voiding which could be problematic for complications after stress incontinence surgery. She relied on straining to enhance a rather weak detrusor contraction and thereby achieve voiding.

1) Since single coughs are done right from the start of the test for quality check, note whether any causes USI by checking the flow trace;

2) Stop filling at 200 ml (or half the functional bladder capacity [7]) and do a cough series, and a Valsalva;

3) Restart filling; if DO becomes apparent, stop filling, wait for the DO to settle, and repeat the cough series/Valsalva;

4) At cystometric capacity, remove the filling line (if the two-catheter technique is used) and do a cough series followed by a Valsalva if necessary;

5) If 4 is negative, transfer to the standing position and do a cough series and Valsalva if necessary, with direct inspection of the perineum (since the woman is now not above the flowmeter, so leakage will not show on the flow trace);

6) If 5 is negative, still in the standing position, do physical exertion challenge;

7) If 6 is negative, still in the standing position, do positional adjustment of the legs, with cough series and Valsalva; and

8) Return to the seated position in order to do the pressure-flow study (PFS) (remembering the quality check cough before and after the void).

If DO is problematic, i.e. emerges before adequate testing to look for USI has been done and persists despite stopping filling, it will be necessary to transfer from the seated position to supine. This can have a good chance of stabilising the detrusor (Figure 13.7), and thereby allow stress testing (single cough, cough series, and Valsalva) to confirm USI; perineal inspection will be necessary, since the woman will not be above the flowmeter when supine. Note that position may influence the chance of USI occurring for some women and that supine position may make leakage less likely to happen. For woman whose symptom score and bladder diary indicate OAB, testing for USI needs to be planned with some thought, and it will often be necessary to commence USI tests earlier than 200 ml of filling, especially if the typical voided volumes on the diary are low. Sometimes, it will be necessary for a test to be done while taking OAB treatment medication so that chance of DO is kept as low as possible and thereby permitting proper USI testing to identify if the full diagnosis is MUI.

Implications of Pelvic Organ Prolapse for SUI Evaluation

A fifth of women who have surgery for pelvic organ prolapse (POP) may develop symptoms of stress incontinence post-operatively. So, UDS should be considered in symptomatic women prior to undergoing surgery for POP. However, there is no specific guidance on whether UDS should be performed with the prolapse in its native state, or with the prolapse reduced. The aim of prolapse reduction is to reveal 'occult' stress incontinence (SUI) that might be concealed because of urethral kinking, changes in pressure transmission ratios to the proximal urethra, or a falsely elevated maximum urethral closure pressure (MUCP) due to the prolapse. Many studies have reported a significant

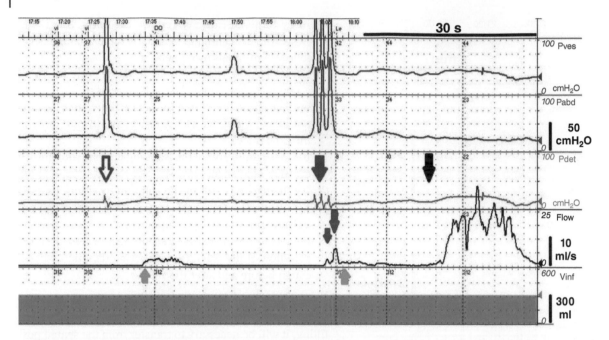

Figure 13.5 Stress provocation testing at the end of filling cystometry and the subsequent pressure-flow study (PFS) in a woman with mixed urinary incontinence. She was asked to do a cough (open purple arrow), which did not lead to urodynamic stress incontinence (USI), but it did provoke detrusor overactivity incontinence (DOI). She then did a sequence of three coughs; the first did not cause a leak, but then a small and a slightly bigger leak is seen (red arrows), and DOI soon afterwards (green arrow). The black arrow indicates permission to void and the PFS follows. This trace illustrates three key points: (i) the attention to detail needed to discern mixed urinary incontinence in someone with USI and stress-provoked DOI, (ii) the importance of a sequence of strong coughs in quick succession for identifying USI, and (iii) the low amplitude of DO that can cause DOI in women with USI – note how the p_{det} pressure change of DOI in this case is almost at the same amplitude as that observed during voiding. (This is an old trace; p_{ves} should not be at the top in modern urodynamics practice.)

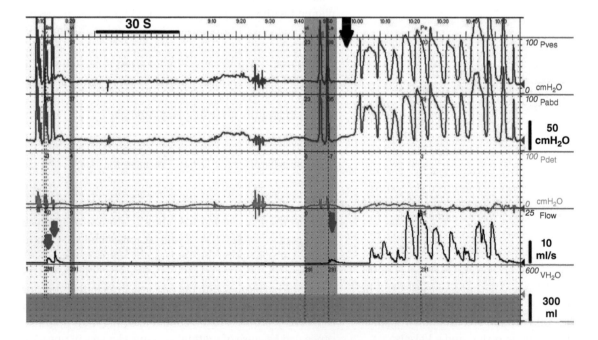

Figure 13.6 Stress provocation testing at the end of filling cystometry and the subsequent pressure-flow study (PFS) in a woman with abnormal voiding. A sequence of three coughs generated two leaks (red arrows) demonstrating urodynamic stress incontinence (USI). Two coughs before the PFS elicited one leak (red arrow). The black arrow indicates permission to void, and the PFS follows. No detrusor contraction is seen, and the intermittent flow pattern is entirely explained by abdominal straining. If this woman underwent surgery to treat USI, there is an extremely high chance she would be unable to void without intermittent self-catheterisation.

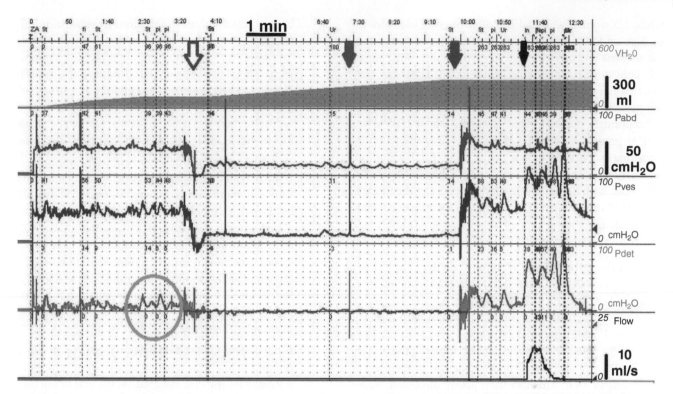

Figure 13.7 Using position change to stabilise the detrusor. This woman developed detrusor overactivity (DO) early during filling, and this persisted despite stopping filling (green circle). She transferred from the seated to the supine position (open purple arrow). Filling was restarted. She experienced stress urinary incontinence with a single cough (red arrow); this had to be detected by perineal inspection during the cough as she was not above the flowmeter when supine. Once filling was completed, she returned to the seated position (closed purple arrow), which immediately led to return of DO. Permission to void was then given (black arrow) for the pressure-flow study.

incidence of occult SUI, using techniques such as ring pessary placement, a vaginal pack, or speculum support. Due to its ease of insertion and widespread availability, the ring pessary is a commonly used method for reducing prolapse prior to urodynamic testing. However, the detection rate of occult SUI in women with higher grades of POP has been variable with ring pessaries. In the Colpopexy And Urinary Reduction Efforts (CARE) trial of women undergoing abdominal sacrocolpopexy for correction of vaginal vault prolapse, prolapse reduction was performed with ring pessaries, and this provided the lowest occult SUI detection rate of 6% compared to 30% with a speculum [8]. Low bladder volume at the time of barrier testing to reposition the prolapse may result in prolapse still masking occult SUI [9]. USI without prolapse reduction has been found to be so uncommon in patients with higher grades of prolapse that it has been suggested that stress testing in these patients should be limited to reduction testing [8]. However, currently available methods for prolapse reduction are not able to predict all the women at risk of developing postoperative SUI after prolapse surgery.

Symptoms of urgency, UUI, and voiding difficulty are commonly reported by women with symptomatic prolapse. In a study of 680 women referred for prolapse management

to a tertiary centre, urgency and urgency incontinence were symptoms reported by 82% and 74%, respectively [10]. A third of all patients described their urgency to be severe, and one-fifth reported severe urgency incontinence. Voiding symptoms were reported by two-thirds of women, while one-third regarded their symptoms as severe. Ten percent of women needed to digitate to empty their bladder.

A significant number of women with prolapse are managed in the community with pessaries. After successful pessary insertion for conservative management of prolapse, improvement may be seen in SUI (45%), UUI (46%), and voiding dysfunction (53%) [11]. There was de novo SUI in 21%, UUI in 6%, and voiding dysfunction in 4%. In our experience, the shelf pessary is useful in women with prolapse who could not retain a ring pessary. Both these pessary types are commonly used in the UK for conservative management of prolapse. Srikrishna et al. [12] performed a ring pessary reduction of prolapse in women having videourodynamics (VUDS) prior to undergoing pelvic reconstructive surgery [12]. The mean ordinal stage of prolapse on the pelvic organ prolapse quantification (POP-Q) system was stage 3. Occult SUI was detected in 10%. Of the 43 women who had no occult USI on the ring test, one developed SUI after pelvic reconstructive surgery (2.3%), while 2/5 women who had USI after the ring test went on to develop SUI after surgery (40%). They concluded that the ring test had poor positive predictive value (40%) but an excellent negative predictive value (98%). However, they inserted the ring pessary only after the cough test and did not perform 'paired' tests.

Accordingly, some thought is needed about UDS when POP is present. Cystocoele can affect urinary function by impeding urinary flow as a result of urethral distortion. Similarly, an advanced vault prolapse (perhaps even a recto-coele) can have the same effect by compressing the urethra. Thus, POP can hide SUI ('occult'/latent incontinence) and/or cause voiding lower urinary tract symptoms (LUTS). There are two key contexts:

1) Does this patient have symptoms attributable to POP, when the POP is at stage 2 (reaching the hymenal ring) or worse? If so, she is likely to be offered POP surgery. In this setting, consider running a UDS test with the POP reduced using a pessary.

   a) If the patient has incontinence symptoms, the pessary UDS will help confirm whether the mechanism is USI or DOI. This can then justify discussion about combining POP and SUI surgery. The National Institute for Health and Clinical Excellence (NICE) Guidelines (Urinary incontinence and pelvic organ prolapse in women: management. NICE Clinical Guideline 123) stipulates, after undertaking a detailed clinical history and examination, to perform multi-channel filling and voiding cystometry before surgery for SUI in women who have anterior or apical prolapse. The SUFU (Society for Urodynamics, Female Pelvic Medicine and Urogenital Reconstruction) guidelines say that multichannel UDS with prolapse reduction may be used to assess for occult stress incontinence and detrusor dysfunction in these women with associated LUTS [13].

   b) If the patient does not complain of incontinence, the UDS test should identify whether occult SUI could be present (see below). If POP surgery is contemplated (usually for patients with symptomatic POP of stage 2 or worse), its implications need to be anticipated, since emergence of symptomatic SUI might then necessitate another operation. Hence, identifying occult SUI in a woman contemplating POP surgery is likely to require discussion about combining POP and SUI surgery.

   c) If the patient has voiding dysfunction (Figure 13.8), the aim is to check whether the voiding returns to normal with the POP reduced. At the end of the test, women with POP, particularly those with advanced stage, may not be able to empty completely. Successful bladder emptying with a vaginal pessary in situ is suggestive of an easily reversible urethral kink rather than a urethral stricture.

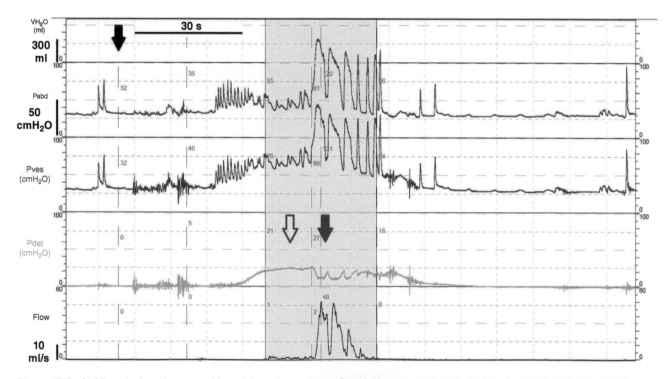

Figure 13.8 Voiding dysfunction caused by pelvic organ prolapse. Permission to void is indicated by the black arrow. She did have a detrusor contraction (open purple arrow), but this generated minimal flow, so she supplemented it with straining (closed purple arrow), which did achieve flow sufficient to enable emptying with only a small post-void residual.

2) Does the patient have no symptoms attributable to POP and/or a prolapse of only stage 1? If so, she is not generally going to be offered POP surgery.

   a) If the patient has incontinence symptoms, the UDS will help confirm whether the mechanism is USI or DOI, and the test will not initially require reduction of POP. However, if incontinence is not demonstrated, and the POP is a cystocoele, there is a possibility that POP may be causing a urethral kink and masking USI. Then, it would be necessary to reduce the POP, using a standard vaginal ring pessary or other physical method to hold the reduction, in order to reveal USI, if present.

   b) If the POP is a cystocoele and she has voiding dysfunction, running the UDS first without the pessary and then with the pessary will help confirm whether the cause of voiding dysfunction is a urethral kink due to the cystocoele. This could inform counselling with regards to surgical POP repair, even for a low-stage prolapse. The differential diagnosis would be a urethral stricture or meatal stenosis, which would not improve, and may worsen, with a pessary in place.

Ideally, a stock of a range of ring pessaries will be available in the urodynamic clinic (Figure 13.9). The starter kit would include at least six to eight of the commonly used sizes, e.g. from 55 to 85 mm. More practically, liaison with a gynaecology service, preferably a co-located one, is important for running the service. The pessary should not be too large; otherwise, it will mask the leakage, particularly if both POP and incontinence are not severe. More advanced POP may be considered for surgery, so the test can appropriately be run with the POP reduced from the start using a pessary as above. This also opens the possibility of an additional approach relevant if the woman strongly reports SUI, but none is seen in the UDS test – which can reflect the limited scope of a UDS test in restricting a patient's position and physical activity potential. Symptoms reported after a one-week home use of a pessary can help anticipate outcome of POP and/or SUI surgery [14].

Up to 22% of women can develop symptomatic SUI following correction of POP, particularly with surgery [15, 16]. It is thought that the prolapse kinks the urethra, therefore masking stress incontinence, which becomes apparent when the prolapse is reduced – i.e. 'occult' or 'latent' SUI. The diagnosis is made by demonstrating USI with the prolapse reduced in a woman who did not report SUI in her initial diagnostic assessment. Several studies have compared different methods to reduce vaginal prolapse at UDS, includ-

Figure 13.9 Pessaries are an important stock item, requiring a range of types and sizes, as an adjunct to control pelvic organ prolapse when undertaking cystometry. Shelf pessaries (not illustrated) are also useful. Pessaries must be fitted with care to avoid discomfort and also to ensure they do not occlude the urethra. *Source:* Marcus Drake.

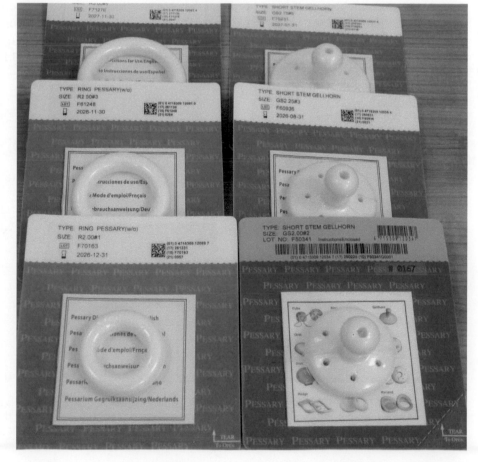

ing pessaries, manual reduction, forceps, swabs, and speculum [8, 12, 17]. There is wide variation in the detection rate of the different reduction methods, and no method is significantly better than others. Overall, they have low sensitivity and high specificity. The diagnosis of occult stress incontinence allows better counselling of women contemplating POP surgery on the risks of post-operative stress incontinence. It should be noted that the prevalence of occult SUI diagnosed urodynamically is higher than the incidence of post-operative de novo SUI after POP surgery [18], suggesting that it is effectively over-diagnosed in UDS.

The role of prophylactic surgery for stress incontinence at the time of surgical correction of prolapse remains uncertain and controversial. For women with POP and asymptomatic (occult) SUI, a meta-analysis confirmed the significantly lower risk of SUI following combined continence and prolapse surgery, compared to only POP procedures (22% versus 52%) [19]. As the number needed to treat, to prevent one woman from developing occult SUI following POP surgery, is three, considerations need to be given towards the risk of a potentially unnecessary SUI surgery and the fact that future repeat SUI surgery may carry lower success rates.

Some centres recommend urodynamic evaluation of women considering surgery for POP even if they do not have LUTS, due to a high prevalence of relevant observations [20]. A finding of USI on UDS in women requesting treatment for prolapse is believed to be important for counselling. Shared decision-making with regards to the use of a continence pessary to address both conditions as a temporary or long-term solution will be more informed. Women keen on avoiding surgery may find a self-managed vaginal continence pessary helpful, particularly if a urodynamically proven leakage is more bothersome during predicted sports activities. For women requesting POP surgery, pre-operative UDS would render counselling more informed when choosing between a concomitant continence procedure, or one done after an interval.

Alternative UDS Techniques for Assessing SUI

VUDS is not necessary for the routine diagnosis of USI, but it is needed to identify ISD (Figure 8.10). This should be considered in women with neurological disease and those who have had previous pelvic surgery. Other urodynamic tests such as urethral profilometry (see Chapter 10) are complementary and may provide useful information supporting the likely situation but cannot be used as the sole basis to diagnose USI if it is not seen during filling cystometry. If, despite carrying out UDS as described above, USI is not demonstrated in patients with the symptom of SUI, and if surgery is strongly being contemplated, then AUDS is the test of choice (see Chapter 9). If no incontinence can be demonstrated with AUDS, then the patient should be told that SUI surgery would not be wise, as the presence and cause of incontinence is unconfirmed. Other conditions such as watery vaginal discharge or a high vesico-vaginal urinary fistula (VVF) (Figure 13.10) may need to be excluded. A VVF

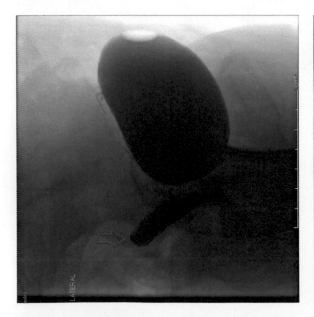 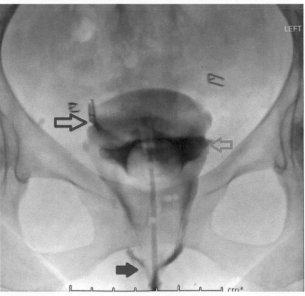

Figure 13.10 Cystogram of a vesico-vaginal fistula after gynaecological surgery. Left image is a lateral view with the patient supine, and right is an antero-posterior view with the patient seated. Contrast has been instilled into the bladder (blue arrow) with a Foley catheter. The open red arrow indicates contrast has gone from the bladder to the upper vagina. From there, gravity takes it to the lower vagina where it leaks out (closed red arrow). *Source*: Marcus Drake.

should be considered in women who have had gynaecological or colorectal surgery within the preceding few months. Sometimes, VVF may follow obstetric complications, or radiotherapy. If suspected, a cystogram (Figure 13.10) or computed tomography scan should be considered.

Recurrent SUI

Women with recurrent or persistent symptoms after previous SUI surgery are an extremely important population for urodynamic assessment. The aim is to establish whether the cause is USI and what type (ISD or hypermobility). This means that VUDS is the more appropriate technique (see Chapter 8). Filling cystometry should be performed in order to assess filling sensation and to establish that the bladder is compliant, does not demonstrate DO, and has a normal capacity [21]. The cystometry should include an assessment in an erect position (seated or standing). If DO or DOI in the erect position makes it difficult to demonstrate USI, lying the patient down in the supine position may help reduce DO so that the presence of USI can be sought – that is, demonstrating mixed symptoms or MUI. Urethral function tests may also have a role with regard to prognosis following surgery and also in planning the most appropriate surgical intervention [22].

When placing the catheters, some relevant feature should be assessed:

- Is the vaginal epithelium healthy? If there is vaginal atrophy, a course of topical oestrogens can be considered [23].

- Is the retropubic space normal? This would make colposuspension or autologous fascial sling a suitable choice.
- Is there any mesh exposure or a significantly tender spot, in a woman who previously had midurethral tape placement? This would need additional surgical planning.

If the cause is pure hypermobility USI, then all the conventional options are probably available to use. If it is ISD, then some compression of the urethra may be needed, for which autologous sling is probably the safest option. Autologous sling can cause voiding difficulty (Figure 13.11), so it is prudent to teach ISC before surgery, thereby ensuring it is possible for the women concerned and would be acceptable to her. Bulking injections to the urethra are an option for either form of USI. The other important thing to identify is whether there is already some voiding dysfunction. If so, careful consideration is needed for the strategy for managing voiding if redo surgery is needed. Two synthetic slings inserted in the same person probably further increases risk of complications and may best be avoided.

Sometimes, DOI is present (Figure 13.12). Clearly, the treatment of that has to address the underlying mechanism. Sometimes, the phrase 'de novo' DO is used; really, this should only be used if the affected person had a symptom score, bladder diary, and UDS which all indicated absence of overactivity. In fact, looking back on these pre-operative evaluations may give some suggestion of OAB, in which case the conversation with a woman struggling with post-surgery DO incontinence can be rather difficult.

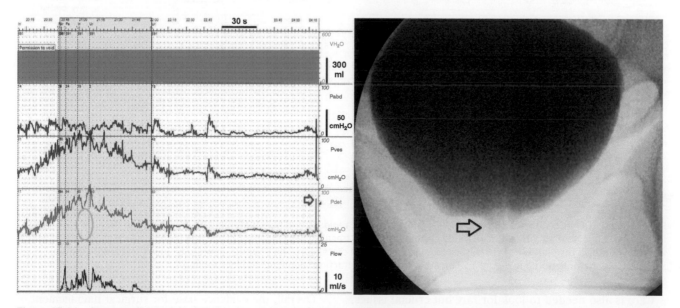

Figure 13.11 Pressure-flow study showing the voiding dysfunction caused by a previous autologous fascial sling. She had a detrusor contraction of high pressure (pink oval) caused by obstruction at the level of the sling (black arrow). She supplemented the detrusor contraction with abdominal straining (yellow oval). The straining is seen in the detrusor line due to poor subtraction, i.e. it is not well picked up in p_{abd}, hence the poor-quality cough subtraction after the conclusion of the PFS (purple arrow). This straining was readily seen with X-ray imaging. *Source*: Marcus Drake.

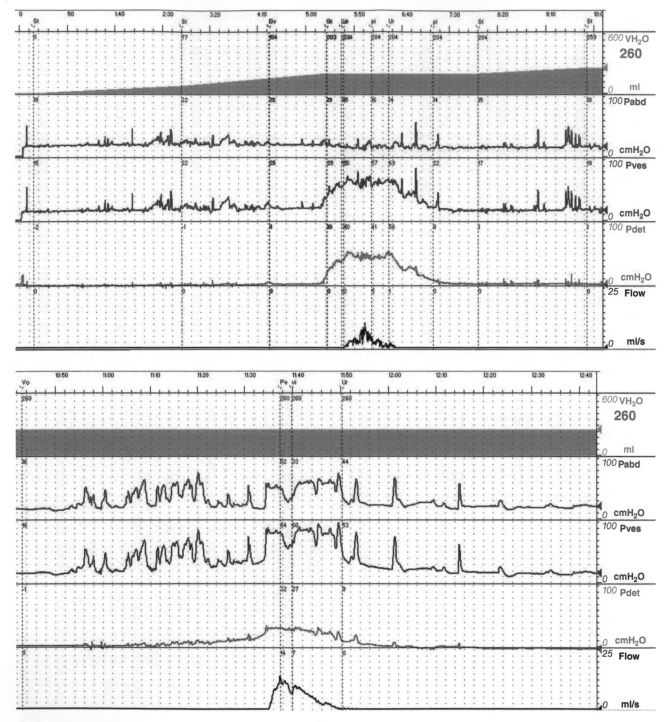

Figure 13.12 DO incontinence in a woman who previously had a midurethral tape placement. She represented because of recurrent incontinence and voiding difficulty. The filling cystometry (upper trace) shows DO incontinence; the high pressure generated for some women with this presentation can be associated with spasm-like discomfort. The pressure-flow study (lower trace) illustrates a situation like that illustrated in Figure 13.11, with a detrusor contraction supplemented by straining.

Care is also needed to look for rare but crucial issues, such as extra-urethral leakage. For example, if a urethral diverticulum was not recognised and SUI surgery done, it could cause the development of a urethro-vaginal fistula.

Overall, the evidence base for surgical management of recurrent SUI is frustratingly limited [24]. For this reason, a large study has recently started in the UK, 'Proper Understanding of Recurrent Stress Urinary Incontinence Treatment in women' (PURSUIT), which is randomising women with recurrent or persistent SUI to surgery or urethral bulking (https://doi.org/10.1186/ISRCTN12201059).

Overactive Bladder

OAB is characterised by urinary urgency, with or without UUI, usually with increased daytime frequency and nocturia, if there is no proven infection or other obvious pathology [25]. In OAB due to DO, increased daytime frequency and urgency may be the first symptoms a woman starts to experience, with UUI developing later. A nulliparous woman can generally use her pelvic floor to prevent leakage during a DO contraction, and in doing so may also shorten its duration (the reason women are given pelvic floor muscle exercises as part of bladder training in OAB) (Figure 13.13). In DO, incontinence occurs because the increased bladder pressure overcomes the combined resistance of the intrinsic urethral muscle plus voluntary contraction of the pelvic floor; where these are strong, high pressures may be generated during a DO contraction. The reduced pelvic floor function commonly seen in parous women places them at greater risk of DOI due to impaired resting tone and voluntary resistance. In this case, leakage may happen at only low pressure (Figure 13.14), and the woman will often report a short interval between urgency

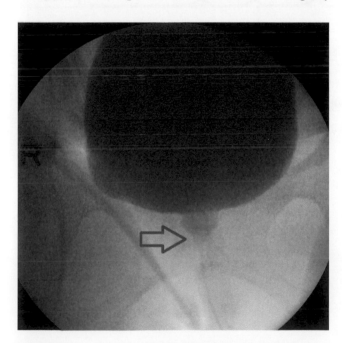

Figure 13.13 A woman who is managing to prevent detrusor overactivity (DO) from causing leakage by contracting her urinary sphincter forcefully (purple arrow). This ability to resist DO can mean that high pressures may be generated in the bladder. Once she eventually relaxes her sphincter, the resulting urinary stream pattern will have a very rapid initial part. *Source*: Marcus Drake.

onset and leakage, making it very difficult to reach the toilet before substantial urine loss has occurred.

Some women have a convincing history of OAB but do not have corresponding DO. This may reflect four scenarios:

- The nature of the urodynamic testing environment, particularly the anxiety many patients experience beforehand, may mask the DO.
- Abnormal muscle activity causing urgency may be present, but it is uncoordinated, and so does not generate detectable pressure change [26].
- The urgency may be because sensory nerve pathways are sensitised, and over-reporting the filling state. This may be more likely when there are also issues with adjacent organs, such as vaginal inflammation or bowel symptoms (Figure 2.20).
- Urethral receptors are being stimulated. This may explain how pre-operative 'urgency' sometimes resolves in some patients following surgery for USI [27].

Conventional UDS tends to show that about two-thirds of women complaining of OAB have DO. When a tightly defined population of women with OAB and UUI and no SUI is studied, AUDS shows the cause of incontinence is almost always DO. Thus, the nature of the presentation and the mode of testing influence how tightly OAB presentations correlate with detection of DO.

There is only limited evidence on the relationship between urodynamic testing and subsequent interventional treatment outcomes for DO. A large UK-based study (Female Urgency, Trial of Urodynamics as Routine Evaluation, 'FUTURE', https://doi.org/10.1186/ISRCTN 63268739) is in progress to evaluate this. Some parameters may anticipate the need for self-catheterisation for those women considering botulinum-A injections (specifically, the maximum flow rate and the projected isovolumetric pressure are significantly lower in patients who require ISC after treatment) [28]. Higher pressure DO is associated with failure of SUI surgery and persistent post-operative urgency [29–31]. Accordingly, the necessity of urodynamic testing in OAB may not be driven so much by evaluating the mechanism, as by detecting whether USI or voiding dysfunction is present, since these would influence treatment choice and outcome. This would only be appropriate for women struggling with ongoing symptoms despite complying fully with conservative therapy as recommended in guidelines [32]. They should also have been offered a proper trial of the best medications available, i.e. more than one antimuscarinic (not solely oxybutynin), and a beta-3 agonist, and potential combination therapy [33]. Where these have been fully trialled and failed, a woman may be keen for interventional therapy, and she will need

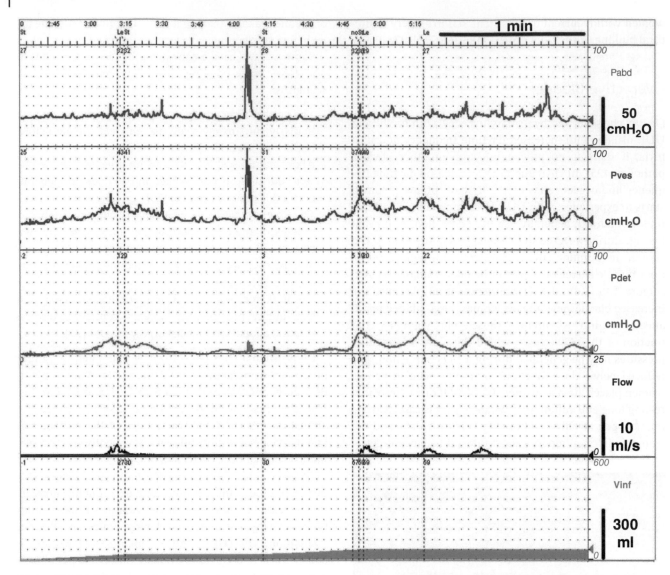

Figure 13.14 A woman who is unable to prevent DO incontinence with her urinary sphincter effectively. Consequently, she leaks when only a small pressure rise has occurred.

to be given good information about the implications of this regarding adverse aspects. Thus, a definitive urodynamic diagnosis may facilitate treatment decisions through better counselling and informed consent.

Increased Filling Sensation

Increased filling sensation ('bladder hypersensitivity') is quite a common urodynamic observation and is used to signify people who, during UDS, experience an early first sensation of filling (FSF) and an early first desire to void (e.g. at only 150 ml), which persists into a normal and a strong desire without a break (Figure 13.15). This contrasts with the general observation that most individuals do not report sensation between FSF and normal desire to void. For people with increased filling sensation, the bladder

diary often shows voided volumes consistently less than 250 ml throughout the day (there may be a larger voided volume on rising in the morning). If the bladder diary does not show this, then a person reporting an early and persisting desire to void in a urodynamic test is probably experiencing urethral stimulation by the catheter, perhaps worsened by the pulsations caused by the filling pump. Attempts to take the patient's mind away from their urinary tract on to other matters may help resolve this issue.

Urethral Relaxation Incontinence

Urethral relaxation incontinence is defined as leakage due to urethral relaxation in the absence of raised abdominal pressure or a detrusor contraction [34]. Leakage without

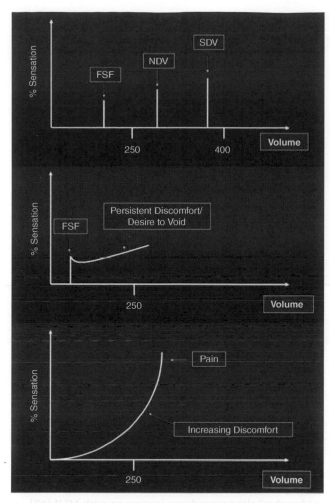

Figure 13.15 Schematic representation of filling sensations for normal lower urinary tract function (top), increased filling sensation (middle), and bladder pain syndrome (bottom). FSF: first sensation of filling; NDV: normal desire to void; SDV: strong desire to void.

change in detrusor or abdominal pressure can really only happen if urethral relaxation occurs. Here, there exists an overlap and some confusion with the previously used term 'urethral instability', which was defined as a fall in urethral pressure of greater than 20 cmH$_2$O recorded when measuring the MUCP, during bladder filling or at capacity. However, it is rare to witness urethral relaxation leading to incontinence whilst doing conventional UDS, and it appears to be an unusual single cause of incontinence. Nevertheless, we have seen the occasional female patient who has flooding incontinence without any prior warning, such as the feeling of urgency. In such patients, if conventional UDS fails to show a cause for incontinence, then it might be helpful to record urethral pressures over a 5–10 minute period, at capacity, to see if the MUCP fluctuates. Alternatively, AUDS can give a greater chance to observe the problem (Figure 13.16).

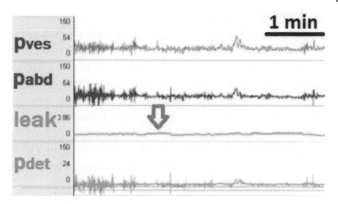

Figure 13.16 Urethral relaxation incontinence during an ambulatory urodynamics study. This lady experienced increasing leakage at the time of the arrow, yet she was not active physically at that time. There was no detrusor overactivity. Accordingly, her urethra must have been inappropriately relaxed.

In some women with USI, urethral pressure fluctuations might make incontinence worse if the fall in urethral pressure corresponds to an increase in abdominal pressure due to coughing or straining.

Bladder Pain Syndrome

This is one of the chronic pelvic pain syndromes described in an International Continence Society (ICS) Standardisation [35]; see Appendix B for the 'fundamentals' summary version [36]. Common complaints include increased urinary frequency (both during the day and the night), urgency, hypersensitivity, pain, pressure, discomfort, pain with filling, hesitancy, intermittency, and feeling of incomplete emptying [35, 37]. Pain/hypersensitivity related to the bladder provides an umbrella for hypersensitive bladder/interstitial cystitis/bladder pain syndrome (BPS) and interstitial cystitis with Hunner lesion [35]. 'Urgency' refers to a compelling need to urinate which is difficult to defer, but the ICS Working Group identified the following adjustments as applying more descriptively, for example, to Interstitial Cystitis/BPS patients: a compelling need to urinate, due to pain or an unpleasant sensation, which is difficult to defer.

The ICS believes that it is unhelpful to put all such patients into the category of 'interstitial cystitis', implying an assumption that this is a single disease, when it seems likely that several disease processes actually contribute to the spectrum of BPS. Bladder pain is a symptom that may warrant further investigations including urine microscopy, cytology, and cystoscopy. However, the value of UDS is doubtful [37], especially as it will usually be a distinctly unpleasant experience for a woman truly affected by BPS. If done, increased filling sensation is present in almost 90% of cases [38]. Flow rates are often reduced; while this prob-

It is also important to enquire about a woman's obstetric history, in particular, number of vaginal deliveries, instrumental deliveries, birthweight, duration of second stage, and use of an episiotomy.

During examination, perianal skin should be carefully assessed, looking for irritation, excoriation or erythema (which may suggest chronic passive soiling), and a patulous anus. Inspection should also include scars from previous surgery, perianal disease such as haemorrhoids or warts, and shortening of the perineal body (which may suggest obstetric trauma [45]). Digital examination should identify rectal content, resting tone, and voluntary and involuntary squeeze pressure.

Affected women undergoing UDS are commonly found to have USI (42%) or DO (37.5%) [46]. Women with mixed urinary and faecal incontinence presented a greater descent of the pelvic floor and more obtuse anorectal angle, suggesting that both urinary and faecal incontinence might be due to pelvic floor denervation [47]. Technical problems with measuring intra-abdominal pressure in women with faecal incontinence are common, as there may be difficulty in ensuring the rectal catheter stays in place during UDS. As a result, this may lead to problems with measuring the intra-abdominal pressure. In such circumstances, clinicians may consider measuring p_{abd} from the upper part of the vagina.

Commonly performed tests to evaluate faecal incontinence include anorectal manometry (described in detail in Chapter 20) and endoanal ultrasonography. Anal manometry involves placing a manometry catheter inside the anal sphincter, below the puborectalis, to measure the muscle strength at rest and during squeezing. An endoanal ultrasound involves placing an ultrasound scanner within the anal canal to assess its anatomy. Additionally, neurophysiological testing, such as electromyography, may be considered. This test evaluates the nerve supply of the anal canal and rectum.

Sequential anorectal physiology and UDS could be considered in women with mixed incontinence, perhaps through joint urogynaecology and colorectal clinics. This approach will allow combined evaluation, which may lead to higher patient satisfaction due to tests being performed in one setting. However, it is important to note that bladder filling and voiding alters intra-anal pressure profiles and anorectal function, therefore potentially affecting interpretation of results.

Primary measures to treat faecal incontinence include identifying contributory factors, excluding treatable causes (e.g. constipation), patient education, and lifestyle advice regarding modifying diet and fluid intake. If there are ongoing symptoms, women should be considered for referral to a specialist bowel dysfunction clinic to consider further management. This may include biofeedback, pelvic floor exercises, and pharmacological treatment.

When considering surgery for women with USI and faecal incontinence, clinicians should identify and treat the most bothersome symptom in the first instance. Concomitant surgery is an option for such women, although this is not common practice in the UK. Persistent post-operative symptoms (either SUI or faecal incontinence) can be challenging to treat. Two-stage procedures may be beneficial and should therefore be discussed with women pre-operatively.

Situational Incontinence; Coital/Orgasm Leakage and Giggle Incontinence

Some women experience incontinence under certain circumstances which can be highly problematic. Coital urinary incontinence (CI) is defined as a urinary incontinence occurring before, during, or after vaginal intercourse [48]. This symptom might be further divided into that occurring with penetration or intromission and that occurring at orgasm [34]. Injury to the pudendal or pelvic nerves, pelvic floor/sphincter incompetence, and DO may contribute to the mechanism [49]. The Bristol database shows that the prevalence of CI in women with LUTS undergoing UDS could be as high as 11.8%, with a younger mean age of 45 years, compared with 53 years for the overall patient population [50]. CI was significantly associated with USI or DO, but not DOI [50] (Table 13.2). In the literature, the prevalence of CI in urinary incontinent women has been reported from 10% to 56% [51]. Obesity (BMI $>30 \text{kg/m}^2$) and parity were significantly associated with CI. In the literature from other centres, the prevalence of CI in urinary incontinent women has been reported from 10% to 56% [51].

Both sphincter weakness and DO can be relevant [49], so this is not a single mechanism responsible for all cases. Our observation that DO without incontinence can be associated with coital incontinence is interesting. It raises the possibility that these women generally remain continent during routine activities by resisting DO with their sphincter (as illustrated in Figure 13.13) but fail to achieve this under the specific circumstance of sexual intercourse. Urodynamic investigations of women suffering from CI revealed that women with incontinence at orgasm have a significantly higher rate of DO (69.4%) compared with women experiencing incontinence during penetration (28.9%) [52]. However, Figures 13.18 and 13.19 demonstrate the complexity of interpretation, since there may additionally be a contribution of inappropriate urethral relaxation.

Giggle incontinence is urinary leakage preceded or accompanied by a sudden urgency to void induced by giggling [53]. It is a rare condition in which extensive emptying or leakage occurs during or immediately after laughing.

Table 13.2 Logistic regression analysis of variables in women with coital incontinence compared with age-matched controls.

Variables	P value	Odds ratio	95% confidence interval
High BMI ($>30\,kg\,m^{-2}$)	0.708	0.968	0.814–1.149
Smokers	0.435	1.077	0.894–1.296
Antidepressants	0.203	1.181	0.914–1.525
Menopausal	0.222	1.158	0.915–1.464
Previous hysterectomy	0.589	1.054	0.871–1.276
Parity[a]	<0.001	1.147	1.076–1.233
Overactive bladder symptoms	0.003	1.293	1.089–1.536
Urinary stress incontinence[a]	<0.001	2.766	1.964–3.896
Normal urodynamics	0.432	1.155	0.806–1.655
Detrusor overactivity	0.324	1.168	0.858–1.589
DOI	0.639	0.938	0.710–1.234
UDSI[a]	<0.001	2.14	1.625–2.818
DOI+UDSI[a]	<0.001	2.814	2.123–3.729
Daytime frequency	0.173	1.020	0.991–1.049
Nocturia episodes	0.237	1.047	0.971–1.129

BMI: body mass index; DOI: detrusor overactivity incontinence; UDSI: urodynamic stress incontinence.
[a] Significant ($P<0.05$). *Source*: Madhu et al. [50].

It may represent a special form of DO, or perhaps an abnormal discharge from the central nervous system, provoked by laughter [54]. It is more often identified in children, but it can be encountered in adults. It is not clear whether the difference is due to resolution of the symptom, or failure to present for medical assessment. Lower urinary tract function is generally normal when there is no laughter [55]. Furthermore, a detailed history and physical examination are normally enough to rule out other reasons of incontinence (at least in children) [56]. Hence, urodynamic testing is not performed routinely for patients with giggle incontinence. Nonetheless, AUDS may play some role in diagnosis,

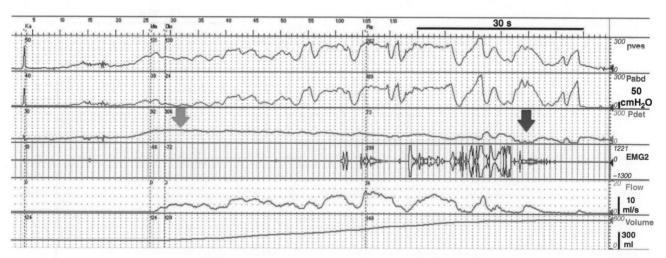

Figure 13.18 Urodynamic trace illustrating orgasm incontinence (non-coital, induced by clitoral self-stimulation) in a 31-year-old nulliparous woman. She had no known neurological problems, and orgasm incontinence was her only symptomatic complaint. Urine leakage (flowmeter reading is plotted in light blue, fifth trace from the top) in the earlier part of the orgasm appears to be a result of detrusor overactivity. The latter half is dominated by very high-amplitude spasmic changes in abdominal pressure (note the scale bar indicating $50\,cmH_2O$). DO has partly abated by this stage (red arrow), and the electromyography recording has declined somewhat, suggesting a contribution of urethral relaxation at this stage.

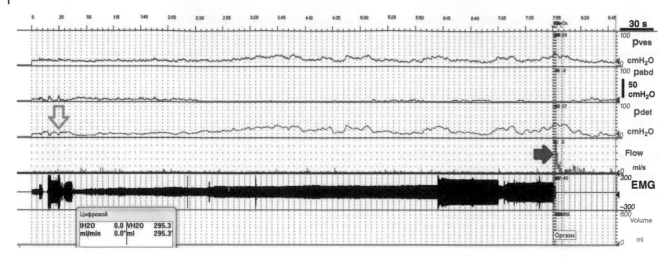

Figure 13.19 Urodynamic trace illustrating orgasm incontinence (non-coital) in a 40-year-old nulliparous operated for myelodysplasia in childhood. Her symptoms were urgency urinary incontinence and orgasm incontinence. Detrusor overactivity is seen early after the start of clitoral self-stimulation (open green arrow) but does not cause incontinence. Incontinence (flowmeter reading is plotted in pink, fourth trace from the top) occurs at the time of orgasm (closed red arrow) and appears to be a result of urethral relaxation, since the electromyographic recording from the pelvic floor abruptly ceases at that point. There is, nonetheless, slight enhancement of the detrusor overactivity at that time.

since this is the test where there is realistically the best chance to capture a giggle incontinence episode and hence establish a mechanism (Figure 13.20). Behavioural modification, biofeedback [57], anticholinergics, antidepressants, methylphenidate [58], or botulinum toxin [59] have been investigated as treatment options for these patients [60], generally with uncertain clinical benefits.

BOO and Detrusor Underactivity (DUA)

BOO

While it is uncommon in women, BOO is clearly a possibility; the basic mechanisms may result from distortion of the outlet, compression of the urethra (structural or functional),

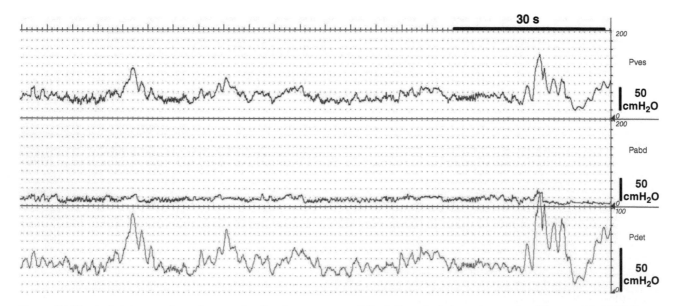

Figure 13.20 Ambulatory urodynamic trace showing detrusor overactivity during giggle incontinence in a 15-year-old girl. High-amplitude detrusor overactivity (118 cmH$_2$O) is prominent. Note the scale of the p$_{ves}$ and p$_{abd}$ traces are up to 200 cmH$_2$O, while p$_{det}$ is plotted to 100 cmH$_2$O.

or occlusion (Figure 13.21). Structural issues can include meatal stenosis (Figure 13.22), urethral stricture, urethral obstruction from POP, and iatrogenic (Figure 13.23). These situations can be compensated physiologically by an increase in detrusor contraction (Figure 13.24); the presence of voiding symptoms presumably becomes an issue if the BOO is severe, or the physiological compensation insufficient (as in neurological disease or ageing). Functional issues include patients found to have abnormally high MUCP (Figure 13.25), of which Fowler's syndrome is the best-known mechanism (Figure 7.55).

Establishing the presence of BOO in women suffers from lack of agreed international consensus on diagnostic parameters. This is because the dynamics of voiding vary more than in men, and there is no equivalent to transurethral resection of the prostate for reliably relieving the problem in women. In order to determine the likelihood of obstruction during a PFS, Defreitas et al. [61] evaluated sensitivity and specificity of various approaches. They established an easily remembered criterion for BOO:

Female BOO is present if flow rate is $\leq 12\,ml/s$, and $p_{detQmax} \geq 25\,cmH_2O$.

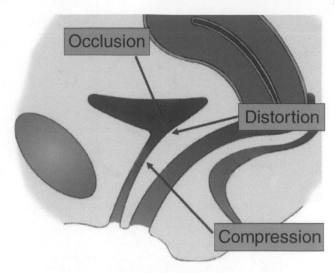

Figure 13.21 Processes that can cause bladder outlet obstruction in women. Occlusion may result from plugging of the internal urethral meatus by a structure such as a bladder stone or a ureterocoele (Figure 8.16). Distortion can be a consequence of iatrogenic problems, such as a tape or sling that is located too proximally or placed too firmly, or a cystocoele affecting the urethra. Compression can result from pelvic organ prolapse pushing onto the back of the urethra.

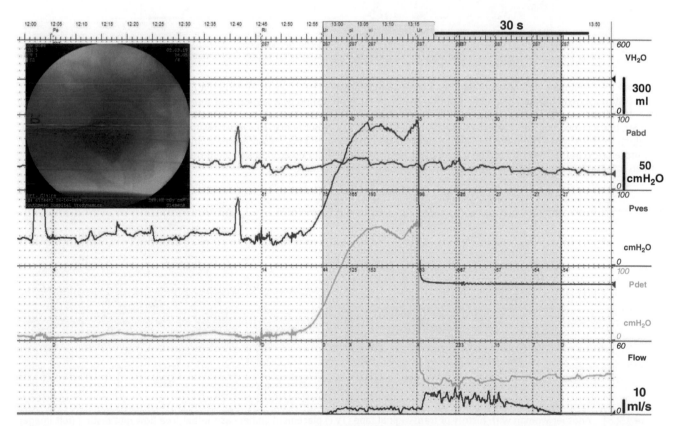

Figure 13.22 Pressure-flow study in a woman with meatal stenosis. The size of the stenosis was very close to the gauge of the double lumen catheter. Consequently, the lumen was largely occluded; this, combined with the inelastic nature of meatal stenosis, meant the bladder outlet was largely 'plugged' by the catheter. This was a comparatively young woman, in her 40s, so her detrusor compensated by generating a very high pressure. This was sufficient to expel the catheter, hence the abrupt drop in p_{ves} and p_{det}. *Source*: Marcus Drake.

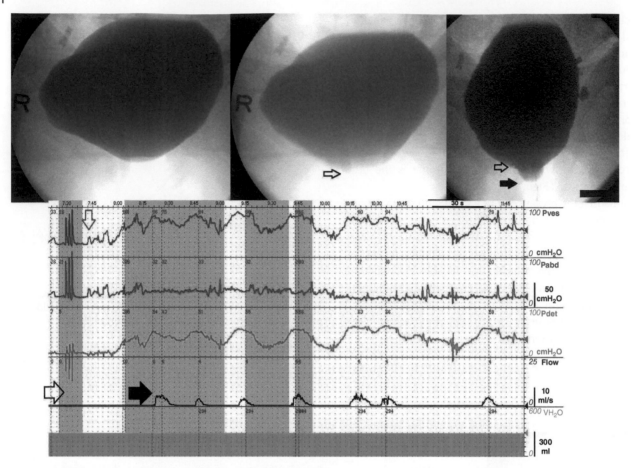

Figure 13.23 A woman with obstruction after a transvaginal tape (TVT) placement. The top left image is taken at rest at the end of filling cystometry. The top middle image is during stress provocation testing by a sequence of three coughs; the open black arrow shows that there was no urethral hypermobility and contrast did not enter the proximal urethra, and in the urodynamic trace below, the open black arrow indicates that there was no urodynamic stress incontinence. This indicates that TVT achieves continence control by reduction of urethral hypermobility. The top right image is taken during the pressure-flow study; permission to void is indicated by the purple arrow in the lower trace. The closed black arrows indicate hold-up at the location of the TVT (image), which is associated with an intermittent urinary stream (urodynamic trace). *Source*: Marcus Drake.

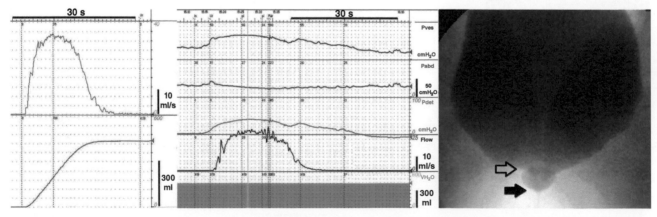

Figure 13.24 Another woman with history of transvaginal tape (TVT) placement. In her case, initial free flow rate testing (left image) showed a normal flow trace. Likewise, pressure-flow study (middle image) indicated a normal flow pattern and speed, generated with a p_{det} of 40 cmH$_2$O (a small amount has to be subtracted from the detrusor pressure value to compensate for a small drop in abdominal pressure during the pressure-flow study). The video urodynamics image (right) showed dilation of the proximal urethra and hold-up at the TVT (closed black arrow), similar to that seen in the woman with clear bladder outlet obstruction shown in Figure 13.23. *Source*: Marcus Drake.

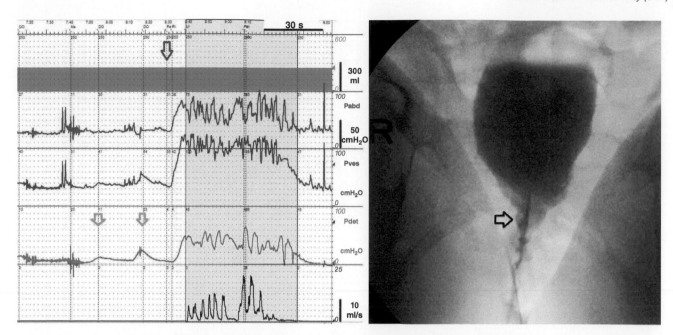

Figure 13.25 A woman with high pressure and slow flow intermittent voiding due to functional hold-up at the urethral sphincter (black arrow). Permission to void is indicated by the purple arrow. The pressure-flow study identifies a detrusor contraction supplemented by straining. This woman also had detrusor overactivity (green arrows). *Source*: Marcus Drake.

Sometimes, the urodynamicist may need to refer to a nomogram, as published by various groups [62, 63]. Comparisons applying these and various approaches developed over the years [64–67] to the same individuals reveal discrepancies, i.e. that a women diagnosed as having BOO with one approach may not with another [68]. This underlines that clinical acumen is important rather than over-relying on uncertain parameters. A practical approach from University College Hospital, London (the Solomon-Greenwell nomogram [62]), uses the female BOO Index (BOOIf):

$$BOOIf = p_{detQmax} - 2.2 \times Q_{max}$$

- If BOOIf is <0, the probability of obstruction is <10%.
- If BOOIf is >5, the probability of obstruction is 50%.
- If BOOIf is >18, the probability of obstruction is >90%.

One of the key necessities to validate an obstruction nomogram is the sensitivity to change in the measured parameter following successful treatment of BOO (i.e. retesting with repeat UDS post-operatively confirms the parameter has shifted from indicating BOO to unobstructed, assuming that surgery successfully resolved the obstruction). This has recently been published for the Solomon-Greenwell nomogram [69].

Underactivity

The term 'detrusor underactivity' (DUA) implies that weakness of the bladder contraction underpins the voiding dysfunction. As a result, an intermittent stream is seen, as the affected woman uses straining to achieve flow (Figure 13.26).

Mere inspection of the PFS trace, seeing a slow and fluctuating detrusor contraction and urine flow, often combined with straining (Figure 13.27), in a woman presenting with voiding symptoms and relevant risk factors (e.g. old age and menopause) can be strongly suggestive. Sometimes, this can be extreme, with no obvious change in detrusor pressure, termed acontractile or 'areflexic' (in neurogenic lower urinary tract dysfunction). This may lead to extremely protracted voiding time (Figure 13.28). Women occasionally undertake considerable physical efforts to initiate or sustain voiding (Figure 13.29). It is worth considering training in ISC for women who have severely protracted voiding time, substantial physical effort to void, or where straining is exacerbating POP.

Two issues should be considered, particularly in women, when scrutinising the detrusor contraction in a PFS:

1) Increasing p_{ves} is hard with a wide outlet, and this can give a misleading impression that the detrusor is not contracting.
2) Recording of p_{abd} is also sometimes unreliable in women, due to impaired pelvic floor function. Consequently, subtraction becomes uncertain, meaning that the plotted p_{det} might be misleading. It is vital to check the cough subtraction before and after voiding to decide whether a plotted p_{det} is representative of actual bladder contraction.

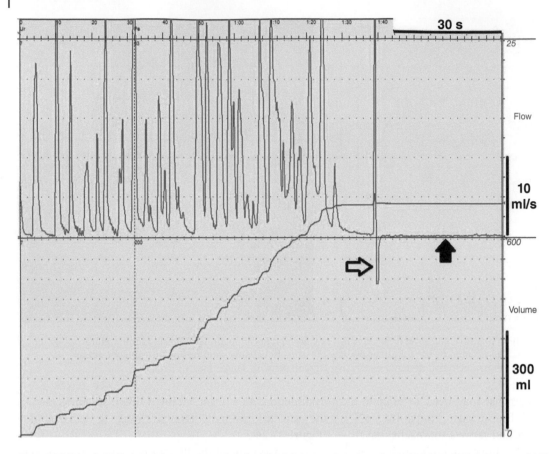

Figure 13.26 Free flow test in a woman, showing the interrupted stream characteristic of straining to void. The high voided volume of 739 ml suggests she has reduced bladder sensation. Post-void residual was 60 ml. The open black arrow indicates a negative value of flow rate, which is an artefact, probably because the flowmeter was knocked. The closed black arrow indicates terminal dribbling.

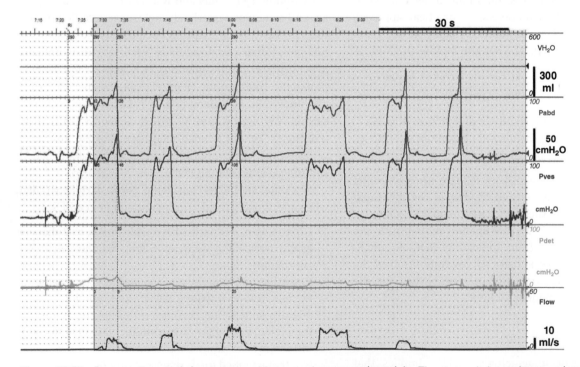

Figure 13.27 Pressure-flow study in a woman with severe detrusor underactivity. The stream is intermittent and mainly generated by straining.

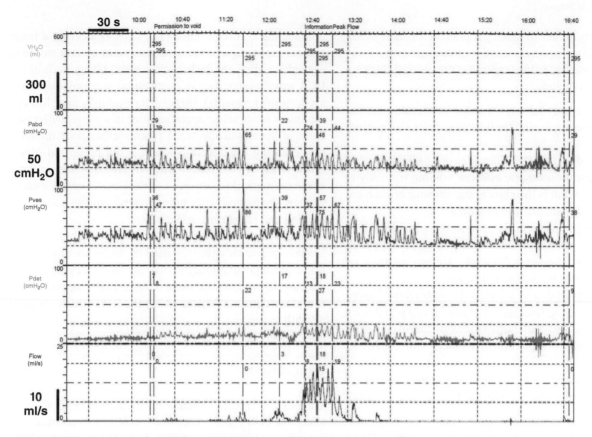

Figure 13.28 Pressure-flow study in another woman with severe detrusor underactivity. The stream is intermittent and mainly generated by straining; flow time is considerable – more than four minutes.

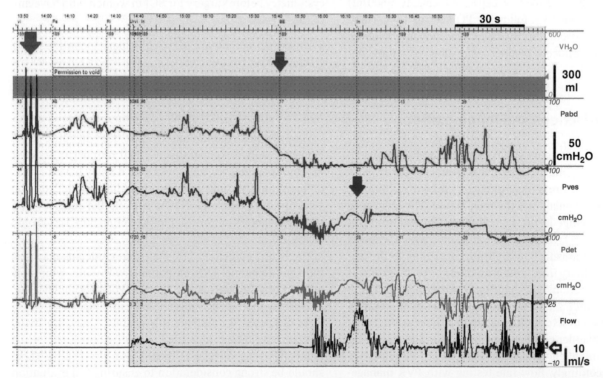

Figure 13.29 Pressure-flow study (PFS) in a woman with severe detrusor underactivity, illustrating the uncertain reliability of pressure recording, and the physical effort women sometimes use when trying to void. The cough test preceding the PFS (red arrow) is very poorly subtracted, indicating that p_{abd} is unreliable. She generated some flow, probably with a detrusor contraction, after permission to void. Beyond the purple arrow, she did a lot of bouncing, shifting from buttock to buttock, lifting her thighs, and straining. This effort did generate some flow but also caused negative flow artefact (as discussed in Figure 13.26) – black arrow indicates zero flow. This physical activity then made the p_{ves} recording unreliable as well (blue arrow).

DUA is even harder to agree parameters for than BOO, and we are still a long way from widespread agreement [70]. Specific discussed questions regarding measure of contractility in women include:

- Which is the optimal cut-off value of female bladder voiding efficiency during uroflow to suspect obstruction or DU?
- Is it right to diagnose DU in females on the basis of prolonged micturition despite efficient voiding (i.e. only a small PVR)? What is the clinical significance of such an observation if there are no symptoms?
- Bladder contractility index is a parameter applicable in men [71]. Nonetheless, it has been used in women, perhaps with rather doubtful intellectual validity. Unfortunately, it is highly influenced by outflow resistance.
- Can pure impaired detrusor vs. pure obstructed voiding be distinguished in females, for example, is it possible to determine the relative contributions of detrusor weakness and outlet obstruction in women with equivocal obstruction?
- Does Valsalva voiding and/or straining in the presence of DU/acontractility have structural or other clinical consequence?

The 'stop test' discussed in Chapter 7 (Figure 7.47) is very rarely used. In clinical practice, a combination of PVR (>200 ml) with large bladder capacity (capacity >600 ml) predicts persistent PVR following POP repair [72]. These may constitute useful thresholds for planning intervention. In addition, reduced bladder sensation is commonly associated [73].

Urinary Infections and Inflammation

Urinary tract infections (UTIs) are common in women, probably due to limited anatomical defences (particularly for women with stress incontinence), and with additional risk for older women after the menopause. The latter may result from change in the vaginal microbial environment, away from the favourable lactobacillus, which enables pathogenic organisms to establish in proximity to the urinary tract. Urinary infections are a mode of presentation of voiding dysfunction. UDS have little part to play, although urine flow studies and ultrasound estimates of residual urine are used to screen older women with recurrent infections. Poor bladder emptying might be relevant, theorising that a PVR might encourage bacterial growth through stagnation. Accordingly, flow rate testing with PVR management should be considered for women presenting with problematic UTI recurrence [74]. DUA as a cause of poor bladder emptying is a recognised issue in elderly women, notwithstanding the lack of consensus on its definition. DUA may be secondary to medications (e.g. opiates or tricyclic antidepressants), surgery (for example, after hysterectomy or other pelvic operations), or neurological disease. Some women with bacterial cystitis experience incontinence during the infection which is not present at other times. This can become a substantial issue for women prone to frequent recurrence of infection. Clearly, for such women, the incontinence management requires a focus on treating and preventing infections.

Bladder inflammation can result from other causes. Notably, pelvic radiotherapy used in cancer treatment can lead to chronic inflammation which may cause progressive scarring. Consequently, some women can develop poorly compliant detrusor (Figure 13.30) and DUA which are very difficult to treat.

Conclusions

The NICE Clinical Guideline for incontinence in women takes a selective line on routine use of UDS, recommending, after undertaking a detailed clinical history and examination, to perform multichannel filling and voiding cystometry before surgery for SUI in women who have any of the following:

- Urgency-predominant MUI, or urinary incontinence in which the type is unclear
- Symptoms suggestive of voiding dysfunction
- Anterior or apical POP
- A history of previous surgery for SUI.

They do not recommend UDS is used in 'pure' SUI. However, only a comparatively small number of women fall into this category, and those who do may have a rather different urodynamic picture from that implied by the symptom [6] (Figure 13.31). As a result, the accuracy of a history diagnosis of pure SUI in predicting pure USI is only 74.4% [6].

The SUFU guidelines [13] state that clinicians may perform multichannel UDS in patients with both symptoms and physical findings of SUI who are considering invasive, potentially morbid, or irreversible treatments.

As discussed throughout this chapter, there are many unexpected findings identified in UDS. Accordingly, while guidelines may advocate limited use, we believe there should be strong consideration to ensuring full evaluation in all cases where any uncertainty is present.

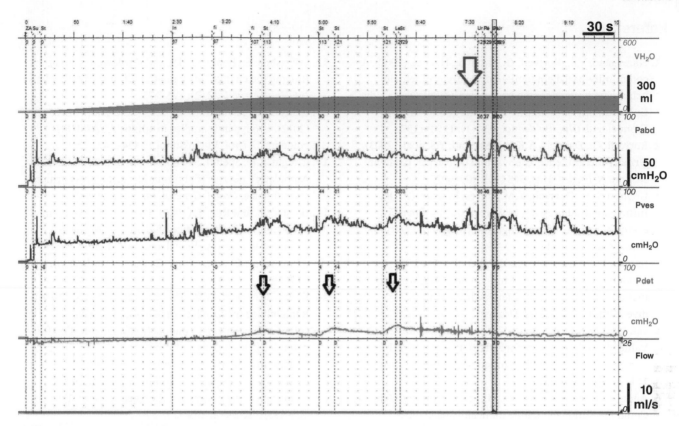

Figure 13.30 Impaired bladder compliance in a woman previously treated with radiotherapy for cervical cancer. The black arrows indicate rising p_{det} associated with running the filling pump. Following permission to void (purple arrow), she used abdominal straining, but there was no detrusor contraction and no flow.

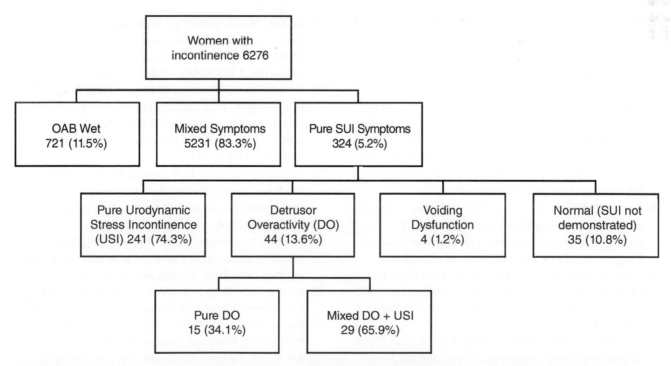

Figure 13.31 An analysis of the history and urodynamic findings for women with incontinence in the Bristol Urological Institute electronic database of urodynamics (UDS). Symptoms were established before conducting the UDS. Strict selection criteria were used to identify patients with pure stress urinary incontinence (SUI), which was identified in only 5.2% of cases. The urodynamic observations below (the third and bottom rows) relate solely to the SUI cases and show that a quarter of them did not have urodynamic stress incontinence as their urodynamic diagnosis. *Source*: Agur et al. [6].

References

1. Hannestad, Y.S., Rortveit, G., Sandvik, H. et al. (2000). A community-based epidemiological survey of female urinary incontinence: the Norwegian EPINCONT study. Epidemiology of incontinence in the county of Nord-Trondelag. *J. Clin. Epidemiol.* 53 (11): 1150–1157.

2. Rortveit, G., Daltveit, A.K., Hannestad, Y.S. et al. (2003). Urinary incontinence after vaginal delivery or cesarean section. *N. Engl. J. Med.* 348 (10): 900–907.

3. Gephart, L.F., Doersch, K.M., Reyes, M. et al. (2018). Intraabdominal pressure in women during CrossFit exercises and the effect of age and parity. *Proc. (Baylor Univ. Med. Cent.)* 31 (3): 289–293.

4. Barratt, R., Malde, S., Pakzad, M. et al. (2019). The incidence and outcomes of urodynamic stress urinary incontinence in female patients with urethral diverticulum. *Neurourol. Urodyn.*

5. van Leijsen, S.A., Kluivers, K.B., Mol, B.W. et al. (2013). Value of urodynamics before stress urinary incontinence surgery: a randomized controlled trial. *Obstet. Gynecol.* 121 (5): 999–1008.

6. Agur, W., Housami, F., Drake, M., and Abrams, P. (2009). Could the National Institute for health and clinical excellence guidelines on urodynamics in urinary incontinence put some women at risk of a bad outcome from stress incontinence surgery? *BJU Int.* 103 (5): 635–639.

7. Henderson, J.W., Kane, S.M., Mangel, J.M. et al. (2018). A randomized comparative study evaluating various cough stress tests and 24-hour pad test with urodynamics in the diagnosis of stress urinary incontinence. *J. Urol.* 199 (6): 1557–1564.

8. Visco, A.G., Brubaker, L., Nygaard, I. et al. Pelvic Floor Disorders N (2008). The role of preoperative urodynamic testing in stress-continent women undergoing sacrocolpopexy: the Colpopexy And Urinary Reduction Efforts (CARE) randomized surgical trial. *Int. Urogynecol. J. Pelvic Floor Dysfunct.* 19 (5): 607–614.

9. Roovers, J.P. and Oelke, M. (2007). Clinical relevance of urodynamic investigation tests prior to surgical correction of genital prolapse: a literature review. *Int. Urogynecol. J. Pelvic Floor Dysfunct.* 18 (4): 455–460.

10. Kapoor, D.S., Thakar, R., Sultan, A.H., and Oliver, R. (2009). Conservative versus surgical management of prolapse: what dictates patient choice? *Int. Urogynecol. J. Pelvic Floor Dysfunct.* 20 (10): 1157–1161.

11. Clemons, J.L., Aguilar, V.C., Tillinghast, T.A. et al. (2004). Patient satisfaction and changes in prolapse and urinary symptoms in women who were fitted successfully with a pessary for pelvic organ prolapse. *Am. J. Obstet. Gynecol.* 190 (4): 1025–1029.

12. Srikrishna, S., Robinson, D., and Cardozo, L. (2011). Ringing the changes in evaluation of urogenital prolapse. *Int. Urogynecol. J.* 22 (2): 171–175.

13. Winters, J.C., Dmochowski, R.R., Goldman, H.B. et al. (2012). Urodynamic studies in adults: AUA/SUFU guideline. *J. Urol.* 188 (6 Suppl): 2464–2472.

14. Chughtai, B., Spettel, S., Kurman, J., and De, E. (2012). Ambulatory pessary trial unmasks occult stress urinary incontinence. *Obstet. Gynecol. Int.* 2012: 392027.

15. Borstad, E. and Rud, T. (1989). The risk of developing urinary stress-incontinence after vaginal repair in continent women. A clinical and urodynamic follow-up study. *Acta Obstet. Gynecol. Scand.* 68 (6): 545–549.

16. Bump, R.C., Hurt, W.G., Theofrastous, J.P. et al. (1996). Randomized prospective comparison of needle colposuspension versus endopelvic fascia plication for potential stress incontinence prophylaxis in women undergoing vaginal reconstruction for stage III or IV pelvic organ prolapse. The continence program for women research group. *Am. J. Obstet. Gynecol.* 175 (2): 326–333; discussion 333-325.

17. Nguyen, J.N., Yazdany, T., and Burchette, R.J. (2007). Urodynamic evaluation of urethral competency in women with posterior vaginal support defects. *Urology* 69 (1): 87–90.

18. Karram, M.M. (1999). What is the optimal anti-incontinence procedure in women with advanced prolapse and 'potential' stress incontinence? *Int. Urogynecol. J. Pelvic Floor Dysfunct.* 10 (1): 1–2.

19. van der Ploeg, J.M., van der Steen, A., Oude Rengerink, K. et al. (2014). Prolapse surgery with or without stress incontinence surgery for pelvic organ prolapse: a systematic review and meta-analysis of randomised trials. *BJOG* 121 (5): 537–547.

20. Asfour, V., Gargasole, C., Fernando, R. et al. (2018). Urodynamics are necessary for patients with asymptomatic pelvic organ prolapse. *Neurourol. Urodyn.* 37 (8): 2841–2846.

21. Smith, A.R., Artibani, W., and Drake, M.J. (2011). Managing unsatisfactory outcome after mid-urethral tape insertion. *Neurourol. Urodyn.* 30 (5): 771–774.

22. Robinson, D., Thiagamoorthy, G., Ford, A. et al. (2018). Does assessing urethral function allow the selection of the optimal therapy for recurrent SUI? Report from the ICI-RS 2017. *Neurourol. Urodyn.* 37 (S4): S69–S74.

23. Rahn, D.D., Carberry, C., Sanses, T.V. et al. (2014). Vaginal estrogen for genitourinary syndrome of menopause: a systematic review. *Obstet. Gynecol.* 124 (6): 1147–1156.

24. Agur, W., Riad, M., Secco, S. et al. (2013). Surgical treatment of recurrent stress urinary incontinence in women: a systematic review and meta-analysis of randomised controlled trials. *Eur. Urol.* 64 (2): 323–336.

25. Drake, M.J. (2014). Do we need a new definition of the overactive bladder syndrome? ICI-RS 2013. *Neurourol. Urodyn.* 33 (5): 622–624.

26. Drake, M.J., Kanai, A., Bijos, D.A. et al. (2017). The potential role of unregulated autonomous bladder micromotions in urinary storage and voiding dysfunction; overactive bladder and detrusor underactivity. *BJU Int.* 119 (1): 22–29.

27. Ward, K. and Hilton, P. (2002). Prospective multicentre randomised trial of tension-free vaginal tape and colposuspension as primary treatment for stress incontinence. *BMJ* 325 (7355): 67.

28. Sahai, A., Sangster, P., Kalsi, V. et al. (2009). Assessment of urodynamic and detrusor contractility variables in patients with overactive bladder syndrome treated with botulinum toxin-A: is incomplete bladder emptying predictable? *BJU Int.* 103 (5): 630–634.

29. Houwert, R.M., Venema, P.L., Aquarius, A.E. et al. (2009). Predictive value of urodynamics on outcome after midurethral sling surgery for female stress urinary incontinence. *Am. J. Obstet. Gynecol.* 200 (6): 649. e641–612.

30. Hsiao, S.M., Chang, T.C., and Lin, H.H. (2009). Risk factors affecting cure after mid-urethral tape procedure for female urodynamic stress incontinence: comparison of retropubic and transobturator routes. *Urology* 73 (5): 981–986.

31. Richter, H.E., Diokno, A., Kenton, K. et al. (2008). Predictors of treatment failure 24 months after surgery for stress urinary incontinence. *J. Urol.* 179 (3): 1024–1030.

32. Lightner, D.J., Gomelsky, A., Souter, L., and Vasavada, S.P. (2019). Diagnosis and treatment of overactive bladder (non-neurogenic) in adults: AUA/SUFU guideline amendment 2019. *J. Urol.* https://doi.org/10.1097/JU.0000000000000309.

33. Drake, M.J., Chapple, C., Esen, A.A. et al. (2016). Efficacy and safety of mirabegron add-on therapy to solifenacin in incontinent overactive bladder patients with an inadequate response to initial 4-week solifenacin monotherapy: a randomised double-blind multicentre phase 3B study (BESIDE). *Eur. Urol.* 70 (1): 136–145.

34. Haylen, B.T., de Ridder, D., Freeman, R.M. et al. (2010). An international urogynecological association (IUGA)/international continence society (ICS) joint report on the terminology for female pelvic floor dysfunction. *Neurourol. Urodyn.* 29 (1): 4–20.

35. Doggweiler, R., Whitmore, K.E., Meijlink, J.M. et al. (2017). A standard for terminology in chronic pelvic pain syndromes: a report from the chronic pelvic pain working group of the international continence society. *Neurourol. Urodyn.* 36 (4): 984–1008.

36. Rana, N., Drake, M.J., Rinko, R. et al. (2018). The fundamentals of chronic pelvic pain assessment, based on international continence society recommendations. *Neurourol. Urodyn.* 37 (S6): S32–S38.

37. Pape, J., Falconi, G., De Mattos Lourenco, T.R. et al. (2019). Variations in bladder pain syndrome/interstitial cystitis (IC) definitions, pathogenesis, diagnostics and treatment: a systematic review and evaluation of national and international guidelines. *Int. Urogynecol. J.* 30 (11): 1795–1805.

38. Kuo, Y.C. and Kuo, H.C. (2018). Videourodynamic characteristics of interstitial cystitis/bladder pain syndrome-the role of bladder outlet dysfunction in the pathophysiology. *Neurourol. Urodyn.* 37 (6): 1971–1977.

39. Shaw, J., Negbenebor, N., Wohlrab, K. et al. (2019). Audiovisual stimulus during urodynamics to provoke detrusor overactivity: a randomized trial. *Low. Urin. Tract Symptoms* 11 (3): 127–132.

40. Gamble, T.L., Botros, S.M., Beaumont, J.L. et al. (2008). Predictors of persistent detrusor overactivity after transvaginal sling procedures. *Am. J. Obstet. Gynecol.* 199 (6): 696. e691–697.

41. Burgio, K.L., Goode, P.S., Locher, J.L. et al. (2003). Predictors of outcome in the behavioral treatment of urinary incontinence in women. *Obstet. Gynecol.* 102 (5 Pt 1): 940–947.

42. Lee, J.K., Dwyer, P.L., Rosamilia, A. et al. (2011). Persistence of urgency and urge urinary incontinence in women with mixed urinary symptoms after midurethral slings: a multivariate analysis. *BJOG* 118 (7): 798–805.

43. Tetzschner, T., Sorensen, M., Lose, G., and Christiansen, J. (1996). Anal and urinary incontinence in women with obstetric anal sphincter rupture. *Br. J. Obstet. Gynaecol.* 103 (10): 1034–1040.

44. Bharucha, A.E., Zinsmeister, A.R., Locke, G.R. et al. (2005). Prevalence and burden of fecal incontinence: a population-based study in women. *Gastroenterology* 129 (1): 42–49.

45. Cooper, Z.R. and Rose, S. (2000). Fecal incontinence: a clinical approach. *Mt. Sinai J. Med.* 67 (2): 96–105.

46. Lacima, G., Espuna, M., Pera, M. et al. (2002). Clinical, urodynamic, and manometric findings in women with combined fecal and urinary incontinence. *Neurourol. Urodyn.* 21 (5): 464–469.

47. Thorpe, A.C., Williams, N.S., Badenoch, D.F. et al. (1993). Simultaneous dynamic electromyographic proctography and cystometrography. *Br. J. Surg.* 80 (1): 115–120.

is not unlike that in women. Thus, the terms referring to prostate histology (such as benign prostatic hyperplasia [BPH]), prostatic size (benign prostatic enlargement [BPE]), and the coexistence of BPE and bladder outlet obstruction (BOO) (benign prostatic obstruction [BPO]) should be employed only when evidence justifies their use in an individual. They should be applied consistently so that clinicians and urodynamicists can communicate clearly about individual patients and groups of patients. The presence of BPH or BPE may have no impact on voiding but BPO does (see Paul Abrams' illustration in the preface), producing the classic urodynamic finding of low flow rate and high voiding pressure.

LUTS is a term which replaces old and misleading use of ambiguous and imprecise terms such as 'BPH', 'symptoms of BPH', or 'prostatism' [2], although even now some practitioners persist in using these terms when referring to LUTS. BPH is a histological term which should only be used in the context of describing the pathological changes. Using BPH and prostatism to describe a patient's LUTS inevitably leads them to conclude the prostate is the cause of the LUTS, when the reality may be nothing of the sort. The same criticism can be applied to evaluating them with the International Prostate Symptom Score, which by its name implies mechanism without actual justification. 'Obstructive' and 'irritative' also suggest mechanism in a way which cannot be justified until investigations have been completed. 'Storage', 'voiding', and 'post-micturition' are categorisations which deliberately focus on justifiable description without unproven implication of mechanism. These are the terms used by the International Continence Society (ICS), and the

sooner the whole urological community can understand the simple but fundamental reasoning, the better.

In men, LUTS are generally due to three main causes:

- Detrusor overactivity (DO);
- Bladder outlet obstruction (BOO); and
- Detrusor underactivity (DUA).

In addition, post-micturition dribble (PMD) is likely to result from pooling in the urethral bulb. Nocturia has to be regarded with caution, as it may well reflect behavioural, sleep, or medical issues. Any of these mechanisms would be incongruous if alluded to as LUTD, and so nocturia may better be termed a systemic symptom [6].

Detrusor Overactivity

During the storage phase of micturition, there should be no activity of the detrusor muscle. Pressure should not rise during filling or should do so to only a small extent. Overactive bladder (OAB) is characterised by urinary urgency, with or without urgency urinary incontinence (UUI), usually with increased daytime frequency and nocturia, if there is no proven infection or other obvious pathology [7]. Urgency and urgency incontinence in men have a strong correlation with the urodynamic finding of DO [8], which is defined as any involuntary contraction during filling cystometry which may be spontaneous or provoked [9], regardless of the amplitude of the contraction (Figure 14.1). When flow accompanies this finding in the storage phase, then DO incontinence (DOI) is diagnosed (Figure 14.2).

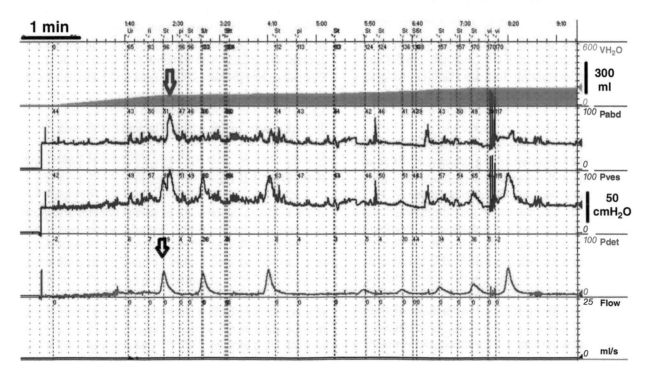

Figure 14.1 Filling cystometry illustrating detrusor overactivity (DO) without incontinence. Multiple phasic waves of increased bladder pressure (first indicated by black arrow). The first DO contraction is followed by a transient change in abdominal pressure (red arrow).

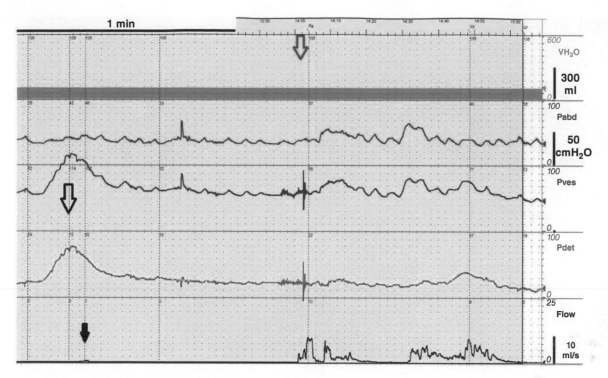

Figure 14.2 Filling cystometry showing detrusor overactivity (open black arrow) causing incontinence (closed black arrow). The right side of the trace is the PFS following permission to void (purple arrow), showing detrusor underactivity.

There is a common misapprehension that DO in men is usually caused by BOO, but this is not supported by evidence [10]. Some key points are:

- Women have a high prevalence of DO which is unrelated to BOO;
- Men can have DO in conjunction with normal or underactive voiding (Figure 14.2); and
- Doing surgery to relieve BOO does not always resolve DO (Figure 14.3).

Storage symptoms constitute the most bothersome for patients; therefore, diagnosing storage problems has a great importance. Furthermore, some of the storage symptoms do not show an improvement after transurethral resection of the prostate (TURP) [11] (urgency improvement in 71%, frequency improvement in 60%, and nocturia improvement in 43.2%), and patients must be aware of this before undergoing an operation.

Bladder Outlet Obstruction

The suspicion of BOO is the most frequent reason for performing UDS in men. In older men, the prostate gland has been traditionally held responsible for many of the symptomatic complaints of male patients, and there has been a tendency to use prostatectomy as a panacea for LUTS. This approach led to a failure rate of TURP of around 30–40%, presumably because the cause of the problem was not the prostate, so operating on it would not be expected to yield

improvement [12] and could well be harmful. The need for objective evaluation was answered by the introduction of pressure-flow analysis of micturition. If conservative treatment has failed and the patient remains symptomatic to the extent that he wishes to consider surgery, then UDS should be considered. Rodrigues et al. [13] reported that pressure-flow study (PFS) predict outcomes after TURP. Decrease in symptom scores and increase in quality of life was noted to be directly related to the degree of BOO. However, a Cochrane analysis could not find sufficient evidence on which to base a conclusion [14]. Thus, a consensus-based approach has been employed by most international urological associations on when to perform PFS [15–18]. In general, most societies recommend performing PFS in patients who will undergo an invasive and potentially morbid procedure [19], and certain situations necessitate the additional information. The European Association of Urology Guidelines on Male LUTS [20] recommends PFS in the following situations:

- Patient cannot void >150 ml;
- Has a maximum flow rate of >15 ml/s;
- Is <50 or >80 years of age;
- Can void but has post-void residual (PVR) urine >300 ml; and
- Had previous unsuccessful (invasive) treatment.

UDS must also be considered where there is suspicion of neurogenic LUTD, or there has been previous radical pelvic surgery.

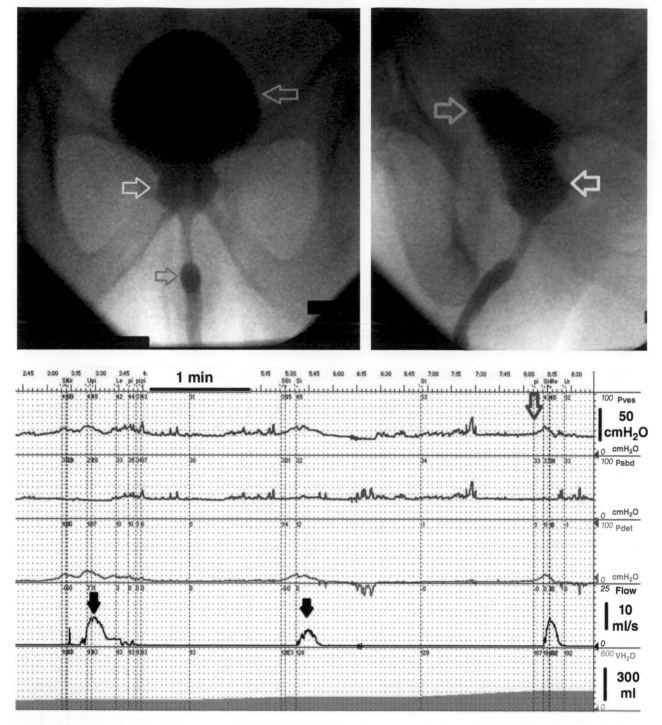

Figure 14.3 Persisting detrusor overactivity (DO) incontinence after transurethral resection of the prostate (TURP). Upper left image showing DO incontinence viewed in postero-anterior projection. The yellow arrow indicates an anatomically excellent prostatic resection. The blue arrow shows the bladder. The orange arrow is included to demonstrate how the bulbar urethra is foreshortened onto itself when seen in two-dimensions using this projection. Upper right image is an oblique projection after permission to void. In the urodynamics trace below, DO incontinence during the filling cystometry is indicated with black arrows, and permission to void at the start of the PFS is shown with the purple arrow. The voiding phase shows a low flow rate with a low p_{det}, suggestive of detrusor underactivity. *Source:* Marcus Drake.

How Is the Diagnosis of BOO Made?

A few urodynamic approaches to diagnosing BOO in men have been described [21, 22], which largely tend to show broad agreement whichever method is used. Accordingly, the diagnosis of BOO is generally made by plotting the maximum flow rate (Qmax) against detrusor pressure at Q_{max} (pdetQmax) into the ICS nomogram (Figure 14.4) [24]. The ICS nomogram and the BOO Index (BOOI) are the modern derivations of the pioneering work of Paul Abrams and Derek Griffiths [25].

If the clinician wishes to describe the degree of obstruction, then the BOOI can be calculated and BOO diagnosed without reference to the nomogram from the simple equation:

$$BOOI = p_{detQmax} - 2Q_{max}$$

It is important to use the corrected Q_{max}, i.e. exclude artefacts to make sure that the value of Q_{max} is representative

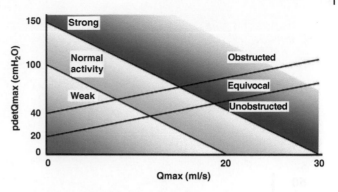

Figure 14.4 Composite bladder outflow obstruction index and bladder contractility index nomogram. *Source:* Hashim et al. [23] © 2007 Elsevier.

of the bladder contraction (Figure 14.5) (rather than meaningless information, such as the flowmeter getting knocked). The p_{det} at that moment is then taken as the $p_{detQmax}$. It is probably sensible to avoid a time when

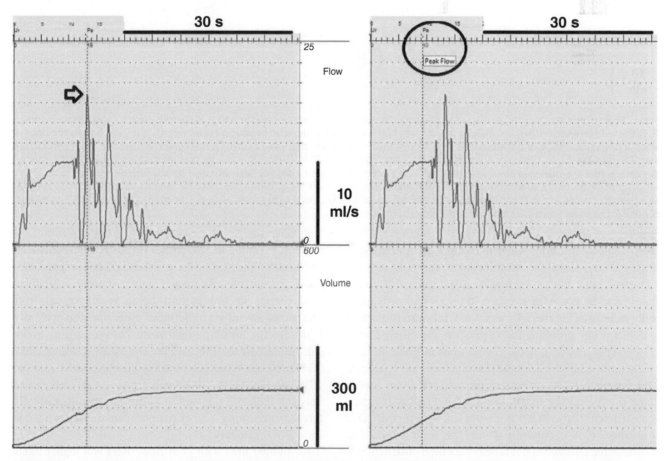

Figure 14.5 Correcting Q_{max}. In a free flow rate test, the machine documents maximum flow rate (Q_{max}) at the time, regardless of the underlying processes. On the left, the spike in pressure indicated by the black arrow was documented as the Q_{max}, at 19 ml/s. This spike was due to a 'squeeze and release', i.e. using a pinch grip with fingers to interrupt the stream which stores up energy, hence the rapid surge of flow when the pinch is released. However, the urodynamicist is trying to interpret the bladder and sphincter function, so needs to look at the underlying curve to see where that has reached its peak. This is done after the test, when it is possible to instruct the machine what is the correct Q_{max}, i.e. 10 ml/s, as has been done on the right.

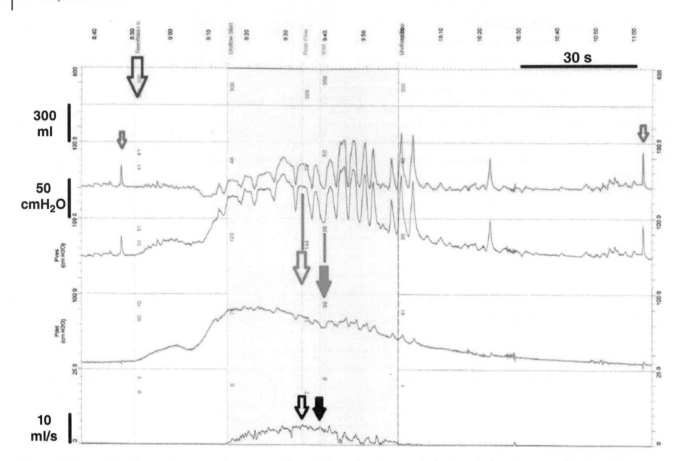

Figure 14.6 Deriving Q_{max} and $p_{detQmax}$. The pressure-flow study begins with permission to void (purple arrow). Coughs before and after the void (orange arrows) are included to confirm both lines were picking up pressures accurately. Q_{max} is indicated by the open black arrow, value 7 ml/s, and there are no artefacts. At that moment, the p_{det} was 71 cmH$_2$O (open green arrow). BOO Index (BOOI) is then 71 − (2 × 7) = 57, i.e. obstructed, and bladder contractility index (BCI) is 71 + (5 × 7) = 106, i.e. normal contractility. The difficulty in this case is that the man was obviously straining at this point; the straining did not have an effect on the flow rate, which in itself suggests BOO; but, were subtraction to be of poor quality, this would affect p_{det}. Hence, the closed arrows have been added to indicate an alternative point where the values could be derived. These give Q_{max} of 6 ml/s and $p_{detQmax}$ of 59 cmH$_2$O, yielding a BOOI of 47 and BCI of 89; the latter value falls into the underactive category.

the patient is straining when deriving Q_{max} and $p_{detQmax}$ (Figure 14.6), since the subtraction of straining may be imperfect, and hence artificially affect p_{det}. Allowance should also be made for any drop in p_{abd}, which will artificially raise p_{det} (Figures 14.7 and 7.42). It is also important to detect if any problem affects pressure recording during the PFS (Figure 14.8). These checks must be gone through by the urodynamicist since the machine does not scrutinise data for plausibility or correct for artefact. Once this is done, the higher the BOOI, the more likely that the man is obstructed. If the BOOI is greater than 40, then BOO is confirmed; if it is between 40 and 20, then obstruction is considered equivocal; if it is below 20, then obstruction is not present.

Generally, a single filling and voiding cycle is done in a UDS appointment. Repeat testing at the same appointment potentially leads to a reduction in $p_{detQmax}$ and Q_{max} in the second filling cycle, with 81% remaining in the same BOOI category assignments (obstructed/equivocal/not obstructed) [23]. Where the BOOI is comparatively low in the obstructed category (BOOI of around 50), there is a chance of the patient being recategorised from obstructed to equivocal between cycle one and cycle two (Table 14.1a). Similar adjustments between filling cycles can be needed for the bladder contractility index (BCI) (Table 14.2a) When comparing baseline with another UDS appointment six months later, the differences between both $p_{detQmax}$ and Q_{max} are not significantly different, and around 70% of patients remain unchanged in their BOOI category [23].

In younger men with poor flow, there is a higher likelihood of bladder neck obstruction (BNO), so video urodynamics may be the investigation of choice, to allow identification of the site of any obstruction (see Chapter 8). For the majority of male patients (older men with LUTS suggestive of BOO), standard (conventional) UDS is the

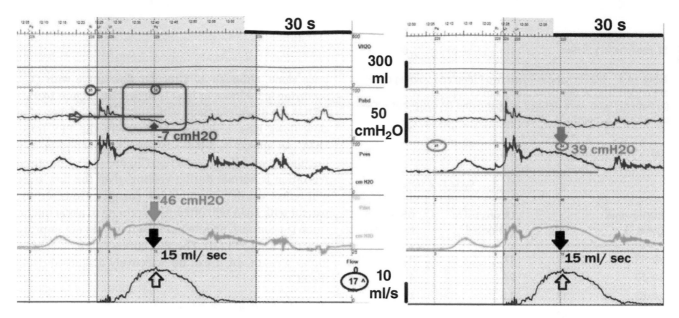

Figure 14.7 Adjustments if p_{abd} changes during the course of a pressure-flow study. If p_{abd} drops, it has the effect of artificially raising the p_{det}, implying a bigger pressure change than the bladder actually generated. Thus, the extent by which the p_{abd} dropped at the time of Q_{max} (purple rectangle and arrows) is taken off p_{det}, as shown to the left. In this case, Q_{max} was corrected from what the machine said (open black arrow, 17 ml/s) because of a small pressure spike. Corrected Q_{max} was thus 15 ml/s. $p_{detQmax}$ was 46 cmH₂O, but this was artificially high, because, by this stage, the p_{abd} had dropped by 7 cmH₂O from its baseline value. Hence, adjusted $p_{detQmax}$ was 39 cmH₂O so that BOO Index was 9 and bladder contractility index was 114. The same result can be obtained by measuring the rise in p_{ves} compared with its baseline value, as shown on the right (orange line and arrow).

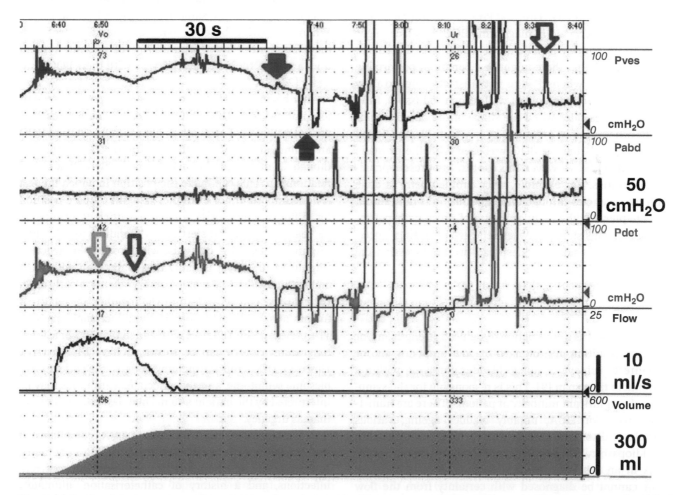

Figure 14.8 Cough tests are done after a pressure-flow study to identify pressure recording problems. In this case, the p_{ves} line failed to pick up the cough (closed red arrow). A series of flushes of the p_{ves} line (first one indicated by the closed blue arrow) was done until eventually the catheter was cleared (open blue arrow). Commonly, the moment at which the p_{ves} catheter blocks is when the bladder is nearly empty, as the bladder lining gets close to the catheter eyehole. An inflection in the line is a hint this has happened, and just such an event is indicated by the open red arrow. Since Q_{max} occurred before that point (green arrow), it is probably acceptable to derive BOOI and BCI from that point, but the report should describe the situation.

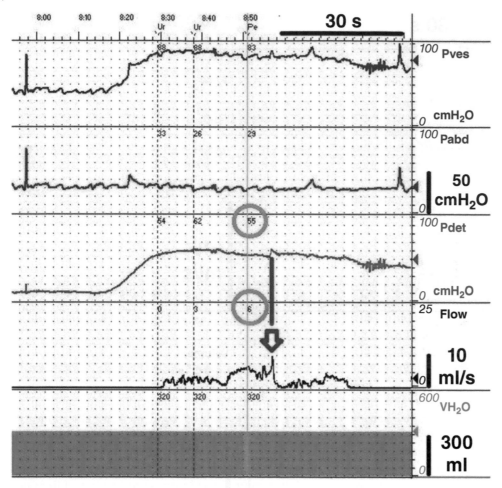

Figure 14.10 A pressure-flow study in which corrected Q_{max} was 6 ml/s and $p_{detQmax}$ was 55 cmH$_2$O (green circles). This gives a BOO Index (BOOI) of 43 (obstructed) and bladder contractility index (BCI) of 85 (underactive). As with previous examples, the machine has taken Q_{max} off the top of a spike as 10 ml/s (red arrow), at which time p_{det} was 54 cmH$_2$O. This would give BOOI as 34 and BCI as 104, i.e. erroneously categorising as equivocal obstruction and normal contractility.

Randomised Evaluation of Assessment Methods) study is the largest study of UDS in men to have been conducted. It is a two-arm trial, set in urology departments of 26 National Health Service (NHS) hospitals in the UK, randomising men with bothersome LUTS for whom surgeons would consider offering surgery, between a care pathway based on urodynamic tests with invasive multichannel cystometry and a care pathway based on non-invasive routine tests. The aim of the trial is to determine whether a care pathway not including invasive UDS is no worse for men in terms of symptom outcome than one in which it is included, at 18 months after randomisation, and whether invasive UDS reduces rates of bladder outlet surgery (principal secondary outcome) [29, 30].

Contrary to a widely held assumption that patients don't want to have UDS, UPSTREAM found satisfaction rates were over 90% (Table 14.3) [31]. UDS was well-tolerated by the participants who had experienced it. However, there was variation in how uncomfortable men found the procedure. Seven reported that it was at least a little painful, with some experiencing severe pain [1]. Eight participants reported short-lived negative after-effects of UDS: stinging when urinating, a small amount of bleeding, a UTI, or disrupted flow/urgency. However, despite these issues, the men said the test was acceptable, and they would willingly have it again if needed. UDS was valued for its perceived accuracy and the information it provided about symptom aetiology and thought to give more insight into LUTS than other tests.

Embarrassment is an important problem for patients in the test environment, and this can be minimised through good communication and privacy: ensuring men knew what to expect, limiting the staff present, introducing staff, and explaining their role. For some men, the

Table 14.2 BCI changes when two filling and voiding cycles are undertaken at the same urodynamics appointment. (a) BCI: first compared to second void cycle.

(a)

BCI cycle 1	BCI cycle 2	n (% of subgroup)
Strong (20)	Strong	9 (45%)
	Normal	11 (55%)
	Weak	0 (0%)
Normal (87)	Strong	5 (6%)
	Normal	62 (71%)
	Weak	20 (23%)
Weak (75)	Strong	0 (0%)
	Normal	3 (4%)
	Weak	72 (96%)

BCI: bladder contractility index.
182 pairs of data (baseline plus six months).
Source: Hashim et al. [23]. © 2007 Elsevier.

gender of the person performing the test was important, with a female clinician preferred [1]. Problems with information provision were reported before, during, and after the test in many hospitals, and there was variability in how and when results were explained and the adequacy of explanations. The finding of variability in the degree of privacy, dignity, discomfort, and information provision experienced by patients undergoing urodynamic testing indicated that staff require training and guidance in these areas, including sensitive conduct of invasive urodynamic testing and associated information provision [1]. Simple considerate behaviour is important; coming into the room without knocking during the procedure is not appropriate. Fundamentally, this is a test about which people are understandably anxious, and which they find intrusive as the test proceeds. Accordingly, the staff need to show empathy and make efforts to ameliorate the impact on the patient. This reflects a basic respect for human dignity, and is also important for ensuring the findings are representative.

UPSTREAM confirms that all components of the pathway (symptom score [Table 14.4], sexual function assessment, flow rate testing with PVR measurement, bladder diary, and urinalysis) bring essential aspects for assessing a man with LUTS, vital for treatment selection and outcome. If all these are done well, suitable selection for surgery can be achieved, and good surgical outcomes obtained. For the men who are found not to be suitable for surgery, symptom improvement is only slight (which is why UPSTREAM had to be a non-inferiority study). Since surgery rates in modern practice are low (just over a third in the UPSTREAM study [32]), it highlights that there are many phenotypes of male LUTS where our treatment options are actually limited – in particular, nocturia. A large part of the problem we have is that the storage LUTS dominate the bother and quality of life impact of LUTS [33]. The voiding LUTS can generally be treated with procedures like TURP, but the outcome in terms of bother improvement is going to be disappointing if the bother is actually a consequence of the type of LUTS that fails to improve with surgery. Interestingly, PMD seems to be a particular problem with a high level of bother for some men [33].

UDS in Younger Men (<55 Years of Age)

Video urodynamics is the investigation of choice after free flow rate testing, since BNO and inadequate urethral relaxation may be more likely in younger men and appear to be functional rather than structural abnormalities. Younger men are less phlegmatic than older men when investigated and require more careful handling. Fainting (vasovagal syncope) is most common in this group, and the UDS team should have the test set up to be able to lie a younger man down at short notice, in order to avoid a faint which could injure the patient and damage the equipment (Figure 14.12). Hence, if the patient goes quiet, looks worried and pale, and starts to sweat, straight away get him to sit down, and, if necessary, lie down. It is wise to stop the filling and allow the patient several minutes to recover. Usually, the patient can then stand and the UDS can be continued. If the patient is very inhibited by the investigation, then it may be necessary to leave him to void alone, in which case the video-imaging part of the study may have to be abandoned.

As with all patients investigated by UDS, each patient should be screened by free flow rate studies for comparison with the PFS; if their flow patterns are markedly dissimilar, the PFS should be repeated.

Younger men may develop voiding and post-micturition LUTS as a result of a stricture (see Chapters 8 and 15), which can also cause difficulties in catheterising. In order to get the best chance of passing the catheter, consider the following:

- Use a generous amount of lubricant.
- Use a small gauge catheter (6 Fr).
- Catheterise gently.
- Use an angle-ended (Coudé or Tiemann) catheter to help steer the catheter tip along the lumen.
- Place a guidewire (passing under vision with a flexible cystoscope to ensure the guidewire enters the distal end of the stricture). A small gauge catheter can be railroaded over the guidewire.

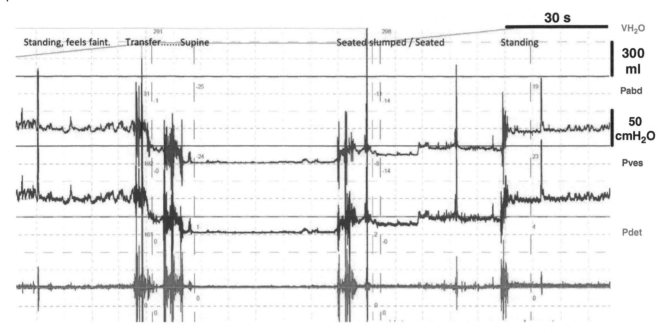

Figure 14.12 A well-recognised issue for younger men being catheterised is the possibility of fainting. It is important to watch out for signs of this starting, and be prepared to transfer the man to the supine or seated position for a few minutes. Most men then recover well enough to allow the test to be completed. In this case, the transducer height was not adjusted according to ICS recommendations, presumably because the urodynamicist was paying close attention to the patient to ensure he did not fall and injure himself.

LUTD after any of these interventions may reflect the proximity of parts of the prostate to the urethral sphincter (distally), the sphincter innervation (peripherally), and the bladder trigone (proximally). Furthermore, the procedures are a notable surgical trauma, with a need for catheterisation in many (which is for several weeks when a vesico-urethral anastomosis has to heal), and a risk of infection and other complications. The trauma and inflammation associated with these interventions are a risk factor for scarring, potentially leading to urethral stricture or bladder neck stenosis. Radiotherapy adds an extra level of complexity to understanding mechanisms and planning treatment. In the short- to medium-term after surgery, indicators like haematuria, leukocyturia, or pain might reflect a surgical complication. Thus, LUTD may be a direct consequence of surgery, on top of any coexisting LUTD already present in this older age group, notably OAB/DO.

Presentations generally fall into storage symptoms, incontinence, or voiding LUTS, either in isolation or combination. It is important to establish whether the symptoms represent a persistence of LUTS that were present before the surgery:

- Persisting voiding LUTS may be a consequence of inadequate resolution of BPO or due to pre-existing DUA. New onset voiding LUTS could reflect the development of a stricture or stenosis, or newly developed DUA, which can occur in radical prostate treatment.
- Storage LUTS may be a result of pre-existing or emerging DO. Major surgery or radical radiotherapy may cause inflammatory sequelae unrelated to DO that could be a factor in the new onset cases post-surgery. UTI must also be excluded.
- For incontinence, again, it must be established whether or not the incontinence was present before operation, along with determining what kind of leakage the patient now suffers.

Voiding LUTS After Prostatectomy

For voiding LUTS, the post-operative complaints of slow stream and hesitancy have in the past often led to repeated transurethral resections, leading to increased likelihood of damage to the intrinsic urethral sphincter mechanism. In fact, the urodynamic results for this group of patients show that generally only a minority of such patients with reduced flow have persistent BOO; the proportion of patients with a slow stream due to DUA is higher (Figure 14.13) [34]. If there is no residual prostatic tissue or demonstrable BOO, then a second prostatectomy will not help the patient. Should there be residual prostatic tissue (Figures 14.14

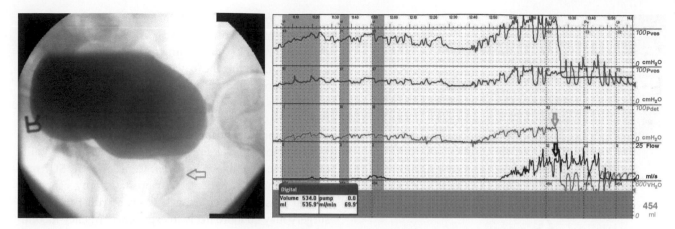

Figure 14.13 A man with voiding lower urinary tract symptoms after transurethral resection of the prostate. The video urodynamics image to the left shows a good prostate resection (green arrow). The pressure-flow study on the right shows a protracted void, with a lot of straining. The p_{ves} catheter is lost slightly before Q_{max}, but taking the values at the points indicated by the black (Q_{max} 10 ml/s) and green ($p_{detQmax}$ 42 cmH$_2$O) arrows gives a BOO Index of 22 (equivocal for obstruction) and a bladder contractility index of 92 (underactive). *Source:* Based on Thomas et al. [34] and Marcus Drake.

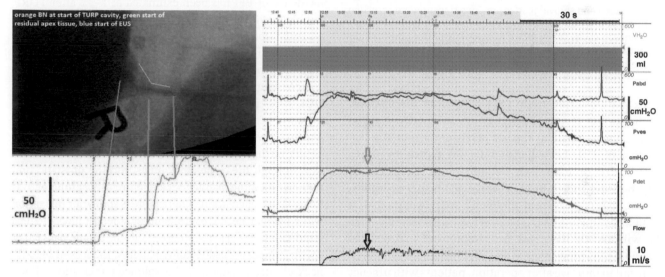

Figure 14.14 A man with voiding lower urinary tract symptoms after transurethral resection of the prostate. The video urodynamics image (upper left) shows a good prostate resection in the region of the bladder neck (orange line), but near the apex (blue line), there is visible tissue, the transition between these two areas being indicated by the green line. This residual tissue shows up in the prostatic plateau of the urethral pressure profile (lower left). The pressure-flow study on the right shows a protracted void with good subtraction and no straining. The black arrow indicates Q_{max} of 10 ml/s, and the green arrow shows $p_{detQmax}$ of 92 cmH$_2$O, giving a BOO Index of 72 (obstructed) and a bladder contractility index of 142 (normal). *Source:* Marcus Drake.

and 14.15), then transurethral resection of the remaining prostatic tissue may improve voiding, even when the detrusor is underactive.

The appearance of new complaints after surgery suggests that a change has occurred in the lower urinary tract. In particular, a significant number of patients may develop DUA after radical prostatectomy [35]. This is probably the effect of denervation of the bladder during the operation and should be considered in patients with post-prostatectomy

voiding problems. The other crucial possibility is development of a urethral stricture or anastomotic stenosis, usually at an interval of a few weeks to months. In the latter case, attempted catheterisation may prove decidedly tricky due to the tightness and distortion.

The symptoms of DO often improve after prostatectomy [11], though the reason for this is not fully clear [10]; it has been suggested that lower voiding pressures after prostatectomy, or the denervation of the bladder

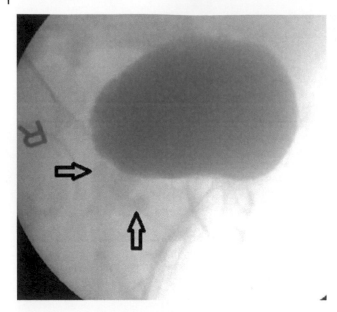

Figure 14.15 Man who was very hard to catheterise for urodynamic assessment of voiding lower urinary tract symptoms (slow stream and spraying) after previous transurethral resection of the prostate. Nodular regrowth was seen, which resulted in a very uneven cavity shape (black arrows). Presumably, the catheter got stuck in the uneven cavity without making it fully to the bladder lumen. *Source:* Marcus Drake.

neck and posterior urethra resulting from surgery, may be important factors, but these are speculative suggestions. Where a patient reports persistent symptoms suggestive of DO, he will generally be shown by filling cystometry to have DO. Patients with symptoms of urgency and UUI, and with severe DO before operation, are at risk of persistent problems after operation. If a patient complains of UUI following prostatectomy, then he will usually have had the symptom of urgency and possible UUI prior to operation. Because these symptoms may fail to improve after operation, patients with urgency prior to operation should be counselled, explaining that although an improvement in urine flow rate is anticipated, one cannot be similarly confident about the symptoms of DO improving. As in pre-operative cases, full UDS in this presentation should be considered once conservative and medical treatment has failed, and invasive procedures (sacral neuromodulation or botulinum toxin injections) are being planned.

Post-Prostatectomy Incontinence

Prostatectomy can be undertaken to treat BPO or prostate cancer. The prostatectomy for BPO is commonly a TURP, or removal of intrusive prostate tissue with a laser, often with incision of the bladder neck. In these patients, the outer part of the prostate (the capsule) is retained, as is the prostatic urethra (after healing of the operation site). For prostate cancer, the entire gland is removed, including the prostatic urethra, and the bladder base is brought downward to be joined to the urethra just above the sphincter. In both types of operation, the absence of the bladder neck enables more direct transmission of changes in p_{ves} down to the sphincter level. Furthermore, there is the possibility of weakened sphincter function. Consequently, SUI may be experienced by patients after prostatectomy, especially radical prostatectomy. Likewise, a man with DO prior to surgery may be more likely to experience urgency incontinence after the operation.

The symptom of incontinence is a considerable issue for patients after surgery. Affected individuals should be asked about the frequency and severity of incontinence and whether or not he suffers social restriction or has to take protective measures to safeguard his clothes. The incidence of PPI has been estimated at 1–3% after TURP, but higher after radical prostatectomy (20–25%). Given the potential complexity, video urodynamic studies (VUDS) are generally the investigation of choice, and urethral pressure profilometry can be very useful.

Incontinence following prostatectomy is principally UUI, stress urinary incontinence (SUI), or mixed urinary incontinence (MUI). It is also important to be aware of climacturia, which is orgasm-associated incontinence that occurs during ejaculation. Male orgasm comprises emission through the ejaculatory ducts into the prostatic urethra, between the bladder neck and urethral sphincter. It is followed by ejaculation, where there is sphincter relaxation while bladder neck closure is maintained (a physiological requirement for ejaculation to enable antegrade passage of sperm). In post-prostatectomy patients, the loss of bladder neck closure means that the sphincter relaxation allows some urine through along with the sperm. It can occur in 20–64% of men who have undergone radical prostatectomy [36]. Limited data of urodynamic studies among male patients with climacturia showed lower functional length of urethra compared to controls [37]. The volume of urine lost in climacturia is small, reflecting the transient duration of the sphincter relaxation. If a large urine volume is lost at the time of orgasm, associated with urgency, the mechanism might be DOI.

The symptom of stress incontinence in neurologically normal male patients is exceptionally rare in the unoperated case. Therefore, the appearance of this symptom following surgery implies per-operative damage to the distal urethral sphincteric mechanism, either directly or by denervation. In urological practice, it is fairly common to see transient stress incontinence following open prostatectomy for benign disease, but much more common after radical prostatectomy for cancer. In male patients, stress incontinence is effectively treated by implantation of an artificial urinary sphincter (AUS), and the male sling is a more recent option.

It is our routine workup to perform multichannel VUDS on all patients before any surgical procedure to treat PPI. The studies need to consider several things, which matter in all cases but especially after radical prostatectomy:

1) What is sphincter function like? This can be evaluated with urethral pressure profile (UPP) and demonstration of USI. Sometimes, USI can be difficult to see emerging from the penile tip due to the length of the urethra and the catheter, but in this case, VUDS screening of the urethral bulb during a cough or Valsalva will demonstrate whether contrast gets below the sphincter (Figure 14.16), confirming USI.

2) Is there DO and is the bladder capacity reduced? Sometimes, these are the principal form of LUTD present, or they may coexist with USI (Figure 14.17). If present, it may affect the symptomatic outcome of surgery [38].

3) What is the state of the bladder outlet? It is important to know if there is significant narrowing or distortion which could make instrumentation or catheterisation difficult. For those men being considered for AUS, scarring will affect where the cuff can be placed, since scarred areas are a high risk of erosion when faced with

the constant compression by an implant. This is discussed in more detail in Chapter 15.

4) Is voiding achieved with an effective bladder contraction? This is perhaps less important in men after radical

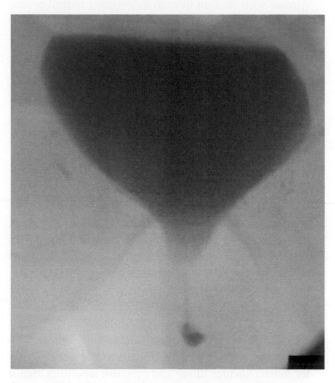

Figure 14.16 A man with history of radical prostatectomy. A small amount of contrast was seen in the urethral bulb during a cough, viewed in postero-anterior projection on this video urodynamics image, confirming urodynamic stress incontinence. *Source:* Marcus Drake.

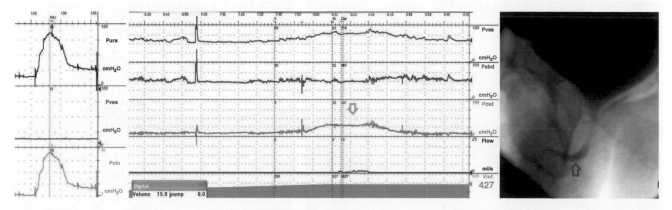

Figure 14.17 A man with history of radical prostatectomy. His urethral pressure profile (UPP) showed a fairly good maximum closure pressure (left) – note the loss of the prostatic plateau and the shape being similar to a female UPP. The filling cystometry in the middle showed detrusor overactivity incontinence (green arrow). VUDS image on the right shows contrast in the urethral bulb during a cough (red arrow – viewed in oblique projection), confirming urodynamic stress incontinence. Hence, the final diagnosis was mixed urinary incontinence. *Source:* Marcus Drake.

prostatectomy, as straining is more likely to be effective in men without a prostate than those with one. Note that the BCI and BOOI were derived using men assessed before and after TURP and therefore have to be interpreted with caution in men following a radical prostatectomy. As for women, there is no validated and generally accepted measure of contractility for men who have undergone radical prostatectomy.

Three practical issues are worth knowing:

- Sometimes, men hold their pelvic floor tight when coughing, and this can make it hard to see stress incontinence. Accordingly, men may need to be told not to 'hold on' during the stress provocation testing (Figure 14.18).
- It can be difficult to demonstrate USI when the filling line is in for a man who previously had a urethro-vesical anastomosis (i.e. after radical prostatectomy) (Figure 14.19). Even a 7 Fr catheter might obscure leaking if the patient has some degree of bladder neck contraction [39, 40]. In this case, the two-catheter technique (standard filling line and a separate 16 G catheter for measuring p_{ves}) is helpful, as the filling line can be removed at cystometric capacity, making observation of USI where present easier and more likely.
- Assessing bladder capacity and DO severity in men with significant USI can be very difficult, as the weak sphincter makes bladder filling and pressure recording almost impossible. In this case, a urethral compression clamp placed on the penis will hold back the contrast (Figure 14.20) and should not occlude the filling line. Thereby, the bladder can be filled to capacity [41]. If this is done, removal of the clamp is likely to lead to an imme-

diate rapid expulsion of the bladder contents, so the flow rate funnel needs to be immediately nearby when about to remove the clamp.

It has been suggested that the presence of DO or DOI on pre-operative UDS does not influence outcome [26, 42, 43]. However, individual cases with high-amplitude DO may well develop contractions of $60 \, cmH_2O$, which is approximately the working pressure within the AUS system, thereby risking DOI forcing its way past the AUS. If there is concern that this could be a problem for someone, it is worth checking whether the man experiences this when using a penile compression device at home. These devices are marketed as a means of urine containment in PPI and achieve compression pressures not dissimilar to those of an AUS [44]. Hence, experience of DO leading to pain or incontinence using one of these devices would indicate caution before proceeding with an AUS placement. Patients who only suffer from DOI, and show a normal sphincteric function, would not receive any benefit from the placement of a device which carries significant risks and costs. This is the case in around 10% of PPI patients [26, 42]. In order to obtain good results with male slings, there has to be some residual sphincteric function. This can objectively be assessed by measuring MUCP and Valsalva Leak Point Pressures (VLLP) [45, 46].

Compliance is an important predictor of outcome following AUS implantation for PPI [38]. This can be impaired after radical prostatectomy and is more likely in men who also had radiotherapy or other relevant features of the post-medical history (notably neurological disease or prolonged catheterisation). The risk here is that the p_{det}

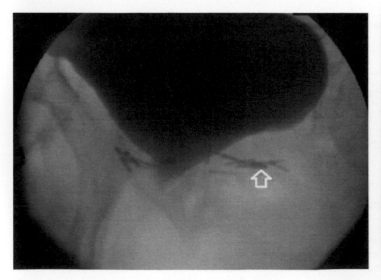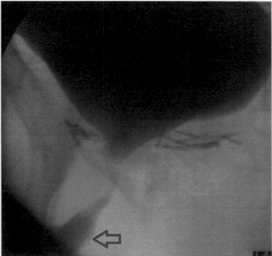

Figure 14.18 Men can often resist stress incontinence by pre-contracting their pelvic floor when about to cough (left image). Asking them not to do this enables identification of urodynamic stress incontinence (right image, red arrow). The yellow arrow indicates surgical clips placed during his previous radical prostatectomy. *Source:* Marcus Drake.

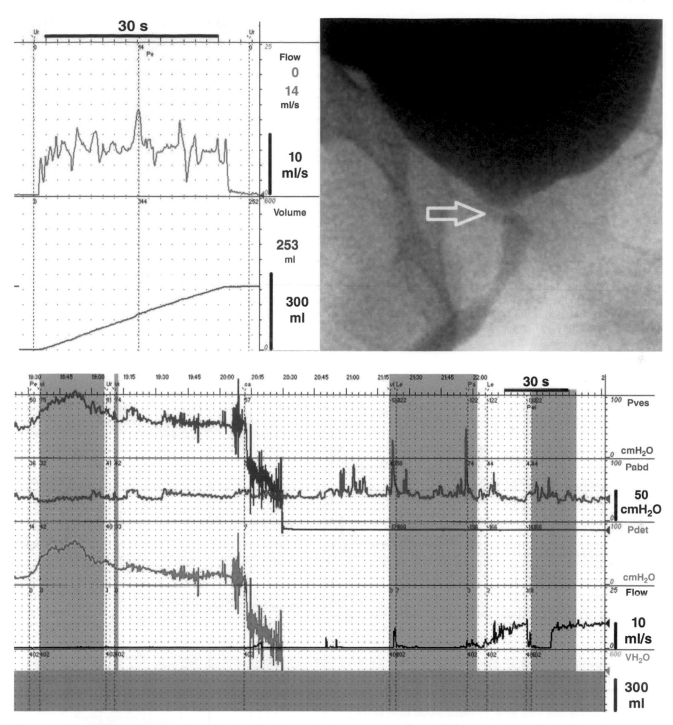

Figure 14.19 Bladder neck stenosis at the site of vesico-urethral anastomosis after radical prostatectomy. Top left: free flow pattern. Top right: Video urodynamics oblique projection showing the stenosis (yellow arrow). Bottom: pressure-flow study. To the left, pressure is generated, but the calibre of the stenosis was similar to the filling line, occluding the lumen and preventing flow. The vesical catheter fell out at 20.30, and after a minute and a half, he managed to initiate flow. *Source:* Marcus Drake.

may climb during filling and reach a pressure decided by the resistance of the AUS. Since a fully functioning AUS generates 60 cmH$_2$O pressure, this may allow the p$_{det}$ to reach values that would be dangerous for renal function (Figure 14.21).

A key thing to be aware of is the fact that recovery of sphincter function after radical prostatectomy can be delayed by many months (Figure 14.22). This is presumably a result of damage to the sphincter innervation where it passes close to the operation site. Regrowth of the nerves

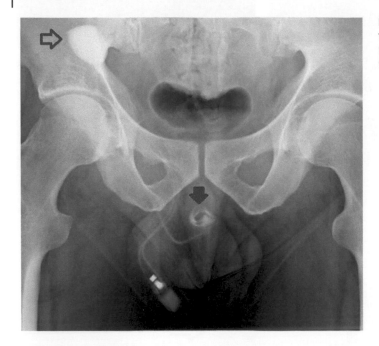

Figure 14.28 The artificial urinary sphincter balloon in this man with recurrent post-prostatectomy incontinence is partly deflated (open red arrow), and there is air in the cuff (closed red arrow). *Source:* Marcus Drake.

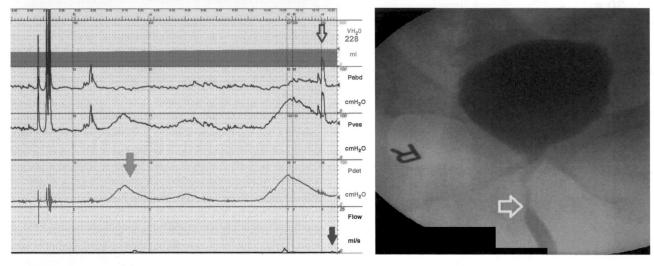

Figure 14.29 A man with incontinence after a male sling. The filling cystometry on the left shows detrusor overactivity incontinence (green arrow) and urodynamic stress incontinence (closed red arrow). The yellow arrow shows the lower extent of the sling, at the start of the urethral bulb.

References

1 Selman, L.E., Ochieng, C.A., Lewis, A.L. et al. (2019). *Recommendations for conducting invasive urodynamics for men with lower urinary tract symptoms: qualitative interview findings from a large randomized controlled trial (UPSTREAM). Neurourol. Urodyn.* 38 (1): 320–329.

2 Abrams, P. (1994). *New words for old: lower urinary tract symptoms for "prostatism". BMJ* 308 (6934): 929–930.

3 Chapple, C.R. and Roehrborn, C.G. (2006). *A shifted paradigm for the further understanding, evaluation, and treatment of lower urinary tract symptoms in men: focus on the bladder. Eur. Urol.* 49 (4): 651–658.

4 Sciarra, A., D'Eramo, G., Casale, P. et al. (1998). *Relationship among symptom score, prostate volume, and urinary flow rates in 543 patients with and without benign prostatic hyperplasia. Prostate* 34 (2): 121–128; discussion 129.

5 Ziada, A., Rosenblum, M., and Crawford, E.D. (1999). *Benign prostatic hyperplasia: an overview. Urology* 53 (3 Suppl 3a): 1–6.

6 Gulur, D.M., Mevcha, A.M., and Drake, M.J. (2011). *Nocturia as a manifestation of systemic disease. BJU Int.* 107 (5): 702–713.

7 Drake, M.J. (2014). *Do we need a new definition of the overactive bladder syndrome? ICI-RS 2013. Neurourol. Urodyn.* 33 (5): 622–624.

8 Al-Zahrani, A.A. and Gajewski, J.B. (2012). *Association of symptoms with urodynamic findings in men with overactive bladder syndrome. BJU Int.* 110 (11 Pt C): E891–E895.

9 Abrams, P., Cardozo, L., Fall, M. et al. (2002). *The standardisation of terminology of lower urinary tract function: report from the Standardisation Sub-committee of the International Continence Society. Neurourol. Urodyn.* 21 (2): 167–178.

10 Thomas, A.W. and Abrams, P. (2000). *Lower urinary tract symptoms, benign prostatic obstruction and the overactive bladder. BJU Int.* 85 (Suppl 3): 57–68; discussion 70–1.

11 Seki, N., Yuki, K., Takei, M. et al. (2009). *Analysis of the prognostic factors for overactive bladder symptoms following surgical treatment in patients with benign prostatic obstruction. Neurourol. Urodyn.* 28 (3): 197–201.

12 Abrams, P. (1994). *In support of pressure-flow studies for evaluating men with lower urinary tract symptoms. Urology* 44 (2): 153–155.

13 Rodrigues, P., Lucon, A.M., Freire, G.C., and Arap, S. (2001). *Urodynamic pressure flow studies can predict the clinical outcome after transurethral prostatic resection. J. Urol.* 165 (2): 499–502.

14 Clement, K.D., Burden, H., Warren, K. et al. (2015). *Invasive urodynamic studies for the management of lower urinary tract symptoms (LUTS) in men with voiding dysfunction. Cochrane Database Syst. Rev.* 4 (4) (Art. No.: CD011179) Wiley.

15 Oelke, M. et al. (2013). *EAU guidelines on the treatment and follow-up of non-neurogenic male lower urinary tract symptoms including benign prostatic obstruction. Eur. Urol.* 64 (1): 118–140.

16 Jones, C., Hill, J., and Chapple, C. (2010). *Management of lower urinary tract symptoms in men: summary of NICE guidance. BMJ* 340: c2354.

17 Nickel, J.C., Herschorn, S., Corcos, J. et al. (2005). *Canadian guidelines for the management of benign prostatic hyperplasia. Can. J. Urol.* 12 (3): 2677–2683.

18 Kaplan, S.A. (2006). *Update on the American Urological Association guidelines for the treatment of benign prostatic hyperplasia. Rev. Urol.* 8 (Suppl 4): S10–S17.

19 Winters, J.C., Dmochowski, R.R., Goldman, H.B. et al. (2012). *Urodynamic studies in adults: AUA/SUFU guideline. J. Urol.* 188 (6 Suppl): 2464–2472.

20 Gratzke, C. et al. (2015). *EAU guidelines on the assessment of non-neurogenic male lower urinary tract symptoms including benign prostatic obstruction. Eur. Urol.* 67 (6): 1099–1109.

21 Donkelaar, S.C., Rosier, P., and de Kort, L. (2017). *Comparison of three methods to analyze detrusor contraction during micturition in men over 50 years of age. Neurourol. Urodyn.* 36 (8): 2153–2159.

22 Schafer, W. (1995). *Analysis of bladder-outlet function with the linearized passive urethral resistance relation, linPURR, and a disease-specific approach for grading obstruction: from complex to simple. World J. Urol.* 13 (1): 47–58.

23 Hashim, H., Elhilali, M., Bjerklund Johansen, T.E. et al. (2007). *The immediate and 6-mo reproducibility of pressure-flow studies in men with benign prostatic enlargement. Eur. Urol.* 52 (4): 1186–1193.

24 Griffiths, D., Hofner, K., van Mastrigt, R. et al. (1997). *Standardization of terminology of lower urinary tract function: pressure-flow studies of voiding, urethral resistance, and urethral obstruction. International Continence Society Subcommittee on Standardization of Terminology of Pressure-Flow Studies. Neurourol. Urodyn.* 16 (1): 1–18.

25 Abrams, P.H. and Griffiths, D.J. (1979). *The assessment of prostatic obstruction from urodynamic measurements and from residual urine. Br. J. Urol.* 51 (2): 129–134.

26 Fang, Q., Song, B., Li, W. et al. (2007). *Role of UPP in evaluating bladder outlet obstruction due to benign prostatic enlargement. Neurourol. Urodyn.* 26 (6): 842–846.

27 Reynard, J.M., Peters, T.J., Lamond, E., and Abrams, P. (1995). *The significance of abdominal straining in men with lower urinary tract symptoms. Br. J. Urol.* 75 (2): 148–153.

28 Madersbacher, S., Pycha, A., Klingler, C.H. et al. (1999). *Interrelationships of bladder compliance with age, detrusor instability, and obstruction in elderly men with lower urinary tract symptoms. Neurourol. Urodyn.* 18 (1): 3–15.

29 Bailey, K., Abrams, P., Blair, P.S. et al. (2015). *Urodynamics for prostate surgery trial; randomised evaluation of assessment methods (UPSTREAM) for diagnosis and management of bladder outlet obstruction in men: study protocol for a randomised controlled trial. Trials* 16 (1): 567.

30 Young, G.J. et al. (2017). *Statistical analysis plan for the urodynamics for prostate surgery trial; randomised evaluation of assessment methods (UPSTREAM). Trials* 18 (1): 455.

31 Lewis, A.L., Lewis, A.L., Lane, J.A. et al. (2019). *Clinical and patient-reported outcome measures in men referred for consideration of surgery to treat lower urinary tract symptoms: baseline results and diagnostic findings of the urodynamics for prostate surgery trial; randomised* *evaluation of assessment methods (UPSTREAM). Eur. Urol. Focus* 5 (3): 340–350.

32 Drake, M.J., Lewis, A.L., Young, G.J. et al. (2020). *Diagnostic assessment of lower urinary tract symptoms in men considering prostate surgery; a non-inferiority randomised controlled trial of urodynamics in 26 hospitals. Eur. Urol.* 78 (5): 701–710.

33 Ito, H., Young, G., Lewis, A. et al. (2020). *Grading severity and bother using the IPSS and ICIQ-MLUTS scores in men seeking lower urinary tract symptoms therapy. J. Urol.*

34 Thomas, A.W., Cannon, A., Bartlett, E. et al. (2004). *The natural history of lower urinary tract dysfunction in men: the influence of detrusor underactivity on the outcome after transurethral resection of the prostate with a minimum 10-year urodynamic follow-up. BJU Int.* 93 (6): 745–750.

35 Chung, D.E., Dillon, B., Kurta, J. et al. (2013). *Detrusor underactivity is prevalent after radical prostatectomy: a urodynamic study including risk factors. Can. Urol. Assoc. J.* 7 (1–2): E33–E37.

36 Fode, M., Serefoglu, E.C., Albersen, M. et al. (2017). *Sexuality following radical prostatectomy: is restoration of erectile function enough? Sex. Med. Rev.* 5 (1): 110–119.

37 Manassero, F., Di Paola, G., Paperini, D. et al. (2012). *Orgasm-associated incontinence (climacturia) after bladder neck-sparing radical prostatectomy: clinical and video-urodynamic evaluation. J. Sex. Med.* 9 (8): 2150–2156.

38 Solomon, E., Veeratterapillay, R., Malde, S. et al. (2017). *Can filling phase urodynamic parameters predict the success of the bulbar artificial urinary sphincter in treating post-prostatectomy incontinence? Neurourol. Urodyn.* 36: 1557–1563.

39 Smith, A.L., Ferlise, V.J., Wein, A.J. et al. (2011). *Effect of a 7-F transurethral catheter on abdominal leak point pressure measurement in men with post-prostatectomy incontinence. Urology* 77 (5): 1188–1193.

40 Decter, R.M. and Harpster, L. (1992). *Pitfalls in determination of leak point pressure. J. Urol.* 148 (2 Pt 2): 588–591.

41 Sharaf, A., Fader, M., Macaulay, M., and Drake, M.J. (2019). *Use of an occlusive penile clamp during filling cystometry in men with symptoms of stress urinary incontinence. Low Urin. Tract Symptoms* 11 (3): 133–138.

42 Majoros, A., Bach, D., Keszthelyi, A. et al. (2006). *Urinary incontinence and voiding dysfunction after radical retropubic prostatectomy (prospective urodynamic study). Neurourol. Urodyn.* 25 (1): 2–7.

43 Thiel, D.D., Young, P.R., Broderick, G.A. et al. (2007). *Do clinical or urodynamic parameters predict artificial urinary sphincter outcome in post-radical prostatectomy incontinence? Urology* 69 (2): 315–319.

44 Lemmens, J.M., Broadbridge, J., Macaulay, M. et al. (2019). *Tissue response to applied loading using different designs of penile compression clamps. Med. Devices (Auckl.)* 12: 235–243.

45 Comiter, C.V., Sullivan, M.P., and Yalla, S.V. (2003). *Correlation among maximal urethral closure pressure, retrograde leak point pressure, and abdominal leak point pressure in men with postprostatectomy stress incontinence. Urology* 62 (1): 75–78.

46 Comiter, C.V., Sullivan, M.P., and Yalla, S.V. (1997). *Retrograde leak point pressure for evaluating postradical prostatectomy incontinence. Urology* 49 (2): 231–236.

47 Fitzpatrick, J.M., Desgrandchamps, F., Adjali, K. et al. (2012). *Management of acute urinary retention: a worldwide survey of 6074 men with benign prostatic hyperplasia. BJU Int.* 109 (1): 88–95.

48 Djavan, B., Madersbacher, S., Klingler, C. et al. (1997). *Urodynamic assessment of patients with acute urinary retention: is treatment failure after prostatectomy predictable? J. Urol.* 158 (5): 1829–1833.

49 Guo, D.P., Comiter, C.V., and Elliott, C.S. (2017). *Urodynamics of men with urinary retention. Int. J. Urol.* 24 (9): 703–707.

50 Abrams, P.H., Dunn, M., and George, N. (1978). *Urodynamic findings in chronic retention of urine and their relevance to results of surgery. Br. Med. J.* 2 (6147): 1258–1260.

51 Thomas, A.W., Cannon, A., Bartlett, E. et al. (2005). *The natural history of lower urinary tract dysfunction in men: minimum 10-year urodynamic followup of transurethral resection of prostate for bladder outlet obstruction. J. Urol.* 174 (5): 1887–1891.

15

Structural Changes of the Bladder Outlet

Michelle Ong[1], Marcus Drake[2], and Devang Desai[3]

[1] *Department of Urology, Toowoomba Base Hospital, Toowoomba, Queensland, Australia*
[2] *Translational Health Sciences, Bristol Medical School, Southmead Hospital, Bristol, UK*
[3] *Department of Urology, University of Queensland, Toowoomba Base Hospital, Toowoomba, Queensland, Australia*

CONTENTS

The principle focus of urodynamics (UDS) is to understand bladder and sphincter function during storage and voiding, and the information is used in most cases to decide on treatment. Clearly, the anatomical context of the lower urinary tract also needs to be considered. This is needed for several key reasons:

- Ensuring urodynamic tests are run safely
- Giving the best chance to gather the necessary information
- Interpreting the findings
- Supporting the treatment recommendations

Many patients attending UDS have had previous lower urinary tract or pelvic surgery, or they may have a disease process or trauma affecting the area. In this chapter, we discuss how such anatomical changes can be identified, and what they can imply for individual patients.

Impaired Blood Supply to the Bladder Outlet

Any trauma (such as a pelvic fracture or surgical operation) or inflammatory process (such as serious infection or radiotherapy) can affect blood supply within the affected anatomical field. Consequently, there is increased scarring and reduced capacity for healing if an operation is subsequently planned. The superior and inferior vesical arteries provide most of the arterial blood supply to the bladder neck, but there are small contributions to the lower part of the bladder from the obturator, inferior gluteal, uterine, and vaginal arteries (in women) [1]. The prostatic artery arises from the inferior vesical artery and divides into urethral and capsular groups. From the urethral group arise the Flock's and Badenoch's arteries (which both supply the transitional zone). Flock's arteries approach the bladder neck at 1 and 11 o'clock and Badenoch's at 5 and 7 o'clock [1, 2]. Venous drainage is via a plexus that converges on the vesicoprostatic plexus in the groove between bladder and prostate in men, or in the base of the broad ligament in females. This drains backwards across the pelvic floor to the internal iliac veins. The penis and urethra are supplied by the internal pudendal arteries. Each artery divides into a cavernosal artery of the penis (which supplies the corpora cavernosa), a dorsal artery of the penis, and the bulbourethral artery. These branches supply the corpus spongiosum, the glans penis, and the urethra.

Stenosis of the External Urethral Meatus

During circumcision, if injury to the glans occurs, then the blood supply of the distal urethra may be compromised, and subsequent urethral ischaemia may occur. This may predispose patients to the development of ischaemic strictures in the future. This is particularly the case where circumcision was needed due to scarring of the prepuce secondary to lichen sclerosus (Figure 15.1). Whilst lichen sclerosus is principally a skin problem, if it is allowed to progress, it is a major offender in the development of strictures, and therefore, this can also lead to the development of strictures in the future. The problem may only become apparent when attempts are made to retract the foreskin, since then it becomes clear that the scarring has caused the prepuce to become tight and hence difficult to retract over the glans (phimosis). This can be especially problematic in obese men with a 'buried penis' (Figure 15.2).

Urethral stenosis in women is predominantly associated with genital lichen sclerosus (Figure 15.3). Other causes include inflammatory (sexual or urinary tract infections),

post-radiation, post-surgical, and trauma (pelvic fracture urethral injuries [PFUI]). The stenosis generally occurs primarily in the mid to distal urethra and historically was also managed with serial/lifelong dilations. Now, the role of buccal mucosal graft urethroplasty is also coming to the forefront of treatment for urethral stenoses in women; however, longer term studies need to be performed in this area [3].

Bladder Neck Stenosis and Urethral Strictures in Men

Bladder neck stenoses may occur in the patient who has had any surgical procedure, i.e. radical prostatectomy for prostate cancer, post-radiotherapy patients, or patients who have had a transurethral resection of the prostate (TURP) [4]. It may also occur secondary to trauma, radiation, or other conditions like Marion's disease (enlarged muscle cells in bladder neck causing obstruction). Clearly, established severe stenosis like that pictured in Figure 15.4 represents an almost impossible challenge for catheterisation when attempting to do UDS. In such a setting, use of a flexible cystoscope is needed to find a way through for a guidewire; a catheter can usually be threaded over the guidewire.

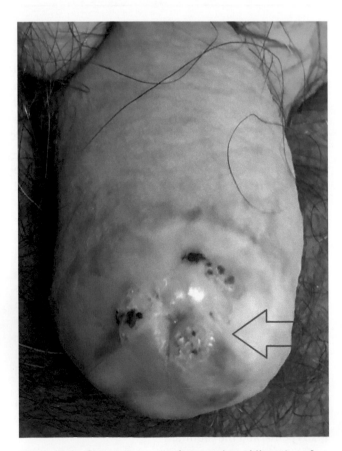

Figure 15.1 Picture demonstrating complete obliteration of the urethral meatus (red arrow) secondary to lichen sclerosus following a circumcision. The white appearance indicates deep scarring and a significant reduction in local blood supply. *Source:* Marcus Drake.

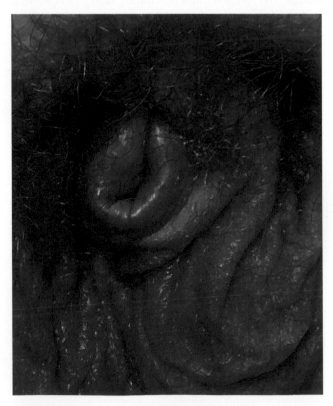

Figure 15.2 A man with a 'buried penis' due to obesity. Attempts to retract the foreskin proved difficult due to phimosis. *Source:* Marcus Drake.

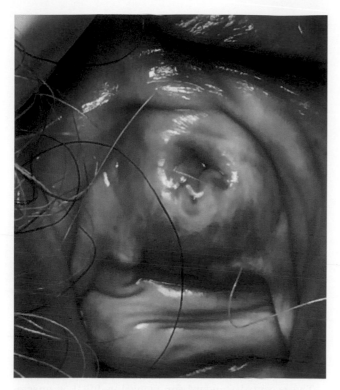

Figure 15.3 Lichen sclerosus affecting the urethral meatus in a woman. This process can extend into the vagina and cause severe structural changes. *Source*: Marcus Drake.

The mechanism of iatrogenic bladder neck stenoses is dependent on the type of procedure that is performed. Endoscopic, laparoscopic, robotic, or open prostate surgery

which disturbs the bladder neck can all predispose patients to bladder neck stenosis or contracture [4]. In endoscopic TURP, the mechanism of bladder neck contracture is not very clear, beyond the involvement of healing and scar formation. Thankfully, with improved technology and equipment, it has become a rare complication of TURP surgery [4, 5]. In radical prostatectomy, bladder neck stenosis and urethral stricture are the result of luminal constriction caused by tissue fibrosis. All wounds are prone to a degree of contraction due to the action of myofibroblasts in the healing process. This is even more relevant in the context of a luminal end-to-end anastomosis, as is needed when the entire prostate is removed. Other contributory factors, such as tissue ischaemia from increased tension at the anastomosis, wound distraction from haematoma, or foreign materials such as clips, increase the risk of a urine leak and therefore increase collagen deposition from the myofibroblasts. This ultimately leads to wound contraction, hypertrophic scarring, and resultant luminal narrowing [4, 5].

In radiation therapy, DNA damage is inflicted by free radical formation with resultant apoptosis. Pro-inflammatory and pro-fibrotic cytokines are activated leading to tissue and vascular injury, and, as such, tissues remain poorly oxygenated with increased collagen deposition, tissue contraction, and scar formation. Consequently, radiation-induced strictures tend to present later than surgical stenoses and in a more insidious fashion (two to three years

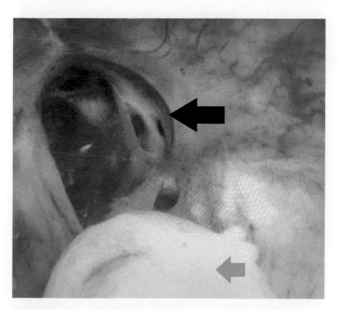

Figure 15.4 Endoscopic view of a severe bladder neck contracture (black arrow) resulting from a previous TURP procedure. The green arrow indicates the verumontanum, which is an anatomical feature relied on by surgeons as a landmark just above the urethral sphincter. *Source*: Marcus Drake.

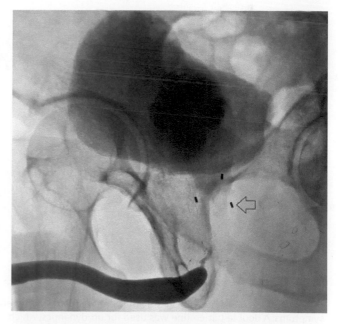

Figure 15.5 Urethrogram demonstrating a membranous and bulbar urethral stricture secondary to brachytherapy. Brachytherapy seeds (red arrow) are seen located within the prostate. *Source*: Marcus Drake.

post-treatment) [4, 5]. Brachytherapy is a form of prostate cancer treatment which involves the implantation of radioactive seeds within the prostate (Figure 15.5). These seeds deliver ongoing radiation to the prostate, serving as a method of treating localised prostate cancer. Seeds can be permanent (low dose rate/LDR) or temporary (high dose rate/HDR) and are placed through the perineum into the prostate using transrectal ultrasound guidance [6].

Brachytherapy can be used in conjunction with external beam radiotherapy (EBRT), which, some studies have shown, can lower the risk of biochemical recurrence of prostate cancer, especially in high-risk patients [7].

Stricture disease is a well-described complication of brachytherapy with studies suggesting the median time to stricture development at 16 months (range of 4–29 months). These strictures are generally identified within the membranous or proximal bulbar urethra. Stricture rates for brachytherapy increase if used in conjunction with EBRT, and essentially double if used in conjunction with radical prostatectomy. Stricture rates are also higher in HDR brachytherapy versus LDR brachytherapy (11% and 2%, respectively) and are higher still in salvage brachytherapy groups (up to 31%) [6–8]. Therefore, a detailed history of previous prostate cancer and treatments for prostate cancer should be obtained prior to performing UDS studies. This is to anticipate problems with running the test and is also useful when deciding on treatment recommendations. Strictures caused by the combination of brachytherapy and

EBRT are often long and severe [9, 10]. In contrast, EBRT strictures are not commonly obliterative and therefore are more amenable to anastomotic urethroplasty [9, 10]. Notably, radiotherapy can affect any normal tissue, potentially including local nerve supply. In the case of prostate brachytherapy, this can influence sphincter innervation (Figure 15.6).

Treatment of Stricture Disease

It is common to dilate or incise a stricture, but recurrence is common. Internal urethrotomy and urethral dilation can also be used; however, these procedures carry a high failure and recurrence rate of up to 40–60% [9]. For a recurrent stricture, further dilation or incision may simply accelerate and exacerbate the process. The current indication of internal urethrotomy is for a short bulbar urethral stricture. It can be performed using a cold blade or a laser fibre [11]. The long-term success of internal urethrotomy is low. It is not advisable to perform repeated endoscopic procedures as the success rate keeps declining on subsequent procedures [12].

The accepted standard for managing PFUI is anastomotic urethroplasty. The technique involves excising the diseased segment, spatulating both ends, and suturing them over a catheter [13]. This requires a stepwise perineal approach and may be combined with an abdominal approach [13]. In the anterior urethra, the indication for

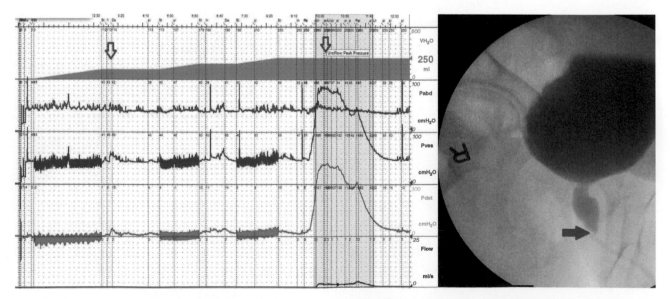

Figure 15.6 A 64-year-old man previously treated with radiotherapy for prostate cancer, with subsequent storage and voiding symptoms. A double lumen line was used for urodynamics, which had pump artefact obvious when the pump was running for filling cystometry. Low-amplitude detrusor overactivity was seen when the pump was stopped (red arrow). Voiding showed high pressure and slow flow rate, i.e. bladder outlet obstruction (open purple arrow). Video urodynamics showed that his urethra was not obstructed by prostate enlargement – the site of obstruction was at the external sphincter (closed purple arrow). Subsequent cystoscopy found no urethral stricture. Hence, this was functional non-relaxing sphincter obstruction. *Source*: Marcus Drake.

anastomotic urethroplasty is for traumatic bulbar urethral stricture [13, 14]. These could be either non-transecting or transecting depending on the degree of spongiofibrosis and the length of the stricture.

Augmentation or substitution urethroplasty involves cutting into the stricture and opening out the defect with a graft or flap. It uses a graft with no blood supply (buccal, lingual, labial, rectal mucosa, and bladder mucosa) or a pedicled flap which brings a blood supply with it (penile skin flap and scrotal flap) to replace or augment a segment of the diseased urethra with an aim to increase the size of the urethral lumen [15]. This can be achieved over a small segment or the entire anterior urethra for panurethral strictures [15]. Given that most strictures are due to lichen sclerosus, there is an increased use of buccal grafts in this procedure [10]. The application of the graft may be dorsal, ventral, or double face with either onlay or inlay techniques [10, 15].

There is currently no consensus on the management of radiation-induced strictures, and the decision between anastomosis or substitution urethroplasty is individualised to the patient. An anastomotic urethroplasty carries a higher risk of incontinence, perhaps due to tissue tension or direct sphincter trauma. The use of a flap or graft brings a higher risk of failure due to poor surrounding tissue blood supply.

UDS and Stricture Patients

For some patients, suspicion for a stricture should be high:

1) The patient who has a classic 'stricture' constrictive pattern on their free flow rate test (Figure 6.13);
2) Someone with a past history of urethral strictures;
3) History of previous stricture surgery, i.e. dilation, self-catheterisation for strictures, urethroplasty, or urethrotomies;
4) Previous instrumentation of the lower urinary tract, i.e. cystoscopy, TURP, or foreign body removal; and
5) Clinical findings of extensive lichen sclerosus with possible meatal stenosis.

Catheterisation can be difficult in this group of patients and can cause avoidable trauma, pain, and bleeding. The following are some measures that can be taken when catheterising a patient for video urodynamics with a potential urethral stricture:

1) Be liberal with the use of lubricant. Note that lubricant should not be forced in – indeed, a severe stricture may cause the lubricant to push back out when trying to instil it.
2) Use a small gauge catheter to start so as to minimise the risk of traumatising the urethra and creating a 'false passage'.

3) Catheterise gently – if you hit resistance, just stop and reassess. Graft perforation occurs with recurrence or when excessive force is used, and avoiding this must be a priority.
4) If catheterisation is unsuccessful and a lot of resistance is met, a guidewire can be used to see if the stricture is traversable with a wire, then a small gauge catheter can be railroaded over the wire to assess the density of the stricture.
5) If catheterisation is not possible at the time of UDS, a urethrogram can be performed distally to assess the location and length of the stricture for operative planning (an 'upogram' – see Chapter 8).

Voiding dysfunction after urethroplasty may result from bladder outlet obstruction secondary to recurrent stricture disease or detrusor underactivity. A thorough history, examination, and detailed review of the past surgical procedure should be undertaken prior to UDS [16]. A prior or on-table retrograde urethrogram would assist in evaluating the site, length of the stricture, and the lumen size [16]. A flexible cystoscopy can also be undertaken if required. In near obliterative strictures, the UDS filling line must be passed gently under visual (fluoroscopic or endoscopic) guidance to make sure the stricture is negotiated to avoid a false passage [16]. Injury to the urethra in a patient who has had previous urethroplasty can result in bleeding, false passages, or damage to the graft. This may lead to recurrent disease or infection [16]. If resistance is felt and catheterisation is not possible, a retrograde urethrogram or voiding micturating urethrogram should be performed prior to further attempts.

Risk of graft perforation is low and is dependent on the type of graft, the location of the graft (penile, bulbar, dorsal, or ventral), the extent of the repair, time post-urethroplasty, and whether the urethroplasty was successful or not. As a rule, dorsal grafts are more successful than ventral and are less likely to be traumatised during catheterisation.

Trauma

Injuries where the urethra is pulled in opposing directions ("distraction") mainly occur in the setting of PFUI (Figure 15.7) [13]. This often results in a membrano-bulbar injury of the urethra (Figure 15.8). is the injury may be far enough away from the sphincter mechanism that continence is often not affected [9]. Incontinence occurs if there is a concurrent bladder neck injury at the time, or post-operatively. If a patient who has had a previous PFUI repaired requires it, an artificial urinary sphincter (AUS) can be placed in the bulbar urethra, away from the anasto-

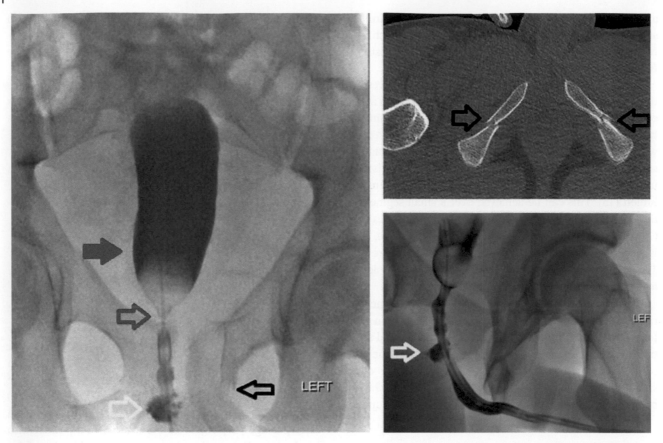

Figure 15.7 Recent pelvic trauma, with fractures of the pubis and ischia (black arrows) which have not yet undergone reduction and fixation. The base of the bladder (open red arrow) has been torn off the prostatic urethra; a catheter has been placed to splint the injury. The inevitable severe bleeding has compressed the bladder into an elongated shape (closed red arrow). Extravasation of contrast is seen from the urethra (yellow arrow). *Source*: Marcus Drake.

mosis. A problem that may be encountered is increased scarring of the urethra at the time of AUS insertion, and to overcome this, the AUS might be placed across the penile erectile mechanism ('transcorporal placement') to give some vascular protection for the urethra [13].

Metal plates used in repairing fractures (internal fixation) can end up extremely close to the lower urinary tract (Figure 15.9). This can make surgical planning difficult, for example, if the patient develops stress incontinence, due to the severe scarring. It is vital to consider this proximity if a patient develops lower urinary tract symptoms (LUTS) and haematuria, as it could indicate the plate, or a fixation screw, has eroded into the urinary tract. This can have disastrous consequences due to the risk of infection of the plate or bones (osteomyelitis).

Hypospadias

Hypospadias is a congenital abnormality in the development of the distal urethra [17]. In hypospadias, the urethral meatus opens on the ventral side of the penis proximal

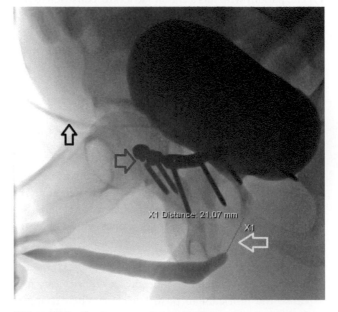

Figure 15.8 Urethrogram demonstrating a stricture following a pelvic fracture urethral injury (yellow arrow). There is contrast tracking along a suprapubic catheter (black arrow). A pelvic internal fixation plate is present (red arrow), which was placed to help healing of the causative fracture. *Source*: Marcus Drake.

to the tip of the glans penis (Figures 15.10 and 15.11) [17]. This occurs in 1 in every 300 male children. Newborns and young children rarely have symptoms related to hypospadias, whilst older children and adults may present with difficulty directing the urinary stream and spraying. Very occasionally, a patient may only present in adulthood because of a downwards curvature, or 'ventral chordee', associated with hypospadias causing difficulties with sexual intercourse. Generally, operations attempting to correct hypospadias are generally done in infanthood [17]. Someone who has had successful surgery may have a scar extending along the penile shaft as far as the location of the meatus at birth, and the newly constructed meatus may be white-edged due to connective tissue healing. Such patients should be catheterised carefully and gently to avoid traumatising the surgical repair – as is the case for urethroplasty patients. 'Traumatic hypospadias' is a term to describe breakdown of the glans in a patient with an indwelling urethral catheter (Figure 15.12). This is a risk in someone with neurological disease (due to lack of sensation) or dementia (due to difficulty with communication).

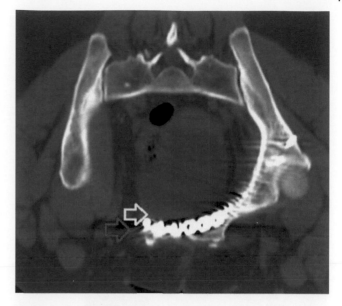

Figure 15.9 A pubic fracture in a woman repaired with internal fixation (red arrow), demonstrating how close the metal foreign body lies to the front of the bladder (yellow arrow). *Source:* Marcus Drake.

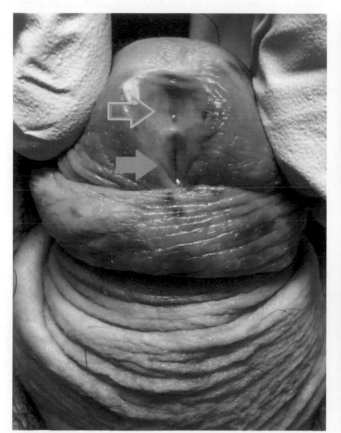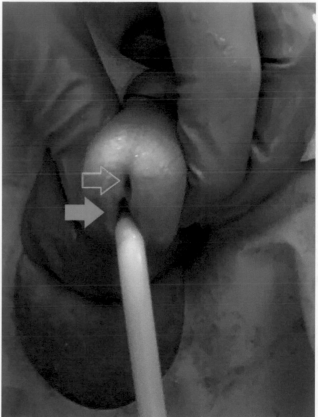

Figure 15.10 Two cases of distal hypospadias, with a urethral meatus located close to the junction between the glans and the penile shaft (closed green arrow). Often, these cases have a shallow pit where the meatus would normally be (open green arrow). Sometimes, the blind pit is deep and can actually look like a meatus (right image, open green arrow) but proves impossible to catheterise as it is blind ending. The proximal hole is more likely to be the actual urethra (closed green arrow). *Source:* Marcus Drake.

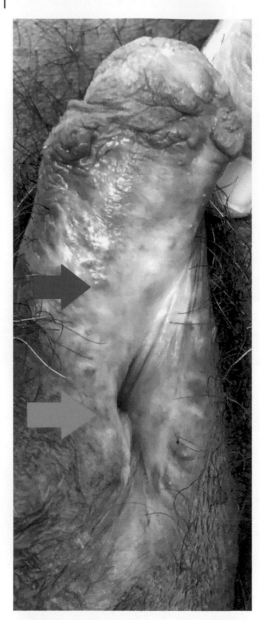

Figure 15.11 Penoscrotal hypospadias (green arrow). This patient had previously undergone several operations aimed at correcting the hypospadias by constructing a penile urethra and meatus on the glans. These had broken down, leaving scarring extensively on the penile shaft (red arrow). *Source*: Marcus Drake.

Mild hypospadias, for which the patient did not seek treatment for as symptoms were minimal, may sometimes be encountered in the UDS clinic. In these cases, the external meatus may be located unusually proximally on the penile shaft, but catheterisation is no different than for someone with a normally located meatus.

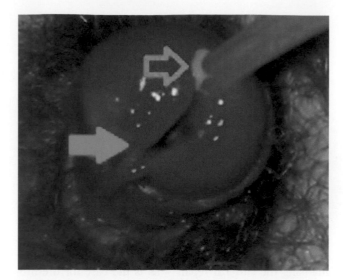

Figure 15.12 Traumatic hypospadias due to an indwelling urethral catheter. The glans has been split down to the penile shaft (green arrow). The blue arrow indicates the purulent exudate resulting from an inflammatory reaction to the catheter. *Source*: Marcus Drake.

A thorough history of childhood operations and urinary issues may be needed in patients with aberrant anatomy. A history of ambiguous genitalia or penoscrotal hypospadias may highlight an underlying syndromic abnormality. The more proximal the hypospadias, the more likely it is to encounter an associated congenital syndrome.

Surgical Mesh

The extensive use of surgical mesh in midurethral tape procedures and pelvic organ prolapse surgery in the recent past means that there is a considerable number of female patients with potentially challenging urodynamic and surgical issues. The tapes can cause several issues with important implications:

1) Scarring, causing cicatrisation;
2) Infection, potentially causing serious soft tissue or bone complications;
3) Chronic pain;
4) Exposure within the urinary tract or vagina (Figure 15.13);
5) Need for removal of mesh, sometimes with several procedures, with important anatomical structures (e.g. the obturator nerve) in proximity;
6) Lower urinary tract dysfunction and dyspareunia; and
7) Psychological trauma and anxiety.

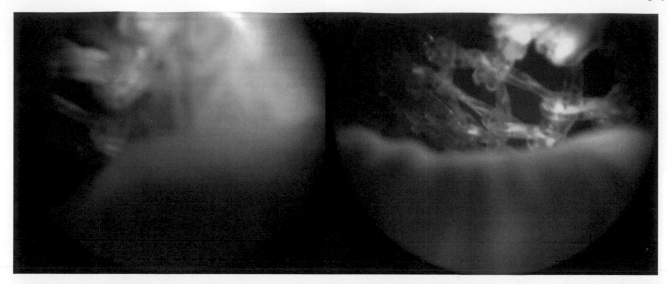

Figure 15.13 Endoscopic view of a midurethral tape which had become exposed in the urethra (left) and extending into the bladder (right). *Source*: Marcus Drake.

Gender Confirmation Surgery

Gender confirmation surgery is undertaken to transition individuals with gender dysphoria to their identified gender. Previously, it was known as sex reassignment surgery or gender reassignment surgery. People who have undergone surgery, or are preparing to undergo it in the future, are sometimes referred for urodynamic evaluation. Everyone presenting in this setting requires an individual approach and considerable experience to plan and undertake testing. Usually, people concerned have a high level of knowledge and are comfortable to discuss the steps in the process that they have completed so far.

Transitioning to another gender may involve:

- A mental health evaluation to look for any concerns that could influence an individual's mental state and to assess a person's readiness to undergo the physical and emotional stresses of the transition;
- A clear and consistent documentation of gender dysphoria;
- Dressing and living in a gender role that is congruent with their gender identity;
- A 'real life' test, taking on the role of the desired sex in everyday activities;

- Taking sex hormones; and
- Surgically removing or modifying genitals and reproductive organs.

Regarding the pelvic organs, male-to-female surgery may include penectomy, orchidectomy, and feminising genitoplasty to create a vagina (maybe using a segment of colon) and labia (by altering the shape of the scrotum). The prostate is not removed (Figure 15.14). Conversely, female-to-male surgery may involve removal of the uterus and ovaries and masculinising genitoplasty based on pedicled flaps and erectile implants. UDS studies of two people awaiting female-to-male gender confirmation surgery are described in Figures 15.15 and 15.16.

Running a UDS test requires a considerate approach and a respectful and professional discussion to describe mechanisms and findings in a matter-of-fact manner. Technical aspects do not differ from conventional filling cystometry and pressure-flow studies except for the differences in the expected structures of the bladder outlet. For someone who has undergone surgery, the possibility of urethral stricture or meatal stenosis should be considered. Someone who is living in a gender role should be addressed as appropriate for that gender, regardless of whether they have yet had surgical procedures.

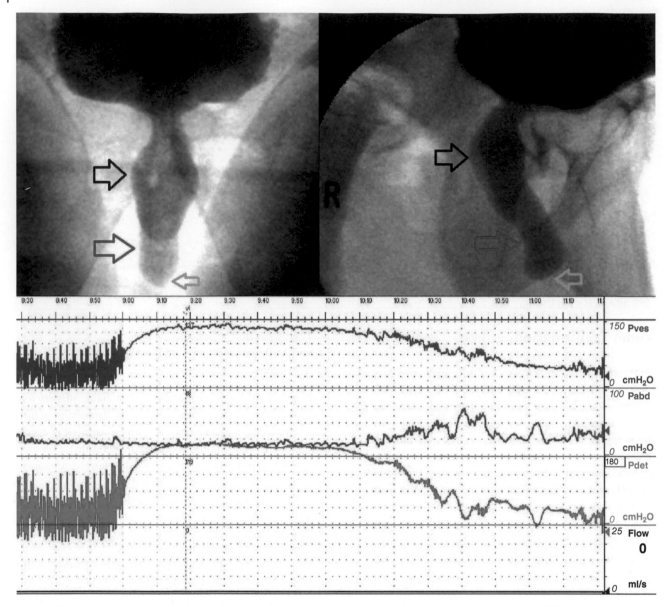

Figure 15.14 A woman who had previously undergone male-to-female gender confirmation surgery. During filling cystometry, she developed severe detrusor overactivity, clearly visible on the pressure trace. This caused marked dilation of the prostatic urethra (black arrows) and the membranous and proximal bulbar urethra (red arrows). Obstruction to flow was present at the new external urethral meatus (green arrows), a common place for narrowing; in effect, the 6Fr double lumen catheter was sufficient to occlude the narrow meatus. There is no obvious prostate enlargement in this patient; the use of feminising hormones means that prostatic enlargement (and hence benign prostatic obstruction) is uncommon. *Source*: Marcus Drake.

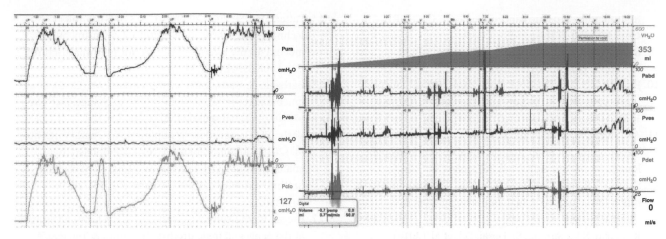

Figure 15.15 A man who was awaiting female-to-male gender confirmation surgery, with voiding dysfunction. The urethral pressure profiles on the left show a high maximum urethral closure pressure; as expected, there was no bladder neck or prostatic plateau on the profile. The filling cystometry and pressure-flow study on the right shows a stable detrusor; when permission to void was given, straining was used, but no flow was achieved.

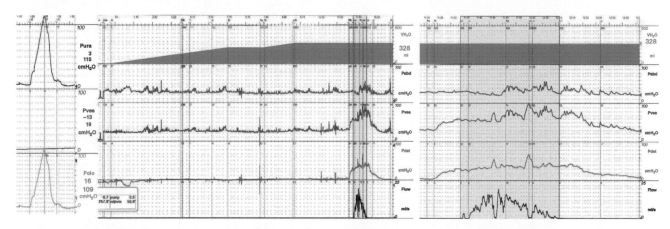

Figure 15.16 Another man who was awaiting female-to-male gender confirmation surgery, with voiding dysfunction. The urethral pressure profile on the left shows a high maximum urethral closure pressure, and no bladder neck or prostatic plateau. The filling cystometry and pressure-flow study in the middle shows a stable detrusor; when permission to void was given (shown in more detail on the right), relatively high pressures generated a comparatively slow flow rate for a person who, at this stage, had a female configuration of bladder outlet.

References

1. McMinn, R. (2014). Abdomen. In: Last's Anatomy, 9e (ed. R. McMinn). London: Elsevier.

2. Smith, J., Howards, S., and Preminger, G. (2012 Chapter 13). Prostate: benign disease. In: Hinman's Atlas of Urologic Surgery, 3e (eds. J.A. Smith, S.S. Howards, G.M. Preminger and R.R. Dmochowski). Philadelphia: Elsevier.

3. Blandy, J.P. (1980). Urethral stricture. *Postgrad. Med. J.* 56: 383–418.

4. Nicholson, H.L., Al-Hakeem, Y., Maldonado, J.J., and Tse, V. (2017). Management of bladder neck stenosis and urethral stricture and stenosis following treatment for prostate cancer. *Transl. Androl. Urol.* 6: S92–S102.

5. Summerton, D.J., Kitrey, N.D., Lumen, N. et al. European Association of Urology (2012). EAU guidelines on iatrogenic trauma. *Eur. Urol.* 62: 628–639.

6. Merrick, G.S., Butler, W.M., Tollenaar, B.G. et al. (2002). The dosimetry of prostate brachytherapy-induced urethral strictures. *Int. J. Radiat. Oncol. Biol. Phys.* 52: 461–468.

7. Hindson, B.R., Millar, J.L., and Matheson, B. (2013). Urethral strictures following high-dose-rate brachytherapy for prostate cancer: analysis of risk factors. *Brachytherapy* 12: 50–55.

8. Elliott, S.P., Meng, M.V., Elkin, E.P. et al. CaPSURE (2007). Incidence of urethral stricture after primary

treatment for prostate cancer: data from CaPSURE. *J. Urol.* 178: 529–534.

9. Mundy, A.R. and Andrich, D.E. (2011). Urethral strictures. *BJU Int.* 107: 6–26.

10. Bhargava, S. and Chapple, C.R. (2004). Buccal mucosal urethroplasty: is it the new gold standard? *BJU Int.* 93: 1191–1193.

11. Al Taweel, W. and Seyam, R. (2015). Visual internal Urethrotomy for adult male urethral stricture has poor long-term results. *Adv. Urol.* 2015: 656459.

12. Santucci, R. and Eisenberg, L. (2010). Urethrotomy has a much lower success rate than previously reported. *J. Urol.* 183: 1859–1862.

13. Kulkarni, S.B., Surana, S., Desai, D.J. et al. (2018). Management of complex and redo cases of pelvic fracture urethral injuries. *Asian J. Urol.* 5: 107–117.

14. Patterson, J.M. and Chapple, C.R. (2008). Surgical techniques in substitution urethroplasty using buccal mucosa for the treatment of anterior urethral strictures. *Eur. Urol.* 53: 1162–1171.

15. Barbagli, G., Sansalone, S., and Lazzeri, M. (2012). Oral mucosa and urethroplasty: it's time to change. *Eur. Urol.* 62: 1071–1073; discussion 1073–1075.

16. Verla, W., Oosterlinck, W., Spinoit, A.F., and Waterloos, M. (2019). A comprehensive review emphasizing anatomy, etiology, diagnosis, and treatment of male urethral stricture disease. *Biomed. Res. Int.* 2019: 9046430.

17. Breyer, B., McAninch, J., and Lue, T. (2013) 41). Disorders of the penis and male urethra. In: Smith & Tanagho's General Urology, 18e (eds. J. McAninch and T. Lue). McGraw Hill.

16

Neurological Disease and LUTS

Marcus Drake[1], Jeremy Nettleton[2], and Mohammed Belal[3]

[1] *Translational Health Sciences, Bristol Medical School, Southmead Hospital, Bristol, UK*
[2] *Department of Urology, Cheltenham General Hospital, Gloucestershire Hospitals NHS Foundation Trust, Cheltenham, UK*
[3] *Department of Urology, University Hospitals Birmingham, Birmingham, UK*

CONTENTS

Lower urinary tract symptoms (LUTS) are significant contributors to the impact of neurological disease. Neurogenic lower urinary tract dysfunction (NLUTD) refers to the extensive potential impact of neurological disease on function and co-ordination of the lower urinary tract (LUT) organs. Specific centres in the spinal cord exert direct control of the muscle groups, and these are overseen by higher centres which organise the reflex activity of storage and voiding. Depending on where in the central nervous system (CNS) the disease is having its effect, the following direct effects on the LUT may be identified:

1) Detrusor overactivity (DO), with or without DO incontinence (DOI) due to loss of bladder inhibition during the storage phase.
2) Detrusor underactivity (DUA) due to loss of bladder excitation during the voiding phase.
3) Stress urinary incontinence (SUI) due to impaired sphincter contraction during the storage phase.

4) Fixed sphincter obstruction due to impaired sphincter relaxation during the voiding phase.

5) Open bladder neck (in men) during the storage phase due to loss of sympathetic regulation.

6) Loss of sensation of the bladder filling during storage, or of urethral flow during voiding. This altered sensation can mean that a person with neurogenic DOI might not experience urgency, and hence the term urgency urinary incontinence (UUI) may not be entirely suitable to describe their NLUTD.

Clearly, neurological disease has a range of additional impacts outside the LUT, with impaired mobility, dexterity, and cognition being particularly important. Consequently, the established symptomatic classification of incontinence (SUI, UUI, and mixed urinary incontinence [MUI]) appropriate for the general population seen in a urodynamic unit does not meet the needs for describing all potential incontinence in NLUTD. Specifically, any detriment of cognitive and brain function potentially affects perception and appropriateness. This is recognised by the development of terminology specific to NLUTD standardised by the International Continence Society (ICS) [1]; the published fundamentals version of this document is given in the appendices. Some of the key additional terms for incontinence in NLUTD are [1]:

- *Impaired cognition urinary incontinence* is periodic urinary incontinence that the individual with cognitive impairment reports to have occurred without being aware of it.
- *Impaired mobility urinary incontinence* is inability to reach the toilet on time for voiding because of physical or medical disability. This inability includes (any combination of) the individual's physical as well as social causes or reasons. Other signs or symptoms of lower urinary tract dysfunction (LUTD) should not be present or should be reported by the professional (as primary or as accessory) (e.g. 'urgency urinary incontinence' with 'mobility impairment'; or 'mobility impairment urinary incontinence' with 'stress urinary incontinence').
- *Voiding dysregulation* is urination in situations which are generally regarded as socially inappropriate, such as while still fully dressed, or in a public setting away from toilet facilities.
- *Involuntary voiding* is both a symptom and a diagnosis of sporadic bladder emptying when awake, without intention to void. Usually, the voiding reflex is preserved, and there is only lack of proper inhibition of the voiding reflex. If that happens when asleep, it is called acquired enuresis.
- *Enuresis* is intermittent incontinence that occurs during periods of sleep. Enuresis is considered different from UUI. Confirming the precise underlying mechanism(s) is often not possible in routine clinical practice.

- *Continuous (urinary) incontinence* means complaint of continuous involuntary loss of urine.

Being specific as to the context of leakage helps ensure treatment choice is logical and prevents inappropriate intervention.

This area of urodynamics (UDS) is complex and requires a strong knowledge base, with the ability to work out processes and solutions logically. It is not appropriate to undertake neurological UDS without a properly established setup and multidisciplinary expertise. The resources need to allow for dealing with the physical limitations (notably wheelchair access, adequate space, supports for transferring, mobile and ceiling-mounted hoists, and video urodynamic equipment) and risks (medications to treat autonomic dysreflexia [AD] or anaphylaxis, and immediate support requirements for acute management of cardiac arrest) for this population.

Impaired Neurological Control of the Lower Urinary Tract: General Principles

The basics of the neural control are described in Chapter 2. In this section, the points are reinforced, emphasising potential deficits and additional clinical features. Neurological diseases tend to have a characteristic lesion distribution in the neuraxis (Table 16.1). For example, dementias mainly affect the cerebral cortex, while multiple sclerosis (MS) can affect any myelinated part of the CNS. This makes it possible to anticipate likely effects of particular diseases and also to surmise the possible site of neurological dysfunction from clinical findings.

Factors that are relevant to the nature of NLUTD include (Table 16.1):

1) Time of onset for the neurological disease (congenital or acquired): with congenital or perinatal lesions, LUT function has never been normal, and so these are particularly significant;

2) Potential for disease progression: many neurological diseases affect more of the nervous system over time, and MS is particularly known for this;

3) Region of the nervous system affected [2]; and

4) Complete or incomplete: incomplete lesions may preserve partial function.

The peripheral nerves and the lower spinal centres are often grouped under the term 'lower motor neurons', as damage to these structures causes loss of contractile function. Elsewhere, the neurological lesions are termed 'upper motor neuron lesions', where the consequences are

Table 16.1 Classification of neurological diseases according to key influences for neurogenic lower urinary tract dysfunction (NLUTD).

	Acquired, non-progressive	Acquired, progressive	Congenital
Suprapontine lesion	Brain tumour Cardiovascular accident	Parkinson's disease	Cerebral palsy
Suprasacral spinal cord/pontine lesion	Prolapsed intervertebral disc	Multiple sclerosis[a]	Spinal dysraphism
Sacral spinal cord lesion	Sacral spinal cord injury	Tethered cord	Spina bifida
Infrasacral (cauda equina and peripheral nerves lesion) lesion	Cauda equina syndrome	Diabetic neuropathy	

The International Continence Society classified NLUTD according to which part of the nervous system is affected [1]. 'Mixed Neuronal Lesion' is used to indicate where patients are affected by lesions of the neural pathway at different levels of the central nervous system concurrently [1].

[a] Potential mixed neuronal lesion picture (lesions of the neural pathway at different levels of the central nervous system concurrently). *Source:* Based on Gajewski et al. [1].

impaired co-ordination and reflex function. However, this is a considerable simplification, and anatomically inaccurate, so the ICS Standardisation working group considers categorisation into lower versus upper motor neuron lesions should no longer be supported [1].

Muscle Contraction in the Lower Urinary Tract

Nerves which are responsible for generation of LUT muscle contraction are located in the lower parts of the spinal cord:

1) Nerves controlling the detrusor are from the parasympathetic division of the autonomic nervous system. They are located in the sacral spinal cord at S2–S4 levels (the intermediolateral horn);
2) The sphincter complex is also controlled by nerves in S2–S4, but in the anterior horn (Onuf's nucleus); and
3) In the male genitourinary tract, the bladder neck is controlled by sympathetic nerves from the thoracolumbar spinal cord (the intermediolateral horn at T11-L2).

Complete loss of function of these parts of the spinal cord, or their associated peripheral nerves, leads to paralysis of the affected structures. This may be reflected in symptoms reported:

- *Straining.* An atonic acontractile bladder incapable of voiding, if the parasympathetic nerves are affected; this means the patient is likely to use abdominal straining for bladder emptying, provided they can contract the relevant muscles voluntarily.
- *Stress incontinence (urinary and/or faecal).* if Onuf's nucleus is affected, due to sphincter dysfunction.

Nerves from the sacral spinal cord also supply the muscles of ankle plantar flexion, so the affected person may have a 'flat' gait; asking a person to rise up on tiptoe one foot at a time is a quick and easy way to screen whether the sacral muscles have preserved control and strength. The skin afferents (dermatomes) of S2–S4 are centred around the anus, so evaluation of the skin sensation in this region is a crucial check.

Two main lesions cause loss of motor function in the LUT:

1) **Sacral spinal cord lesion (SSCL):** There is a loss of parasympathetic control of the detrusor and a somatic denervation of the external urethral sphincter (EUS). Sensory impairment is typically associated with a complete lesion. Some afferent pathways remain intact due to potential preservation of hypogastric afferents. Some patients may have SUI due to sphincter deficiency (loss of Onuf's nuclei).
2) **Infrasacral cauda equina and peripheral nerves lesion (CEPNL):** Acontractile detrusor and/or SUI may be present. Diabetic neuropathy is a lesion of this type in which DO can be seen in combination with the above.

For both these, the consequence will potentially include:

- Weakness of the sphincter (if either of the two Onuf's nuclei cannot function); this will lead to SUI due to intrinsic sphincter deficiency.
- Weakness of the bladder (if either of the parasympathetic [detrusor] nuclei cannot function); this will lead to DUA, and areflexia if extreme. The patient may be unable to void, or may rely on straining to do so.
- Impaired bladder compliance; it is not clear why this should be, but the observation is well-recognised for sacral lesions, notably in spina bifida (meningomyelocele). It does not seem to be the case for peripheral nerve lesions (i.e. nerve damage distal to the spinal cord).
- The anal sphincter may also be weak, leading to flatus leakage and faecal incontinence

- Loss of LUT (bladder and urethra) sensation.
- Loss of skin sensation in the saddle area, including the genitals, with obvious implications for reflex sexual function, such as inability to achieve orgasm.
- Bladder neck function in men may be preserved, provided the sympathetic nucleus (thoracolumbar spinal cord) can still communicate with the periphery.
- Damage to the cauda equina, which carries most of the sacral spinal cord nerve traffic, has similar effects, except that impaired bladder compliance is rare. Incomplete damage to peripheral nerves and the lower spinal centres can result in altered reflex activity and DO [3].

The issue of bladder compliance is not well understood, and there are of course compliance issues associated with bladder fibrosis. However, there is thought to be a neurological element from the sympathetic system T10-L2 which allows receptive relaxation. This is particularly important to understand in patients who have had a neurological injury to the lower spinal cord which may mean receptive relaxation cannot occur. Patients can have poor compliance which may not be recognised until a procedure is performed for stress incontinence. In this situation, the patient has been converted from having a safe wet bladder into a dangerous dry bladder because the pressure rises as the bladder fills.

Co-ordination of the Nerves that Make Muscles Contract

The relevant spinal centres are controlled by the brainstem so that the muscle groups behave synergistically for storage and voiding reflexes. It is the pontine micturition centre (PMC), regulated by higher brain centres, which underpins this co-ordinating function. During bladder filling, the LUT is held in storage mode (bladder neck and EUS are contracted, and the bladder is relaxed). Voiding is initiated by the PMC (bladder contraction with outlet relaxation) when instructed by higher brain centres. The PMC is also responsible for the rather different storage configuration of the male genitourinary tract during ejaculation (bladder and EUS relaxed, bladder neck contraction). Suprasacral spinal cord lesions generally leave the distal cord still functioning, but unregulated and uncoordinated.

Neurological disease may prevent the PMC from communicating with the spinal centres:

a) Most commonly, a lesion in the cervical or thoracic spinal cord interrupting the descending pathways.
b) A lesion in the pons itself is uncommon in practice (because the pons controls functions vital for life, particularly respiratory and cardiovascular functions).

Typically, there will be paraplegia or tetraplegia and loss of sensation, and the LUT urodynamic observations may be:

- DO and DOI, as the PMC is unable to inhibit the detrusor nucleus during the storage phase.
- Detrusor sphincter dyssynergia (DSD), a term that describes a detrusor contraction concurrent with an involuntary contraction of the urethral and/or periurethral striated muscle [1]. In severe NLUTD, this is a storage phase problem (i.e. DOI with a characteristic outlet resistance described below). However, in less severe NLUTD, a person may be able to initiate a detrusor voiding contraction, and experience the same sphincter activity, which can then appropriately be referred to as 'dyssynergic voiding'.
- Inability to initiate voiding, if the pathways that start the processes are fully non-functional.

DSD is not a general term for bladder outlet obstruction (BOO) in neurological disease. DSD explicitly refers to a neurological mechanism in the spine (or brainstem), leading to intermittent flow and a characteristic urodynamic appearance which distinguishes it from straining (Figure 16.1). The neurological features affecting

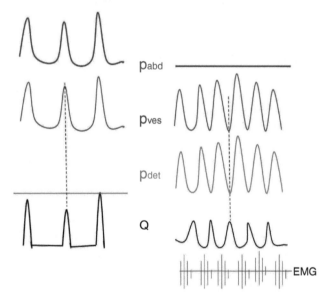

Figure 16.1 Schematic illustration to distinguish straining from detrusor sphincter dyssynergia (DSD). Left side shows straining, where p_{abd} is intermittently raised by a Valsalva manoeuvre, which raises p_{ves}, and this causes flow; hence, the peaks all line up. p_{det} is flat in a well-subtracted pressure-flow study (PFS). Right side shows DSD, which is an appearance that can be seen in filling cystometry or PFS. In DSD, it is p_{abd} that is flat. Since sphincter relaxations are what allows flow, the onset of flow is associated with a drop in p_{ves}/p_{det}, so flow peaks line up with pressure troughs. If an electromyography (EMG) is recorded from the pelvic floor, it would fall quiet during the urine flow.

movement and sensation are invariably very obvious, so absence of these precludes DSD as a likely factor for an individual patient. Figures 16.1 and 16.2 indicate how the characteristic patterns of the pressure and flow recordings are sufficient to make the diagnosis. However, needle-electrode electromyography (EMG) recording from the pelvic floor can reinforce the certainty of diagnosis.

In the ICS classification [1], this situation is classified as a **suprasacral spinal cord/pontine lesion** (SSL). Bladder

sensation may be somewhat preserved (incomplete lesions), but voluntary control of the micturition reflex arc is lost. Altered function of the sympathetic spinal centre in the thoracolumbar spinal cord may alter blood pressure control. Complete SSL above T6 may be associated with AD (see below) when there is residual sympathetic nucleus function; this should be included in the description of the lesion.

Such activity (DSD, DOI, and dysreflexia) is clear if the SSL is a complete spinal cord injury (SCI). In other

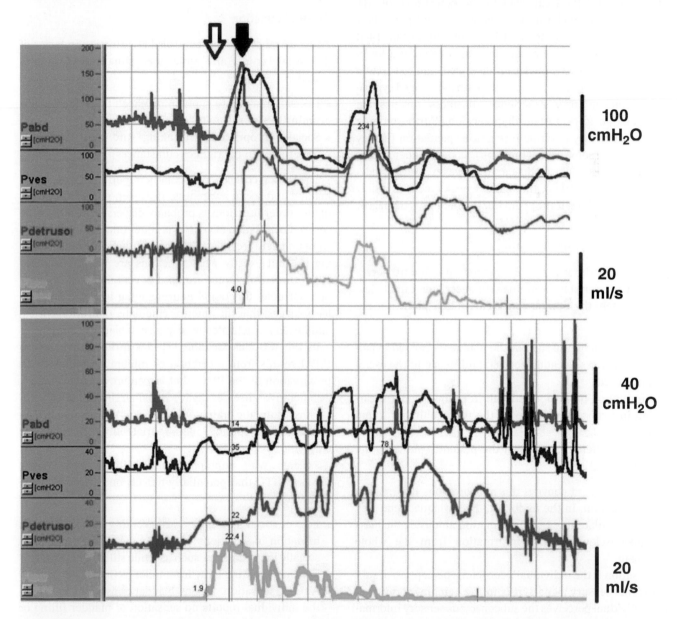

Figure 16.2 Pressure-flow study (PFS) traces from two men with neurological disease, showing intermittent flow patterns through different mechanisms. Flow is plotted in green and p_{det} in pink, unlike most traces in the book. Top PFS: straining. The open black arrow shows the raised abdominal and bladder pressure responsible for the flow. However, the p_{abd} line is soon almost fully expelled (closed black arrow), meaning that p_{abd} is not now recorded to subtract out p_{ves}. Consequently, p_{det} looks like there is detrusor activity, but this is misleading. Losing one of the recording catheters is quite common in neuropathic patients, since reduced sphincter tone is common. The alignment of peaks (orange line) is the key pointer towards underlying straining. Lower PFS: characteristic detrusor sphincter dyssynergia pattern, showing the alignment of flow peak with p_{ves}/p_{det} trough, and concurrently no activity in p_{abd} (orange line).

neurological conditions which can affect nerve transmission in the spinal cord, such as partial SCI or MS, the precise manifestation varies, but any of these elements can occur. In MS, DSD can arise [4], but it is rarely seen to have the severity present in complete SCI.

It is important to understand whether the SSL has left the sympathetic nucleus in the thoracolumbar spinal cord intact, as it is responsible for blood pressure control. Normally, the pons controls this very closely. An SSL above T6 spinal cord level can lead to the emergence of AD, which is an acute elevation of blood pressure potentially reaching life-threatening severity [5] due to an intact but unregulated sympathetic nucleus. For an SSL at a lower level, the sympathetic nucleus is damaged, and so vascular 'tone' is impaired. Hence, a patient with a damaged sympathetic nucleus may experience dizziness on position changes due to orthostatic hypotension. Furthermore, a male patient may describe retrograde ejaculation (if they have retained some sexual function), as the bladder neck is unable to close, described as a 'dry orgasm'. During videourodynamics (VUDS), the bladder neck (men) is visibly open during filling if the sympathetic nucleus is damaged.

Sensory Nerves and Sensation

LUT sensory information is carried in afferent nerves entering the vertebral column at the sacral and lumbar levels to reach the spinal cord. Three key pathways are present:

- Information on the state of the bladder is carried in pelvic nerves to the cauda equina, and hence to the sacral spinal cord.
- Information on noxious stimuli from the bladder is carried in hypogastric nerves to the thoracolumbar spinal cord.
- Urethral afferents travel via the pudendal nerve to the sacral spinal cord.

The spinal cord conveys this subconscious information to the midbrain. In the midbrain, the periaqueductal grey (PAG) assimilates the LUT information alongside the mass of subconscious sensory information from the whole organism.

Sensation is the individual's conscious perception of subconscious sensory signals; it is in the cerebral cortex that the individual perceives the subconscious sensory information to derive the sensations they attribute to the LUT. If the subconscious signal is not generated, interrupted in transit, or not processed centrally, then the person will not experience sensation related to the structure affected. Absent sensations may thus be a feature of central or peripheral neurological deficits. Absence of LUT sensation

may be described by patients using phrases like 'I never know how full my bladder is', or 'I have to listen to the sound of the urine in the toilet to know when I am passing urine'. A patient with a sacral spinal cord or cauda equina problem may use these phrases, and they may also report that they experience an uncomfortable or painful sensation when the bladder is very full (because the lumbar route for noxious sensory information is still intact).

Cerebral Function

The cerebral cortex also controls LUT function in terms of the social context and anticipated situations. Examples include:

- Decision-making (e.g. planning ahead to decide on best timing to visit the toilet);
- Social appropriateness (making sure that voiding is undertaken in the right circumstances).

The frontal cortex is particularly important for decision-making and social awareness. However, regulation of the higher-order functions is probably dispersed widely in the cortex. Localisation of centres is better understood with the comparatively recent availability of functional brain imaging [6], but exactly what functions are being visualised when these techniques are used is very complex to interpret. Of note, functional neuroimaging in normal volunteers suggest that the anterior cingulate, prefrontal cortex, and insula are activated in response to bladder filling [7].

In the ICS classification [1], a **suprapontine lesion** (SPL) results from a cerebral or midbrain problem with preservation of the PMC, that is, cerebrovascular disease, degenerative disease, hydrocephalus, intracranial neoplasms, traumatic brain injury, etc. This may lead to inability to initiate voiding, inappropriate timing of bladder emptying, DO, and DOI.

Patients with suprapontine conditions have rather diverse LUTD that potentially reflects one or more of the following:

- Loss of social appropriateness. Voiding dysregulation is urination in situations which are generally regarded as socially inappropriate, such as while still fully dressed, or in a public setting away from toilet facilities [1].
- Altered sensation. absent bladder sensation, in which the individual reports no sensation of bladder filling or desire to void [8] can occur, and some patients may report absent urethral sensation.
- Loss of decision-making. some people go into retention as they are unable to transmit the conscious decision to void from their prefrontal cortex to the PMC, meaning that the PMC stays in storage mode.

- Loss of top-down inhibition; normally, the brain suppresses PMC and spinal centres during urine storage. Suprapontine neurology can allow the emergence of neurogenic DO. At a more extreme level, it can lead to involuntary voiding defined as a symptom and a diagnosis of sporadic bladder emptying when awake, without intention to void [1]. Usually, the voiding reflex is preserved, and there is only lack of proper inhibition of the voiding reflex.

Understanding the Neurological Situations

Trauma, inflammation, or degeneration cause loss of nerve function. If there is damage affecting a motor nucleus, the associated muscle will be weakened, leading to paralysis if all the motor nerves are lost; damage to the nerve fibres running from the nucleus to the muscle will have the same effect. If there is damage to the sensory nerves, the organ or area will be numb (no sensation can be experienced if the sensory information from which it is derived is lacking). This will also mean a reflex which relies on the relevant sensory input cannot happen. When a structure whose role is co-ordinating a reflex becomes damaged, or the nerve fibres connecting it to the relevant parts of the spinal cord, the nuclei stop co-operating and their congruous action becomes inefficient and counterproductive. Finally, brain problems place a person at risk of complex issues affecting decision-making, social appropriateness, or conscious sensation.

The nature of changes seen for a given patient rapidly give a feel for where the key issues lie, and this is further clarified by noting deficits in other body functions (especially skin sensation in dermatomes, areas of muscle weakness, and altered reflexes), since it is rare for neurological processes to be super-selective for a specific organ system. Commonly, patients experience inexplicable fatigue (out of keeping with the amount of physical activity), headaches, and generalised aches. Where brain functions are affected, they may include:

- Cranial nerves issues. for example, double vision, blurred vision, and slurred speech. An altered voice may indicate impaired neural control of the larynx (which is predominantly controlled by the vagus nerve), which might be an issue in UDS, since the person affected may be unable to cough;
- Problems with the cerebellum. notably impaired co-ordination, stumbling, and clumsiness;
- Autonomic dysfunctions ('dysautonomia'). e.g. palpitations (altered cardiac function), unexplained sweating (altered sweat gland control), and blacking out when standing up quickly (loss of control of blood vessel tone);
- Muscle control. e.g. stiffness and tremor may indicate problems with muscle regulation; and
- Cognition. a range of functions including memory.

Many of these issues are poorly localised and may have developed slowly, so their implication may not have been properly appreciated. Neurological impairment in the spinal cord links more directly and obviously to localised loss of movement and skin sensation changes. Where lower limbs are affected, this can restrict ability to get to the bathroom, or transfer on to the toilet. There is also a risk of ulcers developing in an insensate area of skin. Where the trunk is affected, the affected person may struggle to maintain an upright posture, which is important for intermittent self-catheterising (ISC). Where the upper limbs are affected, impaired manual dexterity will affect ability to adjust clothing for toilet use and also hamper ability to do ISC.

Life-Threatening Issues in NLUTD

Renal Dysfunction

Some patients with NLUTD are at risk of renal damage for several potential reasons:

- A thick-walled bladder can make it hard for the ureters to pass urine fully into the bladder, leading to hydronephrosis and urinary stagnation in the renal collection system;
- Vesicoureteric reflux (VUR) is backwards flow of urine from the bladder to the kidney, indicating that the valve effect of the vesicoureteric junction has been lost. It means there is no protection of the upper urinary tract against bladder pressures, which is especially problematic where there is chronic bacterial colonisation;
- A poorly compliant bladder may allow the resting vesical pressure to exceed a safe value, making it impossible for the ureters to empty. The threshold at which this becomes relevant is probably $25\,cmH_2O$, and it is certainly unsafe at $40\,cmH_2O$;
- DSD and fixed sphincter obstruction may allow damaging high pressures to develop, whether or not there is VUR;
- Immobility causes leaching of calcium from the skeleton, leading to increased risk of kidney stones; and
- Kidney function is also at risk due to wider health aspects seen in neurological disease, such as chronic decubitus ulcers (pressure sores), and a tendency for people to stay dehydrated when they have LUTD.

A principal role of clinical assessment in these patients is therefore to identify those at such risk in order to take steps to prevent renal deterioration starting or progressing. Urinary tract ultrasound is a common evaluation in NLUTD (at initial presentation and during follow-up), as it can identify hydronephrosis, which indicates established VUR or ureteric obstruction. VUDS can pick up VUR at an earlier stage (Figure 8.17), when less invasive treatment may still be possible. VUDS is not useful for detecting ureteric obstruction, so if there is hydronephrosis without VUR, renogram assessment will be more appropriate.

Renal function blood tests are usual practice. However, serum creatinine is a by-product of muscle function. In patients with reduced muscle mass, which applies in many neurological diseases due to paralysis, the body is making less creatinine. Consequently, laboratory reference ranges will be misleading for people with neurological disease, since they are derived from the healthy population with normal muscle mass. This risks a false reassurance if someone with low muscle mass is seen to have a creatinine level within the laboratory reference range (but lying near the higher end of the range). In low weight patients, a normal serum creatinine may reflect decreased production rather than normal renal elimination, and that patient's estimated glomerular filtration rate (eGFR) will appear falsely high. A practical way to allow for this in low weight patients is to multiply the patient's eGFR by an adjustment factor of 0.69 [9]. The need to gain a true insight into an individual's renal function reflects the importance of acting early to minimise progressive renal deterioration and other significant issues such as calculating drug doses – notably aminoglycoside antibiotics.

Autonomic Dysreflexia

AD is a syndrome resulting from upper thoracic or cervical SCI above T6, elicited by a stimulus in the field of distribution of the autonomous sympathetic nucleus, characterised by unregulated sympathetic function below the lesion and compensatory autonomic responses [1]. It is a potential clinical emergency in people with an established SCI [5], where the injury level is T6 or higher. Key features are acute elevation of arterial blood pressure and bradycardia. An increase in systolic blood pressure from baseline of more than 30 mmHg is a practical threshold deciding whether a dysreflexic episode is in progress. Arterial blood pressure in people with SCI generally runs 20 mmHg lower than in healthy people, so this threshold can be crossed with a relatively low blood pressure in absolute terms. The episode may be asymptomatic (increase of blood pressure without any other symptoms), or cause a headache, but a severe attack is potentially a life-threatening emergency, as systolic blood pressure may reach as high as 300 mmHg, where there is a substantial risk of intracranial haemorrhage. The mechanism is driven by uncontrolled sympathetic nucleus activity, since normally the PMC will prevent such severe blood pressure elevation. It is triggered by a stimulus below the injury level, causing the sympathetic nucleus to drive a powerful vasoconstriction. Constriction of the gut blood vessels rapidly and substantially increases the effective circulating volume, underpinning the blood pressure increase. A visible feature is that the patient's skin goes pale below the injury level. As the blood pressure rises, some compensatory mechanisms respond, including bradycardia (since the heart rate is regulated by the vagus nerve, so still functional). There is also vasodilation of the skin above the level of the injury. The risk of severe AD is greater if the SCI is complete and at a higher level in the spinal cord.

Prevention is crucial, so far as possible. AD is triggered by a stimulus below the injury level, and catheterisation for UDS is an important potential cause – for which reason, catheter placement should be done carefully and with local anaesthetic instillation (even though the patient will not experience discomfort if anaesthetic is omitted, due to their SCI). UDS investigations in these patients should be done with blood pressure measurement available, and it should be checked frequently (every five minutes). If the patient starts to complain of a headache, the test may have to be stopped, the bladder emptied, the catheter removed, and the measures described below will need to be started. For everyday life, NLUTD is often managed with catheters (ISC or indwelling), so these people are at risk of a dangerous AD episode at home [10]. How to deal with risky situations, such as catheter blockages, must be planned for accordingly.

The initial management of an acute AD episode [11] is to place the person in the upright position, in the hope of an orthostatic reduction in blood pressure. Tight clothing should be loosened, to encourage blood pooling in dependent areas. This procedure allows further blood pooling in vessel beds below the level of injury and removes possible triggers for peripheral sensory stimulation. Frequent blood pressure checks must be maintained until the subject is stable. The precipitating stimulus must be eliminated; in the urodynamic setting, if bladder emptying and catheter removal does not sort out the problem, bowel impaction irritated by the abdominal line placement might have been a factor. An antihypertensive drug may be needed if systolic blood pressure remains above 150 mmHg. Different centres vary in the medication they use. Two options often used are:

1) Nifedipine 5–10 mg; the capsule is pierced with a pin and squeezed under the tongue, and the capsule is then swallowed. This will remain active after the cause has been treated and eliminated, so the patient may go hypotensive.
2) Glyceryl trinitrate (GTN) spray (400 µg), 1 or 2 sprays sublingually.

3) GTN transdermal patches (0.2 mg/h) applied to a non-hairy area of the vasodilated skin above the level of injury. This skin will feel warm, and if the skin is not pigmented, it will appear pink. Skin that is cold to the touch probably has reduced blood supply, so will not disperse the drug. GTN patches can be taken off once the AD is resolved. GTN must not be used if the patient has recently used a phosphodiesterase inhibitor (e.g. Viagra or Cialis).

It is crucially important that the urodynamicist anticipates the occurrence of AD and the urodynamic suite is prepared to handle such a life-threatening emergency, including immediate availability of a 'crash trolley' with the relevant medications, catheters, and support staff.

Latex Allergy

Latex is potentially associated with severe anaphylactic reactions, with spina bifida patients being at particular risk for this type of reaction [12]. A generalised latex hypersensitivity reaction can be precipitated in UDS, potentially progressing to bronchospasm. This may be presaged by sneezing or a cough a few minutes before the reaction [13]. Due to the severity of reaction that can be set off by even a tiny amount of latex, we maintain all our UDS suites latex-free. We also have protocols for prevention and treatment prominently displayed in the department.

Assessment of LUTS in Neurological Disease

NLUTD must be assessed in the overall context, especially in terms of personal loss of general function (e.g. reduced mobility, and hence difficulty reaching the toilet, or getting from a wheelchair on to the toilet seat), and the social and care support available. This then advises treatment options, ensuring that the facets of NLUTD are addressed directly and that adaptations are made to help with the wider situation as necessary.

History

All aspects of the patient need to be considered, including the neurological condition and non-urological factors.

1) LUTS
   a) What symptoms are present and how much bother are they causing?
   b) If the patient is able to void, can they do so when they wish, or is it only when a sense of urgency has already developed? This would imply they are using DO as the means of bladder emptying; these people would be at risk of going into acute retention if their DO is suppressed with medications
   c) Urinary incontinence. categorised into SUI, UUI, MUI, voiding dysregulation, involuntary voiding, impaired mobility urinary incontinence, impaired cognition urinary incontinence, enuresis, and situational incontinence (e.g. sexual activity urinary incontinence, giggle incontinence, incontinence associated with epileptic seizures)
   d) Urinary tract infections (UTIs). Patients with neurological disease may not experience the typical symptoms of dysuria/loin pain, due to impaired sensory nerve function
   e) Current and previous bladder management methods, including medications and catheterisation (indwelling, ISC or intermittent catheterisation [IC] by a relative or carer)
   f) Risk factors for LUTS in the healthy population, e.g. obstetric history in women, prostate enlargement in men.

2) Neurological features
   a) Classification
      i) Time of onset (congenital or acquired)
      ii) Potential for progression
      iii) Region of the nervous system affected
      iv) Complete or incomplete lesion
   b) Motor skills; mobility, transferring, muscle spasms, contractures, hand function, and balance
   c) Cognitive function
   d) Autonomic features, such as blood pressure problems. Whether dysreflexia occurs, and what provokes it.

3) Function of other pelvic organs
   a) Bowel function. frequency, urgency, faecal incontinence, constipation, loss of rectal sensation, need to strain, and loss of control over flatus
   b) Sexual function. whether they are sexually active, or wish to be, whether they have had or wish to have (more) children, whether genital sensation is preserved.
      i) Men – erectile dysfunction, loss of ejaculation/premature ejaculation, dry orgasm, loss of orgasm
      ii) Women – loss of arousal and lubrication, loss of sensation and orgasm, incontinence, dyspareunia.

4) General medical and social history
   a) Medical conditions and surgical history
   b) Current medication
   c) Allergies
   d) Home situation and carer(s)
   e) Employment.

Examination

This focuses on establishing whether there are any risk factors or limitations for management options:

1) The neurological level has generally already been mapped by the neurology team, but not always. In the urodynamic unit, it is worth confirming findings on sacral examination. S1 motor can be checked through the strength of plantar flexion (Figure 16.3). Sacral sensation can be checked via the dermatomes (back of thigh and perianal). The anocutaneous reflex is the reflexive contraction of the external anal sphincter upon tactile stimulation of the perianal skin. The bulbocavernosus reflex is an anal sphincter contraction in response to squeezing the glans penis or clitoris. Both reflexes confirm integrity of the sacral spinal cord (S2–S4) in someone who cannot voluntarily contract their anal sphincter.

2) Dexterity, mobility, contractures, transfer skills, and balance. Problems with any of these may make either toilet use or IC very difficult. Some of these problems can be addressed; for example, wrist drop in a partial

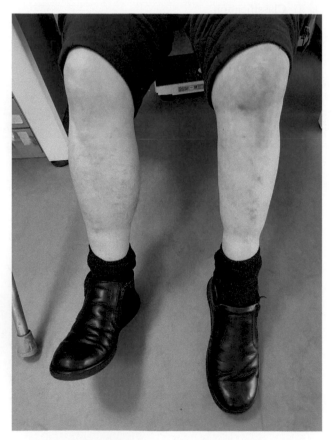

Figure 16.3 Asymmetry of the leg muscles due to neurological deficit in the sacral spinal cord principally affecting the left leg. He had weak plantar flexion and a foot drop on that side. *Source:* Marcus Drake.

tetraplegic may be splinted sufficiently to restore some usable hand function.

3) Urological assessment
   a) Distended bladder
   b) Loss of saddle area sensation may increase the risk of ulceration in incontinent patients and may make the area slow to heal after an incision. For this reason, insensate perineum is a contraindication for a perineal incision to place an artificial urinary sphincter (AUS), as device exposure and hence infection is an increased risk.
   c) External genitalia. skin problems due to urinary or faecal incontinence and any pressure sores.
   d) Pelvic examination

      i) Pelvic floor support. chronic straining in someone with reduced muscle function can lead to pelvic organ prolapse (POP) (especially where upper torso/limbs are strong)
      ii) Pelvic tone. resting and voluntary
      iii) Incontinence. urinary/faecal
      iv) Anal sensation, anal tone and voluntary squeeze, rectal contents, prostate. Bulbocavernosus and anal reflexes.

Initial Investigations

Dipstick urinalysis, midstream urine (MSU), or catheter specimen of urine (CSU) samples are commonly used. They are needed, since altered sensory function may make UTI symptom descriptions unclear (patients may report smell or feeling run-down, but typical dysuria may be absent). However, interpretation must consider that inflammation and bacteriuria might reflect use of ISC or chronic colonisation rather than acute infection.

Serum creatinine and eGFR are suitable without adjustment in people with normal body weight and muscle mass. In underweight patients, multiply the patient's eGFR by an adjustment factor of 0.69 [9]. If this suggests renal dysfunction, formal 24-hour creatinine clearance or renography (99 m DTPA clearance) may be required for an accurate assessment in some cases.

A baseline urinary tract ultrasound is needed to assess for hydronephrosis, scarring and stones, and chronic post-void residual (PVR). Renography may be required in selected patients to assess renal scarring, split function, and renal drainage.

The decision to perform UDS is driven by two major considerations:

1) Assessing the risk of upper tract damage developing in the future

2) Management of LUTS refractory to conservative and medical therapy in a person healthy enough to consider interventional therapy.

Some patients have a high risk of renal damage, e.g. SCI [14] or spina bifida, and so VUDS is generally used in initial assessment – regardless of the nature or severity of the patient's symptoms. Potentially, it is needed during ongoing surveillance in these groups, for example, if LUT or renal function changes, or hydronephrosis develops. In the neurological patient, symptoms may be altered or absent even though marked vesico-urethral dysfunction exists. For example, in SCI or meningomyelocele, there can be changes in bladder behaviour that threaten kidney function even though the patient notices little in the way of LUTS.

Other conditions, notably MS, are associated with a comparatively low risk of renal complications. VUDS is therefore not a routine requirement at initial assessment [15], and its use will be more focussed on LUTS treatment selection. Here, the target is to ensure continent bladder storage, and 'balanced bladder emptying' – the latter defined by the ICS as bladder emptying with physiological detrusor pressure and low residual as perceived by the investigator (and should be defined in the UDS report) [1]. It is important in these patients to confirm that:

- There is a treatment available that has a realistic chance of helping;
- That the patient would genuinely consider undergoing the treatment, having discussed clearly the potential benefits and risks;
- That the patient's overall medical condition does not place them at undue risk. For example, respiratory function is often impaired in neurological disease, with implications for anaesthetic choice;
- That disease progression is not anticipated to be rapid, i.e. making information gained now out-of-date in the near future.

Unless all these points apply, VUDS has only a marginal role in LUTS management and might actually bring nuisance and some risk greater than any benefit.

Urodynamic Observations

Neurogenic Detrusor Overactivity

Neurogenic detrusor overactivity (NDO) is a urodynamic observation characterised by involuntary detrusor contractions during the filling phase which may be spontaneous or provoked, in the setting of a clinically relevant neurologic disease [1]. There are no real differences in urodynamic appearances between NDO and idiopathic DO, as described in previous chapters.

NDO is subcategorised by the ICS [1]:

- Phasic DO is defined by a characteristic wave form and may or may not lead to urinary incontinence.
- Terminal DO is defined as involuntary detrusor contraction occurring near or at the maximum cystometric capacity, which cannot be suppressed, and results in incontinence or even reflex bladder emptying (reflex voiding).
- Sustained DO is defined as a continuous detrusor contraction without returning to the detrusor resting pressure.
- Compound DO is defined as a phasic detrusor contraction with a subsequent increase in detrusor and base pressure with each subsequent contraction.
- High-pressure DO is defined as a phasic, terminal, sustained, or compound high maximal DO with the high detrusor pressure perceived by investigator to be potentially detrimental to the patient's renal function and/or health and the value should be defined in the report.
- Neurogenic DO incontinence is incontinence due to involuntary NDO.

Phasic DO is not always accompanied by any sensation, or may be interpreted as a filling sensation, or normal desire to void. In neurogenic LUTD, it may elicit AD or abnormal bladder sensation. Terminal DO is generally associated with reduced bladder sensation. It can occur, for example, in an elderly stroke patient when urgency may be felt very shortly before the need for voiding. In complete SCI patients, there may be no sensation whatsoever. Hence, incontinence can occur with or without any sensation of urgency or awareness. Detrusor Overactivity Leak Point Pressure is defined as the lowest detrusor pressure rise with DO at which urine leakage first occurs in the absence of voluntary detrusor contraction or increased abdominal pressure (Figure 16.4).

Poor Compliance

Bladder compliance during filling cystometry describes the relationship between change in bladder volume and change in detrusor pressure [1]. It is calculated by dividing the volume change (ΔV) by the change in detrusor pressure (Δp_{det}) during that change in bladder volume ($C = \Delta V / \Delta p_{det}$). It is expressed in ml/cmH$_2$O (Figure 16.5).

The ICS recommends that three standard points are used for compliance calculations, with pressure and volume taken in the absence of any detrusor contraction.

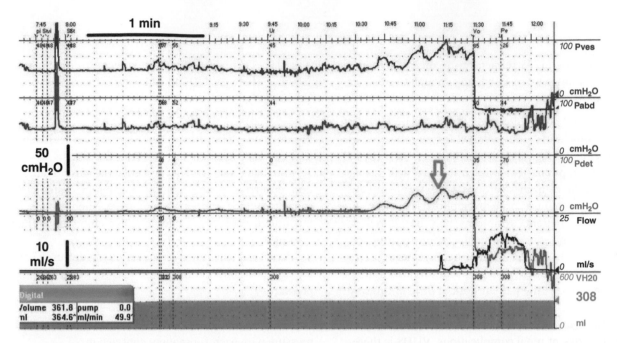

Figure 16.4 Filling cystometry showing neurogenic detrusor overactivity (DO) in a man with lumbar spinal cord injury. The orange arrow indicates the DO leak point pressure (approx. 35 cmH$_2$O in this case). The sudden drop in p$_{ves}$ and p$_{det}$ shortly afterwards is because the vesical catheter was expelled.

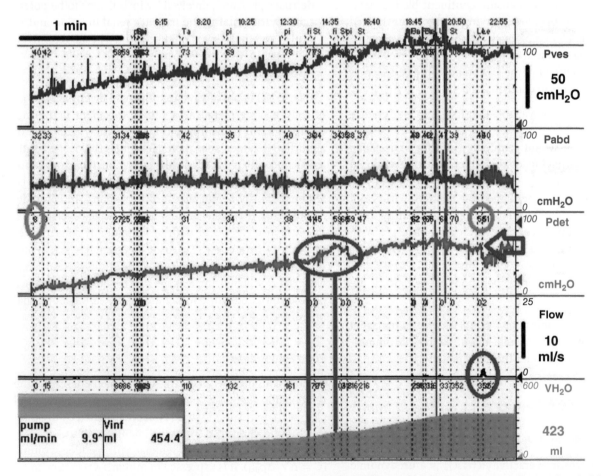

Figure 16.5 Filling cystometry in a man with sacral spinal cord injury, filling at 10 ml/min. Pressure at start and end of filling is indicated by orange circles; the pressure change was 61−8 = 53 cmH$_2$O. Volume change was 0−423 ml, so compliance was 423/53 = 7.98 ml/cmH$_2$O, which is best rounded up to 8. The red circle indicates a leak, which determines the detrusor leak point volume (423 ml) and detrusor leak point pressure (red arrow; 61 cmH$_2$O). The purple oval indicates a p$_{det}$ change which superficially resembles detrusor overactivity but actually illustrates the hugely important influence of filling rate. The pressure change was actually a consequence of a transient increase in filling rate to 20 ml/min, as indicated by the purple lines, the pressure dropping back down when filling was stopped. No vesicoureteric reflux was seen (not shown). This is an old study; nowadays, p$_{ves}$ would not be plotted as the uppermost trace. *Source*: Based on Ukkonen et al. [4].

1) The detrusor pressure at the start of bladder filling and the corresponding bladder volume (usually zero);

2) The detrusor pressure at the bladder volume when the bladder pressure rises significantly and decreased compliance commences, i.e. p_{det} at the 'low compliance starting volume' (Figure 7.36); and

3) The detrusor pressure (and corresponding bladder volume) at cystometric capacity or immediately before the start of any detrusor contraction that causes significant leakage (and therefore causes the bladder volume to decrease, affecting compliance calculation).

Urodynamicists could legitimately use additional points if there is any time at which both pressure and volume are clear and the detrusor is stable. Poor compliance leads to a detrusor pressure which climbs during slow bladder filling (10 ml/min) and stays static (or declines only slightly) when the pump is stopped. This rate is thus suitable as the standard filling rate for VUDS in NLUTD; the rate can slowly be accelerated if the detrusor line stays flat, but it should be brought back down to 10 ml/min if the line starts to climb. If filling is undertaken at a faster rate, stopping the pump might mean the detrusor line declines (towards the pressure it would have been at if 10 ml/min had been used), and this would be regarded as an artefactual rise in p_{ves}. This might be confused with DO, but the linkage of the pressure trace to the pump activity is the giveaway (Figure 16.5).

A complete description of the situation also includes assessment of three additional parameters:

- Detrusor Leak Point Pressure (DLPP) is defined as the lowest detrusor pressure at which urine leakage occurs in the absence of either a detrusor contraction or increased abdominal pressure (Figure 16.5) [4];
- Detrusor Leak Point Volume is defined as a bladder volume at which first urine leakage occurs, either with DO or poor compliance [1]; and
- VUR: If severe VUR occurs, it means that the vesical line is actually measuring entire urinary tract pressure, not simply bladder pressure. In this situation, it is almost impossible to decide if the bladder is compliant. Hence, the wider clinical picture needs to be considered, such as the nature of the neurological problem, and identification of a thick-walled bladder on imaging. In those circumstances, the risk to renal function is potentially very high, and active treatment measures should be planned.

It is vital to appreciate the implications of impaired filling compliance in the context of everyday life for the affected person. A short period with a high detrusor pressure (as in the duration of a VUDS test) is not a particular issue, but it is widely accepted that significant amounts of time spent with a detrusor pressure above $40\,cmH_2O$ is a threshold for unacceptable risk to renal function. Indeed, a safer threshold of $25\,cmH_2O$ may be more appropriate in NLUTD. This leads to some extremely important implications for management decisions. If the detrusor pressure clearly exceeds the safe threshold at a certain bladder volume, therapy has to prioritise measures to prevent this happening:

- An indwelling catheter on free drainage, to prevent bladder filling;
- Increased frequency of ISC, to reduce the chance of reaching the critical volume (for most patients, this is not going to be a reliable approach [16]);
- Improving compliance, using augmentation cystoplasty or other reconstruction of the LUT using bowel (Figure 16.6). Some investigators have used botulinum-A injections, but these have to be repeated often, and improved pressures should be confirmed by VUDS six weeks after the injections. It is far from established that botulinum-A is safe and effective in this context [17];
- Preventing the bladder pressure exceeding the threshold pressure. The aim of sphincterotomy is to assist bladder emptying using reflex micturition or abdominal straining into a penile sheath appliance, thus protecting the

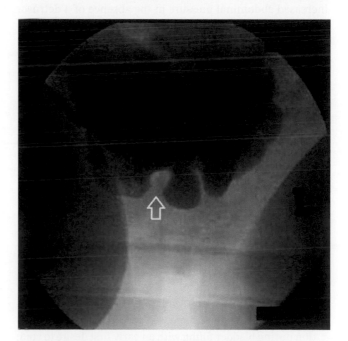

Figure 16.6 Image during video urodynamics of a reconstructed lower urinary tract. Caecum has been used to fashion a bladder reservoir, as indicated by yellow arrow pointing at deep infolds (which anatomically are separating the colonic 'haustra'). The fact that these are present at the base of the bladder indicates this reservoir is not connected to the urethra, i.e. must be drained by intermittent self-catheterisation via a non-urethral channel (Mitrofanoff). *Source*: Marcus Drake.

upper urinary tract. Endoscopic sphincterotomy has been the technique of choice for patients who cannot or do not want to do IC. However, it is invasive, irreversible, and the patient has no adaptation period [18]. Hence, sphincterotomy is very rarely used in current practice, and only in male patients;

- Avoiding measures to increase outlet resistance. These potentially increase the DLPP, and hence increase the chance of bladder pressure staying above the danger threshold for longer. This applies to procedures like autologous sling or AUS placement, so they must only be done in conjunction with other measures in NLUTD with impaired compliance.

Incontinence

As described in Chapter 7, UDS aims to reproduce symptoms, linking them to provocations in such a way that they reflect trigger mechanisms of leakage in everyday life. For NLUTD, urodynamic stress incontinence (USI), DOI, and involuntary voiding can be observed in UDS. USI can be identified with physical activity and a series of Valsalva manoeuvres. This enables some quantification of severity using the Abdominal Leak Point Pressure, defined as the intravesical pressure at which urine leakage occurs due to increased abdominal pressure in the absence of a detrusor contraction [1].

Dysregulated voiding and enuresis cannot be identified in UDS, since the conditions in which they occur do not apply in conventional UDS testing. This is a limitation which must be stated clearly in the UDS report. Sometimes, it is tempting to assume that an observation in UDS must explain everyday symptoms, but this can be unreliable, and the consequences of proceeding if the link was actually mistaken might be serious.

Sensations During Filling and Cystometric Capacity

Regarding sensation in UDS, the ICS NLUTD standardisation identifies situations applicable in this patient group:

- *Absent Bladder Sensation.* The patient reports no bladder sensation during filling cystometry
- *Bladder oversensitivity.* Increased perceived bladder sensation during bladder filling with an early first desire to void; an early strong desire to void, which occurs at low bladder volume; a low maximum cystometric bladder capacity; and no abnormal increases in detrusor pressure
- *Abnormal sensations.* Awareness of sensation in the bladder, urethra, or pelvis, described with words like 'tingling', 'burning', or 'electric shock', in the setting of a clinically relevant neurologic disorder (e.g. incomplete spinal cord lesion)
- *Non-specific bladder awareness.* Perception of bladder filling as abdominal fullness, vegetative symptoms, spasticity, or other 'non-bladder awareness', in the setting of a clinically relevant neurologic disorder (e.g. incomplete spinal cord lesion)

In NLUTD, deciding whether cystometric capacity has been reached has to be decided pragmatically. In the absence of sensation, the cystometric capacity is the volume at which the clinician decides to terminate filling [1]. The reason(s) for terminating filling should be defined in the report, for example, high detrusor filling pressure, large infused volume, or pain. If there is uncontrollable voiding/bladder emptying, cystometric capacity is the volume at which this begins.

In the presence of severe sphincter incompetence, the cystometric capacity may be significantly increased by occlusion of the urethra. For male patients, a penile clamp can be used to do this (Figure 16.7). For a female patient, a Foley catheter balloon may be used. This then enables a check of functional capacity, bladder compliance at the higher volumes, VUR emerging at higher volumes, and terminal DO. Checking for these features is important if planning surgical therapy of USI to avoid doing an operation that subsequently exposes the patient to another NLUTD issue.

Bladder Outlet Obstruction

BOO in NLUTD has complex potential underlying mechanisms. Usually, it is due to the NLUTD, but an older man with an enlarged prostate might have benign prostatic obstruction (BPO) as the explanation. Considerable caution must be applied in deciding if BPO is the cause, backed up by VUDS imaging to pinpoint the prostatic hold-up during a voluntary void, and identification of normal function of the rest of the bladder outlet. Only with scrupulous attention to these points is it appropriate to label BOO as BPO, and hence consider prostatic surgery.

Formal diagnosis of BOO generally requires the patient to have the ability to initiate voiding voluntarily, meaning that PMC drives a bladder contraction co-ordinated with sphincter/outlet relaxation. The presence of high pressure and slow flow rate then points to an anatomical obstruction. Measuring detrusor pressure during DO is not appropriate for people with normal neurological control, as the natural reaction to DO is to resist leakage by voluntarily contracting the sphincter, leading to a functional obstruction which is purely behavioural and not significant for renal function. In contrast, NLUTD can give rise to difficulty initiating voiding voluntarily and/or relaxing the

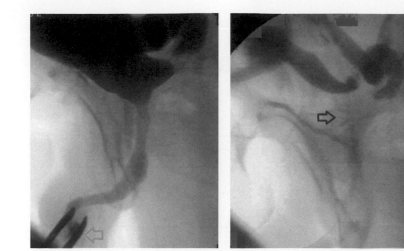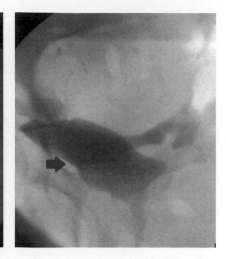

Figure 16.7 Video urodynamic study showing how a penile clamp (green arrow) can be used to control leakage and thereby increase the volume instilled, which may be essential for full understanding of how the urinary tract might behave if some form of outlet surgery was done later. At the end of the pressure-flow study (middle image), they had fully emptied the bladder (open blue arrow). Because this patient had severe vesicoureteric reflux, another X-ray taken soon afterwards showed contrast in the bladder (closed blue arrow, left image), i.e. a 'pseudo-residual' (Figure 8.32). *Source*: Marcus Drake.

sphincter. The need then is to identify whether there is a functional (muscular) obstruction which is driven by the neurological problem, and or an anatomical obstruction such as BPO. In that situation, DOI can be used to study the sphincter behaviour and indicates whether there is a significant functional obstruction in women or men.
The following patterns are recognised:

1) DSD: describes a detrusor contraction concurrent with an involuntary contraction of the urethral and/or periurethral striated muscle. Occasionally, flow may be prevented altogether. This produces an interrupted flow pattern, with intermittently high voiding pressure (during flow interruptions) (Figures 16.1, 16.2, and 16.8). DSD can be present in people with a suprasacral/pontine lesion. Indeed, since DSD reflects a problem of co-ordination of spinal centres by the PMC, the term DSD must only be applied to people with neurological disease of the spinal cord or brainstem. If a similar voiding pattern is seen in someone without such a lesion, the appropriate term is dysfunctional voiding.
2) Non-relaxing urethral sphincter (Figure 16.9) is characterised by a non-relaxing, obstructing urethral sphincter resulting in reduced urine flow. This is recognised in SSCLs, e.g. meningomyelocele. In non-relaxing urethral sphincter obstruction, the patient may strain to overcome the functional obstruction, which would increase p_{abd} accordingly. This is not generally seen in DSD.
3) Delayed relaxation of the urethral sphincter is characterised by impaired and hindered relaxation of the sphincter during voiding attempt resulting in delay of urine flow. This can happen in Parkinson's disease (PD).

Studying the visual configuration of the outlet in men can further help identify key aspects, bearing in mind the features described in Chapter 8 (Figures 8.18–8.21). In men, the bladder neck may be a cause of a functional obstruction, and this will be clear from VUDS imaging. If this is seen, it makes it very hard to assess the behaviour of the sphincter. Accordingly, bladder neck incision may achieve no beneficial effect, if it consequently emerges that the sphincter is now able to take over as the cause of functional obstruction. Furthermore, it may be that the sphincter on its own might be unable to resist DO, meaning that the man could become at risk of severe DOI.

DO can be elicited by progressive bladder filling. For some people, initiated reflex bladder emptying is used. This is an artificially elicited LUT reflex comprising various manoeuvres (exogenous stimuli) performed by the patient or the therapist, resulting in complete or incomplete bladder emptying [1]. Any patients using this technique to manage their bladder can be asked to do it during a VUDS test (Figure 16.10). VUDS is also used to back up the pressure and flow traces with imaging to identify the anatomical location of the functional hold-up.

Detrusor Underactivity

Neurogenic DUA is defined as a contraction of reduced strength and/or duration, resulting in prolonged bladder emptying and/or a failure to achieve complete bladder

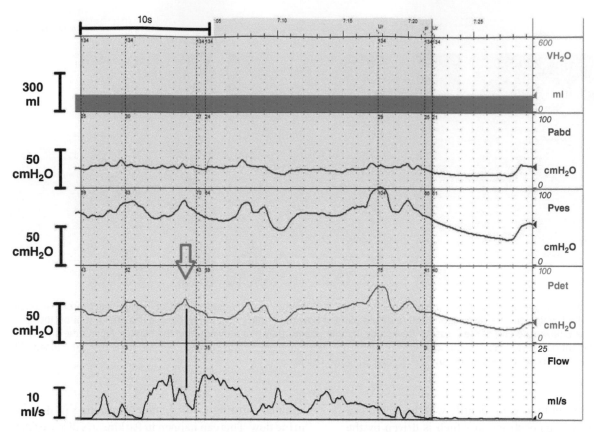

Figure 16.8 Filling cystometry showing detrusor sphincter dyssynergia during detrusor overactivity incontinence in a woman with a partial thoracic spinal cord injury. As illustrated in Figure 16.1, the key aspect is alignment of peaks and troughs in the p_{det} and flow traces respectively (orange arrow).

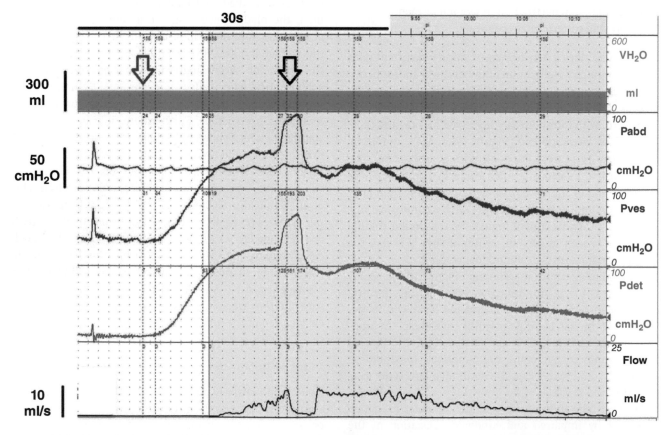

Figure 16.9 Non-relaxing urethral sphincter causing partial obstruction in a man during pressure-flow study (permission to void indicated by purple arrow). This is characterised by high pressure and slow flow. A flow interruption resulted from a non-voluntary increased sphincter contraction (black arrow).

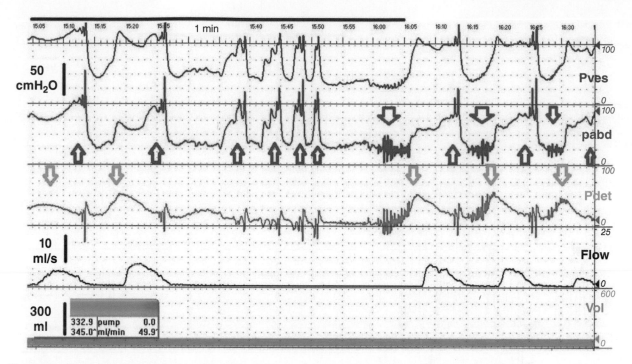

Figure 16.10 Suprapubic 'tapping', i.e. sharp percussive thumps (purple arrows) delivered to the lower abdomen to trigger detrusor overactivity incontinence (green arrows). Each purple arrow indicates three or four such thumps, which caused more marked artefact in the p_{abd} line than the p_{ves} line. This man used 'tapping' to conclude his bladder emptying. Red arrows indicate straining, which he used at the end of each detrusor overactivity (DO) wave to try and perpetuate the flow. He also did four strong strains in the middle, which he had thought might trigger DO, but since they did not, he used tapping thereafter.

emptying within a normal time span in the setting of a clinically relevant neurologic disorder [1]. Neurogenic acontractile detrusor is one that cannot be demonstrated to contract during urodynamic studies in the setting of a clinically relevant neurologic lesion (Figure 16.11). Contributory factors may include:

1) The impaired efferent innervation, so the muscle is weaker;
2) Impaired afferent innervation so that the spinal cord has only limited information about the bladder volume and urethral flow; and
3) Secondary changes resulting from the patient's overall health status.

Urodynamic Technique in the Neurogenic Patient

The International Consultation on Incontinence suggests that antibiotic prophylaxis should be considered for invasive urodynamic testing in NLUTD [18].

Whether to Empty the Bladder Before Filling

Generally, the bladder is emptied before a UDS test. This may be important to prevent causing a UTI in someone who may be at risk of chronic bacteriuria. It is also the most logical way of obtaining full information about the NLUTD, since many such patients use ISC. However, for some patients, ISC is not possible, and in these patients, it may be more appropriate not to empty the bladder for the test, so as to gain insight into likely function in real life for that person. Here, it may be better to fill slowly on top of the residual. The decision is individualised, and having a subjective aspect to the decision means there is currently no consensus on standard practice. It is also important to remember that contrast is used during VUDS, and if it mixes with a large volume of residual urine, then it may get diluted so that image quality may be poor. Therefore, it may be best to partially empty the bladder in those who do not routinely empty their bladders in real life.

Filling Rate

For reasons that are poorly understood, the neurogenic bladder is particularly sensitive to the speed at which it is filled. Hence, fast filling tends to produce artefactual poor compliance. A flexible approach needs to be taken. From the patient's frequency-volume chart and knowledge of the patient's residual urine (usually from ultrasound estimates), a policy for that patient can be defined. Generally, filling should start at 10 ml/min [18]. Medium fill rates (20–30 ml/min) can be used in patients who are known to

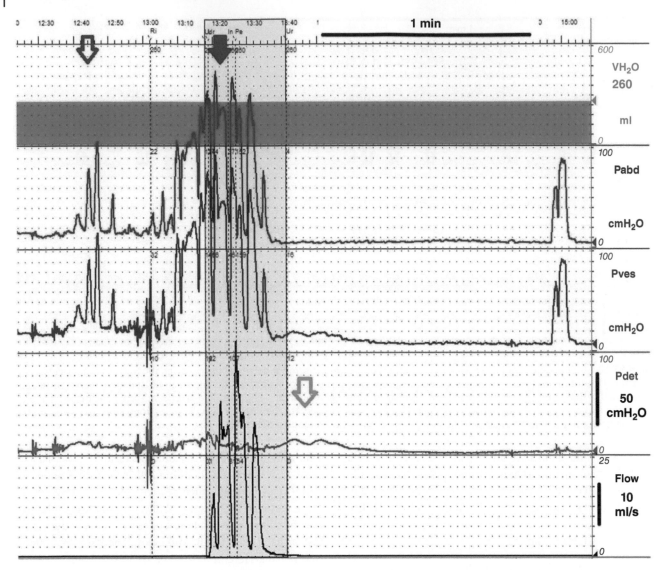

Figure 16.11 Underactive/acontractile detrusor seen during pressure-flow study in a 53-year-old woman with multiple sclerosis. She did some abdominal straining, reaching 100 cmH$_2$O (open red arrow), but this did not lead to emptying. She then went on to do some high-amplitude strains (closed red arrow), which did lead to emptying. Soon after, there was some detrusor activity (green arrow), but this did not cause emptying. The high amplitude of straining she needed to use is physically exhausting in someone with neurological disease (and consequent muscle weakness), and damaging to the pelvic floor (which does not have the muscle tone to resist the force); she may be suitable for considering intermittent self-catheterisation.

have a normal or high functional bladder capacity where compliance is seen to be normal in the early phases of a test [5]. However, if detrusor pressure then begins to rise, filling should be stopped until the pressure has settled, and then restarted at 10 ml/min. In the neuropathic child, the filling rate should be slower, typically 2–5 ml/min.

Patient Position

Many neuropathic patients will not be able to stand, and often they will be unable to sit, either to be filled or to void. Fortunately, for UDS testing, in neurological disease, blad-

der behaviour is less dependent on patient position. So, if the patient has to lie down throughout filling and voiding, this is acceptable for obtaining appropriate information. With the patient lying down, the voiding phase presents problems. In male patients, urine can be voided so that it flows down a collecting gutter or pipe to reach the flowmeter. This means there will be a delay before the flow is eventually registered by the flowmeter, so this has to be compensated for if trying to match the flow pattern to the pressure traces (Figure 16.12). Special problems exist in the neurogenic patient, such as muscle spasms and contractures, which produce particular difficulties during VUDS.

Leg spasms in spinal injury patients may make it difficult to pass the catheters, but usually spasms settle during the investigations. A significant tremor can cause problems in catheterising and observing the pressures (Figure 16.13).

Which Tests to Do?

Symptom scores, voiding diary, urinalysis, and diagnostic imaging are fundamental evaluations. Urodynamic techniques evaluate multiple functional parameters in NLUTD, aiming to define bladder and outlet function during bladder filling and emptying. The core dataset for SCI (and largely applicable in other forms of NLUTD) comprises [19]:

- Bladder sensation during filling cystometry;
- Detrusor function and compliance during filling cystometry;
- Sphincter function during bladder filling;
- Detrusor/sphincter function during voiding;

- DLPP in patients with impaired detrusor compliance; and
- Cystometric bladder capacity and PVR.

VUDS offers suitable testing to identify these parameters in most patients, since it offers visualisation of bladder and outlet, including pelvic floor support, to provide anatomical and functional information during filling and voiding (see Chapter 8). Such testing is informative regarding risk factors for upper urinary tract problems, mechanism(s) of incontinence, and mechanism(s) of voiding dysfunction [18]. VUDS are the investigation of choice in view of the higher incidence of anatomical abnormalities, such as VUR and prostatic duct reflux. VUDS also make it easier to study any abnormalities of co-ordination between the detrusor and the urethra, for example, DSD. As VUDS are required, if the patient needs to be investigated in the supine position, the couch has to be suitable for X-ray investigation.

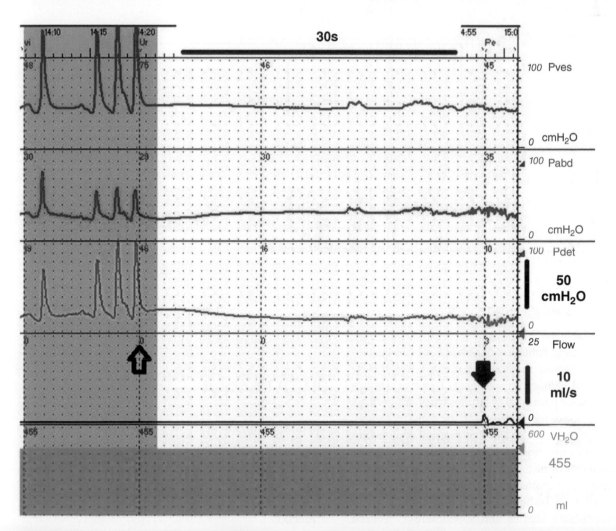

Figure 16.12 Considerable delay between the cough which provoked urodynamic stress incontinence and the recording of the leak by the flowmeter. Confirmation that the two events were linked required videourodynamic screening.

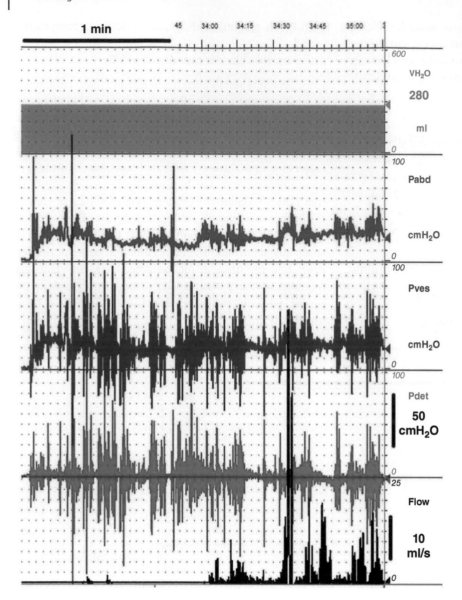

Figure 16.13 Filling cystometry in a male patient with Parkinson's disease showing the effect of a severe tremor. This caused severe oscillations, especially in the p_{ves} recording, and even sufficient to generate artefact in the flowmeter trace.

Supplementary Tests of Muscle and Nerve Function

EMG of the urethral sphincter or pelvic floor can be considered as a diagnostic method in patients with NLUTD and neurological urinary incontinence. However, surface electrodes produce poor-quality studies (they are perhaps most suitably used for biofeedback in some patients). Concentric needle-electrode EMG of external anal or urethral sphincter is the more sensitive technique for detecting abnormalities of sacral root innervation. Changes of reinnervation are characteristic of cauda equina syndrome and can occasionally be helpful in confirming this.

Nerve conduction studies and somatosensory evoked potentials are neurophysiological techniques that can be useful in the further differentiation of the nerve deficits in cases of a suspected neurological cause for bladder dysfunction [18]. Sympathetic skin responses are also another potential consideration [18].

NLUTD Treatment

Goals of therapy are to:

- Preserve or improve upper urinary tract function;
- Enable storage with low intravesical pressure and normal compliance;
- Facilitate continence and social acceptance of LUT function;
- Enable voiding to completion at low intravesical pressure;

- Minimise occurrence and severity of UTIs; and
- Control symptoms.

Summaries of general assessment and treatment were developed as algorithms for initial assessment and specialised care by the International Consultation on Incontinence (Figures 16.14 and 16.15).

When it comes to treatment, behavioural therapy is suitable, provided the person has motor control of the pelvic floor, and cognition or carer support to help with habit intake modification (Table 16.2). Medications employ the agents used for the neurologically intact population (Table 16.3). Bladder reflex triggering comprises various manoeuvres performed by the patient or the therapist to elicit reflex bladder emptying by exteroceptive stimuli (relating to, being, or activated by stimuli received from outside of the bladder) [1]. The most commonly used manoeuvres are suprapubic tapping (Figure 16.10), thigh scratching, and anal/rectal manipulation. Triggered bladder emptying can only be recommended for patients whose situation has proven to be urodynamically safe and stable, and who can manage reflex incontinence [18]. It can be considered for patients after procedures aimed at reducing outlet resistance, in order to improve spontaneous reflex voiding. Patients using this method must reliably be followed up. Bladder expression refers to various compression manoeuvres aimed at increasing intravesical pressure to facilitate bladder emptying. The most commonly used manoeuvres are abdominal straining (Valsalva manoeuvre) and exerting manual suprapubic pressure (Crede's manoeuvre [Figure 16.16]). As with reflex triggering, abdominal straining requires proof that the LUT is urodynamically safe. Contraindications to straining include VUR, POP, hernias, urethral pathology, and symptomatic UTIs. Crede's manoeuvre is now only rarely used. Sometimes, a Queen's Square bladder stimulator (Figure 16.17) can facilitate bladder emptying by vibrating the bladder dome suprapubically and thence increasing pressure – in some cases by triggering DO.

In general, clean IC is considered the appropriate means of achieving complete bladder emptying in most patients with NLUTD and impaired bladder emptying [1] (Table 16.4). IC in NLUTD is effective and safe for short and long-term use. Nevertheless, complications (notably UTI) are regularly seen and seem to be related to both the catheterisation itself and the pre-existing LUT condition. Urethral and bladder complications seem to accumulate with protracted use. Frequency of IC is recommended according to individualised assessment, ensuring non-traumatising technique, and suitable materials [1]. There are no guidelines or consensus on suitable intervals for

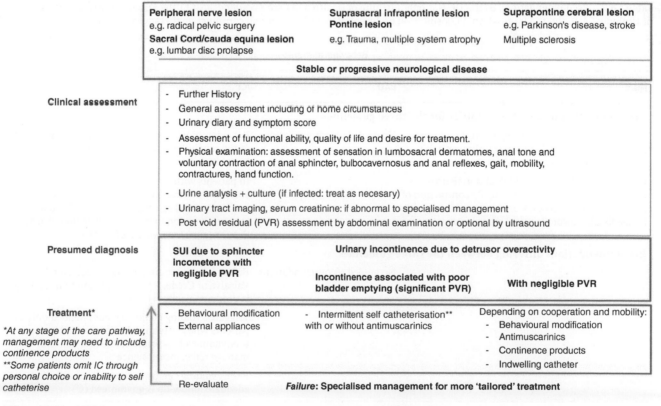

Figure 16.14 Initial assessment and therapy of neurogenic lower urinary tract dysfunction.

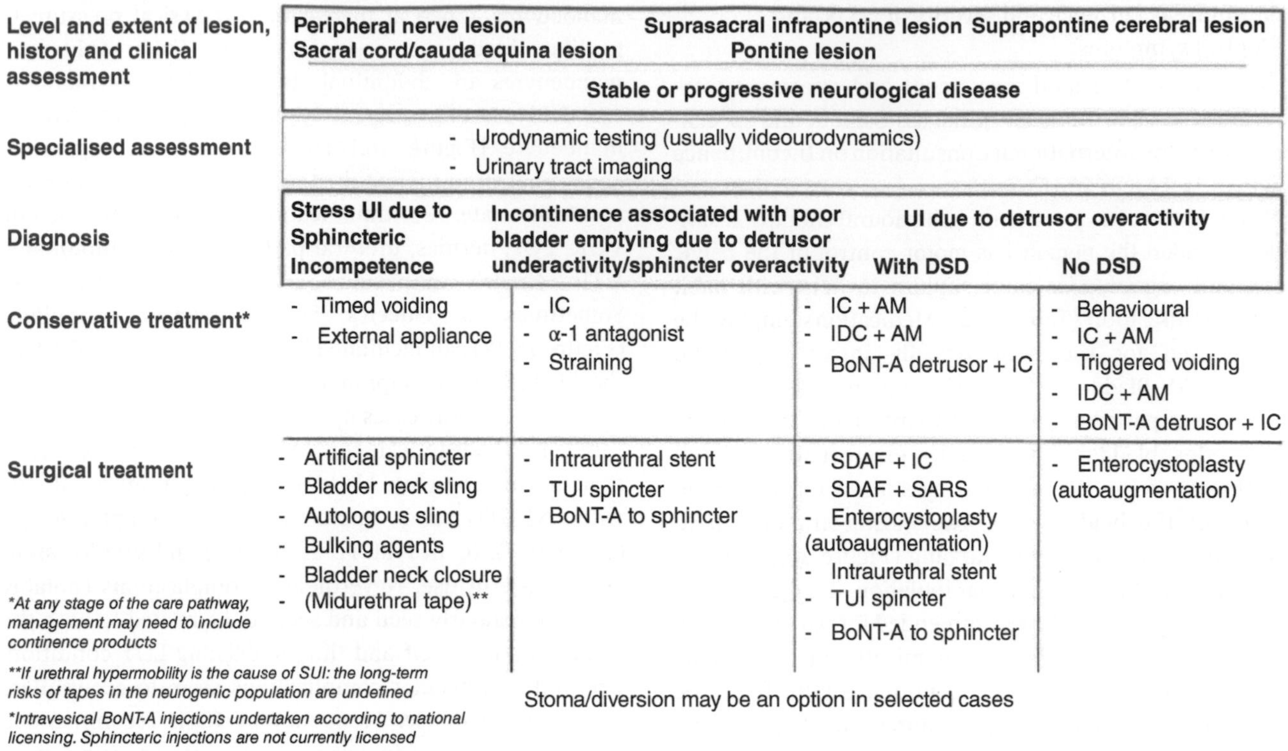

Level and extent of lesion, history and clinical assessment	Peripheral nerve lesion Sacral cord/cauda equina lesion	Suprasacral infrapontine lesion Pontine lesion	Suprapontine cerebral lesion	
	Stable or progressive neurological disease			
Specialised assessment	- Urodynamic testing (usually videourodynamics) - Urinary tract imaging			
Diagnosis	Stress UI due to Sphincteric Incompetence	Incontinence associated with poor bladder emptying due to detrusor underactivity/sphincter overactivity	UI due to detrusor overactivity	
			With DSD	No DSD
Conservative treatment*	- Timed voiding - External appliance	- IC - α-1 antagonist - Straining	- IC + AM - IDC + AM - BoNT-A detrusor + IC	- Behavioural - IC + AM - Triggered voiding - IDC + AM - BoNT-A detrusor + IC
Surgical treatment	- Artificial sphincter - Bladder neck sling - Autologous sling - Bulking agents - Bladder neck closure - (Midurethral tape)**	- Intraurethral stent - TUI spincter - BoNT-A to sphincter	- SDAF + IC - SDAF + SARS - Enterocystoplasty (autoaugmentation) - Intraurethral stent - TUI spincter - BoNT-A to sphincter	- Enterocystoplasty (autoaugmentation)

*At any stage of the care pathway, management may need to include continence products

**If urethral hypermobility is the cause of SUI: the long-term risks of tapes in the neurogenic population are undefined

*Intravesical BoNT-A injections undertaken according to national licensing. Sphincteric injections are not currently licensed

Stoma/diversion may be an option in selected cases

Figure 16.15 Specialised assessment and therapy of neurogenic lower urinary tract dysfunction. AM: antimuscarinics; BoNT-A: botulinum neurotoxin-A; DSD: detrusor sphincter dyssynergia; IC: intermittent catheterisation; IDC: indwelling catheter; PVR: post-void residual; SARS: sacral anterior root stimulator; SDAF: sacral deafferentation; TUI: transurethral incision.

Table 16.2 Recommendations by the UK National Institute of Health and Care Excellence (NICE), the European Association of Urology (EAU), and the International Consultation on Incontinence (ICI) regarding conservative therapy in NLUTD.

	Behavioural therapy	
NICE	**EAU**	**ICI**
Recommendations which are similar for the three guidelines		
Consider a behavioural management programme (e.g. timed voiding, bladder retraining, or habit retraining) for people with NLUTD	No graded recommendations	Behavioural techniques are a suitable component of the rehabilitation programme for each individual (C)
Consider PFMT in SCI and MS and in neurological conditions where voluntarily contraction of pelvic floor is preserved. Consider combining with biofeedback and/or electrical stimulation		In patients with incomplete denervation and some voluntary contraction of the pelvic floor muscle and the striated sphincter, electrical stimulation may be an option to improve pelvic floor function, thus improve incontinence (C/D)
Recommendations differing between the three guidelines		
	No graded recommendations	Before recommending bladder expression by Valsalva or Credé, it must be proven that the LUT is urodynamically safe (B)
		Triggered voiding could be recommended only for patients whose situation has proven to be urodynamically safe and stable and who can manage reflex incontinence
		Reflex voiding can be recommended only if an adequate follow-up is guaranteed (C)

PFMT: pelvic floor muscle training: SCI: spinal cord injuries: MS: multiple sclerosis; NULTD: neurogenic urinary lower tract dysfunction.
Source: Jaggi et al. [20].

Table 16.3 Recommendations by NICE, the EAU, and the ICI regarding medications for LUTD in neurological disease.

NICE	EAU	ICI
Oral pharmacotherapy		
Recommendations which are similar for the three guidelines		
	Use antimuscarinic therapy as the first-line medical treatment for NDO (A)	Antimuscarinic drugs should be recommended for the treatment of NDO (A)
	Prescribe α-blockers to decrease BOO resistance (A)	For decreasing BOO in NGB a-adrenergic antagonists may be used (B/C)
Recommendations differing between the three guidelines		
Offer antimuscarinics to people with spinal cord disease (e.g. MS or SCI) and symptoms of OAB	Maximise outcomes for NDO by considering a combination of antimuscarinic agents (B)	
Consider antimuscarinic drug treatment in people with conditions affecting the brain (for example, cerebral palsy, head injury, or stroke) and symptoms of OAB	Do not prescribe drug treatment in neurogenic SUI (A)	
Consider antimuscarinic drug treatment in people with urodynamic investigations showing impaired bladder storage	Do not prescribe parasympathomimetics for underactive detrusor (A)	
Do not offer alpha-blockers for bladder emptying problems caused by neurological disease		

SCI: spinal cord injuries: MS: multiple sclerosis; SUI: stress urinary incontinence; OAB: overactive bladder; NDO: neurogenic detrusor overactivity; NICE: National Institute of Health and Care Excellence; EAU: the European Association of Urology; ICI: International Consultation on Incontinence. *Source*: Jaggi et al. [20].

Table 16.4 Recommendations by NICE, the EAU, and the ICI regarding catheter use in neurological disease.

NICE	EAU	ICI
Catheterisation and appliances		
Recommendations which are similar for the three guidelines		
When discussing treatment options, tell the person that IDUC may be associated with higher risks of renal complications (such as kidney stones and scarring) than other forms of bladder management (such as intermittent self-catheterisation)	Use IC, whenever possible aseptic technique, as a standard treatment for patients who are unable to empty their bladder (A)	IC is first choice treatment for inability to empty the bladder adequately and safely in neurogenic voiding dysfunction (A)
	Avoid IDC and SPC whenever possible (A)	Long-term IDC should be the last resort and may be safe only if a careful check-up of urodynamic, renal function, and upper and lower tract imaging are performed (B)
Recommendations differing between the three guidelines		
In people for whom it is appropriate, a catheter valve may be used as an alternative to a drainage bag		Short-term IDC during the acute phase of neurological injury is a safe management for neurologic patients (B)
		Regular bladder emptying with low bladder pressures and low post-void residual should be confirmed with condom catheters and external appliances (B)

IDC: indwelling catheterisation: IDUC: indwelling urethral catheterisation: SPC: suprapubic catheterisation: IC: intermittent catheterisation; NICE: National Institute of Health and Care Excellence; EAU: the European Association of Urology; ICI: International Consultation on Incontinence. *Source*: Jaggi et al. [20].

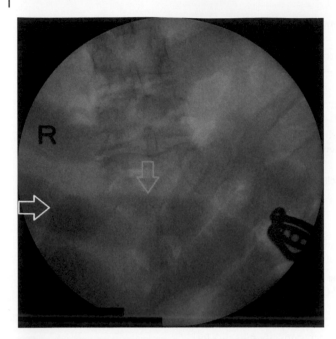

Figure 16.16 Manual suprapubic compression (Crede's manoeuvre) using both hands to push hard down onto the bladder and attempt to squeeze it empty; one finger of the right hand is indicated by the white arrow, and there is a ring on the ring finger of the left hand. The top of the bladder is indicated by the blue arrow. Since considerable force is needed to do this, Crede's manoeuvre is now rarely used. *Source*: Marcus Drake.

bladder emptying. They should ideally be derived from the voiding diary and other related factors (bladder volume, fluid intake, PVR urine volume, and urodynamic parame-

ters) [1]. The schedule needs to consider the cognitive situation, which could be affected by the neurological disease. Generally, IC is strongly favoured, but it must be recognised that the commitment involved for a patient who already has a considerable burden to deal with might hamper their willingness to comply with an intense IC schedule. This might explain why IC is not necessarily the best method for protecting renal function in SCI patients [2]. Indwelling catheters are often needed and can stabilise renal function which has shown deterioration when using other methods [2]. The catheter chosen should use the largest luminal diameter possible that does not traumatise or damage the urethra [1]. Note that the insensate LUT means that a catheter may be traumatically malpositioned without the patient realising (Figure 16.18), so increasing the potential damage. A silicone catheter tends to have a relatively larger luminal size for the calibre, which may help delay blockage. Frequency of change largely depends on time to blockage, which is influenced by catheter materials and lumen, patient factors, and infection. Suprapubic catheter is preferred to urethral catheter if long-term catheterisation is needed [1]. Penile sheath appliances facilitate urinary containment of incontinence in some male patients with NLUTD. Complications may be less if technique, state of the penile skin, hygiene, replacement, and maintenance of low bladder pressures are optimised [1].

The minimally invasive and surgical options are summarised in Tables 16.5 and 16.6. For patients with neurogenic USI, they include:

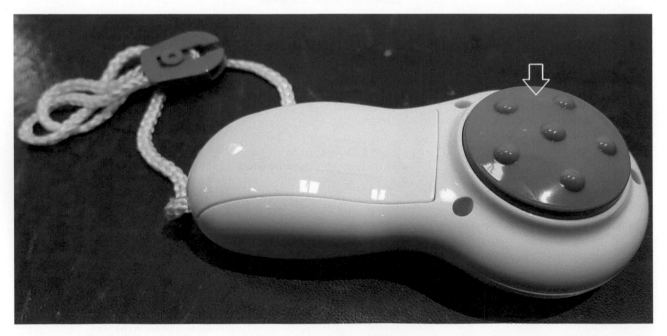

Figure 16.17 Queen's Square bladder stimulator. The vibratory surface (white arrow) is placed suprapubically to stimulate the bladder dome. *Source*: Marcus Drake.

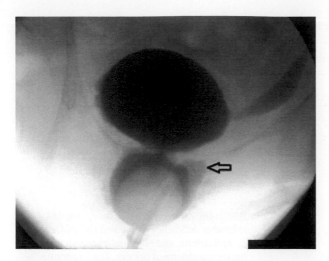

Figure 16.18 Malpositioned urethral catheter, with the balloon inflated in the prostatic urethra. This must have been a chronic problem, since the urethra has become a cavity, with part of the cavity accommodating the catheter tip (black arrow). This situation arises in people with markedly reduced lower urinary tract sensation. *Source*: Marcus Drake.

1) Autologous slings, with ISC/IC to facilitate voiding. The use of synthetic slings and tapes is not supported by an adequate evidence base, and safety concerns are considerable.
2) AUS can be used, with a high grade of recommendation [1]. AUS infection is a major problem which necessitates removal of the device and is more likely to occur in patients with NLUTD than in the general population. Some AUS patients undertake ISC for bladder emptying; this requires specific training and could represent a risk factor for AUS complications.
3) Bulking agents can be used when there is a demand for a minimally invasive treatment, but the patient should be aware that the technique has a low success rate.
4) Bladder neck closure should only be offered where alternative treatments have either failed or are likely to fail.

For neurogenic DO, the options include:

1) Onabotulinumtoxin-A injection into the detrusor muscle improves clinical and urodynamic parameters and

Table 16.5 Recommendations by NICE, the EAU, and the ICI regarding minimally invasive therapies.

	Minimally invasive procedures	
NICE	**EAU**	**ICI**
Recommendations which are similar for the three guidelines		
Offer bladder wall injection with BTX-A to patients with spinal cord disease (e.g. MS or SCI) and with symptoms of OAB and in whom antimuscarinic drugs have proved to be ineffective or poorly tolerated	Use BTX-A injection in the detrusor to reduce NDO in MS or SCI if antimuscarinic therapy is ineffective (A)	
Offer bladder wall injection with BTX-A to adults with spinal cord disease and with urodynamic investigations showing impaired bladder storage and in whom antimuscarinic drugs have proved to be ineffective or poorly tolerated		
Recommendations differing between the three guidelines		
	Alternative routes of administration (i.e. transdermal or intravesical) of antimuscarinic agents may be used (A)	BTX-A should be offered as a treatment option for incontinence associated with NDO (A)
		BTX-A may be considered for DSD in SCI patients (B)
		If pharmacotherapy fails to relax the overactive detrusor, electrical neuromodulation; SNM, anogenital stimulation, pudendal nerve stimulation, dorsal genital nerve stimulation, percutaneous tibial nerve stimulation, magnetic stimulation, and deep brain stimulation) may be optional in patients with neurogenic DO (C/D)

BTX-A: botulinum toxin A: SNM: sacral neuromodulation: SCI: spinal cord injuries: MS: multiple sclerosis; NDO: neurogenic detrusor overactivity; NICE: National Institute of Health and Care Excellence; EAU: the European Association of Urology; ICI: International Consultation on Incontinence. *Source*: Jaggi et al. [20].

Table 16.6 Recommendations by NICE, the EAU, and the ICI regarding surgical management of NLUTD.

Surgical procedures		
NICE	**EAU**	**ICI**
Recommendations which are similar for the three guidelines		
Consider autologous fascial sling surgery for people with SUI		Autologous stings can be used to neat SUI (B)
Do not routinely use synthetic tapes and stings in people with SUI because of the risk of urethral erosion		Artificial urinary sphincter can be used to treat SUI (A)
Consider surgery to insert an AUS for people with SUI only if an alternative procedure, such as insertion of an autologous fascial sling, is less likely to control incontinence		Due to the limited evidence base, possible sphincter deficiency, perceived risk of complications, and potential consequences on future management options, the Committee is unable to recommend routine use of synthetic slings and tapes to treat SUI in neurogenic patients (D)
Recommendations differing between the three guidelines		
Consider augmentation cystoplasty using an intestinal segment for people with non-progressive neurological disorders and complications of impaired bladder storage (e.g. hydronephrosis or incontinence)		Any segment of the gastrointestinal tract may be used for bladder augmentation, but the ileum seems to give the best results in terms of ease of use. Risk of complications and efficacy (B)
For people with neurogenic lower urinary tract dysfunction who have intractable, major problems with urinary tract management, such as incontinence or renal deterioration consider ileal conduit diversion	Place an autologous urethral sling in female patients with SUI who are able to self-catheterise. (B)	Synthetic tapes could be recommended in older women with stable neurological conditions and SUI due to urethral hypermobility (C)
	Insert an AUS in male patients with SUI (A)	Bulking agents can be used to treat SUI when there is a demand for a minimally invasive treatment (D)
		Bladder neck reconstruction can be used to treat SUI (D)
		Bladder neck closure should be offered to patients who have persistent neurogenic stress incontinence where alternative treatments have either failed or are likely to fail (B)
		Non-continent urinary diversion is the last resort for patients with NGB (A)
		Ileal conduit urinary diversion has the best long-term results for non-continent diversion, if the following pro- and perioperative precautions are taken (B)
		Where clean IC is not possible, the use of a urethral stent is possible in DSD (B)
		Although surgical sphincterotomy is the accepted reference treatment for neurogenic DSD, analysis of the literature highlights the lack of reliable efficacy and reproducibility criteria for the technique (B)
		In certain situations, dorsal rhizotomies can be undertaken in association with ventral root stimulators (Brindley's technique) or even with continent cystostomy (B)

SUI: stress unitary incontinence: AUS: autologous unitary sling; NDO: neurogenic detrusor overactivity; NGB: neurogenic bladder: DSD: detrusor sphincter dysynergia: IC: intermittent catheterisation; NICE: National Institute of Health and Care Excellence; EAU: the European Association of Urology; ICI: International Consultation on Incontinence. *Source*: Jaggi et al. [20].

has been approved as second-line treatment for urinary incontinence associated with NDO in patients with inadequate response to or intolerance of an anticholinergic. Repeat intradetrusor injections of onabotulinumtoxin-A generally provide sustained clinical benefits. It is a safe procedure. Increased PVR and need for posttreatment ISC/IC are very common in NLUTD [21]. It may be considered for intrasphincteric injection to treat DSD in SCI.

2) Bladder augmentation involves cutting the bladder in half and sewing a bowel patch (ileum) into the defect. Patients will need to use ISC or IC afterwards. The most frequent and serious complications are bladder calculi and perforation at the bladder/bowel junction, usually caused by over-distension of the reservoir. Bladder augmentation may have sequelae, such as intestinal transit disorder, and patients should be informed of this before surgery.

3) Sacral neuromodulation (SNM) and percutaneous tibial nerve stimulation do not have established places in treatment of NLUTD. Additional research is needed to ascertain their potential contribution in routine practice, but some benefit has been reported in MS patients. Since magnetic resonance imaging (MRI) scanning is so important for neurology follow-up, this can contraindicate SNM therapy. However, new SNM devices are now MRI compatible, so there will perhaps be increased use of this modality for treatment of neurogenic patients in the future.

Urinary reconstruction of diversion for severe intractable NLUTD is a considerable step, from the point of view of the operative challenges, post-operative complications (notably chest infection, thrombosis, and pressure sores), and the difficulty of recovering mobility and bowel function. An orthotopic neobladder uses a large amount of bowel which is reconfigured to create a reservoir, which is drained by catheterisation along the urethra. Since the bowel is a peristaltic organ, it can generate a lot of activity (Figure 16.19), which can cause leakage or kidney problems. Continent cutaneous diversion methods (Figure 16.6) require the construction of a continent catheterisable abdominal channel and require multidisciplinary evaluation (urologist, neurologist or rehabilitation doctor, stomatherapy nurses, etc.). The channel will be made from appendix or reconfigured ileal segment, which is implanted into the bladder wall and runs to the umbilicus or lower abdomen. Unfortunately, operating on the thick-walled neuropathic bladder can prove to be problematic with a high chance of complication (Figure 16.20), so a bowel segment may be needed to augment bladder capacity in addition. Non-continent cutaneous diversion (e.g. ileal conduit) is the last resort in NLUTD. A non-radical ('simple') cystectomy should be considered at the same time because of the risk of later complications from the defunctioned bladder, especially pyocystis [3]. It is crucial to identify the optimal location for the stoma site pre-operatively, with wheelchair test if necessary. Ongoing follow-up is needed to enable monitoring of the upper urinary tracts, electrolyte and metabolic abnormalities, and vitamin deficiencies and to have a better idea of the long-term results of the various procedures [1].

Specific Neurological Diseases

Whenever considering anticipated NLUTD consequences from a given neurological disease, it is worth matching the predominant site of neurological impairment with the ICS lesion classification (Table 16.1) [1].

Multiple Sclerosis

MS is a demyelinating disease of the CNS usually affecting adults aged between 20 and 50 years, with a twofold higher incidence in women than in men. The classic description of

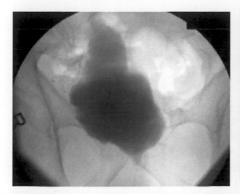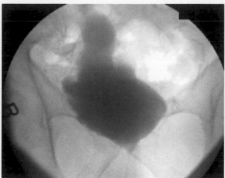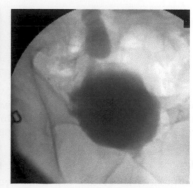

Figure 16.19 A sequence of pictures during video urodynamics for a person with a neobladder constructed from a large section of ileum; the obvious shape changes indicate active peristaltic activity. *Source*: Marcus Drake.

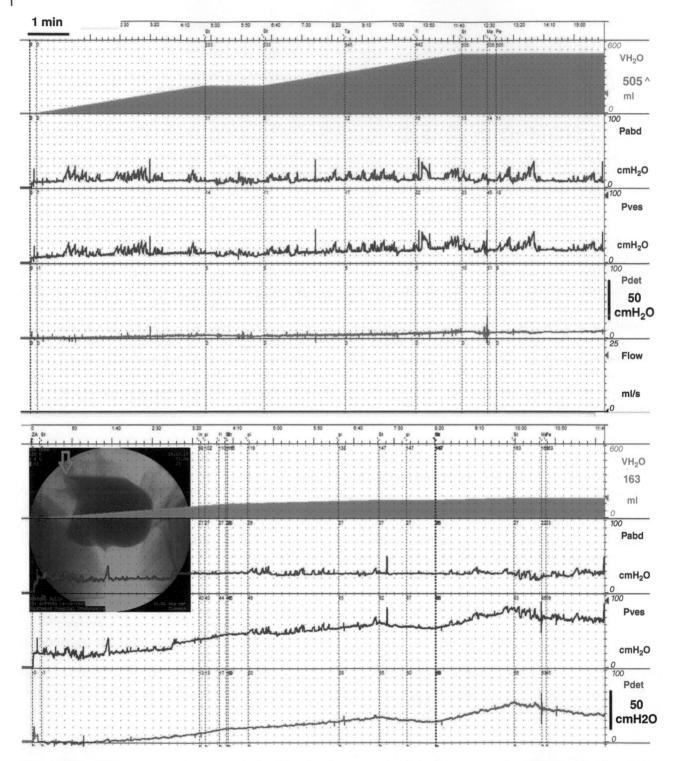

Figure 16.20 Filling cystometry in a woman before (above) and one year after (below) surgery creating a Mitrofanoff catheterisable channel, without an augmentation cystoplasty. The distortion in the bladder wall where the Mitrofanoff channel was implanted is indicated by the orange arrow. The compliance changed from 72 to 3 ml/cmH₂O, and bladder capacity dropped from 505 to 163 ml.

lesions disseminated in time and space means that the cumulative effect leads to a mixed neuronal lesion. However, the clinical course is very varied. MS is very important in the urodynamic setting, as it is a condition which can present with LUTS before the neurological diagnosis has been made (see Chapter 1) [22]. LUTS may be the initial complaint in up to 15% of MS patients [23]. It should be suspected where there is sudden onset severe LUTS (storage more than voiding) in a young- to middle-aged person. In our experience, there is usually some additional subtle feature on examination, such as altered speech or gait. If suspected, the response must be early referral direct to neurology, and imaging should <u>not</u> be requested (the neurologists will attend to that so that the right scans are done, and the appropriate radiologists review them). This referral is important, since early detection may allow disease modification treatment to reduce risk of MS progression.

MS is the major cause of non-traumatic disability in young adults, with prevalence of 83 per 100 000 in Europe [24]. LUTS are reported by 34–99%, correlating with the degree of spinal cord involvement and the level of disability [25, 26]. NLUTD affects many aspects and may progress over time. Overactive bladder (OAB) symptoms are most common, while voiding dysfunction becomes more of an issue with progression [27, 28]. The urodynamic findings in MS patients tend to be [29]:

- DO: 86%
- DSD: 35%
- DUA: 25% (Figure 16.21).

Nonetheless, a range of mechanisms may be identified since MS can affect any part of the nervous system (Figure 16.22).

Conservative treatment of NLUTD in MS patients includes behavioural therapy, antimuscarinics, or mirabegron [30] to decrease DO, with or without ISC/IC (Figure 16.23) [31–33]. Medicinal cannabinoids are being evaluated, with some improvements of NLUTD reported [34]. MS was one of the index conditions for the licencing trials of onabotulinumtoxin-A injection therapy for neurogenic DO. Unfortunately, progression of MS leads to a limitation of therapy options (Figure 16.24).

Parkinson's Disease

PD is a movement disorder resulting from degeneration of dopaminergic neurons in the substantia nigra and a loss of dopamine-containing nerve terminals in the basal ganglia. PD is the second most prevalent neurodegenerative disease after Alzheimer's disease. Prevalence rate estimates range upwards from 65.6 per 100 000, and annual incidence estimates range from 5 per 100 000 to 346 per 100 000 [35]. Patients with PD present with tremor (Figure 16.13), rigidity, postural changes, and a decrease in spontaneous movements. Comorbidities such as anxiety, depression, fatigue, and sleep disorders may well be observed prior to the diagnosis of PD [36]. These CNS changes also have influence on autonomic function, including constipation, blood pres-

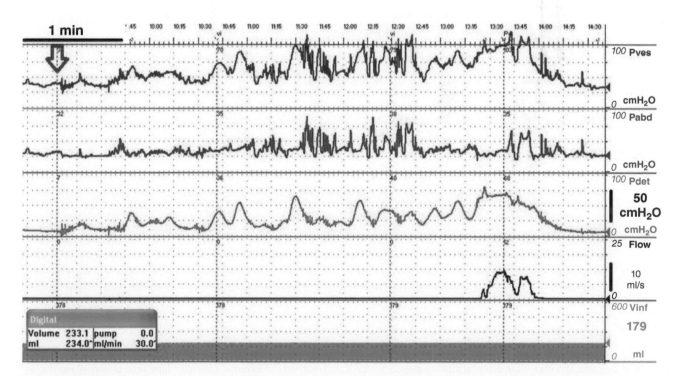

Figure 16.21 Pressure-flow study of a male patient with multiple sclerosis reporting voiding symptoms. Permission to void is indicated by the purple arrow. A delay of more than four minutes resulted while his bladder mounted transient insufficient detrusor contractions, until finally flow resulted. The severe hesitancy and fluctuating detrusor contraction makes this functionally underactive, though actually his bladder contractility index is above the threshold of 100 for normal contractility.

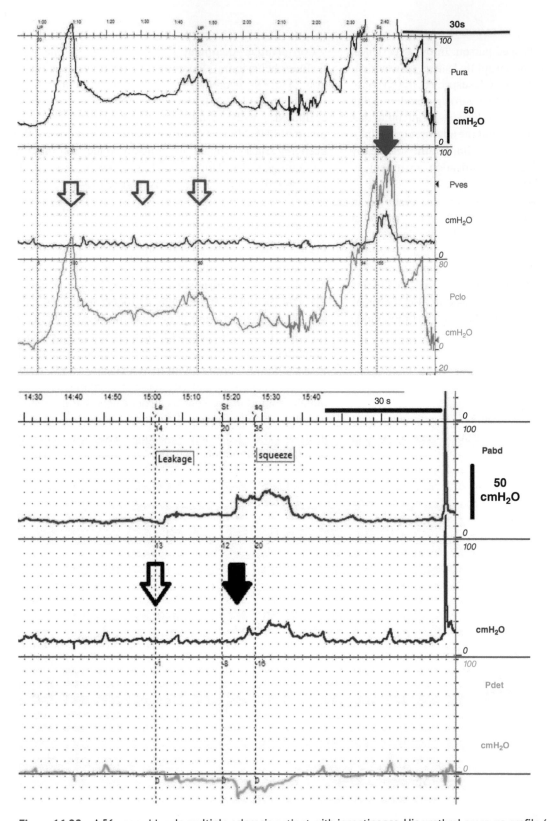

Figure 16.22 A 56-year-old male multiple sclerosis patient with incontinence. His urethral pressure profile (above) showed a remarkably high pressure as the catheter was withdrawn across the bladder neck (blue arrow), a low-pressure prostatic plateau (purple arrow), and low maximum urethral closure pressure once it had reached the external sphincter (open red arrow). When the catheter was returned to the sphincter and he was asked to do a pelvic floor squeeze, there was an excellent voluntary increment in the pressure (closed red arrow). His filling cystometry (below) was then undertaken, also done in the supine position. Incontinence was visualised by direct inspection, as the flowmeter could not be placed to catch it with him in the supine position. Leakage started (open black arrow) with no concurrent exertion and no detrusor overactivity due to his low resting closure pressure. His good voluntary pelvic floor contraction enabled him to stop the leakage (closed black arrow). Hence, the most appropriate urodynamic diagnosis to apply for his incontinence was urethral relaxation incontinence, but the actual mechanism was sphincter weakness rather than acquired relaxation of the sphincter.

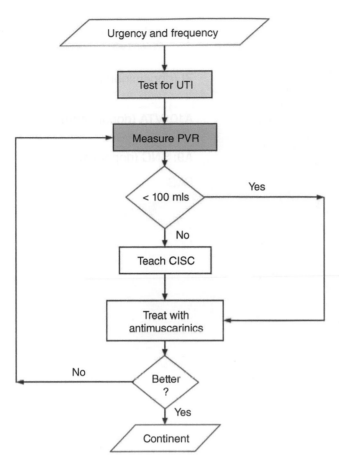

Figure 16.23 Management algorithm for patients with multiple sclerosis presenting with urinary tract symptoms. CISC: clean intermittent self-catheterisation; PVR: post-void residual volume; UTI: urinary tract infection. *Source*: Fowler et al. [15].

sure control, and altered sweating. The movement disorder symptoms are often treated with levodopa. The effects of levodopa, the major drug to treat motor dysfunction, on the bladder in PD vary significantly, and add-on therapy is

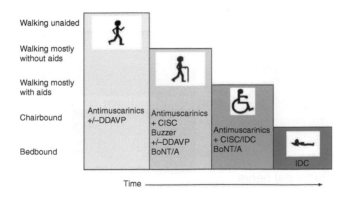

Figure 16.24 Bladder management options with progression of disabilities in multiple sclerosis. BoNT/A: botulinum toxin A; 'buzzer': suprapubic vibration device; CISC: clean intermittent self-catheterisation; DDAVP: desmopressin; IDC: indwelling catheter. *Source*: Fowler et al. [15].

often required [37]. Modern-day therapy can include deep brain stimulation as an option for the movement disorders, and this can be beneficial for urinary symptoms in some patients [38].

The prevalence of urinary symptoms correlates with severity of the disease, but not with the duration of illness. The majority of patients have onset of the bladder dysfunction after the appearance of motor disorder, though LUTS can be the actual presenting feature (see Chapter 1). Storage LUTS affects about a quarter of PD patients, voiding LUTS 11% (though usually with a low PVR), and both types a fifth of them. Nocturia is the most prevalent LUTS, though the underlying mechanism may well be systemic. OAB in PD reflects lesions in the brain, e.g. in the prefrontal-nigrostriatal D1 dopaminergic bladder-inhibitory pathway [39], i.e. an SPL (Figure 16.25). DO is a common feature identified during filling cystometry for someone with PD (Figure 16.26). DO in PD patients can be treated with antimuscarinic drugs, but being cautious with regards to cognition, movement disorder, and increased PVR. Once urinary incontinence occurs, it is often in conjunction with faecal incontinence, whereas no significant relation is seen with sexual dysfunction. SUI surgery should not be offered to patients with significant DO.

Non-relaxing urethral sphincter is characterised by an obstructing urethral sphincter which stays partly contracted, resulting in reduced urine flow. This applies to people with neurological disease affecting muscle relaxation, such as PD or spinal bifida. The urethra opens except for the area of the striated muscle sphincter, at pelvic floor level. This condition produces a continuous obstruction with reduced flow rates. Patients often suffer from stress incontinence owing to sphincter incompetence during bladder filling, as well as from obstructed voiding due to the failure of urethral relaxation.

One feature of treated PD is the dramatic effect medication can have on movement disorders and the speed with which it can change as drug effects kick in or wear off. Motor fluctuations (i.e. changes in the nature of the movement effects of the condition) usually happen when an anti-Parkinsonian drug is wearing off, particularly levodopa. Sometimes, this can happen quickly (over a few minutes), often referred to colloquially as 'switching off'. Hence, being 'on' is when a person's symptoms are controlled and when they feel at their most capable. In contrast, being 'off' is when movement abnormalities are most obvious. As Parkinson's progresses, each drug dose tends not to last quite so long, so fluctuations can become more unpredictable. Medications can also contribute to emergence of dyskinesia, which are involuntary movements such as jerks, twisting, or writhing of the arms, legs, or torso. This might be when levodopa is at its highest level in

nucleus, and cerebellum. Many people affected by MSA experience dysfunction of the autonomic nervous system, which commonly manifests as orthostatic hypotension, impotence, loss of sweating, dry mouth, and urinary retention and incontinence.

MSA is exceptionally important in the urodynamic setting, as it is one of the conditions which can present with LUTS before the neurological diagnosis has been made [22]. We have raised suspicions of undiagnosed MSA on the basis of middle-aged men presenting with rather severe LUTS, who also reported disproportionate fatigue and who had preceding erectile dysfunction when questioned (Figure 16.27). Neurological referral is needed in this case to make the diagnosis so that prognosis can be identified (rather than attempting disease modification treatment). Urogenital indicators which indicate MSA may be the actual underlying cause include urinary symptoms preceding or presenting with Parkinsonism; urinary incontinence and PD; significant PVR urine volume; erectile failure preceding or presenting with Parkinsonism; and worsening bladder control after urological surgery [44]. While MSA is described as Parkinsonian-like, there are a couple of key differences between MSA and PD relevant in the UDS unit:

- Timing of emergence of LUTS. an early feature in MSA, later in PD
- Severity of incontinence. severe in MSA, less so in PD
- PVR. raised in MSA, usually normal in PD
- Male bladder neck. may be open during bladder filling in MSA, usually closed during and difficult to open (bradykinetic) in PD

OAB and urinary retention are both potential problems in MSA, reflecting potential neurological dysfunction in the cerebellum and the brainstem [39]. As the disease progresses, symptoms may change from urinary urgency and frequency to those due to incomplete bladder emptying. Approximately 60% of patients with MSA develop urinary symptoms, either prior to or at the time of presentation with the motor disorder [45]. Among 53 patients with both urinary and orthostatic symptoms, those who had urinary symptoms first (48%) were more common than those who had orthostatic symptoms first (29%), and some patients developed both symptoms simultaneously (23%) [45]. Urinary symptoms of incontinence are caused by neurogenic DO and external sphincter weakness (SUI) [3]. Sphincter EMG abnormalities are seen in a high proportion.

Due to the complex dysfunction and progressive nature of the disease, aggressive treatment and LUT surgery (e.g. TURP) are not recommended. The treatment of choice in men with increased PVR is alpha-blocking agents and IC. OAB is treated with fluid advice, bladder training, and standard medications.

Stroke/Cerebrovascular Accident (CVA)

CNS infarction is 'brain, spinal cord, or retinal cell death attributable to ischaemia, based on neuropathological, neuroimaging, and/or clinical evidence of permanent injury' [46]. CNS infarction includes ischaemic stroke, where there are overt symptoms, while silent infarction causes no identified symptoms. Stroke also includes intracerebral haemorrhage and subarachnoid haemorrhage [46]. Cerebrovascular accident (CVA) is thus the result of impaired blood supply to the brain, mainly due to thrombosis, embolism, or haemorrhage. It is categorised by the specific blood vessel blocked. People at risk for stroke include those who have high blood pressure, high cholesterol, diabetes, and smokers. Reported incidence of stroke in Europe is 450 cases/100000/year, being associated with 10% of cardiovascular mortality [47].

At the time of maximal impairment following a CVA, 41% (46% of females, 37% of males) develop urinary incontinence [48, 49]. For patients seen within seven days of their stroke, the presence of urinary incontinence may be a more powerful prognostic indicator for poor survival and eventual functional dependence than a depressed level of consciousness. Urinary incontinence with impaired awareness of bladder sensation seems to be associated with poorer outcome than UUI with preserved bladder perception [50]. Six months after stroke, 16% of patients experience urine loss, and monthly occurrence appears to be a threshold at which incontinence is perceived [51]. Voiding dysfunction affects a quarter of patients. Nocturia affects a third, but not necessarily due to the stroke – perhaps instead due to the condition that predisposed the patient to stroke.

Prior to the findings of functional brain imaging studies, all that was known about the cortical control of the bladder was based on clinical studies of patients with brain lesions. The classical description of frontal lobe incontinence is a patient with severe urgency and frequency of micturition and urgency incontinence, without dementia, the patient being socially aware and embarrassed by the incontinence [52]. Micturition is not dyssynergic, indicating that the lesion is in the higher (cerebral) control of these processes and that the PMC is still able to regulate LUT synergy. UDS is relatively rarely done in stroke patients, but if undertaken, DO is a common finding.

Urinary incontinence in stroke patients is usually interpreted as the loss of central inhibition. However, loss of bladder perception as a concomitant factor may also be relevant. Deficit of bladder sensation seems to be associated with poorer general outcome. Such patients have more parietal lobe but less frontal lobe impairment than patients with UUI and preserved bladder sensation [53].

Proper urological and multidisciplinary care is needed to prevent major complications in stroke patients. For those

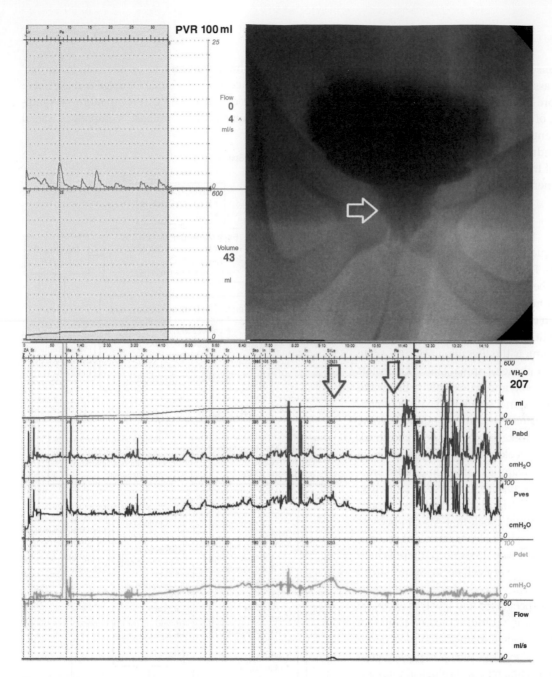

Figure 16.27 A 43-year-old man with longstanding mild lower urinary tract symptoms. Four years ago, he developed occasional urgency incontinence, and was treated with tamsulosin and solifenacin with no real effect. He reported progressively worsening stream, with post-void residual. Previous urological carer did bladder neck incision, after which he went into acute retention, 800 ml volume. One year later, he was treated with onabotulinumtoxin-A bladder injections but had not been taught intermittent self-catheterising (ISC) until six months later. Still not improving, with leakage and flow rate problems, and started using pads due to worsening leakage. The following symptoms were also reported; nocturia 5–8 times per night, worsening and sometimes nocturnal enuresis, and also nocturnal frequency with small trickles. He was referred to another urological centre, where a transurethral resection of the prostate was done. This made no real difference, and, in fact, symptoms became worse. Now he is sore with some physical resistance to ISC and bleeding. Painful bladder spasms (he fights them off, but ends up with faecal urgency). He can achieve more complete bladder emptying in the seated position, still with poor stream. He gets recurrent UTIs, confirmed bacteriologically, with resistance now emerging. Spinal magnetic resonance imaging was normal (requested by urologist). He is awaiting neurology review. He does not get diplopia, headaches or loss of vision but he does get dizzy in the evening – he attributes this to sleep deprivation. He has had erectile dysfunction for five years – difficulty gaining and sustaining erection, and is dependent on Viagra now. On examination, raised BMI, poor gait were found. Intermittent low volume free flow rate (top left). Easy to catheterise, residual 100 ml. Pressure profile showed low sphincter pressure and very weak voluntary squeeze (not shown). Filling: clear and even prostate resection cavity (top right, white arrow). No vesicoureteric reflux. Mild pelvic floor descent with cough/strain. Poor compliance leakage (possible superimposed detrusor overactivity but this is not certain), with a leak point volume of Detrusor Leak Point Pressure of 32 cmH$_2$O (red arrow). After permission to void (purple arrow), he was unable to pass urine – straining was the only contributor to increased bladder pressure when trying to void. Emptied by ISC, 230 ml. CONCLUSION: high likelihood of neurological basis due to severity of onset, broad spectrum, and associated erectile dysfunction. Weak sphincter and poorly compliant bladder during filling, with acontractile bladder and straining during voiding. Likely to need assessment of brainstem. FOLLOW-UP: neurological evaluation included cerebral imaging and confirmed diagnosis as multiple system atrophy (MSA).

who present with urinary retention, IC is regarded as the favoured approach for assisted bladder emptying [54]. This may be in men with pre-existing BOO, who can consider standard management of BOO if they achieve satisfactory general recovery. Prevention of early UTI, especially during the acute phase of indwelling catheterisation, is needed. Thereafter, behavioural training and OAB medications are the mainstays of treatment.

Spinal Cord Injury

SCI is usually a consequence of direct trauma, associated with vertebral fractures. However, the spinal cord is a fragile structure which can be affected by other processes, such as surgery, inflammation, and compressive lesions, with rather similar long-term consequences. In the acute phase, management of the additional injuries inevitably resulting from such a severe trauma is the lifesaving priority. Acute traumatic SCI leads to a phase of spinal shock characterised by loss of sensory, motor, and reflex activity below the level of injury. NLUTD in spinal shock is usually a temporary complete painless urinary retention and is generally managed by indwelling catheterisation. Once spinal shock has resolved (after a few weeks), reflex activity generally returns below the injury, meaning that DO and reflex erections can occur. This is because the nerves are still alive, thanks to the anatomical distribution of the blood supply. It is after recovery from spinal shock that AD can become an issue. In a spinal stroke, caused by occlusion of anterior spinal artery (e.g. in acute aortic dissection), there is neuronal death and no reflex recovery will occur. Spinal stroke thus is not a risk for AD.

Management of SCI is specialised and involves extensive experience and an excellent multidisciplinary team. An overview algorithm of urological management was developed by UK specialist centres [14], which is presented in Figure 16.28. In these patients, regular urological monitoring, at least annually, is appropriate to detect complications and to adjust bladder management. Urinary tract management has to be adjusted according to results of urological evaluation and emergence of complications.

VUDS is the expected evaluation for any urodynamic assessment of a spinal cord problem, due to the diverse range of potential mechanisms, and the impossibility of relying on symptoms where someone has impaired sensory nerve function. An example is given in Figure 16.29.

Cauda Equina Syndrome

Below the lowest point of the spinal cord, at the lower border of the L1 vertebra, the nerve roots of L2 to S4 form a tightly packed bundle referred to as the 'cauda equina' from a resemblance to a horse's tail. Damage to these nerve roots produces a characteristic CEPNL pattern of symptoms. Central lumbar disc prolapse compresses sacral

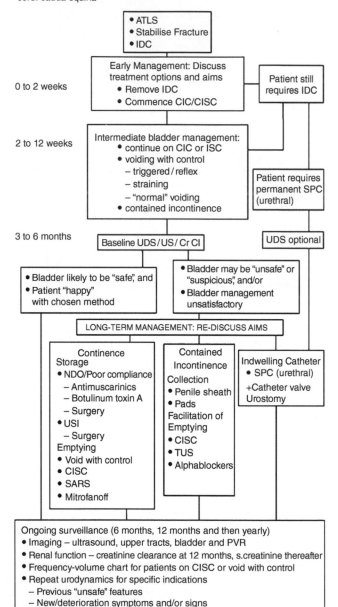

Figure 16.28 Management of NLUTD in SCI. *Source*: Abrams et al. [14]. SCI: spinal cord injury; IDC: indwelling catheter; CI(S)C: clean intermittent (self) catheterisation; NDO: neurogenic detrusor overactivity; TUS: transurethral sphincterotomy; SARS: sacral anterior root stimulator; USI: urodynamic stress incontinence; PVR: post-void residual volume; SPC: suprapubic catheter; NLUTD: neurogenic lower urinary tract dysfunction.

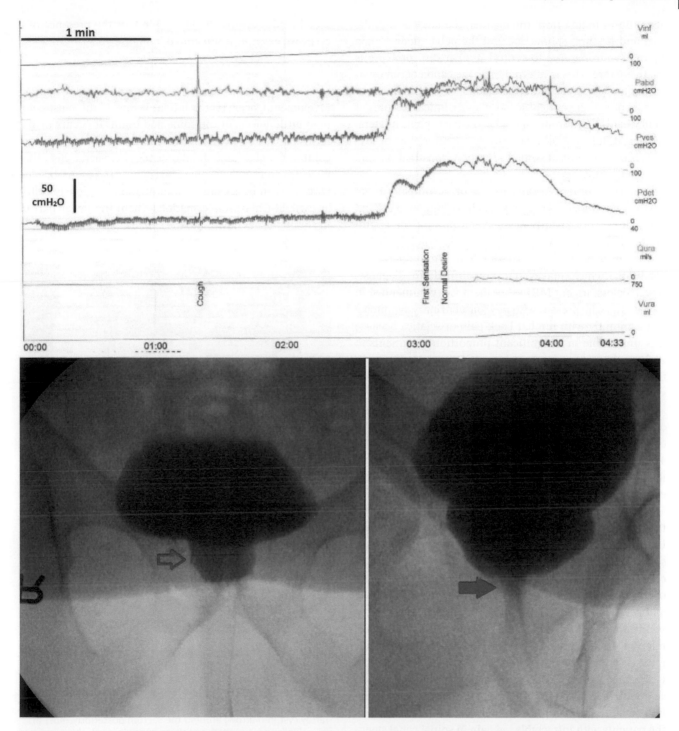

Figure 16.29   The upper illustration is from a urodynamics study done on a man with a background of spinal cord damage caused by 'the bends' during a diving accident. The test was done three years previously at another centre, with no X-ray screening. Based on this trace, they had presumed he had bladder outlet obstruction (BOO) caused by prostate enlargement, and transurethral resection of the prostate (TURP) was done. However, there is no permission to void annotated on the trace, and no video urodynamics (VUDS), making this presumption unreliable. Subsequently, he experienced ongoing voiding and storage symptoms (slow stream and incontinence) and was referred to us. Our VUDS imaging showed a good TURP cavity (open red arrow) obvious during filling cystometry (lower left). Pressure-flow study is shown in the lower right image (oblique view), with the closed red arrow indicating the external sphincter; massive dilation of prostatic urethra above the sphincter and slow trickle of contrast beyond the sphincter indicates this as the site of BOO. Hence, this man's BOO was due to neurological sphincter dysfunction. *Source*: Marcus Drake.

nerve fibres to and from the bladder, the large bowel, the anal and urethral sphincters, and the pelvic floor. Cauda equina syndrome due to central lumbar disc prolapse is relatively rare. This is referred to as the cauda equina syndrome and is associated with bladder, bowel and sexual dysfunction, and perineal sensory loss. Clinical features of cauda equina syndrome include low-back pain, bilateral sciatica, saddle anaesthesia, urinary retention, loss of urethral sensation, loss of genital sensation, constipation, and erectile dysfunction.

Urinary disorders usually follow or accompany more obvious neurologic symptoms, such as lumbar pain and perineal sensory disturbances, which prompt the appropriate diagnosis. However, sometimes, voiding disturbances may be the only or the first symptom of this condition, which makes it more difficult to diagnose. Nevertheless, urgent MRI assessment is recommended in all patients who present with new onset urinary symptoms concomitantly with lumbar back pain or sciatica because it is impossible in a significant proportion of patients to exclude the diagnosis of prolapsed intervertebral disc in the context of referral with suspected cauda equina syndrome.

Emergency surgical decompression increases the chance of recovery in patients with cauda equina syndrome due to central lumbar disc prolapse, with a target of maximum 48 hours after onset. Acontractile detrusor may be irreversible, and if it has not recovered at a year after onset, the chance of subsequent recovery is minimal.

Spinal stenosis (or narrowing) is a common condition that occurs when the vertebral canal becomes compressed. Usually, the narrowing is caused by osteoarthritis of the spinal column and discs. It may also be caused by a thickening of the ligaments in the back, as well as by a bulging of the discs. Symptoms of spinal stenosis often start slowly and get worse over time. Pain in the legs may become so severe that walking even short distances is unbearable, referred to as spinal claudication. Frequently, sufferers must sit or lean forward to temporarily ease pain. Patients with spinal stenosis, especially at lumbar levels, may present with bladder and bowel involvement – urinary retention/incontinence and faecal incontinence. About half of the patients with intractable leg pain in spinal canal stenosis also have bladder symptoms – voiding dysfunction with high PVR and reduced flow rate and/or stress incontinence indicating effects on the cauda equina. Such symptoms, including urinary incontinence, usually improve after surgical decompression.

Quite a diverse range of mechanisms can affect this part of the spinal cord, from tethering (leading to problems worsening with growth) to impingement (such as a prolapsed lumbar intervertebral disc pushing back into the

sacral cord roots that lie just behind, or the presence of a cyst). An example is illustrated in Figure 16.30.

Spina Bifida

Myelomeningocele (spina bifida) is one of the most common birth defects of the spine and brain. It occurs in 1–2 births per 1000, potentially involving all levels of the spinal column (lumbar 26%, lumbosacral 47%, sacral 20%, thoracic 5%, and cervical spine 2%) (Figure 16.31). Associated with this can be a Chiari malformation, previously called an Arnold-Chiari malformation, where the lower part of the brain pushes down into the spinal canal. This is seen in

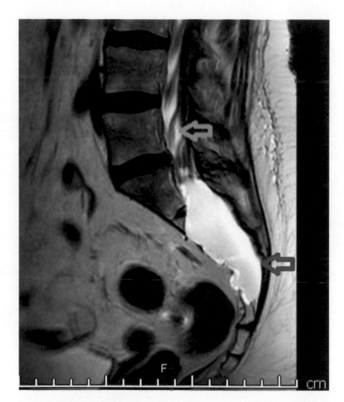

Figure 16.30 Tarlov cysts are perineural sacral nerve root cysts, representing dilations of the nerve root sheaths and filled with cerebrospinal fluid (CSF) that can cause a progressively painful radiculopathy (nerve pain) and loss of sacral nerve root function. This magnetic resonance imaging scan shows a large, lobulated Tarlov cyst (red arrow) eroding the sacrum posteriorly. Most of the midsacrum is eroded, and there is only a small thin rim of cortical bone remaining anteriorly. There are no sinister features, but there appears to be compression of the sacral nerve roots mainly at the mid to distal sacrum. The green arrow shows the normal appearance of lumbar nerve roots crossing the CSF. This patient did have cauda equina dysfunction, with hesitancy, slow stream, interrupted voiding, altered bladder sensation, and stress urinary incontinence. Similar symptoms were experienced for gut function. On examination, her bladder was not palpable at presentation. She had reduced sensation in the saddle area, poor discrimination of pinprick, though she could feel light touch. *Source*: Marcus Drake.

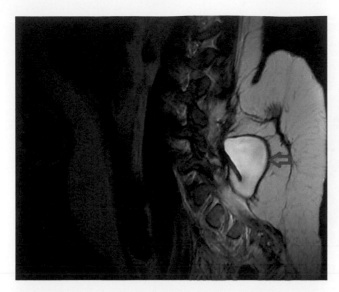

Figure 16.31 Magnetic resonance imaging scan showing a myelomeningocoele (red arrow) and considerable distortion of the lower back. *Source*: Marcus Drake.

85% of children with spina bifida, often requiring ventriculoperitoneal shunting (Figure 16.32) of cerebrospinal fluid (CSF) to avoid secondary deterioration due to altered pres-

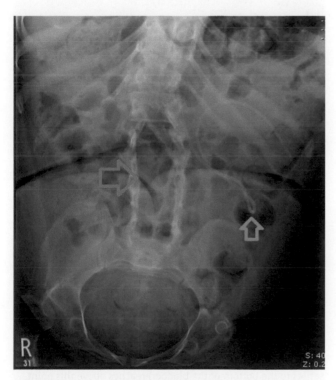

Figure 16.32 Plain abdominal X-ray of a patient with spina bifida, showing the substantial defect in lower vertebral bodies, where the spinous processes are missing (orange arrow). A ventriculoperitoneal shunt is present (blue arrow), which is commonly needed for treating hydrocephalus. *Source*: Marcus Drake.

sures in the spinal cord CSF (syringomyelia) and brain CSF (hydrocephalus). Ingestion of folic acid prior to conception and during the first trimester of pregnancy has significantly reduced the incidence of spina bifida. The neurologic defect produced is quite variable and cannot be totally predicted by the vertebral level of the lesion. Additionally, the fibrosis associated with myelomeningocele closure may tether the cord, leading to subsequent deterioration in NLUTD, bowel function, and lower limb function with growth (especially at the time of growth spurts such as adolescence). Tethered cord syndrome and syringomyelia must be considered at any age for a spina bifida patient reporting a change in function.

The incidence of urethrovesical dysfunction in myelomeningocele is high – perhaps over 90%. Similarly, anorectal dysfunction is very common. Major consequences of the NLUTD include impaired compliance and hydroureteronephrosis (perhaps due to thick-walled bladder often present in these patients (Figure 16.33)), which can occur early or later in life. Significant upper tract deterioration is rare after puberty, but ongoing follow-up into adult life is appropriate. Urodynamic findings may predict the patients at risk of upper tract deterioration, notably poor detrusor compliance, especially where the DLPP is high [55]. VUDS is the appropriate test (Figure 16.34), since VUR is common, and it helps define the level of neurological deficit and identifies additional structural aspects. Filling cystometry may show impaired compliance and DUA (Figure 16.35).

Early initiation of conservative measures (clean IC and antimuscarinic medication) generally provides protection of the upper urinary tract. Renal ultrasound is an important part of follow-up surveillance, assessing renal growth, development of scarring, and hydroureteronephrosis. Repeat UDS and ultrasound may have a role in this patient population; however, recommendations for timing and frequency of these studies still need to be elucidated. Extensive surgery is reserved for failed conservative treatment. The following might be considered:

- Augmentation cystoplasty (due to poor compliance);
- Mitrofanoff procedure (to facilitate ISC); and
- AUS placement (to treat USI) – usually placing an intrabdominal rather than a perineal cuff due to the risk of device erosion in someone with insensate perineal skin.

Normal-Pressure Hydrocephalus

Normal-pressure hydrocephalus (NPH) is important in the urodynamic setting, as it is one of the conditions which can present with LUTS before the neurological diagnosis has been made [22]. Population-based MRI studies suggest that

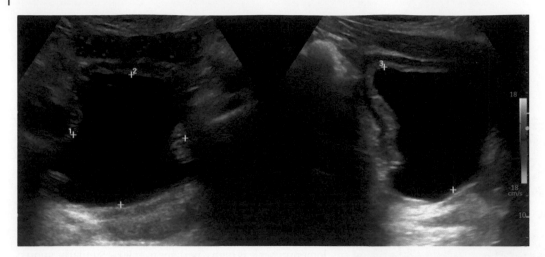

Figure 16.33 The bladder can be very thick-walled in spina bifida, resulting in an increased risk of poor detrusor compliance. *Source*: Marcus Drake.

the incidence of NPH or asymptomatic enlargement of the CSF ventricles is around 1% of the general population over 65 years of age [56]. Thus, it is likely there is significant underdiagnosis, hence the importance in UDS units. Since there is a surgical shunt therapy for NPH, early diagnosis of NPH in patients with OAB is important.

NPH is characterised by a clinical presentation of gait disturbance, memory deficit, and urinary incontinence, combined with dilated cerebral ventricles and normal CSF pressure [57]. The clinical triad of this disorder is like those of vascular dementia or cerebral white matter disease. The neurological treatment is diversion of CSF flow by a shunt. Diagnosis of NPH may comprise:

a) Possible features: gait, cognitive, and urinary disorders with typical ventricular dilatation in brain imaging;
b) Probable features: improved clinical symptoms by 30 ml withdrawal of the CSF by a lumbar tap (the Tap test); and
c) Definite: improved clinical symptoms by ventriculoperitoneal shunt surgery, etc.

LUTS urinary urgency and frequency (OAB) affect a high proportion of idiopathic NPH patients [58]. Urodynamic findings of 42 NPH patients by Sakakibara and colleagues included low Q_{max} (<10 ml/s) in 40%; increased PVR (>30 ml) in 43%; low volume at first sensation (<100 ml) in 33%; decreased bladder capacity (<200 ml) in 57%; and DO in 95% [58]. In patients with NPH, DO can be temporarily improved by a lumbar puncture and later abolished by a shunt operation [59]. Urodynamic testing after lumbar puncture may predict the outcome of a shunt operation in these cases [60].

Dementia

Dementia is a neurodegenerative disease leading to progressive decline in cognitive and functional abilities. The

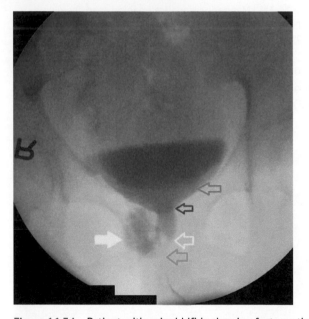

Figure 16.34 Patient with spinal bifida showing features that can be visible on screening during video urodynamics (VUDS), in this case during filling cystometry. The green arrow is the level of the urethral sphincter, and stress incontinence was not seen. The open yellow arrow is pointing to a small filling defect in the lower end of the prostatic urethra, the verumontanum (see Chapter 2). This is where the ejaculatory ducts enter the urethra, and, on the right, reflux is seen into the seminal vesicle (closed yellow arrow). The blue arrow points to the bladder neck, which is open; this indicates some dysfunction of the sympathetic nervous system. The orange arrow is pointing to the approximate level of the left ureteric orifice; the point here is that a VUDS attempting to identify any vesicoureteric reflux (VUR) must ensure that contrast (which is dense and hence settles to the bottom of the bladder) reaches above this point. This patient was filled without having emptied his post-void residual, so there was significant volume already in his bladder (not visible). This has a reasonable chance of excluding VUR caused by high bladder pressure disrupting the antireflux function of the vesicoureteric junction. It does not exclude a high-lying ureteric orifice being responsible for VUR, but that situation is not so common as the cause of VUR in the neuropathic bladder. *Source*: Marcus Drake.

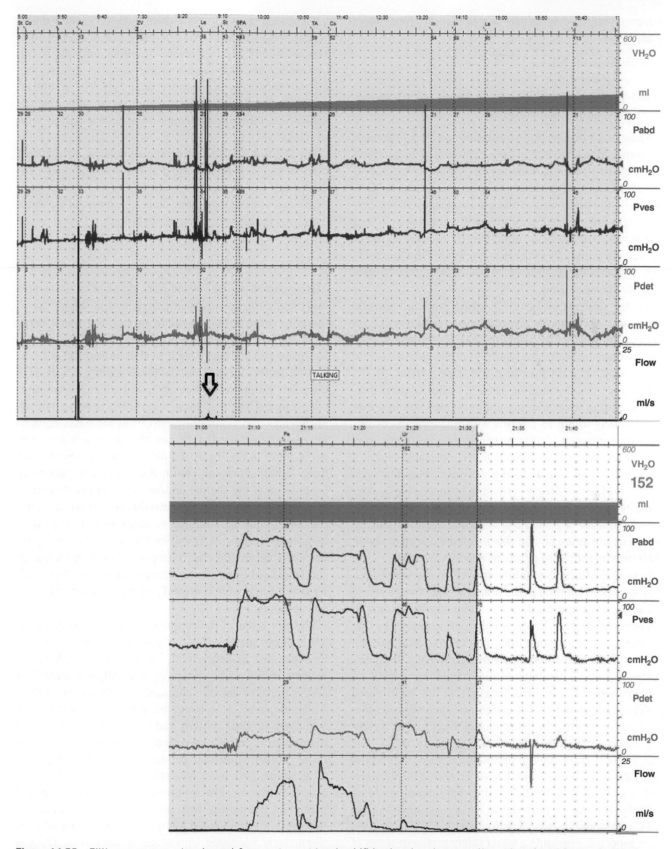

Figure 16.35 Filling cystometry (top image) for a patient with spina bifida, showing that compliance is reduced for a volume of 113 ml, the pressure changed by 24−2 = 22 cmH$_2$O, so the compliance was 5 ml/cmH$_2$O. At several points, it looks like there is low-amplitude detrusor overactivity, but, generally, this appearance was due to transient drops in the p$_{abd}$ reading rather than an actual bladder contraction. The pressure-flow study from the same patient (lower image) indicates that voiding was by straining; the fact that a small change in p$_{det}$ appears to be present during each strain is due to slightly impaired recording by the p$_{abd}$ catheter. These difficulties with p$_{abd}$ recording are quite common in spina bifida, due to the weak anal sphincter and pelvic floor.

dementias can be classified according into four major groups [61]:

1) Alzheimer's disease
2) Vascular dementia
3) Lewy body disease (LBD) and dementia of Parkinson's
4) Frontotemporal dementia

Alzheimer's disease is the most common form of dementia, comprising up to 80% of cases. The clinical hallmark of Alzheimer's disease is memory impairment. A sense of memory failure, detected by the patient or a close relative, is usually the presenting symptom. Language and recognition skills are affected early in the disease course. Motor and sensory symptoms are absent until late in the course of the disease even early in the presentation. Alzheimer's disease is gradually progressive, typically extending 10 years from diagnosis to death.

For the urodynamicist, LUTS could precede dementia diagnosis. LUTS usually precedes severe cognitive deficits in LBD and in vascular dementia [61]. In Alzheimer's disease, urinary incontinence typically correlates with disease progression, i.e. it is a feature of late-stage disease.

LUTS are usually multifactorial [61]. Behavioural therapy, including toilet training and prompted voiding, may be especially useful in patients with unawareness of urinary incontinence. Antimuscarinics are frequently prescribed to dementia patients and are especially useful in LBD and in vascular dementia. However, they may also help in bladder training programmes by increasing bladder capacity in other types of dementia. It is possible that antimuscarinics are of greater benefit to less impaired individuals, who are aware of, and able to tell the caregiver about, their urinary sensation or incontinence [61].

Central cholinesterase inhibitors (which decrease degradation of acetylcholine in the brain) and glutamate receptor antagonists are used to treat memory symptoms of Alzheimer's disease. There is still some controversy that the central cholinesterase inhibitors might exacerbate urinary incontinence in those patients. Conversely, the possibility that OAB antimuscarinics could contribute to development of cognitive impairment in predisposed patients is reported [62]. Current evidence suggests that antimuscarinics can be associated with cognitive worsening due to the blockade of M1 receptors (CNS side effects) [61]. Thus, the use of antimuscarinics that do not easily cross the blood–brain barrier or more M2/M3 selective agents should be taken into consideration. More recently, the use of mirabegron (beta-3 agonist) to treat OAB symptoms in elderly patients with CNS lesions has been reported, providing a better safety profile in terms of cognitive function [63].

Many elderly patients and their caregivers seek medical care for dementia and OAB together. Clinical trials of combining central cholinesterase inhibitors and peripheral anticholinergics for ameliorating both cognition and incontinence have been undertaken [64]. The combined use of a 'central' cholinesterase inhibitor and a 'peripheral' muscarinic receptor antagonist may be considered with caution [65].

For ambulatory patients, prompted voiding, behavioural therapy, and oral anticholinergics seem to be the treatment of choice. Interventional treatment of incontinence in Alzheimer's disease patients should be reserved for those with good general status and ambulation.

Peripheral Neuropathy

LUT dysfunctions can occur from damage to the nerves innervating the pelvic organs, anywhere in the course of these nerves through the cauda equina, the spinal nerve roots, the sacral plexus, or to the various individual nerves. Extensive pelvic surgery, such as abdominoperineal resection for rectal cancer or radical hysterectomy, can damage the pelvic parasympathetic nerves to the bladder and genitalia. Surgical 'nerve-sparing' approaches have been developed which aim to minimise effect, but some risk remains inherent. Pelvic irradiation can also detrimentally affect nerve fibres in the irradiated fields. Bladder, erectile, and faecal dysfunctions can result. Focal injury to peripheral innervation of the bladder and/or sphincter results in denervation referred to as 'decentralisation'. Detrusor acontractility (requiring straining to void) and/or sphincteric deficiency (causing SUI) will be the result, depending on the exact nerves affected. Iatrogenic faecal incontinence can be caused by sphincter damage caused during childbirth and surgery for anorectal problems, trauma, fistulae, and abscesses.

Diabetes is one of the commonest causes of neuropathy. 'Diabetic cystopathy' affects a significant proportion of insulin-dependent diabetics, with no sex or age differences. Patients with diabetic cystopathy generally can have OAB and/or impaired detrusor contractions with increased PVR, while recurrent UTIs might be a long-term problem. A Scandinavian study showed that in patients who have had diabetes for 10 years, the prevalence of diabetic cystopathy in those who were insulin-dependent was 2 to 4 per 1000 and in those on oral hypoglycaemic agents was 1 to 3 per 1000 [66]. The correlation between diabetic cystopathy and peripheral neuropathy was very high. Diabetes duration, treatment type, peripheral neuropathy, and retinopathy are significantly associated with severe incontinence. There is no specific treatment for diabetic cystopathy.

Autonomic Dysfunction

Autonomic dysfunctions are quite commonly seen in neurological disease, and they hugely affect quality of life. Rarely, they can also occur as a primary condition without a neurological disease. For example, autoimmune autonomic ganglionopathy is a result of circulating ganglionic acetylcholine receptor antibodies. Pure autonomic failure is a degenerative post-ganglionic autonomic disorder. Nocturia and voiding dysfunction are common, and bladder emptying is often affected. Bladder diaries may demonstrate nocturnal polyuria. UDS may demonstrate DO in some patients [67]. Bladder and erectile dysfunction are well-recognised in acute idiopathic autonomic neuropathy (acute pandysautonomia). Urinary retention and voiding difficulty are common, reflecting underlying detrusor areflexia. Constipation is another feature.

Alongside storage and voiding dysfunction, the range of functions potentially at risk includes:

- Vision. light sensitivity due to poor iris control
- Stomach. gastroparesis, requiring enteric feeding
- Vascular. severe hypotension on standing, due to loss of vascular tone so that blood pools in dependent parts
- Thermoregulation. loss of sweating and temperature control
- Salivation. dry mouth
- Auditory. excessive noise sensitivity
- Gastrointestinal. constipation

Assisting Neurology and Neurosurgery Teams in Defining the Neurological Lesion

A detailed knowledge of the precise deficits in the urinary tract can help refine the functional aspects of a neurological case, and this can help where CNS imaging is not corresponding with the clinical features, or where neurosurgeons need to establish baseline function prior to a high-risk operation. Urodynamic evaluation gives potential insight into, for example:

- Bladder motor function (storage and voiding)
- Urinary sphincter motor function (storage and voiding)
- Bladder sensations. normal and noxious
- Voluntary pelvic floor muscle function and reflexes
- Spinal cord reflexes. bulbocavernosus and anal
- Perineal dermatomes
- Sympathetic function in men. bladder neck state during bladder filling
- Erectile function

Obviously, every case is distinct and requires a dialogue between the teams to ensure the most pertinent information is considered. The case shown in Figure 16.30 was first referred to us by the neurosurgeons requesting identification of baseline functions, and another example is given in Figure 16.36.

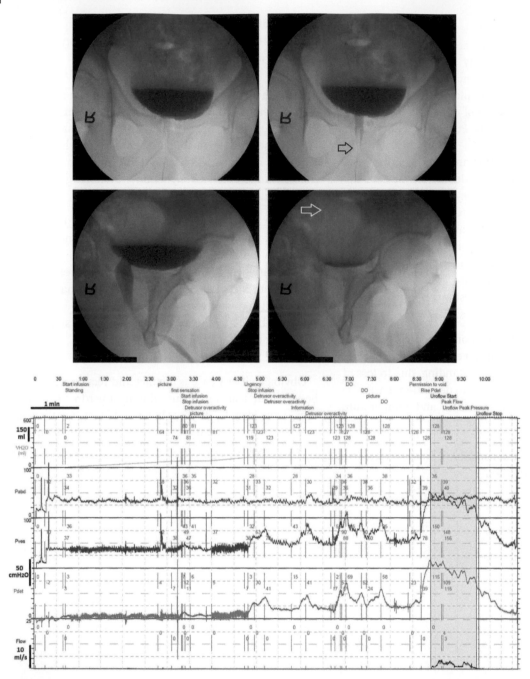

Figure 16.36 Urodynamic evaluation of a man awaiting spinal surgery to treat tethered cord syndrome, where the neurosurgeons wished to identify specific aspects of his neurological deficit and to record baseline prior to surgery. On history, he reported urinary urgency and frequency, with slow stream – rather varied symptoms; no incontinence; normal sexual function (erection and ejaculation). Sometimes, he uses sound of flow rather than feeling to identify passage of urine. On examination, he had reduced perianal sensation (pin prick), more obvious on right side than left. Urethral sensation: he described 'cold' rather than stinging when local anaesthetic antiseptic jelly was placed, suggesting change in sensory nerves. Initial free flow, slow stream, modest volume but with a post-void residual of 270 ml once catheterised. He was slightly difficult to catheterise due to a kink (not a stricture) in the penile urethra from previous minor trauma. This prevented us from doing a urethral pressure profile, as we had to use a Tiemann-tip double lumen catheter. There was clear detrusor overactivity (DO) during filling cystometry. The bladder neck was competent during the DO, until high-amplitude DO overcame the bladder neck, at which point the sphincter was able to resist leakage. Voiding: quite high pressure, suggesting bladder outlet obstruction, but imaging did not show a clear hold-up at bladder neck, prostate or sphincter, or a stricture, so this observation may have been due to the 6Fr catheter rather than real obstruction. SUMMARY: Sympathetic nervous system appears intact. Afferent nerves: partially impaired sacral dermatome and urethral sensation. Motor: sphincter is probably well innervated, but he does report occasional stress incontinence. This is more likely to be post-micturition dribble than sphincter weakness. Anal sphincter tone seemed reduced. Detrusor: overactive bladder during storage, due to reduced inhibition. Normal activity (high pressure but probably not reflecting true obstruction) during voiding. *Source*: Marcus Drake.

References

1. Gajewski, J.B., Schurch, B., Hamid, R. et al. (2018). An International Continence Society (ICS) report on the terminology for adult neurogenic lower urinary tract dysfunction (ANLUTD). *Neurourol. Urodyn.* 37 (3): 1152–1161.

2. Swain, S., Hughes, R., Perry, M., and Harrison, S., Guideline Development Group (2012). Management of lower urinary tract dysfunction in neurological disease: summary of NICE guidance. *BMJ* 345: e5074.

3. Podnar, S., Trsinar, B., and Vodusek, D.B. (2006). Bladder dysfunction in patients with cauda equina lesions. *Neurourol. Urodyn.* 25 (1): 23–31.

4. Ukkonen, M., Elovaara, I., Dastidar, P., and Tammela, T.L. (2004). Urodynamic findings in primary progressive multiple sclerosis are associated with increased volumes of plaques and atrophy in the central nervous system. *Acta Neurol. Scand.* 109 (2): 100–105.

5. Khastgir, J., Drake, M.J., and Abrams, P. (2007). Recognition and effective management of autonomic dysreflexia in spinal cord injuries. *Expert Opin. Pharmacother.* 8 (7): 945–956.

6. Fowler, C.J. and Griffiths, D.J. (2010). A decade of functional brain imaging applied to bladder control. *Neurourol. Urodyn.* 29 (1): 49–55.

7. Fowler, C., Griffiths, D., and de Groat, W. (2008). The neural control of micturition. *Nat. Rev. Neurosci.* 9: 453–466.

8. Abrams, P., Cardozo, L., Fall, M. et al. (2002). The standardisation of terminology of lower urinary tract function: report from the Standardisation Sub-committee of the International Continence Society. *Neurourol. Urodyn.* 21 (2): 167–178.

9. Khuu, T., Bagdasarian, G., Leung, J. et al. (2010). Estimating aminoglycoside clearance and creatinine clearance in underweight patients. *Am. J. Health Syst. Pharm.* 67 (4): 274–279.

10. Vaidyanathan, S., Soni, B., Oo, T. et al. (2012). Autonomic dysreflexia in a tetraplegic patient due to a blocked urethral catheter: spinal cord injury patients with lesions above T-6 require prompt treatment of an obstructed urinary catheter to prevent life-threatening complications of autonomic dysreflexia. *Int. J. Emerg. Med.* 5: 6.

11. Krassioukov, A., Warburton, D.E., Teasell, R., and Eng, J.J., Spinal Cord Injury Rehabilitation Evidence Research Team (2009). A systematic review of the management of autonomic dysreflexia after spinal cord injury. *Arch. Phys. Med. Rehabil.* 90 (4): 682–695.

12. Ausili, E., Tabacco, F., Focarelli, B. et al. (2007). Prevalence of latex allergy in spina bifida: genetic and environmental risk factors. *Eur. Rev. Med. Pharmacol. Sci.* 11 (3): 149–153.

13. Schneck, F.X. and Bellinger, M.F. (1993). The "innocent" cough or sneeze: a harbinger of serious latex allergy in children during bladder stimulation and urodynamic testing. *J. Urol.* 150 (2 Pt 2): 687–690.

14. Abrams, P., Agarwal, M., Drake, M. et al. (2008). A proposed guideline for the urological management of patients with spinal cord injury. *BJU Int.* 101 (8): 989–994.

15. Fowler, C.J., Panicker, J.N., Drake, M. et al. (2009). A UK consensus on the management of the bladder in multiple sclerosis. *J. Neurol. Neurosurg. Psychiatry* 80 (5): 470–477.

16. Drake, M.J., Cortina-Borja, M., Savic, G. et al. (2005). Prospective evaluation of urological effects of aging in chronic spinal cord injury by method of bladder management. *Neurourol. Urodyn.* 24 (2): 111–116.

17. Horst, M., Weber, D.M., Bodmer, C., and Gobet, R. (2011). Repeated Botulinum-A toxin injection in the treatment of neuropathic bladder dysfunction and poor bladder compliance in children with myelomeningocele. *Neurourol. Urodyn.* 30 (8): 1546–1549.

18. Drake, M.J., Apostolidis, A., Cocci, A. et al. (2016). Neurogenic lower urinary tract dysfunction: clinical management recommendations of the Neurologic Incontinence committee of the fifth International Consultation on Incontinence 2013. *Neurourol. Urodyn.* 35 (6): 657–665.

19. Biering-Sorensen, F., Craggs, M., Kennelly, M. et al. (2008). International urodynamic basic spinal cord injury data set. *Spinal Cord.* 46 (7): 513–516.

20. Jaggi, A., Drake, M., Siddiqui, E., and Fatoye, F. (2018). A comparison of the treatment recommendations for neurogenic lower urinary tract dysfunction in the national institute for health and care excellence, European Association of Urology and international consultations on incontinence guidelines. *Neurourol. Urodyn.* 37 (7): 2273–2280.

21. Ginsberg, D., Gousse, A., Keppenne, V. et al. (2012). Phase 3 efficacy and tolerability study of onabotulinumtoxin A for urinary incontinence from neurogenic detrusor overactivity. *J. Urol.* 187 (6): 2131–2139.

22. Wei, D.Y. and Drake, M.J. (2016). Undiagnosed neurological disease as a potential cause of male lower urinary tract symptoms. *Curr. Opin. Urol.* 26 (1): 11–16.

23. De Ridder, D., Van Der Aa, F., Debruyne, J. et al. (2013). Consensus guidelines on the neurologist's role in the management of neurogenic lower urinary tract dysfunction in multiple sclerosis. *Clin. Neurol. Neurosurg.* 115 (10): 2033–2040.

24. Pugliatti, M., Rosati, G., Carton, H. et al. (2006). The epidemiology of multiple sclerosis in Europe. *Eur. J. Neurol.* 13 (7): 700–722.

17

Urodynamics in Older People

Su-Min Lee[1] and Emily Henderson[2]

[1] *Department of Urology, Royal United Hospital, Bath, UK*
[2] *Population Health Sciences, Bristol Medical School, University of Bristol, Senate House, Bristol, UK*

CONTENTS

Many patients we investigate are over the age of 65 years; lower urinary tract symptoms (LUTS) in this group are a major cause of morbidity and affect the quality of life in both older men and women. As an individual ages, the urinary tract changes, even in the absence of pathological disease. The consequences may include a decline in detrusor function and bladder capacity, leading to increased urinary frequency, voiding LUTS, and poor bladder emptying in both men and women. Urodynamic findings in older people tend to demonstrate detrusor overactivity (DO), even in individuals that do not spontaneously report symptoms or bother [1].

Along with the other factors described in this book, decision-making in the surgical context for an older person specifically needs to factor in physiological changes that occur with ageing. Furthermore, any relevant comorbidity must be identified. Overall, it is important to determine the degree to which the patient is susceptible to harm versus the anticipated benefits of invasive investigations and a subsequent potential surgical approach. In these patients, use of urodynamics must be considered carefully, as a diagnosis may be of only passing interest rather than real value if subsequent treatments are unavailable due to the associated risk. Since urodynamics may be uncomfortable or upsetting for patients, carries a risk of urinary tract infection, and can be challenging for urodynamic staff, its use

should be justifiable. However, whilst older people are more vulnerable to negative outcomes, they potentially have a lot to gain from intervention, and therefore, this should never be denied simply on the basis of age. There is opportunity with effective investigation and treatment to mitigate negative health outcomes that are associated with incontinence, such as a sense of shame [2], falls and fractures [3], and functional deterioration [4]. Therefore, in the absence of using age criteria to guide investigation and treatment, what is the best approach to evaluating urological symptoms older people?

Understanding and Evaluating Frailty

Frailty is a multidimensional syndrome that confers an excess risk of negative outcomes. Whilst it is associated with age, it is not an inevitability of ageing, per se. People living with frailty lose physiological reserve, and consequently, the ability to cope with acute stressors may be compromised. In terms of everyday life, the progression can be indicated by the size of the spatial area a person purposely moves through in his/her daily life, as well as the frequency of travel within a specific time frame (known as their 'life space' [5]). With advancing age, this life space may become considerably more confined, leading to

---

decreased physical activity and social engagement, accelerated deconditioning, and exacerbated decline in physiological reserve, contributing to the development of clinical frailty and subsequent mortality [6].

Two approaches have been advocated to conceptualise frailty, with both being effective for prognostication. The 'deficit accumulation' method advocates summing a person's illnesses and disabilities [7] which in turn reproducibly predicts adverse outcomes and mortality [8]. This work has been the basis for the development of the pictorial Clinical Frailty Scale (CFS) which provides a semi-quantitative measure that can easily be applied in non-geriatric care settings [8]. The physiological approach to frailty classifies individual as robust, pre-frail, or frail on the basis of low grip strength, low energy, slowed waking speed, low physical activity, and unintentional weight loss [9]. Frailty is a dynamic state, and whilst a proportion of older individuals do progress from being pre-frail to frail, the trajectory is not necessarily linear, nor is it inevitable.

When clinicians 'eyeball' an older adult and determine frailty status, they are likely making their determination based on walking speed, weight, and potentially the burden of comorbidities and functional impairment from clinical examination and history taking. Whilst some frailty scales are lengthy and useful only in research settings, others such as the CFS and Timed Up and Go (TUG) [10] are accessible and quick. During a TUG, an individual is asked to stand up from a seated position in a chair, walk 10 ft at a normal pace (using a device like a walking stick if needed), turn around, walk back to the chair, and then sit back down. A time taken of 12 seconds or more may be considered slow and serves as an indicator of frailty. Whilst no standard tools are in routine use, measurement of frailty status will likely have utility not only in informing perioperative risk but also facilitating pre-habilitation and optimisation pre-surgery.

The Management Pathway in Older People

The fundamentals for managing older people are the same as for the others described in the book. Thus, each person needs history and examination (evaluation of LUTS [severity and bother], risk factors, and indicators to suggest serious underlying conditions), urinalysis, symptom scores, bladder diary, and flows with post-void residual (PVR) measurement, according to the nature of presentation. Specific attention should however be given to assessing the effect of LUTS on daily life, associated functional impairment as well as the wider psychosocial context. Conservative interventions are trialled before re-evaluating and considering whether more interventional therapy may be indicated. One key aspect for older adults is to take a clear-thinking line on the likelihood that the LUTS are multifactorial. If the LUTS are clear-cut and an individual is physically and cognitively robust and willing to consider intervention, then suitable treatment options, including surgery, should be pursued.

Urinalysis is routinely done in most clinics. However, bacteriuria and/or pyuria cannot confirm the diagnosis of a urinary tract infection because of high prevalence of asymptomatic bacteriuria in older people regardless of presentation [11]. Urine flow studies and assessment of PVR volumes are often helpful. Flow studies and PVR can help identify likelihood of significant outlet obstruction or detrusor underactivity (DUA). If a substantial PVR is seen, then it may be beneficial to treat this by intermittent self-catheterisation (or occasionally indwelling catheterisation), considering in parallel an individual's cognitive ability and dexterity when recommending this approach. Many older people may be troubled by recurrent infections made worse by failure to achieve proper bladder emptying; knowledge of the PVR in these patients will aid treatment. The bladder diary is a helpful way to identify key influences, notably fluid intake. Advice around fluid intake should always consider concurrent issues prevalent in older adults, such as heart failure and/or postural hypotension.

Initial management of LUTS should include a thorough history and examination, placing emphasis on reversible comorbidities, including infections, delirium, impaired mobility, bowel habits, and social and environmental factors. A holistic approach is absolutely paramount in older adults, recognising that the aetiology of LUTS is more often multifactorial. Several trials have combined pelvic floor training with physical interventions such as walking and cognitive interventions, with the positive effects extending to gait and cognition as well [12, 13].

Older individuals frequently have comorbid conditions, and the drugs used to treat them can impair continence via direct effects on lower urinary tract function or indirectly via influences on urine production or the central nervous system. Urinary incontinence might be precipitated by benzodiazepines, antidepressants, and antipsychotic medications, as a consequence of cognitive impairment, sedation, and instability. Hormone replacement therapies can occasionally be associated with urinary incontinence in postmenopausal women. Urinary retention can be a risk with use of anticholinergic drugs, tricyclic antidepressants, antipsychotic medications, and opioids. Some associations have also been reported between urinary incontinence and use of antihistamines, beta receptor agonists, angiotensin II receptor, and anticonvulsants (noting that a causal relationship was not

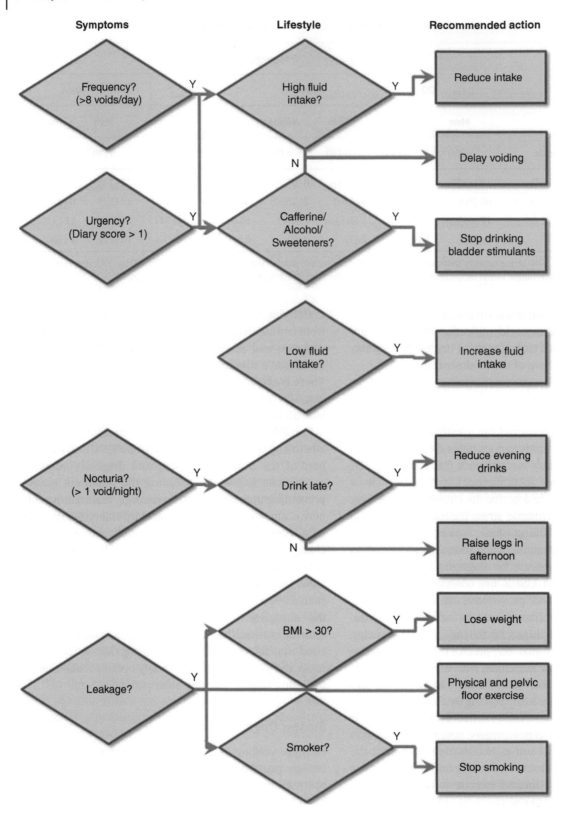

Figure 17.2 Flowchart of evidence-based self-managed action given on the basis of patient symptoms and lifestyle. This flowchart is intended for patients without pain, haematuria, pregnancy, heart disease, postural hypotension, or other medical issues. *Source:* Gammie [19]. © 2020, Wolters Kluwer Health, Inc. [19].

that BOO tends to present with. DUA increases in prevalence with ageing [22], and many guidelines advocate urodynamic testing in older men to exclude this possibility when considering surgery [23]. DUA may coexist with DO in many of these patients [22]. Thus, in patients with refractory symptoms, or previous episodes of urinary retention, urodynamics is an important adjunct. Voiding symptoms alone do not correlate well with diagnosis of BOO, largely due to overlap with DUA. Therefore, those suitable for surgery benefit from urodynamics to formalise this diagnosis. Patients with proven BOO have better outcomes following surgery, including transurethral resection of the prostate (TURP). Similarly, a diagnosis of OAB in the obstructed patient enables the clinician to appropriately counsel the patient regarding chances of symptom benefit and risk of postoperative urgency incontinence.

Therapy Decisions

LUTS in older people are multifactorial and related to physiological changes associated with ageing, urological diseases, neurological conditions, and polypharmacy. In the range of issues already affecting older people, the addi-

tional presence of LUTS can further decrease quality of life [24]. The therapeutic approach should be holistic, recognising where therapy focussed on the lower urinary tract can help, as opposed to the wider health and social circumstance of the individual. Comprehensive geriatric assessment (CGA) is a framework in which this can be successfully undertaken; it is a multidimensional, multidisciplinary diagnostic and therapeutic process to determine the medical, psychological, and functional capabilities of an older person and develop a coordinated and integrated plan for treatment and follow-up [25]. For example, people with dementia have LUTS even more frequently [26], but attempting to treat LUTS in isolation, without addressing mobility, function, fall risk, environment, care partner support, and prognosis is inadequate and unsatisfactory.

In terms of considering the utility of urodynamics in older people, the key issue is determining whether the outcomes will genuinely influence treatment that might lead to benefit. The LUTS-FORTA study reviewed the efficacy and safety of drugs used to treat LUTS in older patients, looking at 25 clinical trials that evaluated the use of 16 drugs of interest [27]. No drug was rated as indispensable. Only three were considered beneficial in frail older people: the 5α-reductase inhibitors dutasteride and finasteride and the antimuscarinic fesoterodine. Most drugs should be used with caution. Drugs that should be avoided in older people include alfuzosin, doxazosin, oxybutynin in standard dose/immediate release formulations, propiverine, and terazosin. Oxybutynin in extended-release and transdermal formulations can be used with caution, but studies in older adults are lacking, and there remains some concern about cognitive side effects. The specific issue with anticholinergics used to treat OAB is the cumulative anticholinergic burden on top of other medications, which increases the risk of dementia. This risk may be small overall [28], but more vulnerable individuals can experience a marked cognitive decline when initiated on one of these drugs. The few trials that have performed cognitive testing in healthy older people taking antimuscarinics suggest that oxybutynin can adversely affect cognition, while darifenacin, trospium, solifenacin, and tolterodine appear to have lower risk [29]. Caution is essential for people with early cognitive impairment or pre-existing dementia. In addition, increased risk of falls is reported [30], given the association between gait instability and cognitive function. Mirabegron does not place cognitive function at specific risk [31], but cardiovascular side effects should be considered in prescribing mirabegron for older people.

Our approach advocates the use of conservative measures before moving to a selective use of medications, only then considering invasive diagnostic testing specifically

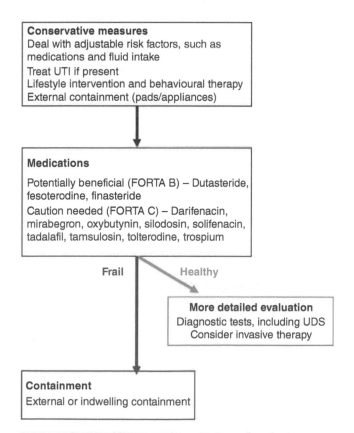

Figure 17.3 Considerations when treating incontinence in patients older than 65.

Part V

Running a Urodynamics Unit

18

Troubleshooting During Urodynamics

Laura Thomas[1], Rachel Tindle[1], and Andrew Gammie[2]

[1] *Urodynamics & Gastrointestinal Physiology, Southmead Hospital, Bristol, UK*
[2] *Bristol Urological Institute, Southmead Hospital, Bristol, UK*

CONTENTS

Urodynamic procedures are invasive and should only be used when the outcome is likely to change the subsequent treatment plan. Given the nature and the role of urodynamic procedures, it is imperative that they are conducted to the highest standard. Quality control checks should be used regularly throughout the procedure to ensure all pressure lines are reading correctly. Problems may emerge when the quality control check fails. Once an issue has been detected, the role of the urodynamic practitioner is to troubleshoot the problem in order to carry out remedial action while it is still possible.

The term 'troubleshoot' refers to the systematic approach of problem-solving. In urodynamics, it requires us to identify the problem, determine the cause, and establish ways to resolve it. Not all artefacts can be readily corrected. Some may have no impact on the overall trace, but in order to understand which ones to resolve, it is important to be able to identify the common patterns. This is a fundamental expectation of urodynamic practice [1–4]. Unfortunately, quality control evaluations identify that quality of testing still needs considerable improvement [5, 6].

This chapter aims to demonstrate some of the more common issues seen that can be resolved during a urodynamic test and present suggestions for the subsequent management of them. This has to be done by the urodynamic practitioner, since automated recognition by the equipment or software is still a long way from being adequate [7] (see below). The process of troubleshooting requires the practitioner to maintain a constant watch for issues. Troubleshooting challenges are described according to the stage of the urodynamic test at which they are most commonly seen. Table 18.1 provides an overall summary and is intended to be a handy guide for clinical use.

Prior to troubleshooting, you must ensure that you have set up your equipment correctly. The essential points to remember are:

- Ensure all channels have their calibration checked and are correctly connected;
- Zero all pressure transducers to atmospheric pressure;
- Ensure transducers are at the height of the symphysis pubis throughout the procedure; and
- Quality control checks should be done throughout the procedure: ensure cough tests are done, observe the fine movements in the pressure traces, and check the resting pressures.

Abrams' Urodynamics, Fourth Edition. Edited by Marcus Drake, Hashim Hashim, and Andrew Gammie.
© 2021 John Wiley & Sons Ltd. Published 2021 by John Wiley & Sons Ltd.

For catheter-tip systems, unequal transmission may be caused by poor positioning or setup of the catheter. In these cases, repositioning, resetting, or replacing the catheter should resolve the issue.

It has been proposed that a cough test can be deemed 'passed' if the smaller pressure response is more than 70% of the larger response (cough test C in Figure 18.1 [5]). This tolerance is sufficient to account for variations in connection tube dimensions and in the precise timing of data acquisition.

Resting Pressures

When the bladder and abdominal muscles are at rest, there should be a steady pressure within the body cavity determined by surrounding muscle tension, body weight, and abdominal organs resting on the pelvic organs. From experience, the normal range of such pressures is 5–20 cmH$_2$O when supine, 15–40 cmH$_2$O when seated, and 30–50 cmH$_2$O in the standing position, for both p$_{ves}$ and p$_{abd}$ [1, 2]. At rest, these pressures should be equal, so p$_{det}$ should be very close (within 5 cmH$_2$O) to zero. If this is not the case, and the cough tests are satisfactory, then further troubleshooting is required. This may involve re-zeroing to atmosphere, check-

ing transducer height, or reviewing the catheters' function or position. Displaced catheters can be detected through variations in resting pressure, often confined to a single line. Figure 18.3 shows a sequence of troubleshooting where this is evident.

If the problem persists despite all troubleshooting, the issue may be that the catheter is affected by proximity to the organ (rather than being free in the lumen). This is quite common when the bladder is empty, in which case starting filling may quickly achieve acceptable pressure transmission (Figure 7.28).

Gradual descent of resting pressures during a test, as seen on Figure 18.4, should not occur. Any such changes may be due to a leak in the system or movement of a catheter-tip system. Alternatively, rectal contractions may remove water from the rectal balloon, reducing contact with the patient. In this case, a flush with water should restore tissue contact and normal pressure readings.

Live Signal

Small variations in pressure on both p$_{abd}$ and p$_{ves}$ should be seen throughout the urodynamic test, since breathing, talking, and other patient activity will cause slight internal

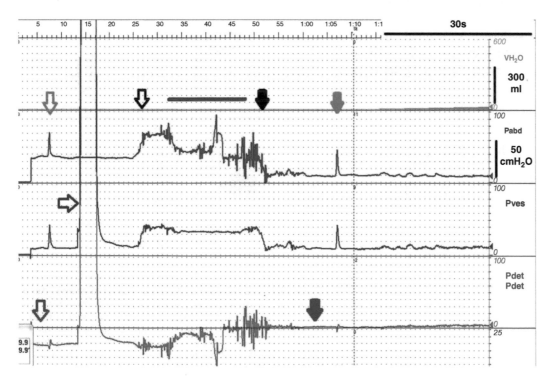

Figure 18.3 Unequal resting pressures are present at the start of the trace with an unacceptable p$_{det}$ reading (open red arrow); p$_{abd}$ is just over 30 cmH$_2$0 and p$_{ves}$ is 10 cmH$_2$0. A cough test (open orange arrow) shows good subtraction and indicates how a cough test alone is sometimes insufficient to indicate a problem with pressure recording. Flushing the p$_{ves}$ line (blue arrow) did not correct this problem, so it was decided to re-site the rectal catheter higher into the rectum, in case the high pressure reading indicated the recording was from the anal canal rather than the rectum. To do this, the patient was asked to stand up open (black arrow), and the catheter was advanced carefully (purple line); the p$_{abd}$ pressure clearly reduced down to the level of the p$_{ves}$ reading during this process. The short sharp frequency spikes indicate movement on the catheter as a result of the manipulation required. The patient then sat down again (closed black arrow). After this sequence of troubleshooting, the resting pressures are equal, producing a p$_{det}$ close to zero (closed red arrow), while a cough test demonstrates good pressure transmission has been maintained (closed orange arrow).

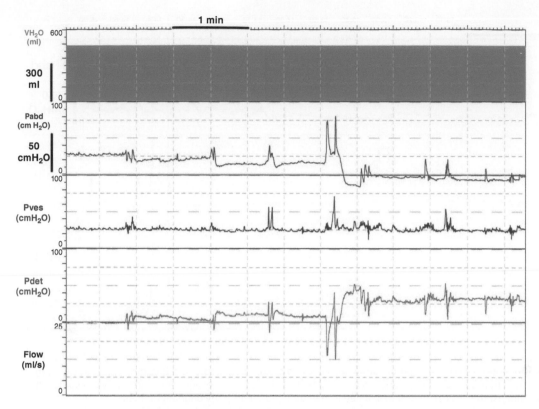

Figure 18.4 Within this section of a filling cystometry, there is a gradual reduction in p_{abd} pressure, to the point where it falls below zero. This results in an apparent p_{det} increase of approximately 25 cmH_2O, but that value is meaningless, since it is not due to bladder contraction. There is nothing physiological that would cause this reduction in abdominal pressure throughout the filling phase, and therefore, the issue needs to be addressed and rectified by checking for any leaks in the abdominal pressure recording apparatus (catheter, connection tubing, connections, etc.), whether the catheter has shifted position, and whether the connection to the flushing syringe has been left open.

pressure changes. Such live signal, being equal on both lines, should be cancelled out when subtracting to obtain p_{det}. If either p_{abd} or p_{ves} stay completely flat, even if within normal resting pressure ranges, this would indicate a problem with pressure transmission from the patient (Figures 18.5 and 18.6). This is normally corrected by flushing the catheter, or occasionally catheter repositioning might be necessary.

Leaks

If flushing with water does not rectify the transmission problem identified by a cough test, the issue may be with leakage from one of the tubing connections. If this is suspected, all connections between catheter, tubing, and transducer should be checked for leaks. A leakage problem may alternatively cause a slow descent in pressure, a situation rectified by dealing with the leak and refilling the system.

Catheter Positioning

If unequal transmission of coughs continues, then catheter positions must be checked. Either the bladder or the rectal catheter may have slipped down into the respective sphincter region, causing a pressure transmission problem. This is rather more common with the rectal catheter, which can be difficult to keep in position, especially in patients with poor anal function. A gradual drifting of the rectal catheter reading is visible in Figure 18.5 and can produce a confusing picture, with p_{abd} falling slowly, leading to an apparent increase in p_{det}. Alternatively, p_{abd} may rise as the balloon approaches the anal sphincter, leading to a fall on the p_{det} trace. Examination of the p_{ves} line will show that intravesical pressure is constant, and this reveals the necessity of dealing with the problematic abdominal line.

A different problem relates to observation of identical pressure readings from the two lines. This may indicate that both catheters are recording in the same space. This is more likely if the vagina is being used for recording abdominal pressure. It could indicate that attempted urethral catheterisation has been unsuccessful, and so the p_{ves} catheter is actually in the vagina (Figure 18.7). It is therefore important that the catheter is visualised going into the urethra on catheterisation, ensuring entry to the meatus, and that it does not spring out when it is advanced. Alternatively, a urethro-vaginal fistula may have allowed the vesical catheter to divert into the vagina. A vesico-vaginal fistula may lead to equalisation of pressures between the two organs, with extra-urethral urinary leakage.

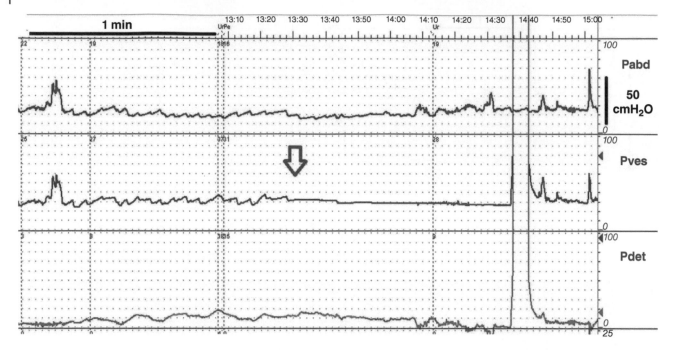

Figure 18.5 The loss of live signal can occur at any point during a urodynamic test. Here, the live signal appears to be lost from the p_{ves} line approximately 13:30 minutes into the test (purple arrow), as indicated by the flattening of the line, having previously been working. The problem is rectified by a flush of the p_{ves} line, which restores the live signal. A subsequent cough test is picked up better by the p_{abd} line than the p_{ves} line, so the vesical recording still needs monitoring to identify any ongoing problem.

The vesical catheter used for pressure recording in urodynamics is very small (6 Fr or less), similar in size to a ureteric stent. Luckily, the direction of entry from urethra into bladder is in the midline, while the ureteric orifices are to the side (Figure 2.1). However, if a nodule or deformation in the bladder outlet causes the p_{ves} catheter to deviate to the side, in theory it can enter the ureter. This is exceptionally rare but is a recognised possibility (Figure 18.8) [8]. When it happens, ureteric peristalsis may be visible, comprising short-duration phasic pressure changes in p_{ves} at intervals of about

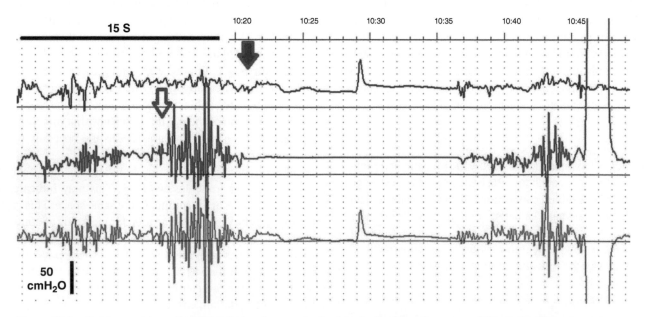

Figure 18.6 Problems arising when the catheters became trapped under the legs of an overweight person. The open red arrow indicates the start of a considerable amount of disruption due to the knocking of the p_{abd} tube from the movement of the patient on the seat. The solid red/blue arrow is the point at which the fine detail was lost from both p_{abd} and p_{ves} recordings as a result of occlusion. The alert urodynamicist identified the problem quickly and so occlusion only lasted about 15 seconds.

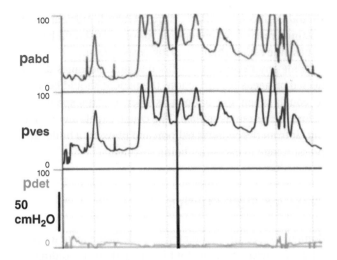

Figure 18.7 The remarkable similarity of p_{ves} and p_{abd} readings on this study is because the p_{ves} catheter had not successfully been placed in the bladder and was actually in the vagina, alongside the p_{abd} catheter.

transmission, the patient will experience excruciating pain radiating to the loin, which immediately indicates the problem. The catheter will have to be repositioned, and the patient may well feel unable to continue with the test.

Empty Bladder Pressure Readings

Poor pressure transmission or unusual resting pressure may be seen when the bladder is empty (see Figure 7.28). If there is no fluid surrounding the catheter tip, or if the bladder wall can press around the catheter, it may not be possible to read true pressure. If there is no other obvious cause for poor transmission at the start of a test, 50 ml should be infused into the bladder and a cough test repeated. If this fails to resolve the issue, the catheter should be replaced.

10–20 seconds. Changes in p_{abd} should not directly be apparent, but if there is associated discomfort, the patient may get restless with pain, leading to indirect change in p_{abd} (Figure 18.8). If the catheter is flushed to improve pressure

Tube Obstruction

Unequal pressure transmission or abnormally high pressures may be observed if the catheter tube or connection tubing is kinked or compressed. This can happen if the wheel of a trolley is squashing tubing externally, if the patient is sat on a tube (Figure 18.6), or if there is a kink –

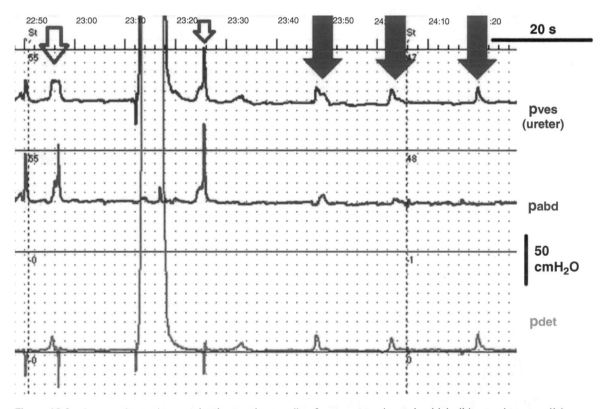

Figure 18.8 A p_{ves} catheter that was inadvertently recording from a ureter. A cough which did not subtract well (open red arrow) led the urodynamicist to flush the catheter. This resulted in severe unilateral loin pain. The cough after the flush (purple arrow) subtracts fairly well, so it is clear that intraureteric recording does pick up abdominal pressure changes. The closed red arrows indicate low-amplitude phasic contractions from ureteric peristalsis; these caused the patient notable pain, so the patient bent over in discomfort, hence leading to an associated small change in p_{abd} (an indirect consequence of ureteric peristalsis).

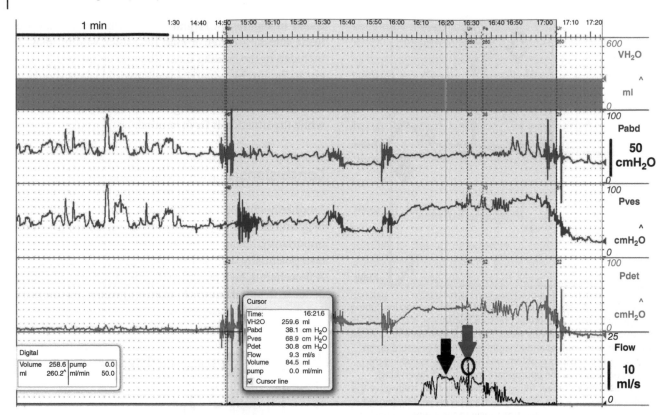

Figure 18.12 Pressure-flow studies are common time for errors to occur due to automatic analyses, where they can badly affect the interpretation of outlet function. In this case, the machine again places Q_{max} on a spike in the flow, as indicated by the red arrow. Consequently, Q_{max} is given a misleading value by the machine, and, furthermore, the machine takes $p_{detQmax}$ at the wrong moment; this double error makes values of indices like the bladder outlet obstruction index unreliable unless properly scrutinised by the urodynamicist. In this case, the Q_{max} was adjusted by the urodynamicist to the location indicated by the black arrow to give a reliable Q_{max} and appropriately timed $p_{detQmax}$.

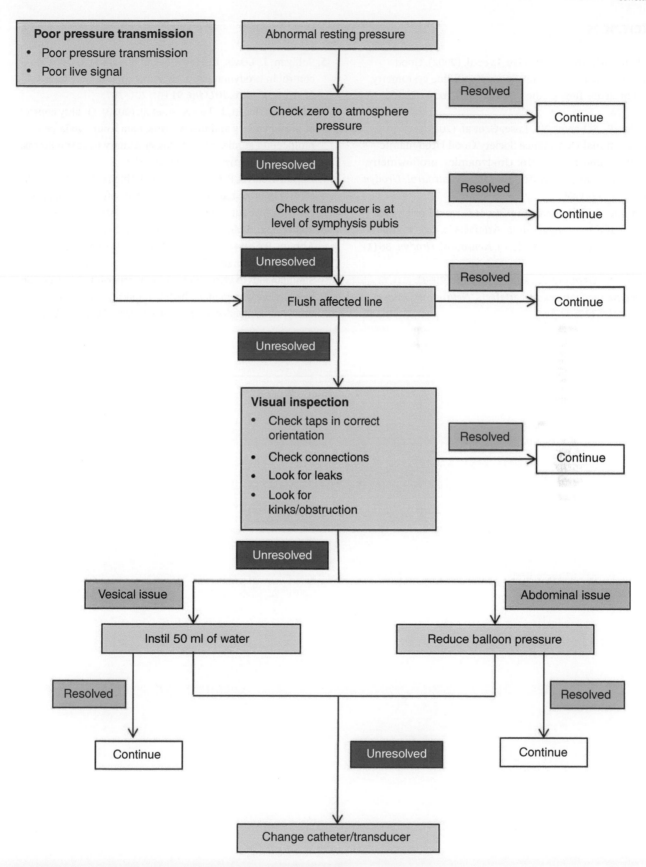

Figure 18.13 A flowchart for troubleshooting during urodynamics.

References

1. Schafer, W., Abrams, P., Liao, L. et al. (2002). Good urodynamic practices: uroflowmetry, filling cystometry, and pressure-flow studies. *Neurourol. Urodyn.* 21 (3): 261–274.

2. Rosier, P., Schaefer, W., Lose, G. et al. (2017). International Continence Society Good Urodynamic Practices and Terms 2016: Urodynamics, uroflowmetry, cystometry, and pressure-flow study. *Neurourol. Urodyn.* 36 (5): 1243–1260.

3. Gammie, A., D'Ancona, C., Kuo, H.C., and Rosier, P.F. (2017). ICS teaching module: Artefacts in urodynamic pressure traces (basic module). *Neurourol. Urodyn.* 36 (1): 35–36.

4. Hogan, S., Gammie, A., and Abrams, P. (2012). Urodynamic features and artefacts. *Neurourol. Urodyn.* 31 (7): 1104–1117.

5. Sullivan, J., Lewis, P., Howell, S. et al. (2003). Quality control in urodynamics: a review of urodynamic traces from one Centre. *BJU Int.* 91 (3): 201–207.

6. Aiello, M., Jelski, J., Lewis, A. et al. (2020). Quality control of uroflowmetry and urodynamic data from two large multicenter studies of male lower urinary tract symptoms. *Neurourol. Urodyn.* 39 (4): 1170–1177.

7. Hogan, S., Jarvis, P., Gammie, A., and Abrams, P. (2011). Quality control in urodynamics and the role of software support in the QC procedure. *Neurourol. Urodyn.* 30 (8): 1557–1564.

8. Malde, S. and Moore, J.A.: Re: Hogan S, Gammie A, Abrams P. (2014). *Neurourol. Urodyn.* 33 (7): 1171–1173.

9. Gammie, A., Abrams, P., Bevan, W. et al. (2016). Simultaneous in vivo; comparison of water-filled and air-filled pressure measurement catheters: implications for good urodynamic practice. *Neurourol. Urodyn.* 35 (8): 926–933.

19

Artefacts in Urodynamics

Andrew Gammie

Bristol Urological Institute, Southmead Hospital, Bristol, UK

A dictionary definition of an artefact is 'something not naturally present, but which occurs as a result of the procedure'. In the context of urodynamics, this means that the signal observed is not simply the pressure or flow generated by the bladder and bladder outlet but contains extraneous features that must be recognised as such and disregarded. The importance of discerning fact from artefact is a fundamental requirement of urodynamics [1–6]; it is crucial for understanding the patient's lower urinary tract function and avoiding spurious conclusions that could have very bad consequences if they lead to inappropriate treatment.

This book tries to give sufficient practical detail to enable the urodynamicist to generate high-quality traces and avoid measurement artefacts. Measurement artefacts are produced by problems in the equipment, somewhere between the tip of the catheters and the display. Setting up the equipment properly will uncover and deal with most of these problems. Modern electronic equipment is reliable, but if there are problems with the transducers or the urodynamic equipment after proper calibration and zero setting procedures have been followed, then the agent or manufacturer will have to help.

Some artefacts that occur during urodynamics must be resolved during the test, and these are described in Chapter 18 on Troubleshooting. There are a number of other artefacts which cannot be easily resolved during the test, and thus may trick the urodynamicist when reviewing the trace. We divide these latter artefacts according to the test in which they occur and their cause, as set out below.

Artefacts During Flow

'Cruising'

An obvious artefact is caused by the patient moving their stream in relation to the central exit from the collecting funnel. This is usually a male patient since the penis enables him to steer the stream around the funnel. Figure 19.1 illustrates some good examples. The 'peaks' occur when the point of impact of the stream is moving down the side of the funnel towards the central exit; that is, the urine being passed is catching up with the urine passed immediately before. The 'valleys' occur when the impact point is moving away from the exit. Usually, the 'peaks' will fit into the 'valleys' in this type of tracing. Manufacturers have attempted to minimise this phenomenon by complex baffles in the funnel, although a better solution might be to paint a target onto the funnel for the patient to aim at.

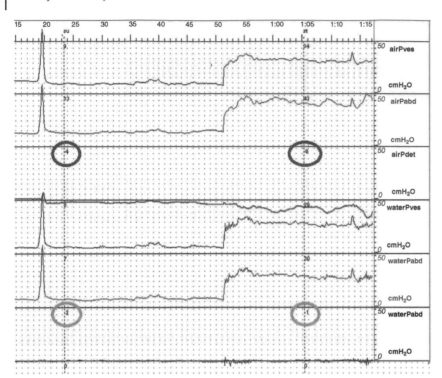

Figure 19.11 A patient with both air-filled (upper three lines) and water-filled (lower three lines) catheters changed position from supine to standing at 50 s. The change in the p_{det} values for air-filled was from $-4\,cmH_2O$ to $-9\,cmH_2O$ (red circles), reflecting the change in the relative positions of the two catheter balloons. The change in the p_{det} values for water-filled was only from $-2\,cmH_2O$ to $-1\,cmH_2O$ (green circles), since in this case the pressures were measured by transducers at the same level, i.e. level with the symphysis pubis.

As with a flush, this high pressure should be ignored, and if necessary, marked to avoid later misinterpretation.

Catheter Movement (Catheter-Tip Transducers)

Since in air-filled and microtip systems, the pressure is measured at the tip of the catheters, any change in position of the tip of the catheter within the patient will affect the reading, even though absolute patient pressures have not changed. Where slippage of the catheter is known to have occurred, an explanatory marker should be placed on the trace so that changes in pressure readings at that point can be ignored. For the same reason, when the patient moves from supine to seated or standing, the relative position of the two catheter tips will change due to rotation of the pelvis, causing an artefactual change in p_{det}, which is exemplified in Figure 19.11. Such a change should be scrutinised carefully in case there is real detrusor activity occurring. If it is judged not to be caused by the detrusor, then the change in resting pressure resulting from the movement must be taken into account when interpreting.

Artefacts During Pressure-Flow Studies

Drop in p_{abd} During Voiding

For reasons not fully understood, the abdominal pressure recorded during voiding can sometimes be seen to drop, an

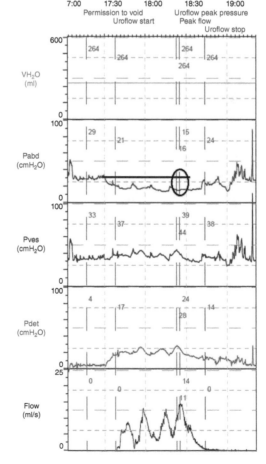

Figure 19.12 The p_{abd} line has dropped by $14\,cmH_2O$ during voiding; thus, p_{det} should be decreased from 24 to $10\,cmH_2O$, since it can be assumed that the p_{abd} drop is local to the balloon and is not involving the bladder as well.

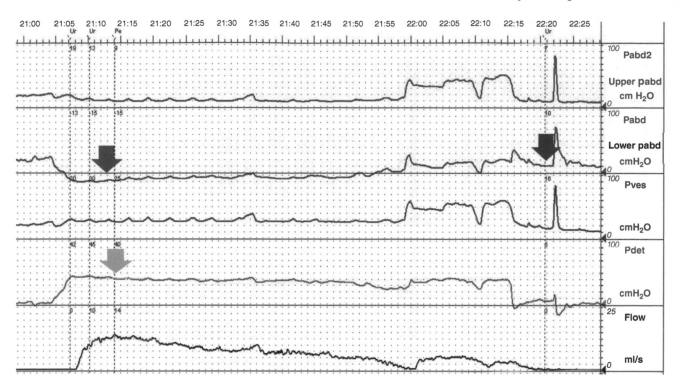

Figure 19.13 A void where two different catheters are measuring abdominal pressure, the upper trace (p_{abd2}) being an extra line that is deeper in the rectum than the lower line (p_{abd}), the latter being used to calculate p_{det}. The lower abdominal trace shows a significant pressure drop during voiding (red arrow), which returns to normal value after voiding (blue arrow) and which is seen in neither the upper abdominal trace nor the vesical line. Hence, we can assume that this drop is local to the lower p_{abd} catheter. This pressure drop should therefore be compensated for when calculating p_{det}. Here, $p_{detQmax}$ is 40 (green arrow), but as the p_{abd} line drops by 35 cmH$_2$O, the true value is only 5 cmH$_2$O. This changes the diagnosis from normal contractility to poor contractility.

example of which is shown in Figure 19.12. This may be due to pelvic floor relaxation, or due to more general changes within the whole abdomen. Current practice is to assume it is a temporary artefact local to the p_{abd} catheter tip. Hence, when calculating $p_{detQmax}$, we should decrease the p_{det} value by the amount p_{abd} has fallen from its value immediately prior to voiding. This approach is supported by the situation in Figure 19.13, where the upper trace shows an abdominal line which is deeper in the rectum than the lower abdominal trace, and which varies less during the void.

Straining

Another issue not fully understood is that the recording of pressure during strained voiding (or during a Valsalva manoeuvre) can be different on the two lines (p_{abd} and p_{ves}). It may be that the rectal pressure is imperfectly transmitted when the balloon is squeezed, or that the position of the rectal wall is changed by the pressure of other organs. Whatever the cause, p_{det} during a significant abdominal strain should not be treated as fully reliable. If the patient

is able to void without straining, they should be asked to do so. Figure 19.14 shows how straining with this artefact makes interpretation difficult.

Expelled Catheter and Loss of Live Signal During Void

During voiding, pressure may be enough to expel one of the catheters from the body (the p_{ves} catheter, if there is a detrusor contraction, and either of the p_{ves} and p_{abd} catheters, if there is straining). The display will show a sudden drop in pressure on that line, after which pressure changes will no longer be recorded, as seen in Figure 19.15. In other cases, it may be that the live signal disappears during the void. This may be recognised, for instance, by the p_{ves} signal appearing flat and unresponsive (Figure 19.16), likely due to occlusion by the bladder wall. If this means that the pressures at the Q_{max} point are not reliable, and if these are vital to answering the urodynamic question, it may be necessary to repeat the pressure-flow study, paying close attention to securing the catheter in position.

surgery such as an anterior resection for bowel cancer. The real skill is in managing expectation, changing the focus of treatment from an operation to behavioural change and all the time having a complete focus on quality of life as the main marker of success.

Anorectal Physiology

Anorectal physiology encompasses a variety of diagnostic tests which assess the function, sensitivity, and autonomic reflexes of the anorectum. The tests provide valuable information for pre-surgical assessments, including potential stoma reversals. But their true strength comes when combined with a thorough clinical history and other diagnostic tests to help guide conservative treatments such as biofeedback.

Tests are performed by registered Clinical GI Physiologists or Clinical Scientists, as well as specialist nursing staff, and provide precise clinical measurements to be used in patient decision-making. Additional to this, those conducting the procedures are involved in a more holistic patient care, involving conservative treatment. Current UK National Institute for Health and Clinical Excellence (NICE) guidelines recommend that patients attend biofeedback therapy prior to any surgical intervention [2], and this change in guidance has resulted in a large increase in referrals. NICE guidelines also recommend biofeedback for patients suffering with obstructive defecation and constipation associated with faecal incontinence. The role of the physiologist has therefore become more varied and now represents core membership within pelvic floor multidisciplinary teams.

Indications for Anorectal Physiology

Anorectal physiology testing is potentially indicated in a range of situations:

1) *Pelvic organ prolapse.* The majority of patients are post-menopausal women who have been through childbirth. The commonest symptom is faecal incontinence. Other evacuatory disorders requiring investigation include constipation, obstructed defecation, pelvic floor dysfunction (anismus and vaginismus), and pelvic pain.
2) *Systemic conditions.* Patients at risk of evacuatory disorders include those with systemic neurological disorders (i.e. multiple sclerosis) and congenital anomalies such as Hirschsprung's disease. More commonly, pregnancy and childbirth can result in neurological damage to the pudendal nerve. The point at which the nerve exits Alcock's canal can result in a disproportionate stretch and cause permanent neurological damage. This results

in denervation to pelvic floor muscles and weakness of the endopelvic fascia that supports them, which contribute to tissue laxity and impair the ability to evacuate effectively. Also, patients with diabetes mellitus and collagen disorders may be at increased risk of developing rectal prolapse or symptoms of obstructed defecation.

3) *Trauma.* Perineal trauma (accidental, obstetric, or surgical) may lead to an evacuatory disorder requiring this investigation. Similarly, a past history of radical pelvic irradiation may result in impaired evacuation.
4) *Adjunctive use in biofeedback therapy.* Increasingly, biofeedback therapy is used in order to retrain the pelvic floor musculature in a conservative, non-surgical manner. Utilising anorectal physiology in order to identify the maximum rectal volume tolerated has been shown to be effective in patients with urge incontinence over regular follow-up sessions.

Anorectal Manometry

Anorectal manometry (ARM) is the most well-known component of anorectal physiology; however, unlike urodynamics for the urinary tract, it is limited by its lack of standardisation. Both equipment and procedure protocols vary across departments, with individual centres using their own normative data. Regardless of this, there are a subset of manoeuvres and tests which have high clinical utility.

Essential components of equipment for ARM include a rectal catheter for insertion (air-filled, solid state, or water-perfused), pressure transducers to measure manometric pressure, and a device on which they can be visualised. Water-perfused catheters require a closed pressurised system (Figure 20.2). Catheter perfusion ports are arranged circumferentially in a spiral configuration, and non-latex balloons are also attached at the distal end. The large number of ports and the catheter configuration means that the profile of the entire sphincter can be built up both radially and longitudinally, requiring less catheter manipulation than is needed for urethral pressure profilometry. The balloon is inflated with either air or water to assess first and urge sensations, as well as the maximum tolerated volume.

To ensure accurate measurements, calibration should be checked regularly. In recent years, there has been a shift to high-resolution anorectal manometry (HR-ARM) as research has demonstrated its strong correlation with standard ARM and superiority in displaying anatomical details [3].

Preparing the equipment and environment is fairly straightforward. Figures 20.2 and 20.3 demonstrate how the water-perfused catheter is attached to the pressure transducers via a Luer-lock system and the type of

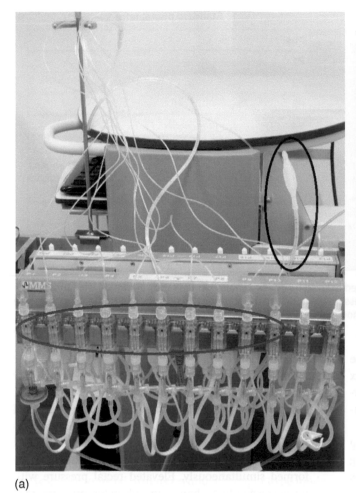
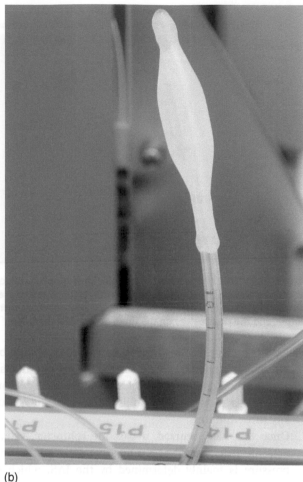

(a) (b)

Figure 20.2 This picture shows a water-perfused system, with the 10-channel anorectal catheter attached to 10 correspondingly numbered transducers (circled in red). These transducers can be easily removed or replaced at regular intervals or if there is any concern about their reliability. At the bottom of the first transducer, it is possible to see the filter (brown circular object); this should also be changed at regular intervals. The tip of the balloon catheter is circled in black and is deflated ready for intubation; it is seen in close-up on the right. *Source*: Marcus Drake.

information generated. It is imperative that this is done correctly to prevent water leaks at the point of connection. Water is perfused, at a set rate, through each of the individual water channels that make up the catheter. Zeroing against atmospheric pressure should be performed before every procedure; this can be done by holding the catheter externally at the anal verge and then selecting the zero function on your device.

Procedure

Prior to any invasive diagnostic procedure, a full clinical history is taken. This provides the clinician with crucial information regarding the patient's symptomatology, allowing investigations to be tailored appropriately. A pre-consultation completed bowel diary and questionnaire is also reviewed, and when ready, full written consent is obtained. Generally, no bowel preparation is required prior

to ARM; however, enemas can be utilised if the rectum is loaded as this can impede intubation.

Digital rectal examination (DRE) is advocated at the beginning of the test to assess resting tone and determine patient comprehension of squeeze and strain manoeuvres. The clinical importance of a DRE in the assessment of resting tone has however been questioned, with little support [4]. Examinations should identify scar tissue, prolapsing mucosa, or stool which may hinder intubation or increase the likelihood of bowel perforation. Any marked external abnormalities such as haemorrhoids or excoriation should be reported.

The International Anorectal Physiology Working Group has developed a standardised testing protocol for HR-ARM procedures which outlines the study protocol, including important periods of rest and recovery [5]. The procedure uses a variety of manoeuvres to review anorectal function, and all comparative 'normal' values are dependent on equipment type used.

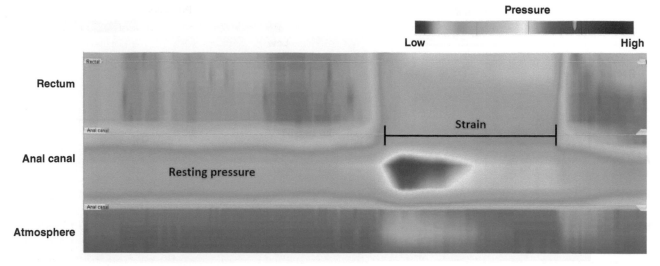

Figure 20.6 During simulated defaecation through straining, the patient produces an increased pressure in their rectum, which should be associated with a fall in anal pressure. In this case, the patient increased the pressure within their anal canal (identified by the red area), so is likely to struggle to empty their bowels efficiently. Patients with this finding often present with symptoms of obstructive defecation. *Source*: Marcus Drake.

Conservative Treatment

There has been an increased demand for conservative methods of managing patients with bowel dysfunctions [2], and therefore, anorectal physiology services have evolved to include bowel management advice, biofeedback, and percutaneous tibial nerve stimulation (PTNS).

Biofeedback

Biofeedback therapy involves ARM-guided pelvic floor retraining. It requires patients to commit to a series of follow-up sessions and uses visual aids to help retrain muscle behaviour. With catheters in situ, the patient is asked to perform manoeuvres and visualise the resulting pressure changes.

Individuals who are unable to reduce anal canal pressure during defecation should be able to visualise the incremental increase in pressure and practice relaxation techniques to counteract it. Recent studies report biofeedback as a treatment tool for reducing symptoms of constipation [13, 14], in turn reducing urinary symptoms in individuals presenting with combined pelvic floor dysfunction [15].

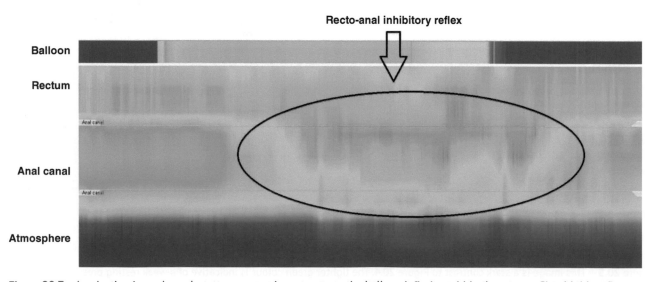

Figure 20.7 A reduction in anal canal pressure occurs in response to the balloon inflation within the rectum. Should this reflex occur prior to a patient's first sensation, then there is a risk of passive faecal incontinence due to the reduced anal canal pressure. The resting pressure returns (green band, right side) once the air has been removed from the balloon. *Source*: Marcus Drake.

Neuromodulation

Sacral neuromodulation (SNM) is an invasive technique widely used in the treatment of faecal incontinence. It involves a test phase, which if successful leads on to the implantation of a permanent lead and battery. A Cochrane review has demonstrated its efficacy through improvements in patient incontinence scores [16, 17]; however, it is associated with high-cost consumables. PTNS is a less invasive method of peripheral neuromodulation which involves inserting a single needle electrode posterior to the medial malleolus on the inner side of the ankle, thus stimulating the tibial nerve. Sessions last for 30 minutes, once a week for 12 weeks. However, a major trial randomising against sham therapy found PTNS given for 12 weeks did not confer significant clinical benefit in the treatment of adults with faecal incontinence [18].

Management of Colorectal Pelvic Floor Patients

Rectocoele

A rectocoele is a protrusion of the rectal wall, usually anteriorly through the posterior vaginal wall, though occasionally it may occur posteriorly. It is a common condition and usually affects postmenopausal women who have experienced vaginal childbirth. Patients may complain of a 'bulge' in the vagina on defecation or incomplete evacuation as stool becomes trapped in the protrusion. The condition may be worsened by chronic constipation, leading to the need to press on ('digitate') the protrusion in order to evacuate effectively. It is essential to assess the impact of this condition on the patient's quality of life, as size of rectocoele does not always correlate with severity of symptoms.

Management of this condition is generally undertaken in the domain of urogynaecology and female urology. Surgical treatment may involve a posterior vaginal wall repair employing direct plication, with or without use of a mesh patch, though most vaginal prolapse mesh kits have been withdrawn from use due to the increasing reports of significant complication. Frequently, however, rectocoele may overlap with other pelvic floor disorders such as vaginal/uterine prolapse, cystocoele, and/or rectoanal intussusception. In these scenarios, therefore, a posterior wall repair may not be sufficient to improve the patient's symptoms, and other surgical treatments may need to be considered. The importance of multidisciplinary working between colorectal surgeons, urogynaecologists, and urologists is imperative for the successful outcome of surgery that affects different compartments of the pelvic floor.

Anismus

This failure of the puborectalis muscle to relax during defecation is more common in the younger, female population. Anismus or dyssynergic defecation is thought to be an acquired behavioural problem with an unclear aetiology. Patients will usually complain of constipation, straining, and incomplete evacuation, sometimes requiring digitation. In one-third of patients, symptoms began in childhood.

Management involves pelvic floor investigations which may include a detailed history, stool diaries, careful DRE, defecating proctogram, ARM. Examination under anaesthetic may be required if examination in clinic is not possible. This ensures that rectoanal intussusception (Figure 20.8) is ruled out as a possible cause.

A holistic approach to care is vital for this group of patients. There is a high degree of overlap with other conditions, notably other GI problems (e.g. irritable bowel syndrome) and mental health disorders such as anxiety. It is advisable to assess patients jointly with a dietician and/ or a clinical psychologist. First-line treatment should include dietary recommendations to improve stool consistency so as to aid evacuation – adequate hydration, dietary assessment, fibre supplements, and use of enemas/laxatives as necessary.

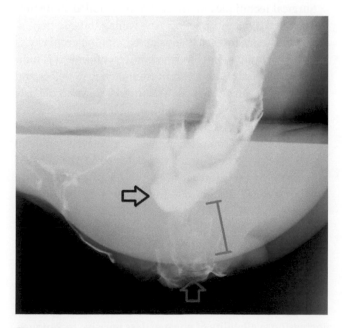

Figure 20.8 Proctogram showing the rectum (black arrow), anal canal (orange bar), and a rectoanal intussusception with external prolapse (red arrow). *Source*: Marcus Drake.

Targeted biofeedback is a useful adjunct with the aim of retraining the bowel in effective relaxation. Surgery is not recommended for this condition, although some centres have had success with injection of botulinum toxin [19].

External and Internal Rectal Prolapse

Rectal prolapse refers to the full-thickness protrusion of the lower rectal wall through the anus. It is a socially debilitating condition and is more common in postmenopausal women. Internal rectal prolapse refers to the prolapse of mucosa and/or muscle within the rectum, which is thought to be a precursor to the development of external rectal prolapse. It may be diagnosed clinically or radiologically (fluoroscopy and dynamic magnetic resonance imaging [MRI]) and classified using the Oxford Rectal Prolapse Grade from I (high rectal, prolapse descends no lower than top of rectocoele) to V (external rectal prolapse through anus) [20]. Symptoms include obstructed defecation, excessive straining, and faecal incontinence.

Traditionally, surgery has involved an abdominal approach (posterior rectopexy) or perineal procedures such as Delorme's/Altemeier's procedures (plication/resection of the protruding muscle). One study has reported no difference in outcomes between these techniques [21], but elsewhere recurrence rates of up to 50% have been reported [22]. More recently, improved recurrence rates have been seen with laparoscopic ventral mesh rectopexy introduced by the Leuven, Oxford, and Bristol groups [23]. This technique involves laparoscopic abdominal surgery with anterior dissection of the rectal prolapse to the level of the perineal body. A mesh, which may be synthetic or biological, is sutured to the perineal body and fixed to the sacral promontory (Figure 20.9). The rectovaginal septum and uterosacral suspensory mechanism are restored using this technique, and it has the advantage of reduced inci-

dence of nerve damage and post-operative constipation compared with the previous techniques. Their potential for mesh complications must be considered. It is beyond the remit of this book to look at the full range of available treatments for pelvic organ prolapse.

Faecal Incontinence

The mechanisms controlling continence are complex and multifactorial. Incontinence may be due to changes in the consistency of the stool, abnormalities of the mucosal lining of the rectum/colon, neurological disorders, trauma, or may develop in time with pelvic floor dysfunction. Most patients are women who have been through vaginal childbirth. Vaginal deliveries are associated with a 50% incidence of anal sphincter injury [24].

Patients with faecal incontinence require a careful evaluation process, including a detailed history, assessment of symptom severity, assessment of quality of life, and pelvic floor examination. Initial investigations concentrate on assessment of the lower GI tract to exclude organic disease. A colonoscopy would be appropriate if the patient is medically fit or a plain computed tomography scan of the abdomen and pelvis if the patient is frail. The next step involves ARM, defecating proctogram, and endo-anal ultrasound scan. The challenge in treating this group of patients is that objective assessment such as ARM may not correlate with symptom severity and quality of life. As a result, treatment options require an individual, patient-centred approach.

Surgical techniques in the past have included sphincteroplasty and dynamic graciloplasty. Failing these, a permanent colostomy might be considered. Sphincteroplasty is the only technique that has stood the test of time. It is indicated for patients with a recent traumatic EAS defect and symptoms of incontinence. Traditionally, gynaecologists use an overlapping technique to repair anal sphincter defects sustained in traumatic vaginal deliveries. Colorectal surgeons use the same technique as a delayed repair in occult EAS defects that are not detected at the time of childbirth. In the short term, two-thirds of patients have excellent/ good results, but this reduces to half in the longer term [25].

SNM has gained popularity worldwide in the treatment of faecal incontinence due to external sphincter dysfunction. A recent meta-analysis has demonstrated that overall long-term results are similar vin efficacy to sphincteroplasty, with 53% of patients demonstrating good results [26]. Techniques for neuromodulation are evolving, with increasing availability of cheaper, less invasive techniques, including PTNS, but the evidence for efficacy must be established.

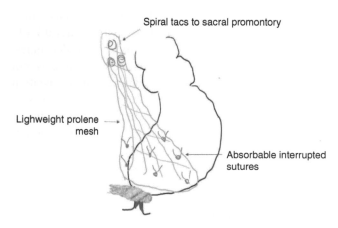

Figure 20.9 Position of mesh in laparoscopic ventral mesh rectopexy.

Bulking agents (biological or synthetic) may be used to treat IAS dysfunction. The internal sphincter may be become weak with age or damaged by previous colorectal surgery or other treatments such as pelvic radiotherapy. Traditionally, these agents have been used in the treatment of stress urinary incontinence. They have gained popularity in the treatment of passive faecal incontinence, where they are injected into the inter-sphincteric space. Although a minimally invasive procedure, this technique may be associated with infection, pain, and anal fistulae. The most recent innovation in sphincter prostheses involves Sphinkeeper, which is an injectable polyacrylonitrile compound aimed at augmenting a deficient IAS [27]. Historically, a high levels of morbidity and surgical re-intervention have been reported with artificial anal sphincter surgery. A Cochrane review evaluating the technique found one randomised controlled trial, which demonstrated a 50% improvement in faecal incontinence in the short term [28]. Long-term data is currently unavailable. The general consensus is that this technique may be considered as a bridging treatment between conservative measures and more complex surgery. Currently, it is only available within a research setting.

Psychological Distress and Quality of Life

Pelvic floor disorders resulting in any of the defecatory symptoms described above are associated with significant psychological distress. This type of distress is proportionate to the symptoms that patients experience. The embarrassing nature of these symptoms can lead to barriers in patients obtaining specialist healthcare. This is turn can lead to detrimental effects on quality of life, as affected patients limit their working and social lives to better cope with embarrassing symptoms.

In addition, several studies have reported a higher prevalence of anxiety, depression, and psychotic diseases [29]. In this group of patients with underlying psychiatric diagnoses, the impact of developing pelvic floor symptoms may be more complex to treat.

A multidisciplinary approach including psychological assessment is highly recommended for patients who exhibit significant psychological distress. It may be challenging for surgeons to elicit which patients have psychological distress as a result of their symptoms and which ones have an underlying psychiatric diagnosis that has been exacerbated by their symptoms. Currently, there is increasing interest in the Emotional Freedom Technique as a therapeutic intervention, which has been shown to improve a broad range of health markers, most notably anxiety and depression [30].

Future Direction of Colorectal Pelvic Floor Surgery

Mesh

The use of intra-abdominal mesh in rectal prolapse surgery gained popularity over the last decade after positive outcomes were reported from high-volume centres (laparoscopic ventral mesh rectopexy) [31]. The technique was considered safe and effective [32], albeit with a significant learning curve for pelvic floor surgeons. It was rapidly adopted worldwide, despite its complexity, because successful outcomes were far more likely than standard prolapse operation such as Delorme's repair. Recent studies have reported a risk of up to 8% mesh erosion rate in long-term follow-up, which needs to be considered in light of the 15% mesh erosion rates seen with vaginally inserted mesh. [33].

An independent review conducted in 2019 in the UK looked into the use of vaginal mesh and concluded that for the foreseeable future mesh should not be used to treat stress urinary incontinence in the NHS or independent sector, based on serious problems identified [34, 35]. Currently, NICE guidelines support the use of laparoscopic mesh rectopexy in the treatment of rectal prolapse for selected patients who have been recommended to undergo this surgery by specialists who are trained in pelvic floor surgery and with governance approvals from their individual hospitals [36]. Despite this, nervousness remains throughout the community in relation to vaginal mesh experience, and the future of mesh use in the treatment of rectal prolapse is currently uncertain.

The Gut Microbiome

The issue of gut microbiota is currently a hot topic in colorectal surgery. Recent advances in stool culture technologies have provided a wealth of information about the diversity, functional capacity, and dynamics of the human microbiome. It has been shown that imbalances in the composition and function of microbes that live in the large bowel are associated with health disorders such as the development of bowel cancer, inflammatory bowel disease, and irritable bowel syndrome. In addition, microbiome imbalances have been linked to wider disease manifestations such as type II diabetes and obesity [37].

It is widely believed that the composition of gut microbiota as a young child is simple and that this early process is instrumental in determining composition of gut microbiota as an adult. Our eating habits and the type of food we

21

Organisation of the Urodynamic Unit

Laura Thomas[1], Alexandra Bacon[1], Joanne Sheen[2], and Andrew Gammie[2]

[1] *Urodynamics & Gastrointestinal Physiology, Southmead Hospital, Bristol, UK*
[2] *Bristol Urological Institute, Southmead Hospital, Bristol, UK*

CONTENTS

The urodynamic unit must respond to the need for patient investigation from a variety of sources and must ensure that the studies are carried out to a consistently high standard. In the Bristol unit, we cover a very diverse range of tests, and this chapter shows how the unit is organised to deliver testing in the specific healthcare system in which we work. Clearly, every unit has its own pattern of referrals and works in a specific healthcare system, so we provide the following discussion as an example of the issues that may need to be considered.

We have identified there is a potential need for three levels of investigation in urodynamics (UDS):

- Routine UDS, including urine flow studies, filling cystometry, pressure-flow studies, and pad testing
- Advanced UDS, including urethral pressure profilometry and video urodynamics (VUDS)
- Complex UDS, including ambulatory urodynamics (AUDS) and neurophysiological testing

The requirements for each level are different, although all have common needs:

- Secretarial staff and administrative support
- Technical/nursing support
- Medical physics or medical engineering backing, including equipment maintenance
- Medical involvement

- Urodynamic records system

The basic organisation of our department can be illustrated by tracing a patient through the department.

Patient Referral

After reviewing the referral letter from the responsible specialist or the patient's general practitioner (GP) (family physician), the patient is assigned to suitable urodynamic tests and prioritised according to the clinical urgency, into the urgent category, or the routine list. Patients are added to a urodynamic waiting list from which they are booked using a partial booking system.

Making the Patient's Appointment

The individual patient's requirements are assessed so that an appointment of appropriate length and timing can be given. Appointment lengths are:

- 75 minutes: for routine or advanced UDS in the neurologically normal patient;
- 90 minutes (or in some extreme cases 150 minutes): for advanced UDS in people with severe mobility issues, for example, some patients with neurological disease. It is

important that the process of referral prompts the referrer to mention any mobility issues; and

- 180 minutes: for ambulatory UDS. The patient is pre-warned they need to set aside two to four hours for the appointment.

For patients who have not had screening uroflowmetry, a separate urine flow clinic appointment is made prior to their UDS. The flow clinic is 180 minutes, and patients are told they will be expected to void twice.

Female patients in whom there is a possibility that AUDS may be needed can be investigated by routine or VUDS in the morning, with a provisional appointment for AUDS in the afternoon. If patients have to travel some distance to reach us, then a late-morning appointment is given out of consideration for the prolonged travel time they will have.

Appointments are booked through a partial booking system. A letter is sent out to the patient asking them to call and arrange a convenient appointment time. Once this is confirmed verbally, a formal appointment letter is sent to the patient, and with this is sent the three-day International Consultation on Incontinence Questionnaire (ICIQ) bladder diary and a symptom questionnaire (International Consultation on Incontinence Questionnaire-Male Lower Urinary Tract Symptoms [ICIQ-MLUTS] or International Consultation on Incontinence Questionnaire-Female Lower Urinary Tract Symptoms [ICIQ-FLUTS]) – for completion before attending their appointment. Both urodynamic patients and flow clinic patients are sent patient information leaflets, which describe the investigation and how it is carried out. In the British system, we can have a problem with 'no-shows' or 'DNAs' (did-not-attends) as we call them: by allowing patients to select a time suitable to them, we have significantly increased our efficiency.

The Patient's Hospital Attendance

On arrival, the patient presents at the clinic reception, and the urodynamic team is notified.

Urodynamic Studies

The patient is collected from the waiting area by the clinician performing their procedure and their identity is confirmed. They are guided to their urodynamic room, which needs to be set up to consider privacy of the patient and ability to run the test efficiently (Figure 21.1). A space to sit and have a conversation is needed, so the test can be explained to the patient in comfort. This enables clarification of the symptom presentation, discussion of the points

raised in the information leaflet, and enables full written informed consent to be obtained.

The following sequence is then followed:

- Urodynamic history. We use a standard proforma which can be followed to guide questioning, and answers are entered directly into our database. If the clinician is new to the urodynamic team, or does not have access to the database, then they can complete a proforma sheet which can be uploaded later that day.
- After the history has been taken, the patient removes their lower items of clothing and changes into a gown. This is done in private behind a curtain.
- Urodynamic examination. The examination as detailed in previous chapters is carried out and recorded. This includes an initial flowmetry into a sterile jug so that screening urinalysis can be undertaken. For some at-risk patients, antibiotic prophylaxis may be needed.
- Urodynamic investigations. After the investigation is complete, the urodynamic traces are reviewed and the data is entered into the database.
- After completing the test, the patient dresses and then the physician explains the finding of the tests to the patient. If possible, the discussion could cover possible management options. However, if the responsible specialist is not present at the test, or if further interpretation of the data is needed, then management discussion will need to be arranged subsequently.
- The patient is advised to drink well for the next 24 hours. They are told about the possible symptoms of urinary tract infection, and how to proceed if they think an infection might be developing.
- Urodynamic report generation. Urodynamic reports are generated from the database. They include the patient demographics, clinical history, urodynamic findings, management recommendations, and finally any arrangement for follow up. The report is sent to the referring clinicians, as well as the patient, other relevant doctors including the GP, and further relevant persons, such as the continence advisor.

Urine Flow Clinic

We set up a dedicated flow clinic, because in regular outpatients, the process was too impractical. As with UDS, we follow a set protocol:

- Patients are sent their appointment in ample time together with a three-day bladder diary and symptom score.
- The patient is asked to drink normally at home on the day of the appointment.
- On arrival at the hospital, the patient is shown the flow room (Figure 21.2) and the tests are explained.

- In large units, permanent medical staff should provide a continuity that ensures good quality control for the studies and enables doctors coming to the department to receive proper training in urodynamic theory and technique; and
- Training-grade doctors may perform many of the tests in departments that are large or in small departments if the consultant is too busy to perform all UDS themselves. Herein lies a danger, because relatively inexperienced doctors require supervision for several months before they are able to report reliably on the urodynamic findings. In many departments, the key personnel will be the technicians, nurses, or scientists who assist with the tests and, like the consultant or other permanent staff, provide a continuity that allows the maintenance of an efficient and effective unit.

Who should assist at UDS? It is not important whether assistance is provided by a nurse, technician, or scientist, as all can bring the same urodynamic experience and training whilst offering a variety of additional skills useful for the running of a UDS department. Our unit started with technicians only but now has a mixture of experienced nurses, technicians, and scientists.

The principle responsibilities of the nurse/technician/scientist are to:

- Maintain and calibrate the urodynamic equipment;
- Ensure proper standards of cleanliness and sterility;
- Be responsible for the general care of patients;
- Work the urodynamic equipment during UDS;
- Potentially, undertake the running of tests without a doctor present, for example, some routine UDS cases and ambulatory UDS;
- Analyse the urodynamic tracing and prepare the report;
- Be responsible for restocking the urodynamic room with disposables, catheters, infusion fluids and sterile gloves, and other logistic essentials; and
- In video urodynamic tests, be responsible for X-ray screening.

What record system should be used? It is now normal practice to use electronic storage for patient letters, test results, and urodynamic traces. Where paper documentation is used, this can be scanned into an electronic file.

Most electronic patient records (EPR) systems allow linking to such electronic data, so the history of a given patient can be easily reviewed. Where an EPR system is not used, it is vital that all paper records are kept together so that this history review is comprehensive.

For urodynamic records, it is important not just to store the diagnosis and report letter but to file the urodynamic trace as well. A mere verbal description can never incorporate all the details of trace pattern and test features that the trace itself contains.

What equipment should you buy? This is discussed in more detail in Chapter 22. The decision as to which system to buy depends on a number of factors:

- First, decide what range of urodynamic tests will be offered.
- It is wise to involve the medical engineering department of your hospital whose help can prove invaluable at times of crisis.
- It is sensible to talk to and visit colleagues who are using the equipment you wish to buy.
- Attend meetings which have trade exhibitions, because you will be able to have a demonstration on how to handle the equipment on the commercial stands.
- Establish what service facility the company can offer. In a busy department, losing some of the diagnostic equipment for a week, due to a breakdown, is highly problematic.
- Ask for a trial in your own hospital so that you can invite colleagues to use the equipment and review.
- Lastly, make a cost-benefit assessment, going for reliability and service rather than equipment with a myriad of computer functions you are unlikely to use.

What relationships should exist with other departments? The urodynamic unit is a service department for other departments. However, as discussed above, the lead specialist and permanent doctors will have or will develop the skills to advise on management. The important relationships will be with:

- Urology, which provides more than 50% of our referrals. In particular, the flow clinic is largely used by male patients;
- Gynaecology, the next largest referral source;
- Neurology/neurosurgery, which refers a significant number of patients with proven or suspected neurological abnormalities associated with vesicourethral dysfunction;
- Paediatrics, since an increasing source of referrals comes from paediatric urologists, paediatric surgeons (for example, problems associated with anorectal anomalies), paediatricians, and paediatric nephrologists (with referrals of children who may have a lower urinary tract cause for renal impairment). Our unit offers a transition clinic as well, for facilitating the move for children reaching the adult age-range where they have to be managed in adult clinics;
- Geriatrics, which seems to be a declining primary source of referral. We have found it useful to screen the elderly in outpatients before requesting UDS;

- Gastroenterology and colorectal, and in particular surgeons with an interest in lower bowel dysfunction who are moving into closer relationships with urodynamic units. They are forming collaborative links with gynaecologists and urologists interested in pelvic floor function. In our department, anorectal physiology measurements and rectal irrigation clinics are carried out by our scientists;
- Nephrology, particularly where patients have renal failure which cannot clearly be attributed to intrinsic renal disease, and who often need to be assessed urodynamically prior to being transplanted;
- Radiology, an important link because it is often necessary to organise additional tests such as urethrography, micturating cystourethrography, pyelography, and isotope scanning (renography); and
- Medical engineering, who are useful friends and allies both for emergencies and for basic maintenance and problem-solving. They can also be useful in discussion with the equipment manufacturers.

The Investigating and Therapeutic Team

In terms of therapy, the team approach should be continued and should consist of:

- nurse continence care staff under the direction of the nurse continence adviser;
- a specialist physiotherapist;
- a urologist;
- a gynaecologist or urogynaecologist;
- a colorectal surgeon; and
- a paediatric urologist, depending on the specific population being served.

The facilities should exist for joint outpatient sessions and joint operating lists, where necessary. Regular multidisciplinary team (MDT) meetings are a valuable approach. These provide opportunities to:

- discuss challenging cases for consensus therapy recommendations;
- increase awareness of what is expected from urodynamic tests, and what is possible; and
- ensure good quality practice [1].

Reference

1. Working Group of the United Kingdom Continence Society, Abrams, P., Eustice, S. et al. (2019). United Kingdom Continence Society: Minimum standards for urodynamic studies, 2018. *Neurourol. Urodyn.* 38 (2): 838–856.

Table 22.2 Essential requirements for uroflowmetry, filling volume measurement, and pressure measurement in clinical urodynamics [1].

Parameter	Guideline value
Flowmeters	
Accuracy for flow rate	± 1 ml/s
Accuracy for voided volume	The greater of $\pm 3\%$ of true value or ± 2 ml
Range for flow rate	0–50 ml/s
Range for voided volume	0–1000 ml
Maximum duration of flow recordable	≥ 120 s
Minimum flow recordable	≤ 1 ml/s
Bandwidth of flow measurement	0 to between 1 and 5 Hz
Filling volume measurement	
Accuracy	The greater of 1–5% of true value or ± 1 ml/min
Range	0–1000 ml
Range of rate of infusion	0–100 ml/min, adjustable during filling
Sample rate of volume measurement	≥ 2 Hz
Pressure measurement	
Accuracy	The greater of $\pm 3\%$ of true value or ± 1 cmH$_2$O
Range	-30–250 cmH$_2$O (water-filled systems), 0–250 cmH$_2$O (other systems)
Bandwidth of pressure measurement (whole system)	0 to ≥ 3 Hz, equal on both channels
Required feature when water-filled catheters are used and patient positions are changed during the test	Equipment must allow reference levels to be reset

Source: Gammie et al. [1]. © 2014, John Wiley & Sons.

Reference

1. Gammie, A., Clarkson, B., Constantinou, C. et al. (2014). *International continence society guidelines on urodynamic equipment performance*. Neurourol. Urodyn. 33 (4): 370–379.

23

Working with Limited Resources

Andrew Gammie[1], Laura Thomas[2], Marcus Drake[3], and Eskinder Solomon[4,5]

[1] Bristol Urological Institute, Southmead Hospital, Bristol, UK
[2] Urodynamics & Gastrointestinal Physiology, Southmead Hospital, Bristol, UK
[3] Translational Health Sciences, Bristol Medical School, Southmead Hospital, Bristol, UK
[4] Department of Urology, Guy's and St Thomas' Hospital, London, UK
[5] Department of Paediatric Nephro-Urology, Evelina London Children's Hospital, London, UK

CONTENTS

There are many places in the world where advanced equipment and highly trained staff are not readily available. In such areas, it is still possible to carry out some urodynamic tests using the following guidelines.

Clinical Issues

For many people, whether to proceed with urodynamics requires an assessment of whether doing the test is likely to give information that could change treatment. This may include key clinical indications, such as neurogenic lower urinary tract dysfunction, certain situations of unexplained renal failure, and young men potentially considering bladder neck incision and more. If the limitation of healthcare resources affects potential availability of treatment, then undertaking the urodynamic test may not be appropriate.

A key aspect of practice is to prioritise safety. Urodynamics carries a risk of urinary tract infection, and so preventive measures should be considered in those at increased risk of infection and those for whom any infection that does occur could have more serious implications. Patients also need to be given advice on signs to look out for and actions to take if they feel an infection might be starting. The possibility of an anaphylactic reaction to latex means that prevention and therapy for anaphylaxis must be available.

Clinically, one of the main reasons to undertake urodynamic studies in neurological disease is to identify people who might be at risk of renal dysfunction. This is a greater risk if there is impaired detrusor compliance, detrusor sphincter dyssynergia (DSD), or vesicoureteric reflux (VUR). Basic urodynamic testing can be contributory in this setting, if video urodynamics is not possible, since impaired compliance can be identified from the filling cystometry and DSD from the pressure-flow study. Ultrasound can be used to give an indicator of whether gross established VUR might be present, based on the presence of hydronephrosis. If this is present, it means that identifying impaired detrusor compliance may well be unreliable, since the pressure recording will include the refluxing upper urinary tract, not solely the bladder. Ureteric obstruction could also cause hydronephrosis, and ultrasound is not sensitive at picking up low-grade reflux.

Urodynamic tests require the patient to describe and replicate symptoms that are usual for them. Privacy is thus essential, so the room in which testing is undertaken must be suitable. For example, windows should not allow viewing from the outside, and doors must be lockable. Sterility must not be compromised during the test, and clean handling of all urethral catheters must be assured. Thus, there should be space for clean and sterile preparation and a way to dispose of materials once used.

Equipment

For flow rate testing, the patient can be asked to time urinary stream with a stopwatch and to record the voided volume. Average flow rate can hence be calculated by dividing the volume voided (in millilitres) by the time taken (in seconds). Urine flow measurement can also be accomplished by scales and chart recorder, with flow rate being calculated manually after the test. The change in volume recorded every second will correspond to the average flow rate during that second. Acoustic uroflowmetry, where the sound of the urine stream hitting water can be used to determine the flow rate using any android or IOS mobile phone, is one option for reliably approximating flow and

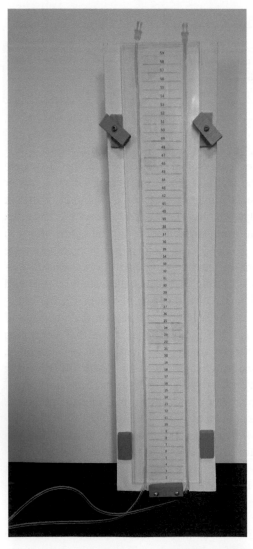

Figure 23.1 A wooden frame holding two vertical water tubes that could be used to display intravesical and abdominal pressure with no electronic equipment. The levels of water in the two tubes can be directly observed and p_{det} calculated from the difference in their heights. *Source*: Marcus Drake.

voided volume. Post-void residual can be measured with in-and-out catheterisation if a bladder scanner or ultrasound machine is not available.

In the absence of a dedicated urodynamic machine, detrusor pressure can still be measured in a number of ways. Water-filled tubes, with the top open to atmosphere, connected to inserted catheters will register pressure (Figure 23.1). The height must be measured from the level of the symphysis pubis vertically to the surface of the column of water, and the detrusor pressure is computed as usual from the difference between the vesical and the abdominal lines. Care should be taken, as usual, in removing all air bubbles from these lines. This method has proven effective in a Himalayan hospital with no special urodynamic equipment at all. Single channel p_{ves} measurement (i.e. not recording p_{abd}) might sometimes be sufficient to assess detrusor overactivity and compliance, especially in unco-operative or minimally mobile patients.

Urethral closure pressure assessment may be performed in the male patient using the retrograde leak point pressure test (RLPP). RLPP is carried out by inserting a catheter into the distal bulbar urethra and the penile urethra is then manually externally compressed (perhaps using tape). The catheter is connected to a saline bag which is then gradually raised vertically until flow begins. The height of bag from the pubic symphysis equates to the column of water pressure required to generate a retrograde leak, indicating the sphincter complex resting pressure. An example indication for RLPP in a resource-poor setting is deciding when bladder neck closure is needed at the same as cystoplasty in neuropathic patients with marked bladder dysfunction.

Invasive blood pressure measurement equipment can also be configured to measure pressures for urodynamics, if two pressure channels are available. If the only pressure measurement apparatus available reads in mmHg, then the figure should be divided by 1.36 in order to produce cmH_2O. A chart recorder or blood pressure monitor could be used to display continuous pressure. Subtraction of abdominal pressure from intravesical pressure during the test would have to be done manually, or it could be done after the test by a computer if the data can be stored electronically.

If a pump is not available for bladder filling, a suspended bag of sterile saline can be used, filling the bladder using gravity. Measurement of volume infused is achieved by using the volume marks on the saline bag or, to be more accurate, by measuring the difference in bag weight before and after filling. A syringe driver may be used for paediatric patients where fill rates are as low as 2 ml/s.

Donated equipment may be reconditioned or may be new. In both cases, it is essential that the user requirements are stated and met before any transfer takes place, as there are countless examples of well-meaning donations becoming junk in a storeroom. The World Health Organisation (WHO) has guidelines for good equipment donation practice (WHO guidelines, http://www.who.int/medical_devices/management_use/manage_donations/en), the core of which is good communication and understanding between donor and recipient. The most critical issue for users of urodynamic equipment will be the technical support of the machine after installation. This will include supply of consumables and spare parts and the availability of maintenance services. This support must be assured before any donation is accepted.

The $100 Urodynamic (UDS) System

The *$100 Urodynamic system* project aims to widen the access to urodynamic investigation to people around the world. The system consists of an Arduino (programmable analogue to digital converter), two pressure transducers, a water circuit to conduct the bladder and abdominal pressure, and two load cells (for flow rate and pump volume measurements) (Figure 23.2). A bespoke open-source software has database, display, analysis, and reporting functions. The details of the system as well as user and technical

manuals will be available at www.urodynamicswithout borders.com. The system components meet International Continence Society urodynamic equipment performance guidelines and may be assembled locally by personnel with minimal technical training and remote assistance from a project team, if required.

Maintenance Requirements

It is a known fact in the field of clinical engineering that most equipment issues arise from user error. It could be damage from transporting equipment, connectors being forced into the wrong place, or dust and water getting inside. Maintenance, therefore, begins with good user training in the care and safe use of equipment. Guidelines are available for free from Engineering World Health (User Care of Medical Equipment: A first-line maintenance guide for end users https://bmet.ewh.org/handle/20.500.12091/83). In summary, cleaning and careful handling will promote long equipment life. This training is best done by the supplier when the equipment first arrives, but regular refresher training in careful use and cleaning is also

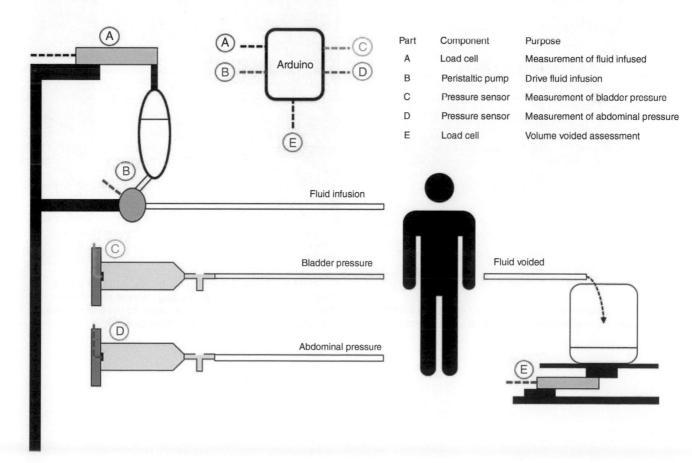

Figure 23.2   A schematic diagram of the $100 urodynamics system.

advised. For good-quality urodynamics, regular checks of calibration are also essential.

Maintenance by technically qualified personnel, whether from the supplier or from the hospital maintenance department, should be done on a regular basis, at least annually. The work required will include computer maintenance and virus checks, pump and motor cleaning and oiling, inspection of transducer integrity, and replacement of worn cables and connectors. Very often, technicians from the local market will be able to solve such issues. Electrical safety must also be assured on a regular basis.

Teaching

Clearly, the challenges of urodynamics are difficult to assimilate by reading alone. Access to face-to-face teaching is invaluable (Figure 23.3), and subsequent advice and ongoing clinical support can be a real asset. It is appropriate to consider adapting teaching methods to suit the environment (Figure 23.4). A sound understanding of measurement principles of urodynamic parameters is especially important in settings with limited resources to enable the confident and accurate use of all alternative/complementary techniques to assess lower urinary tract function. This advanced training requirement with emphasis on urodynamic physics, troubleshooting, and making a urodynamic diagnosis with a limited dataset is perhaps best delivered in small group hands-on teaching (Figure 23.5).

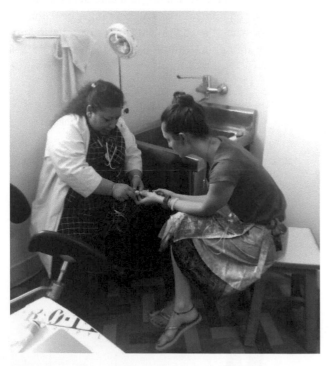

Figure 23.3 Face-to-face discussion is an important aspect of learning the issues of urodynamics. *Source*: Laura Thomas.

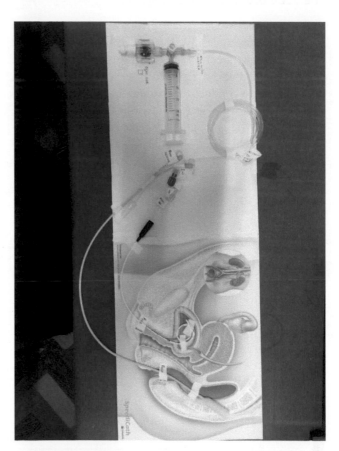

Figure 23.4 A simple teaching aid for the set-up of a fluid-filled p_{ves} catheter system, with a p_{abd} catheter also shown. Often, line drawings alone are not sufficient to communicate a real-world arrangement. *Source*: Marcus Drake.

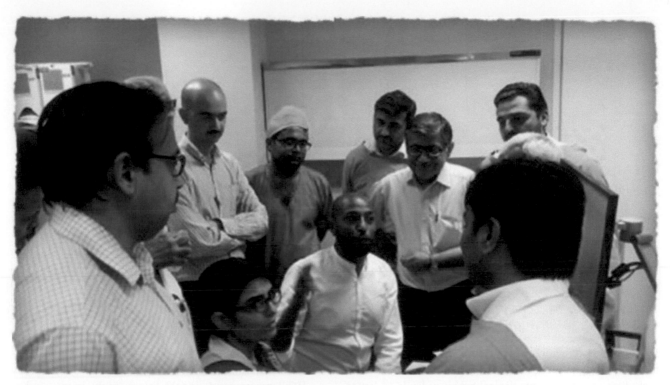

Figure 23.5 Small group urodynamics teaching in Sindh Institute of Transplant and Urology, Karachi, Pakistan.
Source: Eskinder Solomon.

24

Research Evidence on the Clinical Role of Urodynamics

Andrew Gammie[1], Marcus Drake[2], and Hashim Hashim[1]

[1] *Bristol Urological Institute, Southmead Hospital, Bristol, UK*
[2] *Translational Health Sciences, Bristol Medical School, Southmead Hospital, Bristol, UK*

CONTENTS

Evidence-based medicine in current healthcare has led to a focus on urodynamics (UDS), seeking to establish whether including the test in the clinical pathway leads to better outcomes. It is in effect like asking 'if we use this test, will patients get a better result when they go on to have treatment?' [1]. UDS is well established in functional urologic assessment, but its contribution is often questioned. A Cochrane analysis found that UDS changes clinical decision-making in male lower urinary tract symptoms (LUTS), but there was no evidence to demonstrate whether this led to reductions in voiding dysfunction symptoms after treatment [2]. Where such evidence is lacking, other factors come into play, such as clinician opinion, patient preference [3], service delivery, quality of testing [4], quality of treatment, cost, and convenience. The result is that a study in which therapy outcomes are used to justify diagnostic testing have to reflect the whole management pathway, since isolating the urodynamic test as an independent variable is not possible [5]. In the European Association of Urology guidelines on non-neurogenic male LUTS [6], the research evaluated in UDS was only rated as level of evidence C. Naturally, this is an enormously complicated research question, and some of the issues have been comprehensively described in relation to the UPSTREAM (Urodynamics for Prostate Surgery: Randomised Evaluation of Assessment Methods [7]) study. There are some unavoidable issues (confounding factors) which will blur the specific role of UDS in the overall outcomes:

1) Was the UDS test done in line with international standards (usually the International Continence Society [ICS] recommendations)? Interestingly, many studies say they have followed ICS standards, but close scrutiny shows they have not [4].

2) Were the results properly interpreted? Again, there is real concern about how well sites interpret their test results (for example, see [4]).

3) How do the test results translate into treatment? Diagnostic tests are used to select treatment, so there is a systematic influence that certain findings will mean that subgroups are more likely to have certain treatments.

4) What will be the effect of non-treated patients? In UPSTREAM, we identified that some features seen in UDS (e.g. absence of bladder outlet obstruction and presence of detrusor underactivity [DUA]) would mean limited choice of treatment can be offered. Thus, LUTS would not improve, and this could disadvantage the symptom outcomes of people undergoing UDS, counterbalancing the benefit of avoiding "unnecessary" surgery. Hence, the design of the study was to look for non-inferiority of outcome.

5) For those patients having treatment, was it done well? For example, transurethral resection of the prostate (TURP) is not necessarily always done well technically, meaning that outcomes could be poor for a reason unrelated to the preceding diagnostic tests.

Table 24.1 Challenges in the design of a multinational and multicentre urodynamic data collection.

Data agreements	Considerations on which existing registries to include (how to approach them) (obtain contracts and permissions)
Patient consent	This may have been given for the registry to hold the data; consent should also be checked if the data can be used for research by third parties.
Data anonymisation	Minimise risk of reidentification
IT infrastructure and data procurement	Defining storage location of the registry data and secure safe transport of the data
Data access and storage	There are generally two types of data access: (i) a centralised model where the registries provide the data and which can be stored on individual servers or (ii) a federated model where there is access to data in the server and which can only extract aggregated statistics. The servers would need to be multinode CPU, with large memory capacity, and dedicated data management software, such as Hadoop, and statistical software, such as R. Depending on where the data are coming from, there may be restrictions on where they can be stored (for example, EU data will have an EU storage range).
Common data model	Securing the data to enter the registry in a similar format and unit with identical variable names/labels. This will also allow programmers to navigate between datasets with efficiency.
Data protection	The need for support on GDPR EU ruling on data privacy and protection, to ensure data are handled compliantly and legally.

Source: Rademakers et al. [8]. © 2019, John Wiley & Sons.

Thanks to these issues and many others, evidence to say UDS improves outcomes on a population basis is very limited [2]. Such research is also demanding methodologically. For example, some of the challenges relating simply to data handling are listed in Table 24.1.

Failure to understand this type of research properly leads to partial quotation of some clinical trial results which give an impression opposite to the conclusions of the studies quoted – a scientifically inept tendency of the clinical profession graphically described as 'half the message is just mess' [9]. Errors in interpretation have serious potential to mislead. For example, a consensus paper from an expert group [10] pointed out erroneous assumptions from the VALUE trial results [11]. VALUE looked at UDS before stress urinary incontinence (SUI) surgery in women and concluded that 'preoperative office evaluation alone is non-inferior to evaluation with UDS in terms of outcomes at 1 year'. Conclusions that UDS is 'not justified' in this setting have then been extrapolated, with no clinical justification, beyond the confines of the narrow study population. The fact that the VALUE study was focussed only on 'uncomplicated' patients with SUI has often been lost from view, and the very limited message has lost its limitations [9], noting that such patients (uncomplicated SUI) are in the minority [12]. Not only that, the diagnostic value of UDS is often not highlighted – as was seen in subsequent publications from the VALUE study where the test changed management of patients [13]. An appropriate summary of the conclusions of the VALUE study would be that 'UDS is not justified in the small minority of women whose SUI is uncomplicated [9]'. Another factor to consider is the cost effectiveness of UDS balanced against the cost of performing surgery and managing the complications from surgery, which is often not quoted in trials [14, 15]. Oversimplified and incomplete quotation of study conclusions masquerading as a verdict on UDS in its entirety has meant that judgements on the value of this test have been made far too hastily.

The longstanding dearth of robust evidence is set to change. Three current studies looking at specific urodynamic questions are particularly noteworthy for the size and methodological strength, backed up by adequate funding resources, and can be anticipated to yield level 1 evidence:

- UPSTREAM, evaluating men with LUTS considering prostate surgery. The main outcomes of this study have been published [7], and there is also a five-year extension study ongoing.
- FUTURE. Female Urgency, Trial of Urodynamics as Routine Evaluation (https://doi.org/10.1186/ISRCTN 63268739). This is a superiority randomised clinical trial to evaluate the effectiveness and cost effectiveness of invasive urodynamic investigations in management of women with refractory overactive bladder symptoms.
- PRIMUS. PRImary care Management of lower Urinary tract Symptoms in men (https://doi.org/10.1186/ISRCTN10327305) [16]. A study set up for development and validation of a diagnostic and clinical decision support tool. This will develop approaches to diagnosis in primary care which predict outcome of UDS.

These studies have yet to conclude, and they promise to make a considerable difference in the coming decade. For now, what is absolutely vital is to take a much more measured view on population-based research findings into diagnostic tests. In the clinical setting, it is also vital to be crystal clear that UDS can make a huge difference to the individual patient. For an individual, UDS can identify features that make an enormous difference to their personal treatment decisions. Obvious examples include:

- stress-provoked detrusor overactivity incontinence;
- intrinsic sphincter deficiency;
- impaired detrusor compliance;
- vesicoureteric reflux;
- DUA; and
- voiding dysfunction.

These are comparatively uncommon, so do not give a strong signal in population studies, yet missing them potentially leads to a bad situation. Patients are aware of the value of detailed assessment, and for that reason, they are generally perfectly willing to have a UDS test, provided proper information is given to them (both before and after the test) [3]. UDS needs to be viewed as a diagnostic test, and not an outcome measure, which adds to the clinical diagnostic pathway in the management of patients and may change management of patients.

References

1. Drake, M.J., Lewis, A.L., and Lane, J.A. (2016). *Urodynamic testing for men with voiding symptoms considering interventional therapy: the merits of a properly constructed randomised trial.* Eur. Urol. 69 (5): 759–760.

2. Clement, K.D., Burden, H., Warren, K. et al. (2015). Invasive urodynamic studies for the management of lower urinary tract symptoms (LUTS) in men with voiding dysfunction. Cochrane Database Syst. Rev. 28 (4) (Art. No.: CD011179). doi: https://doi.org/10.1002/14651858.CD011179.pub2 Wiley.

3. Selman, L.E., Ochieng, C.A., Lewis, A.L. et al. (2019). *Recommendations for conducting invasive urodynamics for men with lower urinary tract symptoms: qualitative interview findings from a large randomized controlled trial (UPSTREAM).* Neurourol. Urodyn. 38 (1): 320–329.

4. Aiello, M., Jelski, J., Lewis, A. et al. (2020). *Quality control of uroflowmetry and urodynamic data from two large multicenter studies of male lower urinary tract symptoms.* Neurourol. Urodyn. 39 (4): 1170–1177.

5. Bailey, K., Abrams, P., Blair, P.S. et al. (2015). *Urodynamics for prostate surgery trial; randomised evaluation of assessment methods (UPSTREAM) for diagnosis and management of bladder outlet obstruction in men: study protocol for a randomised controlled trial.* Trials 16 (1): 567.

6. Gratzke, C., Bachmann, A., Descazeaud, A. et al. (2015). *EAU guidelines on the assessment of non-neurogenic male lower urinary tract symptoms including benign prostatic obstruction.* Eur. Urol. 67 (6): 1099–1109.

7. Drake, M.J., Lewis, A.L., Young, G.J. et al. (2020). *Diagnostic assessment of lower urinary tract symptoms in men considering prostate surgery: a noninferiority randomised controlled trial of urodynamics in 26 hospitals.* Eur. Urol. 78 (5): 701–710.

8. Rademakers, K., Gammie, A., Yasmin, H. et al. (2020). *Can multicentre urodynamic studies provide high quality evidence for the clinical effectiveness of urodynamics? ICI-RS 2019.* Neurourol. Urodyn. 39 (Suppl 3): S30–S35.

9. Gammie, A. and Kessler, T.M. (2020). *Half the message is just mess: judging the value of urodynamics based on partial or poor-quality results.* BJU Int. 126 (1): 4–5.

10. Finazzi-Agro, E., Gammie, A., Kessler, T.M. et al. (2020). *Urodynamics useless in female stress urinary incontinence? Time for some sense-a European expert consensus.* Eur. Urol. Focus 6 (1): 137–145.

11. Nager, C.W., Brubaker, L., Litman, H.J. et al. (2012). *A randomized trial of urodynamic testing before stress-incontinence surgery.* N. Engl. J. Med. 366 (21): 1987–1997.

12. Agur, W., Housami, F., Drake, M. et al. (2009). *Could the National Institute for health and clinical excellence guidelines on urodynamics in urinary incontinence put some women at risk of a bad outcome from stress incontinence surgery?* BJU Int. 103 (5): 635–639.

13. Sirls, L.T., Richter, H.E., Litman, H.J. et al. (2013). *The effect of urodynamic testing on clinical diagnosis, treatment plan and outcomes in women undergoing stress urinary incontinence surgery.* J. Urol. 189 (1): 204–209.

14. Homer, T., Shen, J., Vale, L. et al. (2018). *Invasive urodynamic testing prior to surgical treatment for stress urinary incontinence in women: cost-effectiveness and value of information analyses in the context of a mixed methods feasibility study.* Pilot Feasibility Stud. 4: 67.

15. Norton, P.A., Nager, C.W., Brubaker, L. et al. (2016). *The cost of preoperative urodynamics: a secondary analysis of the ValUE trial.* Neurourol. Urodyn. 35 (1): 81–84.

16. Pell, B., Thomas-Jones, E., Bray, A. et al. (2020). *PRImary care management of lower urinary tract symptoms in men: protocol for development and validation of a diagnostic and clinical decision support tool (the PriMUS study).* BMJ Open 10 (6): e037634.

Appendix A

Key Patient Assessment Metrics from the International Consultation on Incontinence Questionnaires (ICIQ)

ICIQ-FLUTS

| | | | | | | | ICIQ-FLUTS 08/04 | | | | | | |

Initial number   **CONFIDENTIAL**   DAY   MONTH   YEAR

Today's date

Urinary symptoms

Many people experience urinary symptoms some of the time. We are trying to find out how many people experience urinary symptoms, and how much they bother them. We would be grateful if you could answer the following questions, thinking about how you have been, on average, over the <u>PAST FOUR WEEKS</u>.

1.   **Please write in your date of birth:**   DAY   MONTH   YEAR

2a.   **During the night, how many times do you have to get up to urinate, on average?**

none   0
one   1
two   2
three   3
four or more   4

2b.   **How much does this bother you?**
Please ring a number between 0 (not at all) and 10 (a great deal)

0   1   2   3   4   5   6   7   8   9   10
not at all   a great deal

3a.   **Do you have a sudden need to rush to the toilet to urinate?**

never   0
occasionally   1
sometimes   2
most of the time   3
all of the time   4

3b.   **How much does this bother you?**
Please ring a number between 0 (not at all) and 10 (a great deal)

0   1   2   3   4   5   6   7   8   9   10
not at all   a great deal

4a.   **Do you have pain in your bladder?**

never   0
occasionally   1
sometimes   2
most of the time   3
all of the time   4

4b.   **How much does this bother you?**
Please ring a number between 0 (not at all) and 10 (a great deal)

0   1   2   3   4   5   6   7   8   9   10
not at all   a great deal

Abrams' Urodynamics, Fourth Edition. Edited by Marcus Drake, Hashim Hashim, and Andrew Gammie.
© 2021 John Wiley & Sons Ltd. Published 2021 by John Wiley & Sons Ltd.

ICIQ-FLUTS 08/04

5a. **How often do you pass urine during the day?**

1 to 6 times	0
7 to 8 times	1
9 to 10 times	2
11 to 12 times	3
13 or more times	4

5b. **How much does this bother you?**
Please ring a number between 0 (not at all) and 10 (a great deal)

      0 1 2 3 4 5 6 7 8 9 **10**
   not at all   a great deal

F score: sum scores 2a-5a ☐ ☐

6a. **Is there a delay before you can start to urinate?**

never	0
occasionally	1
sometimes	2
most of the time	3
all of the time	4

6b. **How much does this bother you?**
Please ring a number between 0 (not at all) and 10 (a great deal)

      0 1 2 3 4 5 6 7 8 9 **10**
   not at all   a great deal

7a. **Do you have to strain to <u>urinate</u>?**

never	0
occasionally	1
sometimes	2
most of the time	3
all of the time	4

7b. **How much does this bother you?**
Please ring a number between 0 (not at all) and 10 (a great deal)

      0 1 2 3 4 5 6 7 8 9 **10**
   not at all   a great deal

ICIQ-FLUTS 08/04

8a.	**Do you stop and start more than once while you urinate?**		
		never	0
		occasionally	1
		sometimes	2
		most of the time	3
		all of the time	4

8b.	**How much does this bother you?**
	Please ring a number between 0 (not at all) and 10 (a great deal)

0 1 2 3 4 5 6 7 8 9 **10**
not at all   a great deal

V score: sum scores 6a+7a+8a ☐ ☐

9a.	**Does urine leak before you can get to the toilet?**		
		never	0
		occasionally	1
		sometimes	2
		most of the time	3
		all of the time	4

9b.	**How much does this bother you?**
	Please ring a number between 0 (not at all) and 10 (a great deal)

0 1 2 3 4 5 6 7 8 9 **10**
not at all   a great deal

10a.	**How often do you leak urine?**		
		never	0
		once or less per week	1
		two to three times per week	2
		once per day	3
		several times per day	4

10b.	**How much does this bother you?**
	Please ring a number between 0 (not at all) and 10 (a great deal)

0 1 2 3 4 5 6 7 8 9 **10**
not at all   a great deal

ICIQ-FLUTS 08/04

11a. **Does urine leak when you are physically active, exert yourself, cough or sneeze?**

never ☐	0
occasionally ☐	1
sometimes ☐	2
most of the time ☐	3
all of the time ☐	4

11b. **How much does this bother you?**
Please ring a number between 0 (not at all) and 10 (a great deal)

    0 1 2 3 4 5 6 7 8 9 **10**
  not at all   a great deal

12a. **Do you ever leak urine for no obvious reason and without feeling that you want to go?**

never ☐	0
occasionally ☐	1
sometimes ☐	2
most of the time ☐	3
all of the time ☐	4

12b. **How much does this bother you?**
Please ring a number between 0 (not at all) and 10 (a great deal)

    0 1 2 3 4 5 6 7 8 9 **10**
  not at all   a great deal

13a. **Do you leak urine when you are asleep?**

never ☐	0
occasionally ☐	1
sometimes ☐	2
most of the time ☐	3
all of the time ☐	4

13b. **How much does this bother you?**
Please ring a number between 0 (not at all) and 10 (a great deal)

    0 1 2 3 4 5 6 7 8 9 **10**
  not at all   a great deal

I score: sum scores9a-13a ☐ ☐

Thank you very much for answering these questions.

ICIQ-MLUTS

Initial number

ICIQ-MLUTS 01/06

CONFIDENTIAL

DAY   MONTH   YEAR
Today's date

Urinary symptoms

Many people experience urinary symptoms some of the time. We are trying to find out how many people experience urinary symptoms, and how much they bother them. We would be grateful if you could answer the following questions, thinking about how you have been, on average, over the <u>PAST FOUR WEEKS</u>.

1.   **Please write in your date of birth:**

DAY   MONTH   YEAR

2a.   **Is there a delay before you can start to urinate?**

never ☐ 0
occasionally ☐ 1
sometimes ☐ 2
most of the time ☐ 3
all of the time ☐ 4

2b.   **How much does this bother you?**
Please ring a number between 0 (not at all) and 10 (a great deal)

0 1 2 3 4 5 6 7 8 9 **10**
not at all   a great deal

3a.   **Do you have to strain to <u>continue</u> urinating?**

never ☐ 0
occasionally ☐ 1
sometimes ☐ 2
most of the time ☐ 3
all of the time ☐ 4

3b.   **How much does this bother you?**
Please ring a number between 0 (not at all) and 10 (a great deal)

0 1 2 3 4 5 6 7 8 9 **10**
not at all   a great deal

4a.   **Would you say that the strength of your urinary stream is…**

normal ☐ 0
occasionally reduced ☐ 1
sometimes reduced ☐ 2
reduced most of the time ☐ 3
reduced all of the time ☐ 4

4b.   **How much does this bother you?**
Please ring a number between 0 (not at all) and 10 (a great deal)

0 1 2 3 4 5 6 7 8 9 **10**
not at all   a great deal

ICIQ-MLUTS 01/06

11a. **Do you leak urine when you are asleep?**

never	☐	0
occasionally	☐	1
sometimes	☐	2
most of the time	☐	3
all of the time	☐	4

11b. **How much does this bother you?**
Please ring a number between 0 (not at all) and 10 (a great deal)

0 1 2 3 4 5 6 7 8 9 **10**
not at all   a great deal

12a. **How often have you had a slight wetting of your pants a few minutes after you had finished urinating and had dressed yourself?**

never	☐	0
occasionally	☐	1
sometimes	☐	2
most of the time	☐	3
all of the time	☐	4

12b. **How much does this bother you?**
Please ring a number between 0 (not at all) and 10 (a great deal)

0 1 2 3 4 5 6 7 8 9 **10**
not at all   a great deal

IS: sum scores 7-12 ☐ ☐

13a. **How often do you pass urine during the day?**

1 to 6 times	☐	0
7 to 8 times	☐	1
9 to 10 times	☐	2
11 to 12 times	☐	3
13 or more times	☐	4

13b. **How much does this bother you?**
Please ring a number between 0 (not at all) and 10 (a great deal)

0 1 2 3 4 5 6 7 8 9 **10**
not at all   a great deal

ICIQ-MLUTS 01/06

14a. **During the night, how many times do you have to get up to urinate, on average?**

none ☐	0
one ☐	1
two ☐	2
three ☐	3
four or more ☐	4

14b. **How much does this bother you?**
Please ring a number between 0 (not at all) and 10 (a great deal)

      0 1 2 3 4 5 6 7 8 9 **10**
    not at all   a great deal

© IC*Smale*SF

Thank you very much for answering these questions.

ICIQ-BD

BLADDER DIARY　　　　**YOUR NAME:** _____

Please complete this **3 day** bladder diary. Enter the following in each column against the time. You can change the specified times if you need to. In the time column, please write **BED** when you went to bed and **WOKE** when you woke up.

Drinks Write the amount you had to drink and the type of drink.

Urine output Enter the amount of urine you passed in millilitres (mls) in the urine output column, day and night. Any measuring jug will do. If you passed urine but couldn't measure it, put a tick in this column. If you leaked urine at any time write **LEAK** here.

Bladder sensation Write a description of how your bladder felt when you went to the toilet using these codes

　0 - If you had no sensation of needing to pass urine, but passed urine for "social reasons", for example, just before going out, or unsure where the next toilet is.

　1 - If you had a normal desire to pass urine and no urgency. *"Urgency" is different from normal bladder feelings and is the sudden compelling desire to pass urine which is difficult to defer, or a sudden feeling that you need to pass urine and if you don't you will have an accident.*

　2 - If you had urgency but it had passed away before you went to the toilet.

　3 - If you had urgency but managed to get to the toilet, still with urgency, but did not leak urine.

　4 - If you had urgency and could not get to the toilet in time so you leaked urine.

Pads If you put on or change a pad put a tick in the pads column.

Here is an example of how to complete the diary:

Time	Drinks		Urine output	Bladder sensation	Pads
	Amount	Type			
6am WOKE			350ml	2	
7am	300ml	tea			
8am			✓	2	
9am					
10am	cup	water	Leak	3	✓

DAY 1　**DATE:** _____/_____/_____

Time	Drinks		Urine output (mls)	Bladder sensation	Pads
	Amount	Type			
6am					
7am					
8am					
9am					
10am					
11am					
Midday					
1pm					
2pm					
3pm					
4pm					
5pm					
6pm					
7pm					
8pm					
9pm					
10pm					
11pm					
Midnight					
1am					
2am					
3am					
4am					
5am					

BLADDER DIARY   YOUR NAME: _____

DAY 2   **DATE**: _____ / _____ / _____

Time	Drinks		Urine output (mls)	Bladder sensation	Pads
	Amount	Type			
6am					
7am					
8am					
9am					
10am					
11am					
Midday					
1pm					
2pm					
3pm					
4pm					
5pm					
6pm					
7pm					
8pm					
9pm					
10pm					
11pm					
Midnight					
1am					
2am					
3am					
4am					
5am					

DAY 3   **DATE**: _____ / _____ / _____

Time	Drinks		Urine output (mls)	Bladder sensation	Pads
	Amount	Type			
6am					
7am					
8am					
9am					
10am					
11am					
Midday					
1pm					
2pm					
3pm					
4pm					
5pm					
6pm					
7pm					
8pm					
9pm					
10pm					
11pm					
Midnight					
1am					
2am					
3am					
4am					
5am					

Bladder sensation codes
0 – No sensation of needing to pass urine, but passed urine for "social reasons"
1 – Normal desire to pass urine and no urgency
2 – Urgency but it had passed away before you went to the toilet
3 – Urgency but managed to get to the toilet, still with urgency, but did not leak urine
4 – Urgency and could not get to the toilet in time so you leaked urine

neurourology
Urodynamics

For submission instructions, subscription, and all the latest information, visit http://onlinelibrary.wiley.com/journal/10.1002/(ISSN)1520-6777

Neurourology and Urodynamics

Volume 37   Issue S6   2018

TABLE OF CONTENTS

Neurourology
and Urodynamics

T A B L E   O F   C O N T E N T S

DOI: 10.1002/nau.23791

EDITORIAL COMMENT

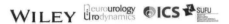

The International Continence Society (ICS) Board of Trustees is glad to present a special supplement of *Neurourology and Urodynamics* which sets out the core knowledge for any practitioner needing to assess lower urinary tract dysfunction (LUTD) in their clinical work. The material will be useful to trainees, allied health professionals, and people working in related disciplines like neurology, primary care, and care of the elderly. The documents are written in a simplified way to offer a helpful source of education and knowledge of several different aspects of LUTD.

A significant motivation for this effort is the need to be concise, explicit, and definitionally correct when using a common lexicon, as with the ICS Standardization documents, that govern the manner in which professionals in our field define their research and report results thereof. A sequence of documents is included which covers;

- Urinary symptoms in general, and in specific patient groups (nocturia; neurological disease; chronic pelvic pain)
- Pelvic organ prolapse quantification
- Urodynamic tests (flow rate testing; filling cystometry with pressure flow studies; videourodynamics)
- The importance of standardization and how the ICS Standards are developed

The knowledge base is drawn from the ICS Standards, which constitute the basis of specialist practice in LUTD, supplemented by practical application. The authors were asked to write succinct and approachable documents, describing what they feel any practitioner really must know for everyday practice, and providing examples. Thus, these documents are derivatives of the many reports and publications that represent the ICS Standards but are not in themselves ICS Standardization documents. Inevitably, the choice of content is subjective, but each document seeks to offer simplicity and clarity. For those working to become specialists in the area, this supplement is a starting point for getting to grips with the comprehensive repository of detailed professional consensus documents established by the ICS over the course of several decades and available on the ICS website (https://www.ics.org/folder/189).

A significant aspect of the knowledge transfer is the education of those who are students or early career clinicians and investigators. Thus, the supplement aims to facilitate clarity, accuracy, and specificity of reports in the fields of urodynamics, neurourology, pelvic floor disorders, and urogenital reconstruction. Health care practitioners and clinicians will benefit from these documents, which give a brief review of those subjects related to LUT dysfunction, and as their knowledge grows, we hope they will feel enthused to engage with the full ICS Standards.

Sherif Mourad
Roger Dmochowski
Marcus Drake

may be reported by a urodynamic machine, but practitioners must check the source traces for plausibility, noting any spikes which the machine may inappropriately have used for deriving those parameters, and moving the cursors to instruct the machine where the values can be taken.

The final report must be carefully phrased, describing whether symptoms reported by the patient were actually encountered during the test, and what was the urodynamic observation at that time (Table 1). Of course, certain symptoms simply cannot be reproduced during a urodynamic test- obvious examples being nocturia, nocturnal enuresis, and coital incontinence. For these symptoms, observations made during urodynamics must not be claimed as the cause of the symptom. The "only report what you see" approach is crucial for safer consideration to making treatment recommendations.

5 | VIDEOURODYNAMICS

Conventional urodynamic tests principally can be used if there is a relatively evident underlying mechanism. The main situations are;

- Post-obstetric stress incontinence in a healthy woman, where urethral hypermobility has been identified on physical examination.
- Voiding LUTS in a man in the right age range, where benign prostate enlargement is identified on rectal examination.

For these individuals, the underlying mechanism can be assumed with reasonable confidence. Thus, if stress urinary incontinence is seen in the first situation, the hypermobility is probably the cause. In the second, if BOO is seen, the prostate enlargement is probably the cause. However, many other presentations throw up more complex possibilities and a range of causes should be considered. Using X-ray contrast as the urodynamic filling medium, and taking images at key moments during the tests ("videourodynamics") allows greater confidence when deciding what mechanism(s) are present, and potentially linking them to symptoms. The additional information that X-ray screening can achieve includes;

1. Instantaneous detection of leakage.
   a) If there is delay for the leakage reaching the flow meter, for example, in men with post prostatectomy incontinence due to sphincter damage.
   b) When evaluating leak point pressures in a patient with neurological disease.

This precision on identifying timing of leakage allows the urodynamicist to know the detrusor pressure at the precise moment when it matters.

2. Identifying the exact location of bladder outlet obstruction; bladder neck (Figure 1a), prostate, urethral sphincter/pelvic floor, stricture. This can be very valuable for establishing the cause of BOO, and hence deciding on treatment.

3. Detecting muscle function deficits in patients with neurological disease.
   a) An open bladder neck may indicate a deficit in sympathetic innervation.
   b) A poorly supported bladder base and proximal urethra, which can be seen to descend on straining, may be due to pelvic floor weakness and may reflect muscle denervation in men, or women with no obstetric history.

4. Explaining difficulty in detecting expected increased pressure change, due to dispersal into a low pressure region.
   a) A large bladder diverticulum (Figure 1b).
   b) Significant vesico-ureteric reflux (VUR).

5. Identifying VUR in its early stages; potentially it may be possible to treat early VUR with a bulking injection of the ureteric orifice.

6. Correlating a patient's reported urgency sensation with urine entering the proximal urethra (Figure 1c); this might help explain why some people with urgency do not gain benefit from medical therapy of OAB.

7. Demonstrating whether the bladder empties fully; a well-timed X-ray taken at the exact end of voiding confirms whether the bladder has emptied fully. This is more accurate than bladder scanning, since the scanner takes a while to get in position, during which time people with VUR may have had enough liquid come back in to the bladder to show up on a scanner- a "pseudo-residual" (Figure 1d).

8. Identifying pooling in patients with post micturition dribbling.
   a) Pooling in the male urethral bulb (Figure 1a).
   b) Vaginal pooling.

6 | CONCLUSIONS

The ICS has pushed a logical and systematic approach to terminology and assessment in lower urinary tract function. In the current review we emphasize the importance of being specific with the language used, the need to justify severity thresholds, the philosophy underlying urodynamic testing and the potential benefits of videourodynamics in patients whose underlying pathophysiology is potentially complex.

ORCID

Marcus J. Drake http://orcid.org/0000-0002-6230-2552

REFERENCES

1. Abrams P, Cardozo L, Fall M, et al. The standardisation of terminology of lower urinary tract function: report from the Standardisation Sub-committee of the International Continence Society. *Neurourol Urodyn*. 2002;21(2):167–178.
2. Drake MJ. Should nocturia not be called a lower urinary tract symptom?. *Eur Urol*. 2015;67(2):289–290.
3. Abrams P, Personal Communication, on behalf of the Working Group on the UK Continence Society Minimum Standards for Urodynamics 2018.

How to cite this article: Drake MJ, Abrams P. A commentary on expectations of healthcare professionals when applying the international continence society standards to basic assessment of lower urinary tract function. *Neurourology and Urodynamics*. 2018;37:S7–S12. https://doi.org/10.1002/nau.23732

Received: 30 April 2018 | Accepted: 2 July 2018

DOI: 10.1002/nau.23768

SOUNDING BOARD

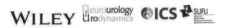

Fundamentals of terminology in lower urinary tract function

Marcus J. Drake[1,2]

[1] Translational Health Sciences, Bristol Medical School, Bristol, UK

[2] Bristol Urological Institute, Southmead Hospital, Bristol, UK

Correspondence
Marcus J. Drake, Bristol Urological Institute, 3rd Floor L&R Building, Southmead Hospital, Bristol BS10 5NB, UK.
Email: marcus.drake@bristol.ac.uk

Aims: To summarize basic definitions in the International Continence Society (ICS) Standardization of Terminology in lower urinary tract (LUT) function and their application.

Methods: Fundamental terminology in the ICS Standardization of Terminology LUT Function was identified and summarized.

Results: Evaluation of LUT requires appreciation of symptoms, signs and urodynamic observations. Symptoms are categorized according to their occurrence during the micturition cycle into storage symptoms (eg, increased daytime frequency [IDF], urgency, nocturia, or incontinence) or voiding and post-voiding symptoms (eg, slow stream or post micturition dribbling). Several problems may be present, giving rise to symptom syndromes, notably overactive bladder (during the storage phase) or underactive bladder (during the voiding phase). Signs may be derived from a bladder diary or may be elicited on physical examination. Urodynamic observations may be made by assessing flow rate, and this is combined with pressure measurement when undertaking filling cystometry and pressure flow studies. Key elements of flow and pressure measurement are described.

Conclusions: The review provides a succinct summary of symptoms, signs, and urodynamic observations as set out in the ICS Standard on LUT Function.

KEYWORDS
LUTS, overactive bladder, standardization, urodynamics

1 | INTRODUCTION

The International Continence Society (ICS) has for many years led the development of standardized definitions of the symptoms, signs, urodynamic observations, and conditions associated with lower urinary tract dysfunction (LUTD). The current document is a summary of core terminology related to LUTD for use in a general medical context. For example, LUTD is commonly encountered by healthcare professionals working in gerontology, neurology, and nephrology. The terminology is also useful for residents in urology or gynaecology preparing for examinations. This document is not intended for subspecialists working in functional urology,

urogynaecology, and neuro-urology, for whom the ICS has developed a range of standardizations (see www.ics.org). These cover the full scope terms in different contexts and patient groups for use in subspecialty research and clinical practice, which are beyond the scope of the current review.

2 | METHODS

Recommendations in the ICS Standard on LUTD[1] were reviewed and summarized, this document being selected as the terminology is applicable to all patients regardless of gender. Definitions of nocturia,[2] underactive bladder,[3] and pelvic organ

Roger Dmochowski led the peer-review process as the Associate Editor responsible for the paper.

prolapse (POP)[4] are those given in subsequent context-specific ICS consultations or documents. Definitions and key terms are generally transcribed verbatim. In the original document, many of the definitions are accompanied by explanatory or exemplary footnotes. The footnotes have been adapted (non-verbatim) in certain cases for the current review, or have been excluded for the sake of brevity, and additional explanatory text is included. Readers should note that in urogynaecology practice, some terms have been updated in the International Urogynecology Association/ICS joint report on the terminology for female pelvic floor dysfunction,[4] where there is some divergence from the reported definitions in the current review. Accordingly, users are advised to specify the source of the definitions they employ when publishing in the area.

3 | LOWER URINARY TRACT SYMPTOMS

Normal lower urinary tract (LUT) function relies on the facility for storage of urine in the bladder, and the ability to pass urine (voiding) at a time to suit the individual. The alternation between these two modes of storage and voiding is known as the micturition cycle (Figure 1). lower urinary tract symptoms (LUTS) are categorized according to the time at which they are experienced in relation to the micturition cycle;

1. Storage symptoms
   a) Increased daytime frequency (IDF) is the complaint by the patient who considers that he/she voids too often by day.[1] There is no minimum voiding frequency serving as a threshold for the symptom, since it is highly subjective, and there is a wide overlap between normal and symptomatic.

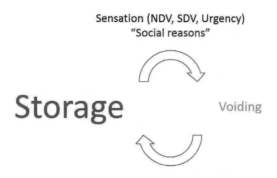

Sensation (NDV, SDV, Urgency)
"Social reasons"

Storage   Voiding

FIGURE 1 The micturition cycle as anchor for categorizing LUTS. Each individual person stores urine until they make an active decision to switch to voiding in response to a sensation or a social reason (eg, anticipation that toilets will be difficult to access in the foreseeable future as a result of a meeting or journey, or when going to bed for sleep). Once voiding is complete, storage mode is re-established. Voiding occupies only a very small part of the cycle (eg, if frequency is six times daily, and duration of each void is 20 s, then only 2 min of 24 h may be in voiding mode). NDV, normal desire to void; SDV, strong desire to void

b) Nocturia is waking at night to pass urine.[2] If a person typically passes urine once per night, they should be documented as having nocturia even if it does not cause them impairment of quality of life.

"Day" and "night" for IDF and nocturia refer to the patient's sleeping pattern, not environmental daylight and night-time.

These symptoms are strongly influenced by fluid intake, and healthcare practitioners need to factor in whether the symptom reflects LUTD, or rather a physiological mechanism dealing with excessive intake of free water or salt, or a pathological consequence of a systemic medical condition (eg, chronic kidney disease).[5]

c) Urgency is the complaint of a sudden compelling desire to pass urine which is difficult to defer.[1]
d) Urinary incontinence is the complaint of any involuntary leakage of urine.[1]

Incontinence is subclassified according to the circumstances most typically eliciting the problem

(i) Urgency urinary incontinence is the complaint of involuntary leakage accompanied by or immediately preceded by urgency.
(ii) Stress urinary incontinence is the complaint of involuntary leakage on effort or exertion, or on sneezing or coughing.
(iii) Mixed urinary incontinence is the complaint of involuntary leakage associated with urgency and also with exertion, effort, sneezing, or coughing.

2. Voiding and post-voiding symptoms
   Voiding symptoms

a) Hesitancy is the term used when an individual describes difficulty in initiating micturition resulting in a delay in the onset of voiding after the individual is ready to pass urine.[1]
b) Slow stream is reported by the individual as his or her perception of reduced urine flow, usually compared to previous performance or in comparison to others.[1]
c) Intermittency is the term used when the individual describes urine flow which stops and starts, on one or more occasions, during micturition.[1]

In addition, a person may report splitting of the stream, or spraying. They may also describe straining to void, which is muscular effort used to either initiate, maintain, or improve the urinary stream.

Post-voiding symptoms are experienced immediately after voiding.

d) Feeling of incomplete emptying is experienced by the individual after passing urine.[1]

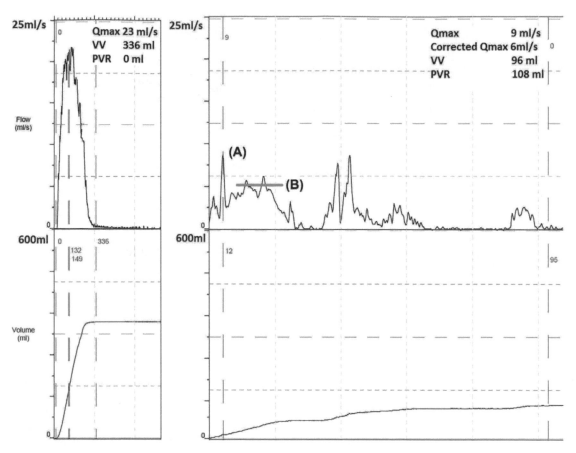

FIGURE 3 Uroflowmetry (free flow rate testing). On the left is a normal flow rate test for a women. It shows a continuous flow, with a good maximum flow rate (Qmax) and complete emptying, with a suitable VV. On the right is an abnormal test suggesting voiding dysfunction. The pattern of flow is interrupted. The Qmax reported by the machine was 9 mL/s, but inspection of the trace shows the machine interpreted a spike (A) as the maximum flow, which will not be indicative of the patient's own urinary tract function, but rather is likely to be an artefact (eg, an aberration of flow delivery to the meter, a strain by the patient, or the patient moving on the commode). By definition, Qmax must be corrected to exclude artefacts.[1] Correcting the Qmax to a part of the curve (B) that is likely to be properly representative of urinary tract function gives a lower Qmax of 6 mL/s. The VV was low, but when the PVR of 108 mL is factored in, the bladder volume can be considered adequate when the flow test was done (96 + 108 = 204 mL)

in the bladder wall (passive and active), and it is calculated by subtracting P_{abd} from P_{ves}.[1] P_{det} is computed throughout filling cystometry and PFS, and is plotted alongside the two measured pressures (P_{ves} and Pa_{bd}) and flow (Q) (Figure 4).

Filling cystometry assesses the storage phase of the patient's micturition cycle. Filling cystometry should be described according to bladder sensation, detrusor activity, bladder compliance, and bladder capacity. Bladder compliance describes the relationship between change in bladder volume and change in detrusor pressure, and is calculated by dividing the volume change by the change in p_{det} during that change in bladder volume[1] (Figure 4). The standards points are (i) p_{det} at the start of bladder filling and the corresponding bladder volume (usually zero) and (ii) the p_{det} and bladder volume at cystometric capacity or immediately before the start of any detrusor contraction that causes significant leakage.

Both points are measured excluding any detrusor contraction. Detrusor overactivity (DO) is a urodynamic observation characterized by involuntary detrusor contractions during the filling phase which may be spontaneous or provoked. Provocative maneuvers are techniques used during urodynamics in an effort to provoke DO, for example, rapid filling, use of cooled medium, postural changes, and hand washing.[1]

Cystometric capacity is the bladder volume at the end of the filling cystometrogram. It is the volume voided, plus any PVR. The PFS starts when "permission to void" is given (Figure 4), or when uncontrollable voiding begins, and ends when the patient considers voiding has finished. PFS is a model of the patient's voiding phase and combines synchronous flowmetry with measurement of p_{ves}. Thus, flow rate testing in PFS differs from free flowmetry by the presence of a fine tube to enable pressure measurement. Normal voiding is achieved by a voluntarily initiated

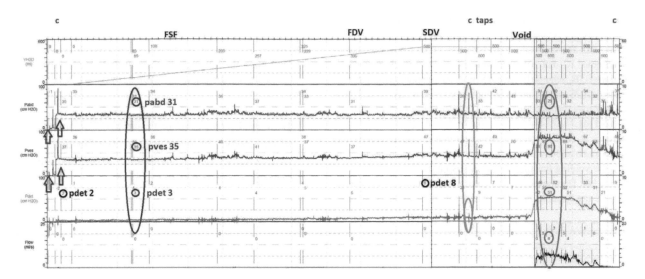

FIGURE 4   Pressure measurement. The record shows continuous tracings of two measured pressures; the abdominal pressure p_{abd} in red, and the vesical bladder pressure p_{ves} in blue. These are continuously subtracted (p_{ves}-p_{abd}) to give the detrusor p_{det}, in green. Also shown are the volume instilled in orange, and flow rate in black. Filling cystometry precedes permission to void (indicated with "void"), and the pressure flow study (PFS) follows it. The zero reference point is atmospheric pressure (purple arrows), so when the transducers are connected to the patient (blue arrows), there is an obvious rise in p_{abd} and p_{ves}, referred to as "resting pressures"—the blue oval indicates the resting pressures for this patient at one timepoint. Coughs (indicated with "c") are used to check that p_{abd} and p_{ves} detect a short spike of pressure (larger green oval), and that the p_{det} has a deflection which is equal above and below the line, the biphasic artefact (smaller green oval). It is important to check pressure recording with a cough at the start of filling, and on each side of the PFS. Normal detrusor function allows bladder filling with little or no change in pressure, and there should be no involuntary phasic contractions despite provocation.[1] In this study, the p_{det} was 2 cmH$_2$O at the beginning of the filling cystometry, and eight at the end; since filled volume was 500 mL, the compliance (change in volume/change in pressure = 100/[8-2]) was 17 mL/cmH$_2$O. Sensations are reported by the patient and annotated on the trace. First sensation of bladder filling (FSF) is the feeling the patient has, during filling cystometry, when he/ she first becomes aware of the bladder filling. First desire to void (FDV) is the feeling that would lead the patient to pass urine at the next convenient moment, but voiding can be delayed if necessary. Strong desire to void (SDV) is a persistent desire to void without the fear of leakage.[1] A provocation was applied to try to elicit DO by making the sound of running water "taps"; no change in p_{ves} or p_{det} was seen, so this patient had a stable detrusor. In the PFS, the key parameters derive from the time of maximum flow rate (Q_{max}). The current patient had a Q_{max} of 8 mL/s and detrusor pressure at Q_{max} of 51 cmH$_2$O, so his BOO Index was 35 and Bladder Contractility Index was 91. P_{abd} did not change at that time, so no allowance has to be made for the effect on P_{det}

continuous detrusor contraction that leads to complete bladder emptying within a normal time span, and in the absence of obstruction. Detrusor underactivity (DUA) is a contraction of reduced strength and/or duration, resulting in prolonged bladder emptying and/or a failure to achieve complete emptying within a normal time span. Bladder outlet obstruction (BOO) is the generic term for obstruction during voiding and is characterized by increased detrusor pressure and reduced urine flow rate.[1] For male patients, BOO and DUA can be quantified using the BOO Index and the Bladder Contractility Index.[8] They rely on measuring Qmax and detrusor pressure at maximum flow, which is the lowest pressure recorded at maximum measured flow rate (see [9]).

6 | CONCLUSIONS

The ICS Standardization provides a logical framework and definitions to describe symptoms, signs, and urodynamic observations in relationship to the micturition cycle.

ORCID

Marcus J. Drake   http://orcid.org/0000-0002-6230-2552

REFERENCES

1. Abrams P, Cardozo L, Fall M, et al. The standardisation of terminology of lower urinary tract function: report from the Standardisation Sub-committee of the International Continence Society. *Neurourol Urodyn.* 2002;21:167–178.

2. Hashim H, Drake MJ. Basic concepts in nocturia, based on International Continence Society standards in nocturnal lower urinary tract function. *Neurourol Urodyn.* 2018;37:S20–S24.

3. Chapple CR. Terminology report from the International Continence Society (ICS) working group on underactive bladder (UAB). *Neurourol Urodyn.* 2018;In press.

4. Haylen BT, de Ridder D, Freeman RM, et al. An International Urogynecological Association (IUGA)/International Continence Society (ICS) joint report on the terminology for female pelvic floor dysfunction. *Neurourol Urodyn.* 2010;29:4–20.

5. Cornu JN, Abrams P, Chapple CR, et al. A contemporary assessment of nocturia: definition, epidemiology, pathophysiology,

6 | EXPLAINING THE PROBLEMS

For anyone with nocturia, a basic interpretation of the bladder diary can be used to categorise likely contributory factors,[10] and thereby guide subsequent evaluation and treatment.[11,12]

- 24-h polyuria; caused by a range of medical problems, such as diabetes insipidus, salt loss, or poorly controlled diabetes mellitus. These people often report constant thirstiness.
- NP; caused by problems such as obstructive sleep apnoea or peripheral oedema.
- LUTD; generally associated with storage LUTS, and with increased bladder sensation scores on the bladder diary.
- Sleep disturbance; should be considered if the patient describes anxiety, restless legs, nightmares, and sleep-walking.

Simple behavioral tendencies should be considered, for example identification of a high fluid intake in someone who does not experience constant thirst. LUTD is actually a relatively uncommon explanation for nocturia in the wider population, so urologists or urogynecologists should identify the other possible situations and avoid urological or gynecological interventions, where not specifically indicated.

7 | ENURESIS

Enuresis is a symptom in which the patient complains of intermittent incontinence that occurs during periods of sleep. It is also a sign of "wetting" while asleep. This is not the same as waking with urinary urgency and having insufficient time to reach the toilet, which is urgency urinary incontinence.

Enuresis may have more in common with voiding dysregulation (urination in situations which are generally regarded as socially inappropriate) or involuntary voiding (sporadic bladder emptying when awake)[13] than nocturia. Thus, they must be clearly distinguished when both nocturia and enuresis are reported by a patient.

8 | CONCLUSION

The symptom of nocturia is present if the patient reports waking at night to pass urine and nocturia is also a sign indicated by the number of times an individual passes urine during their main sleep period. NP is present if the patient reports passing large volumes of urine at night, and this can be quantified with the nocturnal polyuria index. The bladder diary is an important diagnostic tool, helping identify 24-h polyuria, NP, LUTD, and sleep disturbance. Enuresis is distinguished from nocturia, as the patient fails to wake up for passing urine.

CONFLICT OF INTEREST

Dr. Hashim reports personal fees and non-financial support from Ferring, personal fees from Astellas, personal fees from Medtronic, personal fees from Boston, personal fees and non-financial support from Allergan, outside the submitted work. Dr. Drake reports grants, personal fees and non-financial support from Ferring, during the conduct of the study; grants, personal fees and non-financial support from Astellas, grants, personal fees and non-financial support from Allergan, outside the submitted work.

ORCID

Hashim Hashim http://orcid.org/0000-0003-2467-407X
Marcus J. Drake http://orcid.org/0000-0002-6230-2552

REFERENCES

1. Tikkinen KA, Johnson TM, Tammela TL, et al. Nocturia frequency, bother, and quality of life: how often is too often? A population-based study in Finland. *Eur Urol.* 2010;57:488–496.
2. van Doorn B, Blanker MH, Kok ET, Westers P, Bosch JL. Prevalence, incidence, and resolution of nocturnal polyuria in a longitudinal community-based study in older men: the Krimpen study. *Eur Urol.* 2013;63:542–547.
3. van Kerrebroeck P, Abrams P, Chaikin D, et al. The standardisation of terminology in nocturia: report from the Standardisation Sub-committee of the International Continence Society. *Neurourol Urodyn.* 2002;21:179–183.
4. Van Kerrebroeck P, Abrams P, Chaikin D, et al. The standardization of terminology in nocturia: report from the standardization subcommittee of the International Continence Society. *BJU Int.* 2002;90:11–15.
5. Abrams P, Cardozo L, Fall M, et al. The standardisation of terminology of lower urinary tract function: report from the Standardisation Sub-committee of the International Continence Society. *Neurourol Urodyn.* 2002;21:167–178.
6. Abrams P, Avery K, Gardener N, Donovan J. The international consultation on incontinence modular questionnaire: www.iciq.net. *J Urol.* 2006;175:1063–1066. discussion 1066.
7. Abraham L, Hareendran A, Mills IW, et al. Development and validation of a quality-of-life measure for men with nocturia. *Urology.* 2004;63:481–486.
8. Bright E, Cotterill N, Drake M, Abrams P. Developing and validating the International Consultation on Incontinence Questionnaire bladder diary. *Eur Urol.* 2014;66:294–300.
9. Bright E, Drake MJ, Abrams P. Urinary diaries: evidence for the development and validation of diary content, format, and duration. *Neurourol Urodyn.* 2011;30:348–352.
10. Cornu JN, Abrams P, Chapple CR, et al. A contemporary assessment of nocturia: definition, epidemiology, pathophysiology, and management-a systematic review and meta-analysis. *Eur Urol.* 2012;62:877–890.
11. Sakalis VI, Karavitakis M, Bedretdinova D, et al. Medical treatment of nocturia in men with lower urinary tract symptoms: systematic

review by the european association of urology guidelines panel for male lower urinary tract symptoms. *Eur Urol.* 2017;72:757–769.

12. Gratzke C, Bachmann A, Descazeaud A, et al. EAU guidelines on the assessment of non-neurogenic male lower urinary tract symptoms including benign prostatic obstruction. *Eur Urol.* 2015;67:1099–1109.

13. Gajewski JB, Schurch B, Hamid R, et al. An International Continence Society (ICS) report on the terminology for adult neurogenic lower urinary tract dysfunction (ANLUTD). *Neurourol Urodyn.* 2018;37:1152–1161.

How to cite this article: Hashim H, Drake MJ. Basic concepts in nocturia, based on international continence society standards in nocturnal lower urinary tract function. *Neurourology and Urodynamics.* 2018;37:S20–S24. https://doi.org/10.1002/nau.23781

Received: 1 May 2018 | Accepted: 11 June 2018

DOI: 10.1002/nau.23758

SOUNDING BOARD

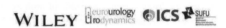

Neurological lower urinary tract dysfunction essential terminology

Jerzy B. Gajewski[1] | **Marcus J. Drake**[2,3]

[1] Dalhousie University, Halifax, Nova Scotia, Canada

[2] Translational Health Sciences, Bristol Medical School, Bristol, UK

[3] Bristol Urological Institute, Southmead Hospital, Bristol, UK

Correspondence

Marcus J. Drake, Bristol Urological Institute, 3rd Floor L&R building, Southmead Hospital, Bristol, BS10 5NB, UK.
Email: marcus.drake@bristol.ac.uk

Aims: To introduce basic concepts and definitions in the International Continence Society (ICS) Standardisation of Terminology in adult Neurogenic Lower Urinary Tract Dysfunction (NLUTD).

Methods: Fundamental terminology in the ICS Standardisation of Terminology of Adult NLUTD was identified and summarized.

Results: NLUTD is often associated with impairment of cognitive, motor, sensory, and/or autonomic functions. Lesions are categorized into suprapontine, pontine/ suprasacral spinal, sacral spinal, cauda equina/peripheral nerve, or mixed lesions. People affected with neurological disease are also at risk of the conditions seen in the general population, such as benign prostate enlargement. Symptoms of NLUTD include alterations in bladder or urethral sensation and incontinence. Loss of urine can result from incontinence, involuntary passing of urine and factors that impair toilet use, incorporating problems such as impaired cognition urinary incontinence, impaired mobility urinary incontinence, and voiding dysregulation. Signs may be discerned by physical examination and recording of a frequency volume chart or bladder diary. Urodynamic observations during filling cystometry may include altered sensations, neurogenic detrusor overactivity, and reduced bladder compliance. During pressure flow studies, there may be detrusor underactivity or bladder outlet obstruction (BOO). BOO may be caused by various forms poorly co-ordinated muscle activity in the bladder outlet. Symptoms, signs, and urodynamic observations may be useful in diagnosing the presence and specific location of neurological impairment.

Conclusion: The review provides a succinct summary of symptoms, signs, and urodynamic observations as set out in the ICS Standard on Adult NLUTD.

KEYWORDS

incontinence, LUTS, neurological disease, standardization

1 | INTRODUCTION

Adult neurogenic lower urinary tract dysfunction (NLUTD) refers to abnormal or difficult function of the bladder, urethra

(and/or prostate in men) in mature individuals in the context of clinically confirmed relevant neurologic disorder. NLUTD is a key subgroup of the broad range of lower urinary tract symptoms (LUTS), due to the severity of the symptoms, and the implications of urinary dysfunction for wider health. The International Continence Society (ICS) categorizes symptoms, signs, urodynamic observations, and conditions

Alan Wein led the peer-review process as the Associate Editor responsible for the paper.

associated with lower urinary tract dysfunction (LUTD) in relationship to the storage and voiding phases of the micturition cycle. Neurological disease brings additional dimensions to the LUTD as experienced in the lives of affected individuals. The current document is a summary of core terminology in NLUTD for use in the wider context of LUTS in people known to have a neurological disease, or suspected of potentially having one which has not yet been diagnosed.

2 | METHODS

Recommendations in the ICS Standard on Adult Neurogenic Lower Urinary Tract Dysfunction[1] were reviewed and summarized. Definitions and key terms are generally transcribed verbatim and highlighted in bold. In the original document, many of the definitions are accompanied by explanatory or exemplary footnotes which have been adapted or excluded for the current review for the sake of brevity. Readers requiring more detailed information are referred to the full ICS Standard, and other documents produced by the ICS Standardisation Steering Committee.

3 | NEUROLOGICAL CONTROL

The nervous system controls many facets that are essential for the normal micturition cycle (storage and voiding). Particularly crucial are cognition (eg, decision making, anticipation, awareness of environment/social context, and conscious perception of sensation), motor functions (eg, mobility, balance, and dexterity), sensory nerve activity, and autonomic functions (eg, regulation of the detrusor and sphincter). The neurological functions act together to make sure that both urine storage and voiding reflect timings and contexts appropriately, with full voluntary control (Figure 1).

Neurological diseases are diverse and differ in terms of the parts of the nervous system affected (eg, the cognitive-predominant effects of dementia) and their behavior (eg, progressive, such as multiple sclerosis, or non-progressive, such as spinal cord injury). Thus, neurological disease may have differing effects on cognitive, sensory, motor, and autonomic functions which manifest in the specific NLUTD experienced by the patient. Inevitably, the consequences of neurological disease extend beyond LUTD, and mean that affected patients have a range of issues that influence treatment potential and health risk. Problems with bowel function, sexual and reproductive function, cognition, mobility, and blood pressure control are particularly relevant.

In describing the features of an individual patient's dysfunction, clinicians should appreciate the distinction between symptoms, signs, and urodynamic observations as set out in the ICS Standardisation of Terminology of Lower Urinary Tract Function[2] (for summary see[3]). A summary of the classification of neurological lesions,[1] including the potential clinical and urodynamic features, is given in Figure 2.

4 | NLUTD SYMPTOMS

People with NLUTD may describe storage, voiding, and post voiding symptoms consistent with the definitions used for the general population.[2,3] Sometimes, a patient may not express that a symptom is present, so it is appropriate to discuss with the caregiver as well when establishing the presenting complaint. Storage symptoms may converge in **Neurogenic Overactive Bladder, which is a symptom syndrome characterized by urgency, with or without urgency urinary incontinence, usually with increased daytime frequency and nocturia in the setting of a clinically relevant neurologic disorder with at least partially preserved sensation**.

4.1 | Bladder and urethral sensation

Neurologically healthy people are intermittently aware of bladder sensations related to filling and voiding, and urethral sensation with voiding. Someone with NLUTD may describe alterations, for example:

Increased bladder sensation: the desire to void during bladder filling occurs earlier or is more persistent than that previously experienced. Reduced: the definite desire to void occurs later to that previously experienced despite an awareness that the bladder is filling. *Absent*: the individual reports no sensation of bladder filling or desire to void. Such patients may have a significant post voiding residual in the bladder, without any sensation of incomplete emptying.

Non-specific bladder awareness: the individual reports no specific bladder sensation, but may perceive, for example, abdominal fullness, vegetative symptoms, urethral sensations, or spasticity as bladder filling awareness or a sign of bladder fullness. This may indicate that the usual sensory nerve pathways are not communicating centrally. Instead anatomical routes which do not usually contribute to everyday sensations may be intact and functional.

In addition, some people report they are unable to feel flow of urine along the urethra. They may report that they can only discern whether bladder emptying is finished by looking, or listening for the splash of urine in the toilet to stop.

4.2 | Loss of urine

Mature CNS regulation ensures storage (detrusor relaxation with outlet contraction) and the transition to voiding (detrusor

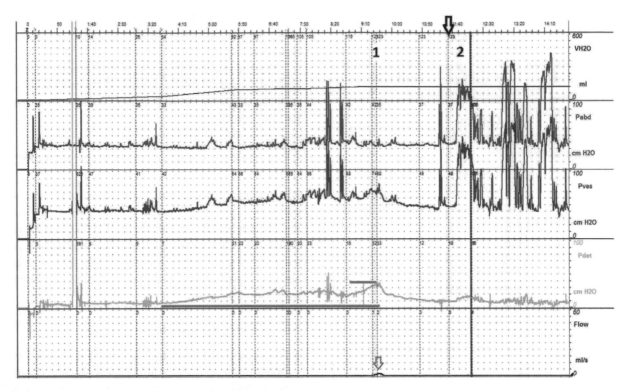

FIGURE 3 Filling cystometry in a sacral spinal cord lesion (SSCL) showing reduced compliance; the lower orange line indicates the phase during which the detrusor pressure (green trace, second from bottom) is climbing, even though the filling rate is slow (10 mL/min). The upper orange line indicates the detrusor leak point pressure. The change in volume over this time was $123-34 = 89$ mL, and the change in pressure was $33-7 = 26$ cm H_2O. Compliance (change in volume divided by change in pressure) was thus $89/26 = 3.4$ mL/cm H_2O. Detrusor Leak Point Volume (DLPV) is defined as a bladder volume at which first urine leakage occurs (1), either with detrusor overactivity or low compliance (orange arrow). The leakage is seen in the flow trace (black, bottom trace), and the leakage causes the elevated detrusor pressure to dissipate. The arrow indicates permission to void. However, there is no flow generated, and the patient does several Valsalva strains, shown by the substantial pressure rises in both abdominal pressure, and hence bladder pressure (2), signifying neurogenic acontractile detrusor. At time of urodynamics, neurological diagnosis had not previously been suspected, and subsequently he was identified to have multiple system atrophy

5.2 | Pressure flow studies

When passing urine, a slow stream may be explained by impaired detrusor contraction, bladder outlet obstruction (BOO), or a combination of both. Potential causes of neurogenic BOO include:

- **Non-relaxing urethral sphincter, characterized by a non-relaxing, obstructing urethral sphincter resulting in reduced urine flow.**
- **Delayed relaxation of the urethral sphincter, characterized by impaired and hindered relaxation of the sphincter during voiding attempt resulting in delay of urine flow.**
- **Detrusor-Sphincter Dyssynergia (DSD), which describes a detrusor contraction concurrent with an involuntary contraction of the urethral and/or periurethral striated muscle.** Occasionally flow may be prevented altogether.

DSD is an indicator that the pontine micturition center is not communicating effectively with the sacral spinal cord, and occurs in people with a suprasacral spinal cord/pontine lesion. The term should not be used in other forms of NLUTD, and it is not a general term for neurogenic BOO.

Other causes of BOO present in the general population, such as benign prostatic obstruction, bladder neck obstruction, or urethral stricture in men, can also be present in people with neurological disease, and videourodynamics may be appropriate to discern the proximal site of BOO.

Impaired detrusor contraction can indicate:

- **Neurogenic detrusor underactivity; a contraction of reduced strength and/or duration, resulting in prolonged bladder emptying and/or a failure to achieve complete bladder emptying within a normal time span in the setting of a clinically relevant neurologic disorder.**

- **Neurogenic acontractile detrusor;** the detrusor cannot be demonstrated to contract during urodynamic studies in the setting of a clinically relevant neurologic lesion (Figure 3).

Balanced bladder emptying is a bladder emptying with physiological detrusor pressure and low residual as perceived by the investigator, and should be defined in the report.

6 | NLUTD CLINICAL DIAGNOSES

- **Spinal Shock Phase is usually temporary following acute neurologic insult or SCI that is characterized by loss of sensory, motor, and reflex activity below the level of injury.** NLUTD in Spinal Shock is usually a temporary complete painless urinary reten`tion.
- **Autonomic Dysreflexia is a syndrome resulting from an upper thoracic or cervical spinal cord injury above T6, elicited by a stimulus in the field of distribution of the autonomous sympathetic nucleus, characterized by unregulated sympathetic function below the lesion and compensatory autonomic responses.** It is potentially a medical emergency characterized by hypertension, bradycardia, severe headaches, and flushing above, with pallor below the cord lesion, and sometimes convulsions. An increase of blood pressure without any other symptoms is called Asymptomatic Autonomic Dysreflexia.

Urinary retention is an inability to properly empty the bladder. Retention may be complete or incomplete:

- **Acute retention of urine is an acute event of painful, palpable or percussable bladder, when the patient is unable to pass any urine when the bladder is full.** Although acute retention is usually thought of as painful, in certain circumstances pain may not be a presenting feature, for example, when due to prolapsed intervertebral disc, post-partum, or after regional anesthesia such as an epidural anesthetic. The retention volume should be significantly greater than the expected normal bladder capacity.
- **Chronic retention is a non-painful bladder, which remains palpable or percussable after the patient has passed urine. Such patients may be incontinent.** Chronic retention, excludes transient voiding difficulty, for example, after surgery for stress incontinence, and implies a significant residual urine.

7 | DIAGNOSING NEUROLOGICAL DYSFUNCTION

In order to understand the full picture of the neurological deficit, the history may be used to identify features which could localize the site of a problem or suggest the causative condition and its behavior. Such observations can be helpful to a patient's neurologist in localising areas of deficit. These features are important in defining a patient's condition, since it guides subsequent testing (such as the anatomical sites and scan protocols for MRI). For example, retrograde ejaculation reported by a man who has not had bladder neck or prostate surgery may indicate a neurological deficit in the thoracolumbar spine or related peripheral nerves; this may be accompanied by visualization of an open bladder neck during videourodynamic filling cystometry. Signs can also help; for example, loss of the anal reflex indicates a lesion affecting the sacral spinal cord or its sensory or motor nerves.

In rare but important cases, urinary dysfunction may present for urological evaluation in a patient with no known neurological background whose ultimate cause may subsequently prove to be a neurological disease. This can occur for example in MS, normal pressure hydrocephalus, multiple system atrophy, and early Parkinson's disease.[4] Key symptoms include erectile dysfunction, retrograde ejaculation, enuresis, loss of filling sensation, or unexplained stress urinary incontinence.[4] If there is any suspicion that an undiagnosed neurological disease could be present, questioning should enquire about visual symptoms, back pain, anosmia, bowel dysfunction and incontinence, or memory loss.[4] Specialist evaluation is likely to be needed.

8 | CONCLUSIONS

NLUTD is categorized into: suprapontine; pontine/suprasacral spinal; sacral spinal; cauda equina/peripheral nerve; mixed lesions. Loss of urine can result from impaired cognition urinary incontinence, impaired mobility urinary incontinence, and voiding dysregulation. Urodynamic observations during filling cystometry may include altered sensations, neurogenic detrusor overactivity, and reduced bladder compliance. During pressure flow studies, there may be detrusor underactivity or bladder outlet obstruction (BOO). BOO may be caused by various forms poorly co-ordinated muscle activity in the bladder outlet. Symptoms, signs, and urodynamic observations may be useful in diagnosing the presence and specific location of neurological impairment.

CONFLICT OF INTEREST

The authors declare no conflict of interest.

ORCID

Jerzy B. Gajewski http://orcid.org/0000-0003-0769-583X
Marcus J. Drake http://orcid.org/0000-0002-6230-2552

REFERENCES

1. Gajewski JB, Schurch B, Hamid R, et al. An International Continence Society (ICS) report on the terminology for adult neurogenic lower urinary tract dysfunction (ANLUTD). *Neurourol Urodyn.* 2018;37:1152–1161.
2. Abrams P, Cardozo L, Fall M, et al. The standardisation of terminology of lower urinary tract function: report from the Standardisation Sub-committee of the International Continence Society. *Neurourol Urodyn.* 2002;21:167–178.
3. Drake MJ. Fundamentals of terminology in lower urinary tract function. *Neurourol Urodyn.* 2018;37:S13–S19.
4. Wei DY, Drake MJ. Undiagnosed neurological disease as a potential cause of male lower urinary tract symptoms. *Curr Opin Urol.* 2016;26:11–16.

How to cite this article: Gajewski JB, Drake MJ. Neurological lower urinary tract dysfunction essential terminology. *Neurourology and Urodynamics.* 2018;37:S25–S31.
https://doi.org/10.1002/nau.23758

Received: 28 May 2018 | Accepted: 1 July 2018

DOI: 10.1002/nau.23776

SOUNDING BOARD

WILEY Neurourology Urodynamics ICS SUFU

The fundamentals of chronic pelvic pain assessment, based on international continence society recommendations

Neha Rana[1] | Marcus J. Drake[2,3] | Rebecca Rinko[1] | Melissa Dawson[1] | Kristene E. Whitmore[1,4]

[1] Division of Female Pelvic Medicine and Reconstructive Surgery, Department of Obstetrics and Gynecology, Drexel University College of Medicine, Philadelphia, Pennsylvania

[2] Translational Health Sciences, Bristol Medical School, Bristol, UK

[3] Bristol Urological Institute, Southmead Hospital, Bristol, UK

[4] Division of Female Pelvic Medicine and Reconstructive Surgery and Urology, Drexel University College of Medicine, Philadelphia, Pennsylvania

Correspondence
Kristene E. Whitmore, Division of Female Pelvic Medicine and Reconstructive Surgery and Urology, Department of Obstetrics and Gynecology, Drexel University College of Medicine, 207 North Broad Street, 4th Floor Philadelphia, PA 19107.
Email:bladder1@aol.com

Aims: Chronic pelvic pain (CPP) is defined as a noncyclical pain that has duration of at least 6 months and can lead to decreased quality of life and physical performance. The pain can be attributed to problems in the pelvic organs and/or problems in related systems, and possible psycho-social attributes may contribute to the manifestation. Due to the complex nature, CPP syndromes are multifactorial and the terminology needs to reflect the setting.

Methods: The current review is a synthesis of key aspects of the recent International Continence Society Standardization for Terminology in CPP Syndromes.

Results: Nine domains can be used for a detailed description of CPP. They include four domains specific to the pelvic organs (lower urinary tract, female genital, male genital, gastrointestinal), two related to other sources of pain which may be perceived in the pelvis (musculoskeletal, neurological) and three which may influence the response to the pain or its impact on the individual (psychological, sexual, and comorbidities). For an individual patient with CPP, each domain should be reviewed in terms of symptoms and signs, noting that positive findings could reflect either a primary cause or a secondary consequence. The findings will guide further evaluations and subsequent treatment.

Conclusion: We present a synthesis of the standard for terminology in CPP syndromes in women and men, which serves as a systematic framework to consider possible sources of pain (pelvic organs or other sources) and the individual responses and impact.

KEYWORDS
chronic pelvic pain, lower urinary tract dysfunction, LUTS, pelvic floor muscle pain, standardization

1 | INTRODUCTION

CPP is defined as a noncyclical pain that has duration of at least 6 months, and it can lead to decreased quality of

life and physical performance.[1] The presentation can be a challenge to assess and treat. This is because the pain can potentially be attributed to several contributory factors, in the context of the varied nature of pain responses manifested by individuals. Healthcare professionals (HCPs) need to consider gynecological, urological, gastrointestinal, musculoskeletal, neurological, or

---

Roger Dmochowski led the peer-review process as the Associate Editor responsible for the paper.

3.2 | Domains related to other causes of pain

Musculoskeletal problems are common, and sometimes are hard to localize for the patient. In CPP, they may be the principle cause of pain, or they may be consequential as the patient makes physical adaptations to deal with their primary problem (Table 5). Features that indicate a primary or secondary musculoskeletal problem include; tenderness, abnormal movement and alterations in the muscle (tone, stiffness, tension, spasms, cramping, fasciculation, and trigger points). Pain may originate from muscles, fascia, ligaments, joints, or bones, so familiarity with the anatomy and approaches to clinical examination is needed. Particularly key regions include;

- Muscular: the pelvic floor[8] (levator ani group/perineum), the lower abdominal wall, or posterior pelvic and gluteal regions.
- Joints, ligaments and bones: Coccyx pain syndrome, sacroiliac or pubic symphysis joints, sacrospinous or sacrotuberous ligaments, or the pubic ramus, ilium, and ischial spine

Where there is an issue in the neurological domain (Table 6), patients commonly use characteristic terms to describe pain (burning, stabbing, throbbing, tingling, stinging, electric shock-like) or they may report paresthesia. Somatic Neuropathic pain is secondary to a specific nerve injury, and is associated with symptoms related to the nerve distribution. In CPP, the relevant nerves could be sacral (Figure 2), pudendal, thoracolumbar, ilioinguinal, iliohypogastric, genitofemoral or obturator. A neuroma secondary to surgery or other trauma may give a localized tender point in the specific location, and if present should be identified and removed.

Complex regional pain syndrome (CRPS)[9] is a situation whose precise etiology is uncertain, but it can be categorized by burning pain and changes in the skin (increased sensitivity, and changes in skin temperature, color, and/or texture). CRPS type 1 is triggered by tissue injury without an underlying nerve injury and CRPS type 2 is attributed to a history of a nerve injury.

Pain in someone with a history of surgery which involved placement of synthetic is a specific issue. It can present as pain during physical activity, dyspareunia, vaginal discharge, and/or exposure of the mesh in the vagina or surrounding tissues.

3.3 | Domains affecting response or impact

Psychological aspects are an important element in the individual situation (Table 7). Patients may report symptoms of anxiety, worry, low mood, sleep disturbances, helplessness, hopelessness, difficulty concentrating, and pain impairing enjoyment. Alternatively, people close to the affected person may observe these features.

Sexual function may be affected by CPP in both men and women, and relationships may be affected (Table 8). Patients may report decreased libido, inability to become aroused, dyspareunia, and difficulty achieving an orgasm, and there may also be partner concerns. Several disorders can be identified;

- Sexual desire disorders; Hypoactive sexual disorder or Sexual aversion disorder
- Sexual arousal disorder
- Orgasmic disorder
- Sexual pain disorder

A comorbidities domain is also included (Table 9), as patients with CPP syndromes have a higher prevalence of problems such as allergies, chronic fatigue syndromes, fibromyalgia, and autoimmune diseases that may affect multiple systems.

4 | CONCLUSIONS

The current document extracts some of the pertinent elements that should be identified in order to understand fully the range of factors potentially present in CPP. The domain structure serves as a checklist to aid consideration of the several issues, and thereby ensure key relevant factors are not overlooked. The approach aids a logical sequence in considering the pelvic organs, other potential sources of pain, and factors that affect individual pain response and its impact.

CONFLICTS OF INTEREST

Drs Neha Rana, Marcus J. Drake, Rebecca Rinko, and Melissa Dawson have nothing to disclose. Dr Kristene Whitmore reports grants from Allergan, grants from Astellas, and grants from Coloplast clinical research during the conduct of the study.

ORCID

Marcus J. Drake http://orcid.org/0000-0002-6230-2552
Kristene E. Whitmore http://orcid.org/0000-0002-0135-1158

REFERENCES

1. Ahangari A. Prevalence of chronic pelvic pain among women: an updated review. *Pain Physician.* 2014;17:E141–E147.
2. Doggweiler R, Whitmore KE, Meijlink JM, et al. A standard for terminology in chronic pelvic pain syndromes: a report from the chronic pelvic pain working group of the international continence society. *Neurourol Urodyn.* 2017;36:984–1008.

3. Bornstein J, Goldstein AT, Stockdale CK, et al. 2015 ISSVD, ISSWSH and IPPS consensus terminology and classification of persistent vulvar pain and vulvodynia. *Obstet Gynecol.* 2016;127: 745–751.

4. Engeler DS, Baranowski AP, Dinis-Oliveira P, et al. The 2013 EAU guidelines on chronic pelvic pain: is management of chronic pelvic pain a habit, a philosophy, or a science? 10 years of development. *Eur Urol.* 2013;64:431–439.

5. Jarrell JF, Vilos GA, Allaire C, et al. Consensus guidelines for the management of chronic pelvic pain. *J Obstet Gynaecol Can.* 2005;27: 781–826.

6. Hanno P, Dmochowski R. Status of international consensus on interstitial cystitis/bladder pain syndrome/painful bladder syndrome: 2008 snapshot. *Neurourol Urodyn.* 2009;28: 274–286.

7. Drossman DA. The functional gastrointestinal disorders and the Rome III process. *Gastroenterology.* 2006;130:1377–1390.

8. Montenegro ML, Mateus-Vasconcelos EC, Rosa e Silva JC, Nogueira AA, Dos Reis FJ, Poli Neto OB. Importance of pelvic muscle tenderness evaluation in women with chronic pelvic pain. *Pain Med.* 2010;11:224–228.

9. Harden RN, Oaklander AL, Burton AW, et al. Complex regional pain syndrome: practical diagnostic and treatment guidelines, 4th edition. *Pain Med.* 2013;14:180–229.

How to cite this article: Rana N, Drake MJ, Rinko R, Dawson M, Whitmore K. The fundamentals of chronic pelvic pain assessment, based on international continence society recommendations. *Neurourology and Urodynamics.* 2018;37:S32–S38. https://doi.org/10.1002/nau.23776

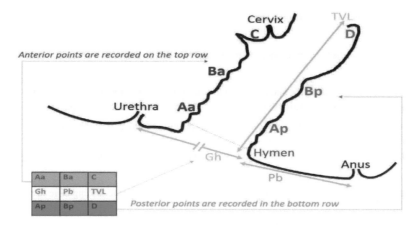

FIGURE 2 How the six defined point and three measurements relate to a 3 × 3 grid used for clinical documentation. Gh, genital hiatus; Pb, perineal body; TVL, total vaginal length

prolapse and which can be confirmed by the woman, by digital palpation or use of a mirror, should be used (left lateral, standing, lithotomy, or standing). Use a Sim's speculum if necessary to retract the anterior and posterior vaginal walls to assess for prolapse. The techniques and positions used should be recorded, as they may influence findings.[7]

Step 2: Measurements ("points to remember") (Table 1, Figure 1):

- There are six defined points (Aa, Ba, C, D, Ap, Bp) that are considered while recording the POP-Q, which are used to report the extent of descent or prolapse of the anterior vaginal wall, vaginal apex, and posterior wall.
- The positions of these six defined points are measured during maximal Valsalva or cough in relation to the hymen. If the point descends to the hymen it is measured as 0 cm, if it remains above the hymen it is measured in centimeters and described as negative integers and if it descends beyond the hymen it is

measured in centimeters and described as positive integers. For example, if point C remains 4 cm above the hymen during Valsalva/cough it is recorded as −4 cm. If point C descends 4 cm beyond the hymen during Valsalva/cough it is recorded as +4 cm.

- There are three further descriptive measurements, which are also recorded independent of the hymen (genital hiatus-point GH, perineal body-point PB, and total vaginal length at rest-point TVL). Of note, all of the POP-Q points are recorded during maximal Valsalva or cough except for point TVL which is recorded at rest with the prolapse reduced.

Step 3: Recording the measurements (Figure 2):

The above measurements are recorded on a 3 × 3 grid. The anterior vaginal wall and the cervix or vault are documented on the top row, the posterior vaginal wall, and the posterior fornix on the bottom row. The descriptive measurements of the genital hiatus, perineal

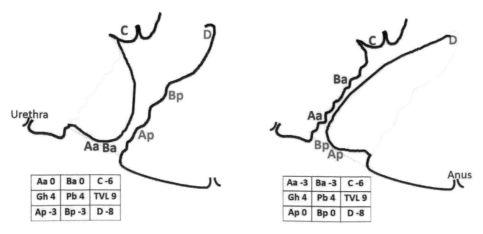

FIGURE 3 POPQ staging of a second stage anterior (left) and second stage posterior (right) vaginal wall prolapse

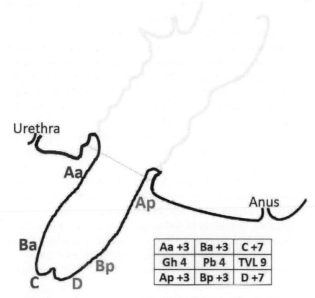

Aa +3	Ba +3	C +7
Gh 4	Pb 4	TVL 9
Ap +3	Bp +3	D +7

FIGURE 4 POPQ staging of a stage 4 pelvic organ prolapse (procidentia)

body, and total vaginal length at rest are recorded in the middle row.

Step 4: Staging of the prolapse

Depending on the measurements, prolapse of each of the compartments is staged based on its relationship to the hymen.

- Stage 0: No prolapse is demonstrated (points Aa, Ba, C, D Ap, and Bp are all $</=-3$ cm).

- Stage I: The most distal portion of the prolapse is more than 1 cm above the level of the hymen (points Aa, Ba, C, D, Ap, and Bp are all <-1 cm).
- Stage II (Figure 3): The most distal portion of the prolapse is situated between 1 cm above the hymen and 1 cm below the hymen (any of the points Aa, Ba, C, D, Ap, and Bp has a value between -1 cm and $+1$ cm).
- Stage III: The most distal portion of the prolapse is more than 1 cm beyond the plane of the hymen, but not completely everted meaning no value is $>/=$ TVL -2 cm (any of the points Aa, Ba, C,D,Ap, Bp is $>/=+2$ and $</=$ tvl -3 cm)
- Stage IV (Figure 4): Complete eversion or eversion to within 2 cm of the total vaginal length of the lower genital tract is demonstrated (any of the Points Ba, C, D, or Bp is $>/=$ to TVL -2 cm).

The steps of performing a POP-Q are summarized in Figure 5 and some examples of POPQ recording and staging of various prolapse are demonstrated in Figures 3 and 4.

4 | DISCUSSION

Since its introduction in 1996, POP-Q has been used variably in peer-reviewed publications.[8] It may be perceived as complex, but it has shown good inter-observer agreement and is the most common system used in peer-reviewed literature.[9–11] It has been criticized as being too complicated, difficult to use, teach, and communicate.[12] Various approaches and tools have been used to teach POP-Q and have all been shown to be effective.[13,14]

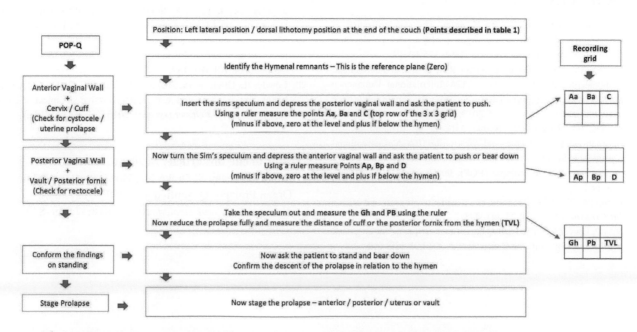

It is standard practice to assess the pelvic floor and perform a bimanual examination to complete the gynaecological examination

FIGURE 5 Practical aspects of performing POP-Q

4.1 | Clinical relevance of POP-Q

Women with POP generally present with several complaints of bladder, bowel, and pelvic dysfunction; however, the symptom of a vaginal bulge is considered specific to prolapse and correlates well with the severity for the prolapse.[15,16] POP is generally considered to be symptomatic when the leading edge of the prolapse is at or beyond the level of the hymen (≥stage 2 POP-Q).[17] Another study suggested that the prolapse becomes symptomatic if it descends lower than a level 0.5 cm above the hymen (≥Stage 2 POP-Q).[18] Genital hiatus size is associated with and predictive of apical vaginal support loss.[19,20] These factors need to be taken in to consideration when diagnosing and offering treatment options to women with prolapse.

5 | CONCLUSION

POP-Q is a useful way of objectively assessing and recording pelvic organ prolapse and helps in better communication of findings. Stage 2 or above POP-Q seems to correlate well with a symptomatic prolapse.

ORCID

Chendrimada Madhu iD http://orcid.org/0000-0002-8571-6117
Marcus J. Drake iD http://orcid.org/0000-0002-6230-2552

REFERENCES

1. Bump RC, Mattiasson A, Bø K, et al. The standardization of terminology of female pelvic organ prolapse and pelvic floor dysfunction. *Am J Obstet Gynecol*. 1996;175:10–17.
2. Haylen BT, De Ridder D, Freeman RM, et al. An International Urogynecological Association (IUGA)/International Continence Society (ICS) joint report on the terminology for female pelvic floor dysfunction. *Int Urogynecol J*. 2010;21:5–26.
3. Haylen BT, Maher CF, Barber MD, et al. Erratum to: An International Urogynecological Association (IUGA)/International Continence Society (ICS) joint report on the terminology for female pelvic organ prolapse (POP). *Int Urogynecol J*. 2016;27:655–684.
4. Bump RC. The POP-Q system: two decades of progress and debate. *Int Urogynecol J*. 2014;25:441–443.
5. Riss P, Dwyer PL. The POP-Q classification system: looking back and looking forward. *Int Urogynecol J*. 2014;25:439–440.
6. Haya N, Segev E, Younes G, Goldschmidt E, Auslender R, Abramov Y. The effect of bladder fullness on evaluation of pelvic organ prolapse. *Int J Gynecol Obstet*. 2012;118:24–26.
7. Visco AG, Wei JT, McClure LA, Handa VL, Nygaard IE. Effects of examination technique modifications on pelvic organ prolapse quantification (POP-Q) results. *Int Urogynecol J*. 2003;14:136–140.
8. Oyama IA, Steinberg AC, Watai TK, Minaglia SM. Pelvic organ prolapse quantification use in the literature. *Female Pelvic Med Reconstr Surg*. 2012;18:35–36.
9. Parekh M, Swift S, Lemos N, et al. Multicenter inter-examiner agreement trial for the validation of simplified POPQ system. *Int Urogynecol J*. 2011;22:645–650.
10. Persu C, Chapple CR, Cauni V, Gutue S, Geavlete P. Pelvic organ prolapse quantification system (POP-Q) – a new era in pelvic prolapse staging. *J Med Life*. 2011;4:75–81.
11. Boyd SS, O'Sullivan D, Tulikangas P. Use of the Pelvic Organ Quantification System (POP-Q) in published articles of peer-reviewed journals. *Int Urogynecol J*. 2017;28:1719–1723.
12. Harmanli O. POP-Q 2.0: its time has come! *Int Urogynecol J*. 2014;25:447–449.
13. Parnell BA, Dunivan GC, Geller EJ, Connolly A. A novel approach to teaching the pelvic organ prolapse quantification (POP-Q) exam. *Int Urogynecol J*. 2011;22:367–370.
14. Geiss IM, Riss PA, Hanzal E, Dungl A. A simple teaching tool for training the pelvic organ prolapse quantification system. *Int Urogynecol J*. 2007;18:1003–1005.
15. Jelovsek JE, Maher C, Barber MD. Pelvic organ prolapse. *Lancet [Internet]* 2007;369:1027–1038.
16. Ghetti C, Gregory WT, Edwards SR, Otto LN, Clark AL. Pelvic organ descent and symptoms of pelvic floor disorders. *Am J Obstet Gynecol*. 2005;193:53–57.
17. Swift SE, Tate SB, Nicholas J. Correlation of symptoms with degree of pelvic organ support in a general population of women: what is pelvic organ prolapse? *Am J Obstet Gynecol* 2003;189:372-7-9.
18. Gutman RE, Ford DE, Quiroz LH, Shippey SH, Handa VL. Is there a pelvic organ prolapse threshold that predicts pelvic floor symptoms? *Am J Obstet Gynecol*. 2008;199:683.e1–683.e7.
19. Medina CA, Candiotti K, Takacs P. Wide genital hiatus is a risk factor for recurrence following anterior vaginal repair. *Int J Gynecol Obstet*. 2008;101:184–187.
20. Lowder JL, Oliphant SS, Shepherd JP, Ghetti C, Sutkin G. Genital hiatus size is associated with and predictive of apical vaginal support loss. *Am J Obstet Gynecol*. 2016;214:718.e1–718.e8.

How to cite this article: Madhu C, Swift S, Moloney-Geany S, Drake MJ. How to use the Pelvic Organ Prolapse Quantification (POP-Q) system? *Neurourology and Urodynamics*. 2018;37:S39–S43.
https://doi.org/10.1002/nau.23740

Received: 23 April 2018 | Accepted: 1 July 2018

DOI: 10.1002/nau.23777

SOUNDING BOARD

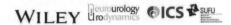

The fundamentals of uroflowmetry practice, based on International Continence Society good urodynamic practices recommendations

Andrew Gammie (iD) | Marcus J. Drake (iD)

Bristol Urological Institute, Southmead
Hospital, Bristol, UK

Correspondence
Andrew Gammie, Bristol Urological
Institute, Southmead Hospital, Bristol BS10
5NB, UK.
Email: andrew.gammie@bui.ac.uk

Aims: To review the recommendations on uroflowmetry in the International Continence Society (ICS) Standardization documents in order to identify a systematic approach to the delivery and interpretation of free flow rate testing in clinical practice.

Methods: Expectations of service and good practice in uroflowmetry described in the ICS standards on Urodynamic Practice, Urodynamic Equipment, and Terminology for Lower Urinary Tract Function were identified and summarized.

Results: Urodynamic centers should provide a suitable uroflowmetry testing environment. Equipment should be calibrated and maintained according to manufacturer requirements. Patients should be well-informed in advance of the test. They should be advised to avoid: knocking the machine; allowing the stream to move; squeezing the urethra; and body movements. It is generally appropriate to get more than one flow trace for each patient. Voided volume should be representative for the patient, for example by comparing with values recorded on a Bladder Diary. Post void residual (PVR) should be measured soon after testing. After the test, the urodynamicist should review the trace and ensure maximum flow rate and end of micturition are correctly identified in case the equipment has inappropriately taken the values from a trace artefact.

Conclusions: The summary provides a systematic approach to ensure a representative, high quality, non-invasive flow test is carried out for individual patients.

KEYWORDS
free flows, standards

1 | INTRODUCTION

Urodynamics is the general term to describe the measurements that assess the function and dysfunction of the lower urinary tract (LUT) by any appropriate method. In

the clinical assessment of LUT symptoms (LUTS), evaluating the nature of an individual's voiding is a fundamental component of the diagnostic pathway, especially for men. Uroflowmetry is a non-invasive urodynamic test in which specific measurements are made of the rate of flow of urine and the volume voided. It is normally followed by an ultrasonically scanned measurement of post void residual (PVR) urine volume, and an interpretation of the flow pattern recorded by the machine over the duration of the void.

The work was undertaken at Bristol Urological Institute, Southmead Hospital, Bristol, UK.

Roger Dmochowski led the peer-review process as the Associate Editor responsible for the paper.

A recent think tank on uroflowmetry[1] recommended that specific, practical guidance be made available to increase the quality of uroflowmetry testing. Accordingly, the current article reviews the recommendations on uroflowmetry in the International Continence Society (ICS) Standardization documents in order to identify a systematic approach to the delivery and interpretation of free flow rate testing in clinical practice.

2 | METHODS

The ICS, through its Standardization Steering Committee (SSC), has an ongoing strategy to standardize LUT terminology and functional assessment, and link it to published evidence.[2] We reviewed key expectations of service and good practice in uroflowmetry described in the ICS standards on Urodynamic Practice,[3,4] Urodynamic Equipment,[5] and Terminology for LUT Function.[6,7] The current document is a synthesis of the key aspects applicable to uroflowmetry.

3 | GENERAL COMMENTS

A good urodynamic practice comprises: a clear indication for, and appropriate selection of, relevant test measurements and procedures; precise measurement with data quality control and complete documentation; accurate analysis and critical reporting of results. These general principles apply to all forms of urodynamic testing, including uroflowmetry.

Departments should develop uroflowmetry protocols on the basis of the ICS Urodynamic standards,[3–5] they should facilitate specific staff training and undertake regular evaluation of performance and adherence.[3] ICS Terminology Standards should be used when alluding to LUT symptoms, signs, and urodynamic observations.[6,7] Equipment should meet the requirements of the ICS guideline on equipment performance.[5]

Uroflowmetry is a test that measures the urinary stream as volume passed per unit time in milliliters per second (mL/s).[4] Maximum flow rate (Q_{max}) and total volume voided must be reported.[4] The PVR should also be reported. This is the remaining intravesical fluid volume determined immediately after completion of voiding. The technique (eg, ultrasound or catheter) used to measure the PVR should be specified.

4 | EQUIPMENT AND ENVIRONMENT

The basic set up for a flow test environment is illustrated in Figure 1. The requirement of a uroflowmeter is that it can continuously measure the flow rate of urine voided and the total volume voided. The method used to make this measurement is not clinically significant. Accuracy need only be to ± 1 mL/s of true flow rate and to $\pm 5\%$ of true volume voided (or ± 2 mL if that is greater than 5%).[5]

Units should regularly check the performance of their system and calibrate according to manufacturer recommendation.[5] Flowmeter calibration can be verified by pouring a precise volume into the flowmeter and checking the recorded volume. Calibration should be verified regularly, for example, at the start of every clinic or week of clinics, and documented. If frequent recalibration is necessary, the flow transducer might need to be replaced.

Uroflowmetry equipment should be placed in a private, quiet environment[3] that can be easily cleaned, with the machine ready for immediate use, as many LUTS patients having flow rate testing will experience urgency. PVR measurement is ideally done in the same room and immediately following the void. A sluice room with connecting door to the flow test room is preferable to an unconnected room.

5 | PREPARATIONS IN ADVANCE OF A UROFLOWMETRY TEST

An explanatory leaflet about uroflowmetry with sufficient information, which uses clear, unambiguous wording, will be appreciated by most patients. To reduce possible waiting time, patients can be asked to attend the clinic with a comfortably full bladder.

When sent the explanatory leaflet, the patient can also be asked to complete a frequency volume chart (FVC) or Bladder Diary. A FVC records the time of each micturition and the voided volumes, while a Bladder Diary also captures symptoms and events such as fluid intake, urgency, pain, incontinence episodes, and pad usage.[6,8] Average and maximum voided volumes, voiding frequency, and day/night urine production can be determined.

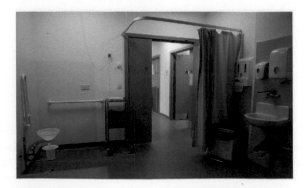

FIGURE 1 A suitable environment for uroflowmetry. The flowmeter can be accessed quickly from the waiting area if the patient experience surgency, achieves privacy (here by having a curtain in addition to a locked doorway), is easy to clean, and has direct access to a sluice room (not in above picture). Female uroflowmetry would have a commode seat in addition to the funnel

6 | FLOW RATE TESTING

Patients should be asked to pass urine when they feel a "normal" desire to void,[4] and should undergo uroflowmetry in their preferred position. Intracorporeal modulations of the flow rate should be minimized, for example, by asking the patient to relax and not to strain.[4] Men should be asked not to move the urine stream around the funnel, and not to squeeze the penis, both of which will affect the flow rate measurement (Figure 2).[7]

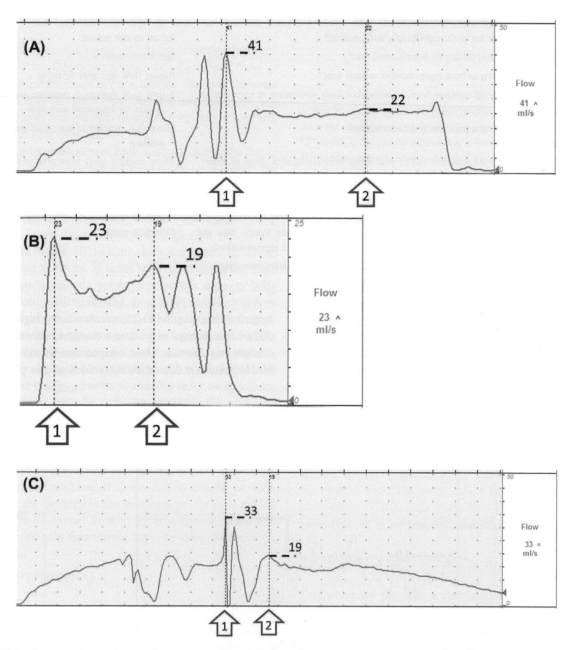

FIGURE 2 Some artefacts encountered in uroflowmetry, and the importance of correcting for the error in Q_{max} to establish the representative parameter. A, A male patient moving the urine stream back-and-forth across the funnel. B, A male squeezing and releasing the urethra at the start of flow, with straining toward the end of flow. C, A "knock artefact" (arrowed), resulting from a patient inadvertently kicking the uroflowmetry machine. In each case, the uroflowmetry machine has given a Q_{max} value which is a result of the artefact, displayed on the right hand side, and taken from the point marked with arrow "1." This is not representative of the patient's own function, so the urodynamicist has scrutinized the trace after the test and selected the highest point in the trace that does appear to result from the patient's own unimpeded bladder and outlet behavior, at the point marked with arrow "2." This means the representative values change, for instance in A from 41 to 22 mL/s, which may well result in a clinically significant difference in interpretation. Before a flow test, the patient should be instructed to keep his stream in the same part of the funnel, not to squeeze his penis, and try to avoid knocking the machine

grants, personal fees, and non-financial support from Allergan, Astellas, and Ferring, personal fees from Pfizer, outside the submitted work.

ORCID

Andrew Gammie http://orcid.org/0000-0001-5546-357X
Marcus J. Drake http://orcid.org/0000-0002-6230-2552

REFERENCES

1. Gammie A, Rosier P, Li R, Harding C. How can we maximize the diagnostic utility of uroflow?: ICI-RS 2017. *Neurourol Urodyn.* 2018. https://doi.org/10.1002/nau.23472
2. Rosier PF, de Ridder D, Meijlink J, Webb R, Whitmore K, Drake MJ. Developing evidence-based standards for diagnosis and management of lower urinary tract or pelvic floor dysfunction. *Neurourol Urodyn.* 2012;31:621–624.
3. Rosier P, Schaefer W, Lose G, et al. International continence society good urodynamic practices and terms 2016: urodynamics, uroflowmetry, cystometry, and pressure-flow study. *Neurourol Urodyn.* 2017;36:1243–1260.
4. Schafer W, Abrams P, Liao L, et al. Good urodynamic practices: uroflowmetry, filling cystometry, and pressure-flow studies. *Neurourol Urodyn.* 2002;21:261–274.
5. Gammie A, Clarkson B, Constantinou C, et al. International Continence Society guidelines on urodynamic equipment performance. *Neurourol Urodyn.* 2014;33:370–379.
6. Abrams P, Cardozo L, Fall M, et al. The standardization of terminology of lower urinary tract function: report from the Standardisation Sub-committee of the International Continence Society. *Neurourol Urodyn.* 2002;21:167–178.
7. Haylen BT, de Ridder D, Freeman RM, et al. An International Urogynecological Association (IUGA)/International Continence Society (ICS) joint report on the terminology for female pelvic floor dysfunction. *Neurourol Urodyn.* 2010;29:4–20.
8. Bright E, Cotterill N, Drake M, Abrams P. Developing and validating the International Consultation on Incontinence Questionnaire bladder diary. *Eur Urol.* 2014;66:294–300.
9. Reynard JM, Peters TJ, Lim C, Abrams P. The value of multiple free-flow studies in men with lower urinary tract symptoms. *Br J Urol.* 1996;77:813–818.

How to cite this article: Gammie A, Drake MJ. The fundamentals of uroflowmetry practice, based on International Continence Society good urodynamic practices recommendations. *Neurourology and Urodynamics.* 2018;37:S44–S49.

https://doi.org/10.1002/nau.23777

Received: 20 April 2018 | Accepted: 1 July 2018

DOI: 10.1002/nau.23773

SOUNDING BOARD

WILEY · Neurourology Urodynamics · ICS · SUFU

Fundamentals of urodynamic practice, based on International Continence Society good urodynamic practices recommendations

Marcus J. Drake[1,2] | Stergios K. Doumouchtsis[3] | Hashim Hashim[2] | Andrew Gammie[2]

[1] Translational Health Sciences, Bristol Medical School, Bristol, UK

[2] Bristol Urological Institute, Southmead Hospital, Bristol, UK

[3] Gynaecology Department, Epsom and St Helier University Hospitals NHS Trust, Epsom, UK

Correspondence

Marcus J. Drake, Bristol Urological Institute, 3rd Floor L&R Building, Southmead Hospital, Bristol BS10 5NB, UK.
Email: marcus.drake@bristol.ac.uk

Aims: To review the recommendations on basic urodynamic testing in the International Continence Society (ICS) standardization documents, specifying key recommendations for delivery and interpretation in clinical practice.

Methods: Fundamental expectations described in the ICS standards on good urodynamic practices, urodynamic equipment, and terminology for lower urinary tract (LUT) function were identified and summarized.

Results: The ICS standard urodynamic protocol includes clinical history, including symptom and bother score(s), examination, 3-day voiding chart/diary, representative uroflowmetry with post-void residual, and cystometry with pressure-flow study (PFS). Liquid filled catheters are connected to pressure transducers at the same vertical pressure as the patient's pubic symphysis, taking atmospheric pressure as the zero value. Urodynamic testing is done to answer specific therapy-driven questions for treatment selection; provocations are applied to give the best chance of reproducing the problem during the test. Quality of recording is monitored throughout, and remedial steps taken for any technical issues occurring during testing. Labels are applied during the test to document events, such as patient-reported sensation, provocation tests, and permission to void. After the test, the pressure and flow traces are scrutinized to ensure artefacts do not confound the findings. An ICS standard urodynamic report details the key aspects, reporting clinical observations, technical, and quality issues. Urodynamic services must maintain and calibrate equipment according to manufacturer stipulations.

Conclusions: The review provides a succinct summary of practice expectations for a urodynamic unit offering cystometry and pressure flow studies (PFS) to an appropriate standard.

KEYWORDS

LUTS, overactive bladder, standardization, urodynamics

Alan Wein led the peer-review process as the Associate Editor responsible for the paper.

2.5 | Practice of cystometry and pressure flow studies

A good urodynamic investigation is performed interactively with the patient.[3] It should be established how the patient's symptoms relate to what they experienced during the test. There should be continuous observation of the signals as they are collected, and assessment of the plausibility of all signals. Direct inspection of the raw pressure and flow data before, during, and at the end of micturition is essential, because it allows artefacts and untrustworthy data to be recognized and eliminated.[4] The flow pattern in a PFS should be representative of free flow studies in the same patient. An overall study trace is illustrated in Figure 1.

Electronic marking of events is important for subsequent analysis; the position of event markers should be adjustable after the test has finished, and the meaning of any abbreviations used for labels should be clear.[5]

2.5.1 | Pressure recording

Zero pressure is the value recorded when a liquid-filled transducer is open to the environment (either disconnected from any tubes, or when the open end of a connected liquid-filled tube is at the same vertical level as the transducer). "Set zero" or "balance" can then be undertaken, making atmospheric pressure the zero baseline for the test. Intravesical pressure (p_{ves}) or abdominal pressure (p_{abd}) is thus the excess pressure above atmosphere at the hydrostatic level of the symphysis pubis. "Set zero" is not done when catheters are already recording from the patient; this is a common mistake in many urodynamic units.

- ICS standard cystometry is performed using liquid filled catheters, with external transducers at the reference level of the top of the symphysis pubis.[2,3,6] To achieve this, most urodynamic machines have a movable platform for the transducers, so they can easily be placed at the same height from the ground as the patient's symphysis.

- Use the thinnest possible transurethral double or triple lumen catheter or a suprapubic catheter. Two-catheter techniques (separate filling and pressure recording catheters) are an acceptable alternative.[2]

- Fix the catheters as close as possible to the anus and urethral meatus with tape, without blocking the urinary meatus.

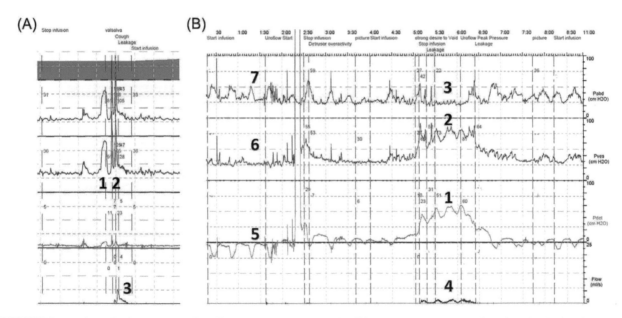

FIGURE 2 Urodynamic observations during filling cystometry. A, USI; the filling pump is stopped, and the patient is asked to do a Valsalva manoeuvre (1) and to do a sequence of 2 or 3 good coughs (2). This patient leaked with the coughs (3), and no DO was present, so the urodynamic observation of USI was documented. B, DO is the presence of a bladder contraction during filling (1), which may be spontaneous or provoked. It is essential to review all the lines in the trace before reporting DO, to confirm there is a bladder contraction (2) and minimal abdominal activity (3; though a small abdominal contraction might be seen if the patient tries to prevent leakage by contracting their pelvic floor). In this case, there is also incontinence (4), so the urodynamic observation here is DO incontinence (DOI). In the same trace, there are also fluctuations in the calculated detrusor pressure (5) which might be misinterpreted as DO. However, these are below the baseline, and there is no change in bladder pressure associated with them (6). Instead, there are phasic pressure changes visible in the abdominal pressure trace (7), indicating the presence of rectal contractions. Practitioners need to recognise that a true change in abdominal pressure shows up in both p_{ves} and p_{abd}; a phasic change in one line which is absent in the other indicates a contraction of the organ containing the catheter tip (bladder or rectum, respectively)

- Rectal placement of a fully liquid filled open catheter, or punctured balloon catheter, to measure p_{abd} is ICS standard. Vaginal or stoma placement is used only if rectal placement is impossible.

Prevention of liquid leaks and air bubbles in the pressure tubing system is needed throughout testing, and should be corrected when identified.[3] Coughs or other abdominal pressure rises are used to ensure that the abdominal and intravesical pressure signals respond equally (see Figure 3).

2.5.2 | Cystometry

Filling cystometry is done in the upright/vertical position (standing or normally seated) whenever physically possible. Detection of detrusor overactivity (DO) and urodynamic stress incontinence (USI) are influenced by the position of the patient; sitting or standing has a higher sensitivity.[2]

2.5.3 | Filling rate

Maximum physiological filling rate is estimated by body weight in kg divided by four,[6] thus typically in the range of 20-30 mL/min. More rapid filling is referred to as non-physiological filling rate.[3]

For a balance between a filling rate that is slow enough to be representative and fast enough to complete the cystometry efficiently, consider a filling rate in mL/min of roughly 10% of the largest voided volume (reported on a FVC; and allowing for PVR).[2]

Diuresis adds bladder volume that is not recorded by the urodynamics system, but that is relevant for interpretation of the results. Cystometric capacity is most reliably determined by calculation of voided volume plus PVR immediately after PFS.[3]

2.5.4 | Sensations

Three sensation parameters are recorded[6]: first sensation of filling (FSF), first desire to void (FDV), and strong desire to void (SDV). The patient also may report sensation(s) suggesting "urgency," which can be marked specifically. When indicating the volumes at which these sensations occurred, the report should make allowance for the fact that the volume instilled into the bladder by the machine is not necessarily the actual liquid volume in the bladder (eg, if the bladder was not empty at the start of the filling cystometry, or if the patient is experiencing diuresis).

1. FSF: "Tell me the moment when you perceive that your bladder is not empty anymore."[2]

2. FDV: "Tell me when you have the sensation that normally tells you to go to the toilet, without any hurry, at the next convenient moment."[6]

3. SDV: "The moment that you would definitely visit the nearest toilet to pass urine." There should be no pain or any fear of losing urine.

The end of filling should relate to a "strong but not uncomfortable need to void," indicated by SDV on the urodynamic graph. A specific marker to indicate permission to void must be used if there is a delay between halting the pump and permission to void. If another reason is chosen for concluding filling, this should be indicated.

Incontinence, fear of leakage, pain, or other signs or symptoms during the test should be specifically marked on the urodynamic graph.

2.5.5 | Provocation

Urodynamic stress test[2] (Figure 2) is used for any physical effort of the person tested, to elevate abdominal pressure during cystometry, with the aim of examining USI. The exact approach to stress testing during urodynamics has not been standardized. Thus, the provocation method, pressure measuring catheter (size) and method, the leak detection method, and the intravesical volume(s) may be reported.

Leak point pressure (LPP)[2] is the pressure (spontaneous or provoked) that has caused fluid to be expelled from the bladder at the moment that it is visible outside the urethra. No ICS (or commonly agreed) standard technique or protocol is available and a variety of terms and techniques are used.

DO (Figure 2) is characterised by involuntary detrusor contractions during the filling phase which may be spontaneous or provoked.[6] Cough-associated DO[2]: Reported when the onset of the DO (with or without leakage) occurs immediately following the cough pressure peak. Cough-associated DO incontinence is a form of DO and must not be confused with USI.

2.5.6 | Pressure-flow studies

The relevance of instruction, position, and privacy while undertaking PFS is equal to uroflowmetry. PFS is done comfortably seated (women, some men) or standing if that is the preferred position (men). Pressure-flow analysis is only validated for voluntarily initiated micturitions and not for incontinence.

- PFS begins immediately after permission to void and ends when the detrusor pressure has returned to the baseline

TABLE 1 Checklist for fundamentals of urodynamic practices

Question	What is the urodynamic question?
	Will patient management change as a result?
	Does the bladder diary/symptom score affect these?
	Does the patient's report match the above?
Setup	
Calibrate	Check that the equipment is registering pressure and volume accurately
Prepare	Fill the domes and tubes with water, and mount them on the transducers
	Catheterise the patient, connect tubes and flush with water
	Level transducers with symphysis pubis bone
Quality	
Zero to atmosphere	Ensure taps are closed to patient, and open to air when zero is pressed.
Check resting pressures are normal	Supine: p_{abd} and p_{ves} 5-20 cmH$_2$O Seated: p_{abd} and p_{ves} 15-40 cmH$_2$O Standing: p_{abd} and p_{ves} 30-50 cmH$_2$O for all positions, p_{det} −5-+5 cmH$_2$O
Continuous monitoring	Check regularly that pressure transmission is equal on both lines, for example, coughs, blowing
	Check that live patient signal is present throughout
	Check that baseline pressures do not drift
	Troubleshoot above during the test, temporarily stopping recording/filling if necessary
	Stop or reduce fill rate if urgency is excessive, or compliance poor
	Change patent position as required (eg, discomfort, stress testing)
	Consider repeating test if urodynamic question not answered
Interpretation	Place markers on the trace frequently, for example, sensation, patient position, stress tests, permission to void
	Adjust positions of markers after completion of test if needed
	Take a when interpreting, for example, rectal contractions, knocking of flowmeter
Report	Bladder during filling Urethra during filling Bladder during voiding Urethra during voiding Reproduction of symptoms Management plan

bubbles in the pressure tubing system should be recognized and reported during post-test analysis, if not identified during the procedure, to prevent mis-diagnosis.[8]

Post-processing automated analysis is an optional extra in urodynamic equipment, and established nomograms and calculated parameters may also be provided. Such analysis could be affected by artefacts (eg, Q_{max} caused by knocking the flow meter, p_{max} from cough),[5] and the urodynamicist must check the trace to be certain that misinterpretation does not result. The user should have the ability to check the values for feasibility and change the relevant ones if necessary. Software should not filter or remove artefacts, but should be able to ignore them for analysis.

2.7 | The urodynamics report

Bladder storage function should be described according to bladder sensation, detrusor activity, bladder compliance, and bladder capacity.[6] The urethral closure mechanism during storage may be competent or incompetent. Voiding is described in terms of detrusor and urethral function and assessed by measuring urine flow rate and voiding pressures. An "ICS standard urodynamic (time based) graph" and an "ICS standard pressure-flow plot" are required elements in the ICS standard urodynamics report.

- Reporting includes the following elements (summarized from GUP2016[2]):

a Overall judgement of the technical quality, clinical reliability, representativeness, and methods of assessment.
b Uroflowmetry: voiding position, Q_{max}, voided volume, PVR.
c Introduction of catheters: sensation, muscular defence, obstruction(s).
d Patient position(s) during cystometry and PFS.
e Patient's ability to report filling sensations and/or urgency and/or urine loss.
f Method of urodynamic stress test and accessory tests (if applicable).
g Diagnoses: filling sensation (with volumes); cystometry; PFS (bladder outflow function, detrusor contraction).

All results and observations should be carefully reported. It is good clinical practice to integrate the urodynamic test results with the history, examinations, and other tests.

Table 1 gives a proposed checklist for Fundamentals of Urodynamic Practice.

3 | CONCLUSIONS

A good study is one that is easy to read and one from which any experienced urodynamicist will abstract the same results and come to the same conclusions (GUP2002). Adherence to the fundamentals of the ICS standards, as synthesized in this review, will enable urodynamic units to ensure the quality of urodynamic studies and compare findings with other units.

CONFLICT OF INTEREST

Dr. Drake reports grants, personal fees, and non-financial support from Astellas, Allergan, and Ferring, outside the submitted work. Dr. Doumouchtsis has nothing to disclose. Dr. Hashim reports personal fees and non-financial support from Ferring and Allergan, personal fees from Astellas, Medtronic, and Boston, outside the submitted work. Dr. Gammie reports other from Astellas and Ipsen, grants from Andromeda, Digitimer, and Laborie, outside the submitted work.

ORCID

Marcus J. Drake http://orcid.org/0000-0002-6230-2552
Hashim Hashim http://orcid.org/0000-0003-2467-407X
Andrew Gammie http://orcid.org/0000-0001-5546-357X

REFERENCES

1. Rosier PF, de Ridder D, Meijlink J, Webb R, Whitmore K, Drake MJ. Developing evidence-based standards for diagnosis and management of lower urinary tract or pelvic floor dysfunction. *Neurourol Urodyn.* 2012;31:621–624.
2. Rosier P, Schaefer W, Lose G, et al. International continence society good urodynamic practices and terms 2016: urodynamics, uroflowmetry, cystometry, and pressure-flow study. *Neurourol Urodyn.* 2017;36:1243–1260.
3. Schafer W, Abrams P, Liao L, et al. Good urodynamic practices: uroflowmetry, filling cystometry, and pressure-flow studies. *Neurourol Urodyn.* 2002;21:261–274.
4. Griffiths D, Hofner K, van Mastrigt R, Rollema HJ, Spangberg A, Gleason D. Standardization of terminology of lower urinary tract function: pressure-flow studies of voiding, urethral resistance, and urethral obstruction. International Continence Society Subcommittee on Standardization of Terminology of Pressure-Flow Studies. *Neurourol Urodyn.* 1997;16:1–18.
5. Gammie A, Clarkson B, Constantinou C, et al. International Continence Society guidelines on urodynamic equipment performance. *Neurourol Urodyn.* 2014;33:370–379.
6. Abrams P, Cardozo L, Fall M, et al. The standardisation of terminology of lower urinary tract function: report from the Standardisation Sub-committee of the International Continence Society. *Neurourol Urodyn.* 2002;21:167–178.
7. Haylen BT, de Ridder D, Freeman RM, et al. An International Urogynecological Association (IUGA)/International Continence Society (ICS) joint report on the terminology for female pelvic floor dysfunction. *Neurourol Urodyn.* 2010;29:4–20.
8. Hogan S, Gammie A, Abrams P. Urodynamic features and artefacts. *Neurourol Urodyn.* 2012;31:1104–1117.
9. Gammie A, Drake MJ. The fundamentals of uroflowmetry practice, based on international continence society good urodynamic practices recommendations. *Neurourol Urodyn.* 2018;37:S44–S49.
10. Wyndaele M, PFWM Rosier. Basics of videourodynamics for adult patients with lower urinary tract dysfunction. *Neurourol Urodyn.* 2018;37:S61–S66.
11. Harding C, Rosier PFWM, Drake MJ, et al. What research is needed to validate new urodynamic methods? ICI-RS2017. *Neurourol Urodyn.* 2018;37:S32–S37.
12. Bright E, Drake MJ, Abrams P. Urinary diaries: evidence for the development and validation of diary content, format, and duration. *Neurourol Urodyn.* 2011;30:348–352.
13. Bright E, Cotterill N, Drake M, Abrams P. Developing and validating the International Consultation on Incontinence Questionnaire bladder diary. *Eur Urol.* 2014;66:294–300.
14. Abrams P. Bladder outlet obstruction index, bladder contractility index and bladder voiding efficiency: three simple indices to define bladder voiding function. *BJU Int.* 1999;84:14–15.
15. Sullivan JG, Swithinbank L, Abrams P. Defining achievable standards in urodynamics—a prospective study of initial resting pressures. *Neurourol Urodyn.* 2012;31:535–540.

How to cite this article: Drake MJ, Doumouchtsis SK, Hashim H, Gammie A. Fundamentals of urodynamic practice, based on International Continence Society good urodynamic practices recommendations. *Neurourology and Urodynamics.* 2018;37:S50–S60. https://doi.org/10.1002/nau.23773

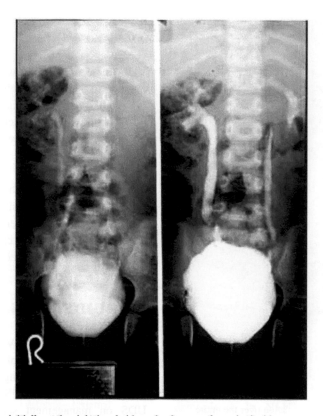

FIGURE 4 Vesico-ureteral reflux initially at the right hand side and subsequently on both sides

TABLE 2 Indications for considering fluoroscopy during the urodynamic evaluation

Neurological findings or history of relevant neurologic disease
(History of) congenital genitourinary anomaly (eg, ectopic ureter, posterior urethral valves, prune-belly syndrome, vesico-ureteral reflux)
Bladder outflow obstruction or urinary retention associated with complex history
History of pelvic radiotherapy or intrapelvic surgery
History of pelvic reconstructive surgery, SUI surgery, urethral stricture repair, POP reconstruction, urethral diverticulectomy
Suspicion of vesico-vaginal or urethro-vaginal fistula
Suspicion of urethral diverticulum
Pre- and post-renal transplant

of patient comfort, making the chance of not representative outcome of studies more likely, especially in patients without neurological disease.

The European Association of Urology (EAU) recommends, based on level 4 evidence, VUDS as the optimum procedure for invasive UDS in neuro-urological patients.[19,20] In male LUTS VUDS are considered applicable if this is needed for the clinician to understand the pathophysiological mechanism of a patient's LUTS although this is also based on experts impressions.[21] The British National Institute for "Health" and Care Excellence (NICE) recommends to offer VUDS to people who are known to have a high risk of renal complications from their LUT function (eg, people with spina bifida, spinal cord injury, or anorectal abnormalities).[22]

The American Urological Association (AUA) and Society of Urodynamics, Female Pelvic Medicine and Urogenital Reconstruction (SUFU) states that, when available, clinicians may perform VUDS in patients with relevant neurologic disease at risk for neurogenic bladder dysfunction, in patients with other neurologic disease and elevated PVR.[23] Clinicians may also perform VUDS in properly selected patients to urodynamically grade and to anatomically localize bladder outflow obstruction, based on this association statement.[23]

5 | CONCLUSION

Medical imaging has developed in a century.[24] Imaging finds its application in healthcare via the evolution of technical possibilities in combination with plausibility, and expert opinion. Randomized prospective studies that demonstrate the effect of diagnosis with and without imaging, on outcome of management have not been published. The development of videourodynamic evaluation is no exception. It is difficult to precisely delineate the indications for the study, as well as to assess its precise surplus for predictive value of the diagnostic strategy, however, it is undoubtedly plausible and useful to combine reliable objective functional physiological measurements (UDS) with anatomical information of synchronous imaging in a proportion of patients with lower urinary tract dysfunction.

ORCID

Peter F. W. M. Rosier (ID) http://orcid.org/0000-0003-0445-4563

REFERENCES

1. Rosier PFWM, Schaefer W, Lose G, et al. International continence society good urodynamic practices and terms 2016: urodynamics, uroflowmetry, cystometry, and pressure-flow study. *Neurourol Urodyn*. 2017;36:1243–1260.
2. Bates CP, Corney CE. Synchronous cine-pressure-flow cystography: a method of routine urodynamic investigation. *Br J Radiol*. 1971;44:44–50.
3. Arnold EP, Brown AD, Webster JR. Videocystography with synchronous detrusor pressure and flow rate recordings. *Ann R Coll Surg Engl*. 1974;55:90–98.
4. Marks BK, Goldman HB. Videourodynamics: indications and technique. *Urol Clin North Am*. 2014;41:383–391, vii-viii.
5. McGuire EJ, Cespedes RD, Cross CA, O'Connell HE. Videourodynamic studies. *Urol Clin North Am*. 1996;23:309–321.
6. Gray M. Traces: making sense of urodynamics testing—part 12: videourodynamics testing. *Urol Nurs*. 2012;32:193–202.
7. Cardozo L, Shakir F, Araklitis G, Rantell A, Robinson D. Narrated video demonstrating the procedure of videourodynamics. *Neurourol Urodyn*. 2018;37:1176–1177. https://www.acr.org/-/media/ACR/Files/Practice-Parameters/cysto-urethro.pdf
8. McAlister WH, Griffith RC. Cystographic contrast media: clinical and experimental studies. *AJR Am J Roentgenol*. 1983;141:997–1001.
9. Giarenis I, Phillips J, Mastoroudes H, et al. Radiation exposure during videourodynamics in women. *Int Urogynecol J*. 2013;24:1547–1551.
10. Galloway NT, Mekras JA, Helms M, et al. An objective score to predict upper tract deterioration in myelodysplasia. *J Urol*. 1991;145:535.
11. Veenboer PW, Bosch JL, Rosier PF, et al. Cross-sectional study of determinants of upper and lower urinary tract outcomes in adults with spinal dysraphism—new recommendations for urodynamic followup guidelines? *J Urol*. 2014;192:477–482.
12. Groutz A, Blaivas JG, Chaikin DC, Weiss JP, Verhaaren M. The pathophysiology of post-radical prostatectomy incontinence: a clinical and video urodynamic study. *J Urol*. 2000;163:1767–1770.
13. Jura YH, Comiter CV. Urodynamics for postprostatectomy incontinence: when are they helpful and how do we use them? *Urol Clin North Am*. 2014;41:419–427, viii.
14. Nitti VW, Lefkowitz G, Ficazzola M, Dixon CM. Lower urinary tract symptoms in young men: videourodynamic findings and correlation with noninvasive measures. *J Urol*. 2002;168:135–138.
15. Nitti VW, Tu LM, Gitlin J. Diagnosing bladder outlet obstruction in women. *J Urol*. 1999;161:1535–1540.
16. Brucker BM, Fong E, Shah S, Kelly C, Rosenblum N, Nitti VW. Urodynamic differences between dysfunctional voiding and primary bladder neck obstruction in women. *Urology*. 2012;80:55–60.
17. Anding R, Rosier P, Smith P, et al. When should video be added to conventional urodynamics in adults and is it justified by the evidence? ICI-RS 2014. *Neurourol Urodyn*. 2016;35:324–329.
18. Drake MJ, Apostolidis A, Cocci A, et al. Neurogenic lower urinary tract dysfunction: clinical management recommendations of the Neurologic Incontinence committee of the fifth International Consultation on Incontinence 2013. *Neurourol Urodyn*. 2016;35:657–665.
19. Stöhrer M, Blok B, Castro-Diaz D, et al. EAU guidelines on neurogenic lower urinary tract dysfunction. *Eur Urol*. 2009;56:81–88.
20. Nosseir M, Hinkel A, Pannek J. Clinical usefulness of urodynamic assessment for maintenance of bladder function in patients with spinal cord injury. *Neurourol Urodyn*. 2007;26:228–233.
21. Gratzke C, Bachmann A, Descazeaud A, et al. EAU guidelines on the assessment of non-neurogenic male lower urinary tract symptoms including benign prostatic obstruction. *Eur Urol*. 2015;67:1099–1109.
22. https://www.nice.org.uk/guidance/cg148/evidence/full-guideline-188123437
23. Winters JC, Dmochowski RR, Goldman HB, et al. Urodynamic studies in adults: AUA/SUFU guideline. *J Urol*. 2012;188:2464–2472.
24. Scatliff JH, Morris PJ. From Roentgen to magnetic resonance imaging: the history of medical imaging. *N C Med J*. 2014;75:111–113.

How to cite this article: Wyndaele M, Rosier PFWM. Basics of videourodynamics for adult patients with lower urinary tract dysfunction. *Neurourology and Urodynamics*. 2018;37:S61–S66. https://doi.org/10.1002/nau.23778

Received: 10 May 2018 | Accepted: 17 May 2018

DOI: 10.1002/nau.23736

EDITORIAL COMMENTS

WILEY · Neurourology Urodynamics · ICS · SUFU

Why ICS standardization of lower urinary tract symptoms matters

Why does as a red traffic light mean "STOP" everywhere? Or why are you able to browse the Internet from anywhere over the world? These are just a few examples from our daily life that illustrate the need for standardization and the use of a common and correct terminology.

Standards make the world a safer place. Our health is dependent on standards, going from the definition of safe drinking water, over the quality of medical equipment to the creation of terminology, standards, and guidelines in healthcare.

Standards and terminology define what is being talked about. This is especially necessary in critical communication, but also to ensure the safe diagnosis and treatment of patients. It is important that the term for a symptom, condition or disease has the same meaning for every healthcare professional on this planet. If you hear of a new development at a congress or in publication, you need to understand it fully in order to adopt it properly into your practice. When talking with patients, both of you need to understand what the other is saying. Achieving this is the aspiration of the International Continence Society (ICS) standardizations.[1] They are a series of evidence based pragmatic documents, some of them developed in partnership with other professional bodies, covering the field of lower urinary tract function and dysfunction, and urodynamic assessment.[2–4]

Similar words can have different meanings in different languages, or translation. Notably an English term in another language can change the linguistic meaning or can have different connotations than in the original language. For example many languages do not make a distinction between urinary urge and urinary urgency. The ICS has clearly defined this difference to make it clear that urgency is pathological, as in overactive bladder, and urge is the normal sensation associated with a strong desire to pass urine. So as to be consistent for inclusion of patients in clinical trials on Overactive Bladder Syndrome potentially being run in several countries, correct interpretation of the inclusion and exclusion criteria is essential. For these trials it is of paramount importance to recruit only patients with urgency, and not those describing the normal sensation of urge. Standards help in managing cultural and linguistic diversity and differences. Such terminology efforts are crucial for the advancement of research and clinical practice.

Standards allow sharing of technology and innovation and information. If we would not use a standardized terminology and a set of standards in urodynamics, results from one center would not be interchangeable with those from another center. This would lead to an unnecessary duplication of examinations, when a patient would be referred to another center. Technology is highly dependent on terminology and standardization.[5] Standards also make information retrievable and speed up research. Every book or published article can be found with internet search engines or through library systems, thanks to unique identifiers that have been attributed according to international standards. Just imagine to have go back in time and to be dependent on an old-fashioned librarian and his reference system on little cards, before you could read an interesting article or book. Standards help tremendously in speeding-up research and interaction between researchers.

We strongly encourage all healthcare professionals to engage with the ICS standardizations, so as to push forward the progress in this field. Once it is in universal use, the ICS terminology offers a backbone for communications between professionals and also with patients.

CONFLICTS OF INTEREST

Dr. De Ridder reports grants from Astellas, grants from Janssen-cilag, grants from Medtronic, other from Coloplast, outside the submitted work.

Dirk De Ridder MD, PhD, FEBU [1]

Marcus Drake BM, BCh, MA(Cantab.), DM (Oxon.), FRCS(Urol)[2]

[1]*Dept. of Urology, University Hospitals KU Leuven, Herestraat 49, 3000 Leuven, Belgium*

[2]*Office C39b, Bristol Urological Institute, University of Bristol, Level 3 Learning and Research Building, BS10 5NB, Bristol, United Kingdom*

*Correspondence

Dirk De Ridder, MD, PhD, FEBU, Department of Urology, University Hospitals KU Leuven, Herestraat 49, 3000 Leuven, Belgium.

Email: dirk.deridder@uzleuven.be

REFERENCES

1. Rosier PF, de Ridder D, Meijlink J, Webb R, Whitmore K, Drake MJ. Developing evidence-based standards for diagnosis and management of lower urinary tract or pelvic floor dysfunction. *Neurourol Urodyn.* 2012;31:621–624.

2. Haylen B, Freeman R, de Ridder D, et al. An international urogynecological association (iuga) − international continence society (ics) joint report on the terminology for female pelvic floor dysfunction. *Neurourol Urodyn.* 2009;28:787.

3. Haylen BT, de Ridder D, Freeman RM, et al. An International Urogynecological Association (IUGA)/International Continence Society (ICS) joint report on the terminology for female pelvic floor dysfunction. *Neurourol Urodyn.* 2010;29:4–20.

4. Toozs-Hobson P, Freeman R, Barber M, et al. An International Urogynecological Association (IUGA)/International Continence Society (ICS) joint report on the terminology for reporting outcomes of surgical procedures for pelvic organ prolapse. *Int Urogynecol J.* 2012;23:527–535.

5. Seth JH, Sahai A, Khan MS, et al. Nerve growth factor (NGF): a potential urinary biomarker for overactive bladder syndrome (OAB)? *BJU Int.* 2013;111:372–380.

How to cite this article: De Ridder D, Drake M. Why ICS standardization of lower urinary tract symptoms matters. *Neurourology and Urodynamics.* 2018;37:S67–S68. https://doi.org/10.1002/nau.23736

Received: 12 April 2018 | Accepted: 5 July 2018

DOI: 10.1002/nau.23779

SOUNDING BOARD

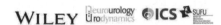

Critical steps in developing professional standards for the International Continence Society

Peter F. W. M. Rosier

Functional Urology, Department of Urology C04.236, University Medical Center Utrecht, Utrecht, The Netherlands

Correspondence
Peter F.W.M. Rosier, MD, PhD, Functional Urology, Department of Urology C04.236, University Medical Center Utrecht, The Netherlands.
Email: P.F.W.M.Rosier@umcutrecht.nl

Aims: Standardization on the basis of systematic assessment of evidence has become an indispensable element of modern healthcare. International Continence Society (ICS) has initiated and produced extremely well cited standardization documents. The process of standardization is recently depicted in a published manuscript, to keep up with modern society healthcare demands.
Methods: A narrative review of the ICS history and current state of standardizations for the terms, assessment and the management of patients with lower urinary tract dysfunction.
Results: This article highlights the philosophy and the historical context of standardization and explains the core elements of modern day standardization. The article also demonstrates the scientific relevance of the ICS standards, on the basis of reference-counts.
Conclusion: The history and the relevance of ICS standards are summarized.

KEYWORDS
health care quality, lower urinary tract dysfunction, systematic assessment and diagnosis

1 | INTRODUCTION

The Mars Climate Orbiter was a space probe launched by NASA on December 11, 1998 to study the Martian climate. However, on September 23, 1999, communication with the spacecraft was lost as the spacecraft went into orbital insertion, due to ground-based computer software which produced output in non-SI units of pound (force)-seconds (lbf/s) instead of the SI units of newton-seconds (N/s) specified in the contract between NASA and Lockheed. The spacecraft encountered Mars on a trajectory that brought it too close to the planet, causing it to pass through the upper atmosphere and disintegrate.[1] SI units are standard units of technical measurement, allowing communication about technical issues. Standardization is relevant, in technical science as well as in medical science. Standard terms, classifications and disease and management patterns were sought, in fact since the early days of healthcare, for example, by Hippocrates. Maybe in the more modern society further standardization began in the 16th century, where parish clerks were asked to classify mortality and standard terms were developed with this aim. This can be seen as the later basis for health epidemiological observations. In the beginning of 20th century a standard nomenclature for diseases was developed that progressed into the nowadays International Classification of Diseases (ICD) and Systematized Nomenclature of Medicine (SNOMED, now SNOMED-CT).[2]

Medical societies are established around (clinical-medical) specialisms to improve knowledge and accountability. The Continence Club was established in Exeter (UK) in 1971, renamed to International Continence Society that same year and had the purpose to ". . . provide a link for the interchange of ideas and results for clinicians and physicists interested in

---

Clinical trial: No.

Roger Dmochowski led the peer-review process as the Associate Editor responsible for the paper.

TABLE 1 "General" (not specific) ICS standardization documents with publication year and between brackets, a double or triple publication are showed

Scopus EXPORT DATE: 15 May 2018 searched quote: "standard* lower urinary tract function"		
Abrams P, Cardozo L, Fall M, Griffiths D, Rosier P, Ulmsten U, Van Kerrebroeck P, Victor A, Wein A. The standardization of terminology of lower urinary tract function: Report from the standardization sub-committee of the international continence society (2002) Neurourology and Urodynamics, 21 (2), pp. 167–178.	2002 (1)	Cited 4360 times.
Bump, RC, Mattiasson, A, Bo, K, Brubaker, LP, DeLancey, JOL, Klarskov, P, Shull, BL, Smith, ARB. The standardization of terminology of female pelvic organ prolapse and pelvic floor dysfunction (1996) American Journal of Obstetrics and Gynecology, 175 (1), pp. 10–17.	"ICS approved"	Cited 2616 times.
Abrams P, Cardozo L, Fall M, Griffiths D, Rosier P, Ulmsten U, Van Kerrebroeck P, Victor A, Wein A.The standardization of terminology in lower urinary tract function: Report from the standardization sub-committee of the International Continence Society (2003) Urology, 61 (1), pp. 37–49.	2002 (2)	Cited 1583 times.
Good Urodynamic Practices: Uroflowmetry, filling cystometry, and pressure-flow studies (2002) Neurourology and Urodynamics, 21 (3), pp. 261–274.		Cited 1006 times.
Abrams P, Blaivas JG, Stanton SL, Andersen JT. The standardization of terminology of lower urinary tract function. The International Continence Society Committee on Standardization of Terminology. (1988) Scandinavian Journal of Urology and Nephrology, Supplement, 114, pp. 5–19.	1988 (1)	Cited 951 times.
Haylen, BT, De Ridder D, Freeman RM, Swift SE, Berghmans B, Lee J, Monga A, Petri E, Rizk DE, Sand PK, Schaer GN. An International Urogynecological Association (IUGA)/International Continence Society (ICS) joint report on the terminology for female pelvic floor dysfunction (2010) International Urogynecology Journal, 21 (1), pp. 5–26.		Cited 771 times.
Abrams P, Cardozo L, Fall M, Griffiths D, Rosier P, Ulmsten U, Van Kerrebroeck P, Victor A, Wein A. The standardization of terminology of lower urinary tract function: Report from the Standardization Sub-committee of the International Continence Society (2002) American journal of obstetrics and gynecology, 187 (1), pp. 116–126.	2002 (3)	Cited 607 times.
Griffiths D, Hofner K, Van Mastrigt R, Rollema HJ, Spangberg A, Gleason D. Standardization of terminology of lower urinary tract function: Pressure-flow studies of voiding, urethral resistance, and urethral obstruction (1997) Neurourology and Urodynamics, 16 (1), pp. 1–18.		Cited 324 times.
Abrams P, Blaivas JG, Stanton SL, Andersen JT. The standardization of terminology of lower urinary tract function recommended by the international continence society (1990) International Urogynecology Journal, 1 (1), pp. 45–58.	1988 (1)	Cited 305 times.
Bates P, Bradley WE, Glen E, Griffiths D, Melchior H, Rowan D, Sterling A, Zinner N, Hald T. The standardization of terminology of lower urinary tract function (1979) Journal of Urology, 121 (5), pp. 551–554..		Cited 233 times
First Report on the Standardization of Terminology of Lower Urinary Tract Function: PRODUCED BY THE INTERNATINAL CONTINENCE SOCIETY, FEBRUARY, 1975 (1976) British Journal of Urology, 48 (1), pp. 39–42.		Cited 215 times.
Austin PF, Bauer SB, Bower W, Chase J, Franco I, Hoebeke P, Rittig Sø, Vande Walle J, Von Gontard A, Wright A, Yang SS, Nevéus T. The standardization of terminology of lower urinary tract function in children and adolescents: Update report from the standardization committee of the international children's continence society (2014) Journal of Urology, 191 (6), pp. 1863–1865.		Cited 193 times.
The standardization of terminology of lower urinary tract function (1990) BJOG: An International Journal of Obstetrics & Gynecology, 97, pp. 1–16.		Cited 118 times.
Glen ES, Bradley WE, Melchior H, Rowan D, Sterling AM, Sundin T, Thomas D, Torrens M, Warwick RT, Zinner NR, Chairman TH. Fourth Report on the Standardization of Terminology of Lower Urinary Tract Function: Terminology related to neuromuscular dysfunction of the lower urinary tract: PRODUCED BY THE INTERNATIONAL CONTINENCE SOCIETY (1981) British Journal of Urology, 53 (4), pp. 333–335.		Cited 90 times.
Abrams P, Blaivas JG, Stanton SL, Andersen JT. The standardization of terminology of lower urinary tract function – Produced by the international continence society committee on standardization of terminology (1989) World Journal of Urology, 6 (4), pp. 233–245.	1998-9 (3)	Cited 52 times.
Austin PF, Bauer SB, Bower W, Chase J, Franco I, Hoebeke P, Rittig S, Walle J.V, Von Gontard A, Wright A, Yang SS, Nevéus T. The standardization of terminology of lower urinary tract function in children and adolescents: Update report from the standardization committee of the International Children's Continence Society (2016) Neurourology and Urodynamics, 35 (4), pp. 471–481.		Cited 47 times.

(Continues)

TABLE 1 (Continued)

Scopus EXPORT DATE: 15 May 2018 searched quote: "standard* lower urinary tract function"		
Bates CP, Bradley WE, Glen ES, Griffiths D, Melchior H, Rowan D, Sterling A, Hald T. Third Report on the Standardization of Terminology of Lower Urinary Tract Function: Procedures related to the evaluation of micturition: Pressure-flow relationships. Residual urine: PRODUCED BY THE INTERNATIONAL CONTINENCE SOCIETY, FEBRUARY 1977* (1980) British Journal of Urology, 52 (5), pp. 348–350.	1977 (3)	Cited 43 times.
Bates P, Bradley WE, Glen E, Griffiths D, Melchior H, Rowan D, Sterling AM, Zinner N, Hald T. Standardization of terminology of lower urinary tract function First and second reports: International Continence Society (1977) Urology, 9 (2), pp. 237–241.	1977 (4)	Cited 34 times.
Abrams P, Blaivas JG, Stanton SL, Andersen JT, Fowler CJ, Gerstenberg T, Murray K. Sixth report on the standardization of terminology of lower urinary tract function. Procedures related to neurophysiological investigations: electromyography, nerve conduction studies, reflex latencies, evoked potentials and sensory testing. The International Continence Society Committee on Standardization of Terminology, New York, May 1985. (1986) Scandinavian Journal of Urology and Nephrology, 20 (3), pp. 161–164.	1985 (1)	Cited 26 times.
Nevéus T, Von Gontard A, Hoebeke P, Hjälmas K, Bauer S, Bower W, Jørgensen TM, Rittig S, Van De Walle J, Yeung, C-K, Djurhuus JC. The standardization of terminology of lower urinary tract function in children and adolescents: Report from the Standardization Committee of the International Children's Continence Society (ICCS) (2007) Neurourology and Urodynamics, 26 (1), pp. 90–102.		Cited 20 times.
Bates P, Bradley WE, Glen E, Melchior H, Rowan D, Sterling A, Hald T. The standardization of terminology of lower urinary tract function (1976) European Urology, 2 (6), pp. 274–276.		Cited 15 times.
Andersen JT, Blaivas JG, Cardozo L, Thuroff J. Seventh report on the standardization of terminology of lower urinary tract function: Lower urinary tract rehabilitation techniques (1992) Scandinavian Journal of Urology and Nephrology, 26 (2), pp. 99–106.		Cited 14 times.
Abrams P, Blaivas JG, Stanton SL, Andersen JT, Fowler CJ, Gerstenberg T, Murray K. Sixth report on the standardization of terminology of lower urinary tract function – Procedures related to neurophysiological investigations: Electromyography, nerve conduction studies, reflex latencies, evoked potentials and sensory testing (1986) World Journal of Urology, 4 (1), pp. 2–5.	1985-6 (2)	Cited 9 times.
Bates P, Rowan D, Glen E. Second report on the standardization of terminology of lower urinary tract function. Produced by the International Continence Society committee on standardization of terminology Copenhagen, August 1976 (1977) European Urology, 3 (3), pp. 168–170.	1977 (2)	Cited 8 times.
Bates P, Bradley WE, Glen E, Melchior H, Rowan D, Sterling A Hald T. First report on the standardization of terminology of lower urinary tract function: Incontinence, cystometry, urethral closure pressure profile and units of measurement (1977) Urologia Internationalis, 32 (2–3), pp. 81–87.	1977 (1)	Cited 7 times.

The third column shows the number of citations to the specific document as obtained from Scopus.com (May 2018).

urodynamic studies ... treating related disorders."[3] To this aim, as a logical consequence, "... to set it [the new society (ICS)] on the way to becoming a professional body"[3] a "standardization of terminology of lower urinary tract function" was developed and published simultaneously in diverse journals.[4] Terms for urodynamic observations were developed since then and refined, together with improvements in the techniques used to objectively measure lower urinary tract functions, independent from the patients expression of symptoms. New ICS standardization documents have been published in the years that followed.

2 | MATERIAL AND METHODS

A narrative review of the evolution of the process of standardization in healthcare, in general and specific for ICS is presented. Scopus—website counts are used to demonstrate the scientific relevance of the published manuscripts of ICS standards.

3 | RESULTS

2.1 | Standard for standards

Early standards in health care have been eloquence based. A group of renowned experts sat together and developed the text of the standard, on the basis of their knowledge. That actual knowledge failed against big data was demonstrated in the late 1960s. A clinical epidemiological book discussed the complexity of medical decision making, and was the starting point for nowadays clinical epidemiology. Clinical epidemiology became a tool to be the more reliable basis for (more) systematic diagnosis and management.[5] This clinical epidemiology, and systematic reviewing of research data were deployed into evidence based medicine later.[6]

Also early ICS standards have been developed in the "good old boys sat around the table" (GOBSAT)—manner. In 2012, however, the ICS standardization committee has published a standard to deviate from GOBSAT and to introduce—evidence based-(healthcare and) ICS standards.[7] This manuscript highlights also that the ICS standardization committee had modernized itself and became a standardizing steering committee, with the aim to oversee and guide (ad hoc) working groups to deliver new ICS standards. The renewed process and structure of standards production were defined, to ensure careful inclusion of evidence in the standard and to explicitly grade evidence and also indicate expert opinion where evidence is lacking. In summary of the earlier published document, the process consists of a proposal stage, a preparatory stage, a committee stage and an approval stage

and has also defined an implementation stage.[7] An idea for a new standard should be proposed to the ICS standardization steering committee who will establish an opinion- and background-balanced working group with a chairperson. The "balance," referred to in the standard[7] includes that the background should as diverse as possible, around the topic of the standardization, not only in opinion and profession but also including partnership of other organizations (outside ICS) when that is deemed potentially rewarding. The working group, when established, searches for relevant evidence and makes summaries of answers for clinical questions associated with the topic of the standard. Terms may also be searched for existence in scientific databases or in the, here above mentioned, international nomenclature—sets, or medical dictionaries, before introduction in the (new) standard.

TABLE 2 The top ranking documents with (clinical OR practice) standard* in the title with the number of citations to the specific document (may 2018) are showed

Scopus EXPORT DATE: 15 May 2018 Search quote: "Standard*"- in Title.	
Standardization of spirometry (2005) European Respiratory Journal, 26 (2), pp. 319–338.	Cited 6495 times.
Standardization of spirometry: 1994 Update (1995) American Journal of Respiratory and Critical Care Medicine, 152 (3), pp. 1107–1136.	Cited 5248 times.
Bone histomorphometry: Standardization of nomenclature, symbols, and units: Report of the asbmr histomorphometry nomenclature committee (1987) Journal of Bone and Mineral Research, 2 (6), pp. 595–610.	Cited 4397 times.
The standardization of terminology of lower urinary tract function: Report from the standardization sub-committee of the international continence society (2002) Neurourology and Urodynamics, 21 (2), pp. 167–178.	**Cited 4360 times.**
The consortium to establish a registry for Alzheimer's disease (CERAD). Part II. Standardization of the neuropathologic assessment of Alzheimer's disease(1991) Neurology, 41 (4), pp. 479–486.	Cited 3495 times.
The standardization of terminology of female pelvic organ prolapse and pelvic floor dysfunction (1996) American Journal of Obstetrics and Gynecology, 175 (1), pp. 10-17	Cited 2616 times.
Lung volumes and forced ventilatory flows. Report Working Party Standardization of Lung Function Tests, European Community for Steel and Coal. Official Statement of the European Respiratory Society. (1993) The European respiratory journal. Supplement, 16, pp. 5-40	Cited 2523 times.
Standard of spirometry- 1987 update. Statement of the American Thoracic Society. (1987) The American review of respiratory disease, 136 (5), pp. 1285–1298.	Cited 2070 times.
Design and standardization of PCR primers and protocols for detection of clonal immunoglobulin and T cell receptor gene recombinations in suspect lymphoproliferations: Report of the BIOMED 2 concerted action BMH4- CT98-3936 (2003) Leukemia, 17 (12), pp. 2257–2317.	Cited 1834 times.
The standardization of terminology in lower urinary tract function: Report from the standardization sub- committee of the International Continence Society (2003) Urology, 61 (1), pp. 37–49.	**Cited 1583 times.**
A Specific Laboratory Test for the Diagnosis of Melancholia: Standardization, Validation, and Clinical Utility (1981) Archives of General Psychiatry, 38 (1), pp. 15-22	Cited 1579 times.
Revised Recommendations of the International Working Group for diagnosis, standardization of response criteria, treatment outcomes, and reporting standards for therapeutic trials in acute myeloid leukemia (2003) Journal of Clinical Oncology, 21 (24), pp. 4642–4649.	Cited 1471 times.
Standardization of uveitis nomenclature for reporting clinical data. Results of the first international workshop (2005) American Journal of Ophthalmology, 140 (3), pp. 509-516	Cited 1435 times.
A working formulation for the standardization of nomenclature in the diagnosis of heart and lung rejection: Heart rejection study group (1990) Journal of Heart Transplantation, 9 (6), pp. 587-592	Cited 1301 times.

When the number of citations to the three versions of the 2002 document are added (4360 + 1583 + 607), 3th not shown, see Table 1), the total of 6650 would rank this document number 1 clinical standard in healthcare. Note also that the number 6 document is an "ICS-collaboration-endorsed" standard.

Objective evidence for management in new standard should be systematically gathered with structured searches of literature and Oxford grading. Theoretically a Delphi process would be applicable for sub-topics where evidence is lacking, however, this procedure is not without pitfalls, for example, has the danger of devaluating to the "old GOBSAT" manner,[8,9] by overestimation of the experts knowledge[8] and underestimation of the existence of evidence. Potential other pitfalls are, for example, imposing preconceptions of a problem and not allowing for the contribution of other related perspectives; poor techniques of summarizing and presenting the group responses; not exploring disagreements and; underestimating the demanding nature of a Delphi.[8] A recent systematic review of reports based on the Delphi method found substantial variation in quality as consequence of lack of rigorousness of the application of the process.[9] Ultimately the (new) standard terms are selected on the basis of arguments made transparent. Sensitive and systematic searching for existing evidence prevents reinvention of knowledge and has to provide the evidence base for the practice recommendations or for the terms. Finally the members and board of the ICS will see the draft standard and control, for process and structure, but also for missed evidence that may change the recommendations. Details of this process are given in the original publication but essentially the draft document is made available for all ICS members via the ICS website, and is also submitted to internal invited peer review and or discussed during an annual society meeting. The finally approved standard is published and, for example, relevant committees can take out relevant elements and make these into educational modules to be published as presentation on the ICS website to enhance implementation of standard good practice and terms by education.

3.2 | Scientific relevance

The International Continence Society has produced one of the most cited standards in healthcare.[10] Table 1 shows the number of citations for the most "general" ICS standards on the basis of the counts given in Scopus.com website on May 15, 2018. Table 2 shows that the number of citations to the 2002 standardization document exceeds all documents with "practice guideline" or "practice standard" in the title when the three versions of the 2002 document (see Table 1) are grouped. (source: scopus.com). The references total of 6650 contains that the document is referred to every single day since its publication.

4 | DISCUSSION

The modern era standards should aim at that level and be the basis for good practice. ICS is still leading in the development of careful objective assessment of lower urinary tract

dysfunction as has been aimed in 1971. Objective assessment of dysfunction meets patients expectations also (or especially?) to date.[11] Modern era healthcare, however, also demands, more than in the early days of ICS, that patients quality of life and well-being are taken into account and that minimal or not invasive management is recommended to them, where possible. Not only terms and techniques for objective assessment and diagnosis should be renewed, in an evidence based fashion, also the assessment of the patients well-being deserves evidence based standardization. Furthermore standards for management may lead the way to improvements. The ICS standard for standardization may become the basis for systematic evidence based documents to enforce the International Consultation on Incontinence management recommendations[12] and may also expand to management of lower urinary tract dysfunctions without urinary incontinence.

5 | CONCLUSION

Standardization prevents miscommunication and therefore mismanagement, also in healthcare. ICS started with standardization, based on scientific progress and development and has continued this, in the lead, for almost 50 years. ICS Standardization is now standardized within the framework of Evidence Based Medicine and apart from further standardization of urodynamic assessment and evidence based objective pelvic floor muscle function evaluation standardization of quality of life assessment as well as standards for management may be future goals.

CONFLICT OF INTEREST

No.

ORCID

Peter F. W. M. Rosier http://orcid.org/0000-0003-0445-4563

REFERENCES

1. https://mars. jpl.nasa.gov/msp98/news/mco990930.html.
2. Chute CG. Clinical classification and terminology: some history and current observations. *J Am Med Inform Assoc.* 2000;7:298–303.
3. Arnold T, Glenn E, Zinner N. *The First 40 Years, History of ICS.* Bristol, UK: Conticom Limited; 2011.
4. No authors listed. First report on the standardisation of terminology of lower urinary tract function. *Br J Urol.* 1976;48:39–42. Report published also in other journals: Bates et al.
5. Feinstein AR. *Clinical Judgement.* Baltimore: Williams & Wilkins; 1967.
6. Sackett DL, Rosenberg WM, Gray JA, Haynes RB, Richardson WS. Evidence based medicine: what it is and what it isn't. *BMJ.* 1996;312:71–72.

7. Rosier PF, de Ridder D, Meijlink J, Webb R, Whitmore K, Drake MJ. Developing evidence-based standards for diagnosis and management of lower urinary tract or pelvic floor dysfunction. *Neurourol Urodyn*. 2012;31(5):621–624.

8. *The Delphi Method: Techniques and Applications*. In: Linstone HA, Turoff M, eds. Addison-Wesley Pub. Co., Advanced Book Program; 1975. University of Michigan, ISBN0201042940, 9780201042948 (digitalized august 27 2007). https://web.njit.edu/~turoff/pubs/delphibook/delphibook.pdf

9. Jünger S, Payne SA, Brine J, Radbruch L, Brearley SG. Guidance on Conducting and REporting DElphi Studies (CREDES) in palliative care: recommendations based on a methodological systematic review. *Palliat Med*. 2017;31:684–706.

10. Abrams P, Cardozo L, Fall M, et al. The standardisation of terminology in lower urinary tract function: report from the standardisation sub-committee of the International Continence Society. *Urology*. 2003;61:37–49. Review. PubMed PMID: 12559262.

11. Makanjee CR, Bergh AM, Hoffmann WA. Healthcare provider and patient perspectives on diagnostic imaging investigations. *Afr J Prim Health Care FamnMed*. 2015;7:art#801.

12. Abrams P, Andersson KE, Birder L, et al. Fourth International Consultation on Incontinence Recommendations of the International Scientific Committee: evaluation and treatment of urinary incontinence, pelvic organ prolapse, and fecal incontinence. *Neurourol Urodyn*. 2010;29:213–240.

How to cite this article: Rosier PFWM. Critical steps in developing professional standards for the International Continence Society. *Neurourology and Urodynamics*. 2018;37:S69–S74. https://doi.org/10.1002/nau.23779

Patient information

In carrying out our day to day activities, including research, we process and store personal information relating to our service users and we are therefore required to adhere to the requirements of the Data Protection Act 1998 and the General Data Protection Regulation (GDPR), which will apply in the UK from 25 May 2018. Some of your data and results may be used for research purposes but none will have any identifiable information.

We take our responsibilities under these acts very seriously. We ensure the personal information we obtain is held, used, transferred and otherwise processed in accordance with applicable data protection laws and regulations.

Flow Studies Pathway

Referred for flow studies by Doctor or Nurse

Contacted by flows co-ordinator (phone or letter)

Flow studies appointment letter sent with bladder diary and quality of life questionnaire

Attend flow study appointment in urology clinic

Test fully explained by a member of staff and bladder diary and quality of life questionnaire collected

Pass urine into flowmeter and have ultrasound scan of bladder – process repeated 2-3 times

Results from your flow studies will be stored on our electronic database and electronic patient records

Results will also be sent to your referring Doctor or Nurse

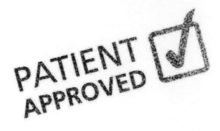

How to contact us:

Flow Coordinator

 Bristol Urological Institute (BUI)
Southmead Hospital
Southmead Road
Westbury-on-Trym
Bristol BS10 5NB

0117 4145000

www.nbt.nhs.uk

If you or the individual you are caring for need support reading
this leaflet please ask a member of staff for advice.

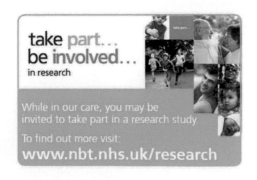

take part...
be involved...
in research

While in our care, you may be
invited to take part in a research study.

To find out more visit:
www.nbt.nhs.uk/research

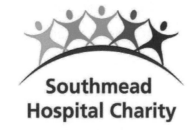

**Southmead
Hospital Charity**

southmeadhospitalcharity.org.uk
Southmead Hospital Charity raises funds for
departments and wards throughout the Trust,
meaning you can support an area close to your heart

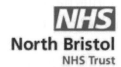

North Bristol
NHS Trust

Service:
Urology

Urodynamics

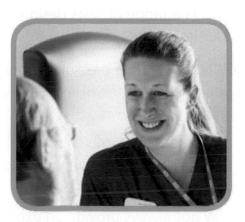

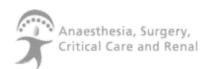

Anaesthesia, Surgery,
Critical Care and Renal

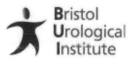

**Bristol
Urological
Institute**

E B U

Certified Centre
EBU-EAU Host Centre for Female Urology and Incontinence

Exceptional healthcare, personally delivered

Standard Urodynamics

You should allow one and quarter hours for the test. Please also let us know if you have any allergies, especially to latex or if you have any problems with your mobility.

What the urodynamics test involves

Before the Test

IMPORTANT: If you feel you may have a urine infection, you should inform the hospital when you receive your appointment so that the necessary arrangements can be made. If you are prone to urinary tract infections please ensure you get your urine checked by your GP surgery five working days before the appointment so that it can be treated prior to the study. We are unable to perform Urodynamics if you have a symptomatic urinary tract infection because we could make your symptoms much worse.

Please let us know if you are currently taking any tablets for your bladder (e.g. Vesicare/Solifenacin, Regurin/Trospium Chloride, Detrusitol/Tolterodine, Oxybutynin, Betmiga/Mirabegron) as you may be asked to stop these a week before your appointment as these can affect your test results.

No special preparations are needed for the test. You can eat and drink as normal, but we would like you to come with your bladder comfortably full. Please complete the Frequency/Volume Chart (ICIQ-bladder diary) and the quality of life questionnaire (ICIQ-LUTS) sent with your appointment letter. It is important that you bring both of them with you to the clinic.

After you arrive, the doctor/nurse performing the test will explain the procedure to you and ask some questions about the symptoms that you have been experiencing. Some questions may be intimate and you may have answered them before, but they are important questions in making a diagnosis of your condition. If you feel that you do not wish to answer some of the questions then please let your doctor/nurse know. You will be asked to sign a Consent Form to ensure that you understand the procedure and any potential side effects.

You will be asked to change and remove all your clothing including underwear/pants (women can keep their brasserie on) and will be given a hospital gown. This will be done in privacy behind closed curtains. This is done to avoid any of your clothing getting wet during the test as the test would involve filling you with saline (salt water) and also avoid urine running onto your socks. If you feel cold during the test then please let the nurse or doctor know and they will provide you with blankets.

The doctor/nurse will then leave you alone to pass urine into a special toilet (flowmeter). This measures how fast the urine flows from you. After you have done this, the doctor/nurse/ urodynamicist may examine you. This will include an internal examination, with a chaperone present, of the rectum and vagina (in women). It may also include inserting a vaginal speculum in women (sometimes this may be cold and the person doing it will warn you before inserting it).

During the test

You will be lying on a couch and one or two small tubes (not measuring more than 3mm in diameter) will be passed into your bladder and another small tube will be placed into your rectum (back passage). If you do not have a rectum because you have had surgery and have a colostomy or stoma then that can be used , or the vagina (in women) can also be used as an alternative to measuring abdominal pressure. These tubes allow us to take pressure measurements both inside and outside the bladder. You will then be asked to sit up or stand and your bladder will be slowly filled with saline (salt water) through the tube until you feel full. If you are unable to sit or stand then you will be allowed to lie down on the couch. You will be asked to cough or strain several times during the test to check the tubes are working. You will also be asked a series of questions such as your first desire to pass urine or whether you experience any urgency. Your bottom half will be covered during the test to conserve your dignity.

If you experience any unusual symptoms during the test then you would need to tell the doctor and/or nurse immediately, especially some young men can get a vaso-vagal response from filling the bladder (this means they feel faint). We would lie you down and offer you water and stop the test until you feel better.

Once your bladder is comfortably full, one of the bladder tubes will be removed. The tube in your rectum and the very tiny tube in your urethra, will be left in. The nurse and doctor will leave the room, and you will be asked to pass urine. The doctor, nurse or technician performing the test will answer any questions you may have and will tell you the results of the test at the end of the procedure, once you are dressed and comfortable. We will provide you with wet wipes and dry wipes in order that you can make yourself comfortable and will give you privacy in which to do this.

A report will be done by the clinical person performing the test and a copy will be sent to your GP, your referring doctor and yourself.

After the test you may experience symptoms of discomfort in

the bladder and urethra for a short time, but these should settle down. We suggest that you drink half to one litre of extra fluid to ensure prompt voiding again to relieve the urethral irritation.

After the test you may experience symptoms of discomfort in the bladder and urethra for a short time, but these should settle down. We suggest that you drink half to one litre of extra fluid to ensure prompt voiding again to relieve the urethral irritation.

Risks associated with the test:

- Urinary Tract Infection (UTI): No matter how careful we are when inserting the tubes, there is a small risk of introducing a UTI anywhere in the urinary tract including the urethra, bladder, testis (in men) and/or kidneys. The risk is about 3% – 4% i.e. 3-4 people in every 100 may get an infection, based on regular auditing of our infection rates every five years. We always advise you to drink plenty of water following the test to help flush the urinary system and reduce the risk of infection. If you think you have developed an infection you will need to contact your GP and tell them you have had this test and they will give you antibiotics. If your urodynamics doctor or nurse believe that you are at a higher risk of getting urinary tract infections e.g. if you are immunosuppressed or immunocompromised, then they may give you antibiotics at the start of the test and/or to go home with

- Bleeding: There is a small chance of bleeding from one of the small blood vessels in the bladder, urethra, rectum or vagina (in women). This is nothing to worry about and will stop within a couple of days. If it does not stop then you would need to contact the urodynamics team and ask them for advice.

It is best to wear loose fitting separate clothes. Ladies may wish to wear a skirt or trousers, and a top. You may want to bring a change of clothes in the event of accidents. Please bring a book or paper to read whilst the test is taking place.

During the Test

On arrival we will once again explain the test to you.

The test involves passing a small tube into your bladder and another small tube is placed in your rectum (back passage). These tubes allow us to take continuous pressure measurements whilst your bladder is filling naturally. These tubes are connected to a small recording device, which is worn discreetly on a belt around your waist for the duration of the test. Your bladder function will be monitored whilst you are walking, exercising and relaxing. You can drink normally during the test. You will be asked to keep a diary of how your bladder feels and how much fluid you have drunk.

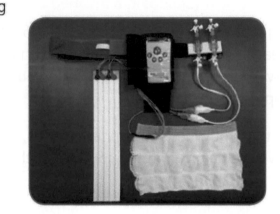

During the test a doctor, nurse, or technician will be available to you. They will answer your questions. When you need to pass urine there will be a specially assigned toilet for you to use, but you will need to let the nurse know when you need to empty your bladder. The portable recording device that you wear will be checked before and after you pass urine.

You will be free to walk around the hospital and the hospital grounds, but we request you to return to the department every hour in order to get the equipment checked. You are free to return at any time should you have any questions or concerns. There is the risk of tubes falling out, especially when you are being very active. Some people do experience some discomfort, but this should settle down. If not, and you are too uncomfortable, then we will remove the tubes and stop the test.

Once you, and the person performing the test, feel that your symptoms have been reproduced the tubes will be removed and you will be able to get redressed and comfortable. You will be given the results of your test. A report will be written and sent to your Consultant, your GP and to you.

After the test

This is the same as that written above for standard Urodynamics. However, if you do have any concerns that have not been covered by us then you can contact your GP or The Urodynamic Department.

Appendix D

Practice, Standards, and Equipment Recommendations

International Consultation on Incontinence 2016; Executive Summary: Urodynamic Testing

Received: 11 June 2018 | Accepted: 1 July 2018

DOI: 10.1002/nau.23903

REVIEW ARTICLE

WILEY Neurourology Urodynamics ICS SUFU

International Consultation on Incontinence 2016; Executive summary: Urodynamic testing

Peter F. W. M. Rosier[1] | Hann-Chorng Kuo[2] | Mario De Gennaro[3] | Andrew Gammie[4] | Enrico Finazzi Agro[5] | Hidehiro Kakizaki[6] | Hashim Hashim[4] | Philip Toozs-Hobson[7]

[1] Department of Urology, University Medical Center, Utrecht, The Netherlands

[2] Department of Urology, Buddhist Tzu Chi General Hospital, Hualien, Taiwan

[3] Department of Nephrology-Urology Pediatric Ospedale Pediatrico Bambino Gesù, Rome, Italy

[4] Bristol Urological Institute, Bristol, United Kingdom

[5] Unit of Functional Urology, Tor Vergata University Hospital, Rome, Italy

[6] Department of Renal and Urologic Surgery, Asahikawa Medical University, Asahikawa, Japan

[7] Department of Gynaecology and Pelvic Floor Medicine, Birmingham Women's and Children's NHS Foundation Trust, Birmingham, UK

Correspondence

Peter F.W.M. Rosier, MD, PhD, P.F.W.M., Senior Lecturer Functional Urology and Neurourology, Department of Urology, University Medical Center, Utrecht, The Netherlands.
Email: rosier@umcutrecht.nl

Aims: The International Consultation on Incontinence has published an update of the recommendations for the diagnosis and management of urine incontinence (ICI2016). This manuscript summarizes the consultations committee—recommendations with regard to urodynamic assessment.

Methods: Expert consensus on the basis of structured evidence assessment has been the basis of the consultations publication and has been summarized by the committee for this manuscript.

Results: Patients that are not satisfied with their initial management on the basis of their reported signs and symptoms of urinary incontinence, as well as all patients with neurological abnormalities that are potentially relevant for the function of the lower urinary tract, may very likely profit from objective diagnosis and staging and grading of their dysfunction, with urodynamic testing, regardless their age, vulnerability and/ or comorbidities. The principles and technical innovations as well as the principal recommendations for the utilization of (invasive) urodynamic assessment for women, men, children, and vulnerable elderly, with or without neurogenic lower urinary tract dysfunction with urinary incontinence are provided in this abbreviated ICI recommendations-document.

Conclusions: The ICI2016 committee on urodynamics presents an executive summary of the most important reasons and recommendations for the use of urodynamic investigations for patients with urinary incontinence.

KEYWORDS

clinical practice guideline, diagnosis, expert review, lower urinary tract dysfunction, neurogenic bladder dysfunction, practice recommendations, urinary incontinence children

1 | INTRODUCTION

The evidence around Urodynamic testing (UDS) for patients with signs and symptoms of urinary incontinence (UI) was reviewed by an expert panel for the 6th International Consultation on Incontinence; held in Tokyo 2016. The conclusions and recommendations from ICI2013 regarding the application of UDS for the following discrete groups; women, men, children, neurogenic lower urinary tract dysfunction (NLUTD) and the frail elderly have been adapted to the new published evidence.[1] We present a summary of the recommendation—updates and selected literature references

when anatomical abnormalities with the NLUTD are not unlikely.

6 | URODYNAMIC TESTING IN CHILDREN WITH URINARY INCONTIENCE

ICI2016 confirmed ICI2013 that within the limits also provided for adults, (i)UDS in children is reliable and reproducible. Non-invasive tests as uroflowmetry are gradually achieving more evidence level, by constructing normative values and more standardized performance of the tests. Although it is plausible and considered useful to reduce filling speed and catheter size in relation to patient size, the exact values cannot be given and the influence of the transurethral catheter size on voiding in children is unknown. The committee has again (ICI2013) concluded that standards for pressure flow analysis in children are lacking. ICI 2016 has also affirmed that the specific demands of children, psychologically as well as physically, are respected before iUDS is carried out as well as during the testing and recommends specialized workers, units and equipment to ensure this. ICI2016 recommends that non-invasive diagnostic tests should be preferred where possible, iUDS should be done only if deemed useful by the results of non-invasive procedures, when the outcome of iUDS can alter management. Clinicians should take into account the effect of the (apparent psychologically stressing) laboratory-situation on the child's behavior and the implications for the results and the representativeness of the tests. A publication of 2015 by the International Children Continence Society provided expert recommendations for the practice of iUDS[27] also practice for VUDS.[28] The indications for UDS evaluation in children with urinary incontinence (or LUTD) are usually, anatomical and/or functional abnormalities and frequently neurological. In children with relevant neurological lesions, UDS is done regardless of (specific) symptoms, to discover conditions causing upper urinary tract risk.

6.1 | Children with neurogenic lower urinary tract dysfunction

6.1.1 | Myelodysplasia and occult spinal dysraphism

iUDS is advised by the ICI2016 in all patients with MMC, on a regular basis throughout the entire life from earliest childhood (3 months), based on ample evidence. iUDS should be considered, apart from routine, by a change of lower body half function and/or clinical change of LUT or UUT function, or when significant management changes have been started. ICI2016 recommended again (ICI2013) that the advantages and disadvantages of the addition of imaging to iUDS

(videourodynamics) should be considered children with MMC on an individual basis, for example, the likelihood of new anatomical abnormalities.

6.1.2 | Spinal cord injury

The committee recommends that iUDS evaluation in children with SCI is done not earlier than 6 weeks after injury, and that follow up is scheduled on an individual basis.

6.1.3 | Cerebral palsy

Some studies have shown that clinically unexpected LUTD can be present in children with cerebral palsy, especially when voiding symptoms are present. Observation and non-invasive testing are helpful, but iUDS should be considered when UTIs or UUT dilation occur.

6.1.4 | Anorectal malformation and sacral agenesis

Diverse studies have shown that a significant proportion of children with ARM has (primary-neuro-anatomical and/or secondary-functional) dysfunction of the LUT and pelvic floor. Clinicians should (grade C) consider iUDS in children with anorectal malformation, imperforate anus, or sacral agenesis when clinical signs of LUTD or when relevant neurologic abnormalities (clinical and or on imaging) exist. Around one third of children with ARM have MMC or tethered spinal cord, with (iUDS demonstrable) and clinically relevant NLUTD. Clinicians should also consider iUDS after (surgery for) sacrococcygeal teratoma.[29]

6.2 | Children with anatomic abnormalities and dysfunctions

6.2.1 | Bladder exstrophy

Once the exstrophied bladder is closed it may be difficult to manage persistent UI, UUT dilation or VUR. UDS for diagnosis and follow up are relevant, also to decide on interventions to improve continence function and/or if augmentation cystoplasty would be required.[30,31,32] UDS remain also helpful to evaluate LUT before (and after) further surgical procedures and for research matters.[33,34,35]

6.2.2 | Posterior urethral valves

In the past iUDS had been essential to understand (functional) outflow obstruction, LUT dysfunction, persistence of UI and UUT (and renal) impairment evolution in boys with PUV.[36,37] Also with early valve ablation, gradual detrusor "decompensation" and/or secondary BOO and finally DU or acontractility may be expected in a proportion of boys. It is reasonable to follow these patients by non-invasive UDS exams and iUDS when clinical progression is noted.[38]

6.2.3 | Vesicoureteral reflux

VUR may be a secondary phenomenon resulting from LUT dysfunction, not (only) from a primary anatomic ureter-ovesical junction abnormality, in a significant proportion of children[39-41] and that for example, DO may lead to VUR in a marginally competent ureterovesical junction mechanism.[42,43] Many clinicians advocate UDS especially for those patients that still have UI, renal damage, or when surgical correction is considered.[44,45]

6.3 | Children with functional disorders of the lower urinary tract

When assessing functional disorders involving the LUT in children, one must take into account the dynamics of the maturing nervous system and the LUT, including the normal learning curve for pelvic floor muscle, bladder, and bowel function, its abnormalities and the social and other positive and negative influences. iUDS has a limited place in diurnal incontinence, before age 5 or 6.[46] Uroflowmetry with PVR determination is the test of choice and results from uroflowmetry (mL) should be compared with information from the patient's frequency voiding charts. Persistent daytime and night-time UI, resistant to conventional therapy may require (V)UDS.[47] It is generally not necessary to conduct UDS for Mono-symptomatic Nocturnal Enuresis. The committee recommends bladder diary, uroflowmetry (with pelvic floor EMG) and PVR assessment in all children with LUTS, UI and with nocturnal enuresis resistant to first line therapy.[48,49] The committee suggests to consider urological assessment in children with chronic constipation and/or fecal incontinence.

7 | URODYNAMIC TESTING OF FRAIL ELDERLY PERSONS WITH URINARY INCONTINENCE

UI in the frail elderly commonly has diverse and multiple coexisting factors. Retrospective single center cohort reports confirm that aging, general health, mobility, medications, and neurologic diseases all have effects on LUT function. ICI 2016 concludes again (ICI2013) that also in the frail elderly, symptoms, and signs are unreliable to predict the type and grade of LUT dysfunction. Especially, but not exclusively, as an example, male elderly patients with central neurological disease, can also have urologic disease (eg, prostatic BOO) as a cause for UI or other LUTD.

Frail elderly with UI should be evaluated by a clinician skilled in the care of those patients. All contributing factors

are managed, before further urological diagnostics are performed. ICI2016 recommended that (standard) UDS should be offered to all elderly patients with signs and symptoms or LUTD not responding to relevant initial management regardless of the age and/or comorbidity if specific invasive treatment is deemed appropriate and/or possible. Every invasive procedure can cause harm but there is no published evidence that iUDS cause significantly more harm in the vulnerable elderly.

"Simple" bedside UDS (observing fluid level in a vertically placed bladder-catheter tube) has an inherent unreliability that very likely does not outweigh its "simplicity." PVR measurement (by ultrasound) is, as earlier (ICI2013), recommended before institution of pharmacological or surgical treatment of UI and should be repeated to monitor the effect of such treatment. Uroflowmetry should be used to screen for voiding abnormalities prior to invasive treatment in the elderly. If its inherent (but unknown) unreliability is taken into account, simple cystometry can be considered as a "screening test" for consideration of non-invasive low risk treatments, when a urethral or suprapubic catheter is already present for management. ICI2016 recommends however offering iUDS to all elderly with due consideration to any co-morbidity, who have not responded to management of relevant contributing factors and/or behavioral or pharmacological therapy and in whom further invasive therapy is considered.

7.1 | Urinary urgency incontinence in frail elderly patients

In non-systematic reviews it appears safe to pragmatically initiate (oral) medical treatment for OAB-S in the frail elderly.[50-52] In frail elderly women, DO is reported to be the commonest iUDS diagnosis in a large retrospective series of symptomatically referred elderly women.[53] On the other hand cautiousness is needed because OAB-s may represent ineffective emptying[54] With regard to male elderly patients, a total of 185 men who had persistent LUTS after TURP were evaluated with VUDS in one single center study and only 9% had normal function.[55]

7.2 | Stress urinary incontinence in frail male elderly patients

UI in elderly men may be the consequence of ineffective emptying and BOO, commonly referred to as overflow urinary incontinence. "Pure" SUI is almost entirely confined to patients after RRP but approximately 1% of geriatric patients suffers from post prostatectomy (TURP) SUI. The majority of SUI after RRP is caused by surgical damage and not related to the aging. However with iUDS a (secondary) reduced bladder compliance, de novo DO, and DU are commonly observed and UDS may have a role in order to establish appropriate treatment strategy.

7.3 | Evidence that performing urodynamic studies improves clinical outcomes in the geriatric population

iUDS was not able to predict the outcome of SUI surgery in older women in a single center uncontrolled cohort.[56] Regarding the diagnostic evaluation of LUTS in older men, an International Consultation on New Development in Prostate Cancer and Prostate Diseases concluded that the frequency/volume chart is recommended to exclude nocturnal polyuria when nocturia is a bothersome symptom. The use of (i)UDS and also transrectal ultrasound is especially relevant when surgery is considered.[57] DO or LUTD with or without BOO are present in patients with Parkinson's disease.[58]

7.4 | Indications for urodynamic testing in the elderly

ICI2016 recommends PVR urine measurement before management of UI, either by life style adaption, with pharmacotherapy or by SUI surgery. A consistently large PVR is a cause for caution, and careful monitoring of bladder emptying is recommended.[54,59] After intradetrusor BoNT-A injection for OAB-S, the chance of large PVR volume (greater than 150 mL) was significantly higher in the frail elderly group than in the non-frail elderly or younger patient groups[60] and ICI2016 recommends monitoring of PVR. A normal uroflowmetry pattern without much PVR probably rules out significant BOO or DU, but this finding is unusual in the elderly. Uroflowmetry (with PVR measurement) may be a useful screening tool prior to instituting therapy.[61]

After screening with uroflowmetry and PVR measurement, pressure-flow studies may be indicated in older men in whom BOO cannot be ruled out otherwise. There is weak evidence to suggest that prostatectomy may improve continence if iUDS shows BOO in Parkinson's disease patients.[62] ICI2016 concluded that there seems little point in performing surgery (prostatectomy) to alleviate the signs and LUTS if BOO is equivocal or absent.

7.5 | The urodynamic parameters important in various geriatric conditions

UDS can be of relevance to determine the most important cause of the LUTS in the elderly, where central nervous system disease is a prevalent comorbidity and where clinical signs and symptoms of LUTD are regularly more difficult to obtain or to isolate. Brain disorders such as stroke, Parkinson's disease and white matter disease affect LUT function and likely for example, the prevalence of OAB-S in the elderly population.[63]

7.5.1 | Parkinson's disease

The duration and severity of Parkinson's disease were reported not to associate with iUDS results in a prospective observational study.[64] iUDS is therefore recommended to stage the LUT dysfunction in men with Parkinson's disease with LUTD as specific (urological) treatment can improve the LUT function and quality of life.[58]

7.5.2 | Other CNS disorders

Acute urinary retention and/or voiding difficulty are frequently encountered signs of LUTD in stroke patients. The majority of stroke patients ($\pm 60\%$) had remained able to void spontaneously at rehabilitation admission. During rehabilitation this percentage increased, partially because iUDS had provided the arguments to remove the indwelling catheter. At discharge $\pm 20\%$ of the patients depended on intermittent or indwelling catheter or on condom conduit.[65]

8 | CONCLUSION

Patients that are not satisfied with their initial management on the basis of their reported signs and symptoms of urinary incontinence, as well as patients with neurological abnormalities potentially relevant for the lower urinary tract, may very likely profit from objective diagnosis and staging and grading of their dysfunction, with urodynamic testing, regardless their age, vulnerability, and/or comorbidities. This manuscript presents an executive summary of the ICI2016 committees most important recommendations for the use of urodynamic investigations for patients with urinary incontinence.

ACKNOWLEDGMENTS

Prof. Linda Cardozo; Prof. Paul Abrams; Prof. Adrian Wagg and Prof. Alan Wein have, directly and indirectly contributed to the chapter that has been the basis for this manuscript and have been inspiring and indispensable leaders for the International Consultation of Incontinence.

CONFLICTS OF INTEREST

None.

ORCID

Peter F. W. M. Rosier http://orcid.org/0000-0003-0445-4563

REFERENCES

1. Abrams, P, Cardozo, L, Wagg, A, Wein, A. Incontinence 6th Edition (2017). ICI-ICS. International Consultation on Incontinence –International Continence Society, Bristol UK, ISBN: 978–

0956960733. Committee 6: Urodynamic Testing: Chair: Rosier Peter F.W.M. p. 599–670.

2. Abrams, P, Cardozo, L, Khoury S, Wein, A. Incontinence 5th Edition (2013). International Consultation on Incontinence-European association of Urology, Paris, France, ISBN: 978-9953-493-21-3. Committee 6: Urodynamics: Chair: Rosier Peter F.W.M. p. 431–508.

3. Abrams P, Cardozo L, Fall M, et al. The standardisation of terminology in lower urinary tract function: report from the standardisation sub-committee of the International Continence Society. *Urology*. 2003;61:37–49. Review. PubMed PMID: 12559262.

4. Schäfer W, Abrams P, Liao L, et al. Good urodynamic practices: uroflowmetry, filling cystometry, and pressure-flow studies. *Neurourol Urodyn*. 2002;21:261–274. PubMed PMID: 11948720.

5. Rosier PF, Schaefer W, Lose G, et al. International Continence Society Good Urodynamic Practices and Terms 2016: Urodynamics, uroflowmetry, cystometry, and pressure-flow study. *Neurourol Urodyn*. 2017;36:1243–1260.

6. Nager CW, Brubaker L, Litman HJ, et al. A randomized trial of urodynamic testing before stress-incontinence surgery. *N Engl J Med*. 2012;366:1987–1997.

7. Zimmern, N, Albo, F. Mohr McDermott Urinary Incontinence Treatment Network (UITN) Urodynamic inter-rater reliability between local and central physician reviewers for the filling cystometogram in the streee incontinence surgical treatment efficacy trial; Abstract 16 ICS/IUGA 2004.

8. van Leijsen SA, Kluivers KB, Mol BW, et al. Value of urodynamics before stress urinary incontinence surgery: a randomized controlled trial. *Obstet Gynecol*. 2013;121:999–1008.

9. Lee KS, Choo MS, Doo CK, et al. The long term (5-years) objective TVT success rate does not depend on predictive factors at multivariate analysis: a multicentre retrospective study. *Eur Urol*. 2008;53:176–182.

10. Barnard J, van Rij S, Westenberg AM. A valsalva leak-point pressure of >100 cmH$_2$O is associated with greater success in AdVance™ sling placement for the treatment of post-prostatectomy urinary incontinence. *BJU Int*. 2014;114:34–37.

11. Rosier PF, Giarenis I, Valentini FA, Wein A, Cardozo L. Do patients with symptoms and signs of lower urinary tract dysfunction need a urodynamic diagnosis? ICI-RS. *Neurourol Urodyn*. 2013; 33:581–586.

12. Serati M, Cattoni E, Siesto G, et al. Urodynamic evaluation: can it prevent the need for surgical intervention in women with apparent pure stress urinary incontinence? *BJU Int*. 2013;112:E344–E350.

13. Serati M, Braga A, Athanasiou S, et al. Tension-free vaginal tape-Obturator for treatment of pure urodynamic stress urinary incontinence: efficacy and adverse effects at 10-year follow-up. *Eur Urol*. 2016;pii:S0302-2838(16)30527-9.

14. Porena M, Mearini E, Mearini L, Vianello A, Giannantoni A. Voiding dysfunction after radical retropubic prostatectomy: more than external urethral sphincter deficiency. *Eur Urol*. 2007;52: 38–45.

15. Huckabay C, Twiss C, Berger A, Nitti VW. A urodynamics protocol to optimally assess men with post-prostatectomy incontinence. *Neurourol Urodyn*. 2005;24:622–626.

16. Mebust W, Holtgrewe HL. Current status of transurethral prostatectomy: a review of the AUA National Cooperative Study. *World J Urol*. 1989;6:194.

17. Krambeck AE, Handa SE, Lingeman JE. Experience with more than 1,000 holmium laser prostate enucleations for benign prostatic hyperplasia. *J Urol*. 2010;183:1105–1109.

18. Dubbelman Y, Groen J, Wildhagen M, Rikken B, Bosch R. Quantification of changes in detrusor function and pressure-flow parameters after radical prostatectomy: relation to postoperative continence status and the impact of intensity of pelvic floor muscle exercises. *Neurourol Urodyn*. 2012;31:637–641.

19. Lee H, Kim KB, Lee S, et al. Urodynamic assessment of bladder and urethral function among men with lower urinary tract symptoms after radical prostatectomy: a comparison between men with and without urinary incontinence. *Korean J Urol*. 2015;56:803–810.

20. Elliott CS, Comiter CV. Maximum isometric detrusor pressure to measure bladder strength in men with postprostatectomy incontinence. *Urology*. 2012;80:1111–1115.

21. Groen J, Pannek J, Castro Diaz D, et al. Summary of European Association of Urology (EAU) Guidelines on Neuro-Urology. *Eur Urol*. 2016;69:324–333.

22. Abrams P, Cardozo L, Fall M, et al. The standardisation of terminology of lower urinary tract function: report from the Standardisation Sub-committee of the International Continence Society. *Neurourol Urodyn*. 2002;21:167–178.

23. Drake M, Apostolidis A, Emmanuel A, et al. Neurologic urinary and faecal incontinence. In: Abrams P, Cardozo L, Khoury S, et al., eds. *Incontinence*. 5th ed. Paris: ICUD-EAU; 2013:827–1000.

24. Dorsher PT, McIntosh PM. Neurogenic bladder. *Adv Urol*. 2012;2012:816274.

25. DeVivo MJ, Krause JS, Lammertse DP. Recent trends in mortality and causes of death among persons with spinal cord injury. *Arch Phys Med Rehabil*. 1999;80:1411–1419.

26. Tanaka H, Kakizaki H, Kobayashi S, Shibata T, Ameda K, Koyanagi T. The relevance of urethral resistance in children with myelodysplasia: its impact on upper urinary tract deterioration and the outcome of conservative management. *J Urol*. 1999;161:929–932.

27. Bauer SB, Nijman RJM, Drzewiecki BA, Sillen U, Hoebeke P. International children's continence society standardization report on urodynamic studies of the lower urinary tract in children. *Neurourol Urodyn*. 2015;34:640–647.

28. Spinoit AF, Decalf V, Ragolle I, et al. Urodynamic studies in children: standardized transurethral video-urodynamic evaluation. *J Ped Urol*. 2016;12:67–68.

29. Mosiello G, Gatti C, De Gennaro M, et al. Neurovesical dysfunction in children after treating pelvic neoplasms. *BJU Int*. 2003;92: 289–292.

30. Diamond DA, Bauer SB, Dinlenc C, et al. Normal urodynamics in patients with bladder exstrophy: are they achievable? *J Urol*. 1999;162:841–844. discussion 844-5.

31. Burki T, Hamid R, Duffy P, Ransley P, Wilcox D, Mushtaq I. Long-term followup of patients after redo bladder neck reconstruction for bladder exstrophy complex. *J Urol*. 2006;176:1138–1141. discussion 1141-2.

32. Gargollo PC, Borer JG, Diamond DA, et al. Prospective followup in patients after complete primary repair of bladder exstrophy. *J Urol*. 2008;180:1665–1670. discussion 1670.

33. Diamond DA, Bauer SB, Dinlenc C, et al. Normal urodynamics in patients with bladder exstrophy: are they achievable? *J Urol*. 1999;162:841–844. discussion 844-5.

34. Burki T, Hamid R, Duffy P, Ransley P, Wilcox D, Mushtaq I. Long-term followup of patients after redo bladder neck reconstruction for

bladder exstrophy complex. *J Urol.* 2006;176:1138–1141. discussion 1141-2.

35. Gargollo PC, Borer JG, Diamond DA, et al. Prospective followup in patients after complete primary repair of bladder exstrophy. *J Urol.* 2008;180:1665–1670. discussion 1670.

36. Mitchell M. Persistent ureteral dilation following valve resection, in Dialogues in Pediatric Urology. 1982;5:8–10.

37. Glassberg KI. The valve bladder syndrome: 20 years later. *J Urol.* 2001;166:1406–1414.

38. Capitanucci ML, Marciano A, Zaccara A, La Sala E, Mosiello G, De Gennaro M. Long-term bladder function followup in boys with posterior urethral valves: comparison of noninvasive vs invasive urodynamic studies. *J Urol.* 2012;188:953–957.

39. Sillen U, Bachelard M, Hansson S, Hermansson G, Jacobson B, Hjalmas K. Video cystometric recording of dilating reflux in infancy. *J Urol.* 1996;155:1711–1715.

40. Capitanucci ML, Silveri M, Mosiello G, Zaccara A, Capozza N, de Gennaro M. Prevalence of hypercontractility in male and female infants with vesico-ureteral reflux. *Eur J Pediatr Surg.* 2000;10:172–176.

41. Podesta ML, Castera R, Ruarte AC. Videourodynamic findings in young infants with severe primary reflux. *J Urol.* 2004;171:829–833. discussion 833.

42. Khoury AE, Dave S, Peralta-Del Valle MH, Braga LH, Lorenzo AJ, Bagli D. Severe bladder trabeculation obviates the need for bladder outlet procedures during augmentation cystoplasty in incontinent patients with neurogenic bladder. *BJU Int.* 2008;101:223–226.

43. Chandra M, Maddix H. Urodynamic dysfunction in infants with vesicoureteral reflux. *J Pediatr.* 2000;136:754–759.

44. Musquera Felip M, Errando Smet C, Prados Saavedra M, Arano Bertran P, Villavicencio Mavrich H. False postvoid residual volume diagnosed by videourodynamics. *Actas Urol Esp.* 2004;28:792–795.

45. Fotter R, Riccabona M. Functional disorders of the lower urinary tract in children. *Radiologe.* 2005;45:1085–1091.

46. Austin PF, Bauer SB, Bower W, et al. The standardization of terminology of lower urinary tract function in children and adolescents: update report from the standardization committee of the international children's continence society. *J Urol.* 2014;191:1863.

47. Borzyskowski M, Mundy AR. Videourodynamic assessment of diurnal urinary incontinence. *Arch Dis Child.* 1987;62:128–131.

48. Rittig N, Hagstroem S, Mahler B, et al. Outcome of a standardized approach to childhood urinary symptoms-long-term follow-up of 720 patients. *Neurourol Urodyn.* 2014;33:475–481.

49. Sehgal R, Paul P, Mohanty NK. Urodynamic evaluation in primary enuresis: an investigative and treatment outcome correlation. *J Trop Pediatr.* 2007;53:259–263.

50. Kraus SR, Bavendam T, Brake T, Griebling TL. Vulnerable elderly patients and overactive bladder syndrome. *Drugs Aging.* 2010;27:697–713.

51. Staskin DR. Overactive bladder in the elderly: a guide to pharmacological management. *Drugs Aging.* 2005;22:1013–1028.

52. Wagg AS, Cardozo L, Chapple C, et al. Overactive bladder syndrome in older people. *BJU Int.* 2007;99:502–509.

53. Valentini FA, Robain G, Marti BG, Nelson PP. Urodynamics in a community-dwelling population of females 80 years or older. Which motive? Which diagnosis? *Int Braz J Urol.* 2010;36:218–224.

54. Taylor JA, 3rd, Kuchel GA. Detrusor underactivity: clinical features and pathogenesis of an underdiagnosed geriatric condition. *J Am Geriatr Soc.* 2006;54:1920–1932. Review.

55. Kuo HC. Analysis of the pathophysiology of lower urinary tract symptoms in patients after prostatectomy. *Urol Int.* 2002;68:99–104.

56. Sevestre S, Ciofu C, Deval B, Traxer O, Amarenco G, Haab F. Results of the tension-free vaginal tape technique in the elderly. *Eur Urol.* 2003;44:128–131.

57. Abrams P, Chapple C, Khoury S, Roehrborn C, De la Rosette J, International Consultation on New Developments in Prostate Cancer and Prostate Diseases. Evaluation and treatment of lower urinary tract symptoms in older men. *J Urol.* 2013;189:S93–S101.

58. Xue P, Wang T, Zong H, Zhang Y. Urodynamic analysis and treatment of male Parkinson's disease patients with voiding dysfunction. *Chin Med J (Engl).* 2014;127:878–881.

59. Thuroff JW, Abrams P, Andersson KE, et al. EAU guidelines on urinary incontinence. *Eur Urol.* 2011;59:387–400.

60. Liao CH, Kuo HC. Increased risk of large post-void residual urine and decreased long-term success rate after intravesical onabotulinumtoxinA injection for refractory idiopathic detrusor overactivity. *J Urol.* 2013;189:1804–1810.

61. Valentini FA, Robain G, Marti BG, Nelson PP. Urodynamics in a community-dwelling population of females 80 years or older. Which motive? Which diagnosis? *Int Braz J Urol.* 2010;36:218–224.

62. Gormley EA, Griffiths DJ, McCracken PN, Harrison GM, McPhee MS. Effect of transurethral resection of the prostate on detrusor instability and urge incontinence in elderly males. *Neurourol Urodyn.* 1993;12:445–453.

63. Pizzi A, Falsini C, Martini M, Rossetti MA, Verdesca S, Tosto A. Urinary incontinence after ischemic stroke: clinical and urodynamic studies. *Neurourol Urodyn.* 2014;33:420–425.

64. Sakushima K, Yamazaki S, Fukuma S, et al. Influence of urinary urgency and other urinary disturbances on falls in Parkinson's disease. *J Neurol Sci.* 2016;360:153–157.

65. Ersoz M, Erhan B, Akkoc Y, et al. An evaluation of bladder emptying methods and the effect of demographic and clinical factors on spontaneous voiding frequency in stroke patients. *Neurol Sci.* 2013;34:729–734.

How to cite this article: Rosier PFWM, Kuo H-C, De Gennaro M, et al. International Consultation on Incontinence 2016; Executive summary: Urodynamic testing. *Neurourology and Urodynamics.* 2019;38:545–552. https://doi.org/10.1002/nau.23903

Received: 26 November 2018 | Accepted: 28 November 2018

DOI: 10.1002/nau.23909

SOUNDING BOARD

WILEY Neurourology Urodynamics ICS SUFU

United Kingdom Continence Society: Minimum standards for urodynamic studies, 2018

The Working Group of the United Kingdom Continence Society | **Paul Abrams[1]** |
Sharon Eustice[2] | **Andrew Gammie[1]** | **Christopher Harding[3]** |
Rohna Kearney[4] | **Angie Rantell[5]** | **Sheilagh Reid[6]** | **Douglas Small[7]** |
Philip Toozs-Hobson[8] | **Mark Woodward[9]**

[1] Southmead Hospital, Bristol, UK

[2] Cornwall Partnership NHS Foundation Trust, Truro, UK

[3] Freeman Hospital, Newcastle Upon Tyne, UK

[4] St Mary's Hospital, Manchester, UK

[5] King's College Hospital, London, UK

[6] Royal Hallamshire Hospital, Sheffield, UK

[7] Southern General Hospital, Glasgow, UK

[8] Birmingham Women's NHS Foundation Trust, Birmingham, UK

[9] Bristol Royal Hospital for Children, Bristol, UK

Correspondence
Paul Abrams, Bristol Urological Institute, Southmead Hospital, Bristol BS10 5NB, UK
Email: paul.abrams@bui.ac.uk

Funding information
United Kingdom Continence Society

Contents
Introduction

8 Appendices

8.1 Urodynamics antibiotics policy

8.2 Urodynamics patient leaflets for children, women, men, neurological patients, and patients after urodynamics

8.3 Bladder diary and symptom questionnaires (ICIQ-BD – International Consultation on Incontinence Questionnaire Bladder Diary; ICIQ-FLUTS – International Consultation on Incontinence Questionnaire Female Lower Urinary Tract Symptom; ICIQ-MLUTS – International Consultation on Incontinence Questionnaire Male Lower Urinary Tract Symptoms)

8.4 The urodynamics report

8.5 Skills for health competencies

8.6 Training and CPD details for urodynamics staff

8.7 Working Group Members

Organizations that have reviewed and endorsed the document:

> **International Continence Society**
> **Association for Continence Advice**
> **British Association of Paediatric Urologists**
> **British Association of Urological Nurses**
> **British Association of Urological Surgeons (BAUS)**
> **BAUS Section of Female, Neurological and Urodynamic Urology**
> **British Society of Urogynaecologists**
> **Institute of Physics and Engineering in Medicine**
> **Royal College of Nursing, Continence Forum**
> **Royal College of Obstetricians and Gynaecologists**
> **Urogynaecology Nurse Specialist Committee**

Introduction

This publication has been commissioned by the UK Continence Society to replace the Joint statement on minimum standards for urodynamic practice in the UK: Report of the urodynamic training and accreditation steering group, published in April 2009 by the UKCS. The 2009 document has been completely rewritten with the prime aim of providing information, advice, and guidance to help with best practice in urodynamic study services. It is intended for use, by the doctors, nurses, and scientists that provide urodynamic services, and as information to those who commission urodynamic services for their patients across the UK. The document may also help urodynamic services in other countries. However, readers are advised that practices may vary outside the UK.

There is considerable interest in both English versions of the document for use outside the UK, and for foreign version language versions. Therefore, those parts of the document that describe specific information related only to England, and/or the UK, *are shown in italics*.

Document Developed: October 2018
Document Review Due: October 2022

1 Aims of the report

1.1. General Aims

1.1.1 To guide urologists, gynaecologists, clinical scientists, nurses, and technicians in best practice of urodynamic studies (UDS)

1.1.2 To improve the care of patients with lower urinary tract dysfunction (LUTD) by helping to ensure that the UDS used in their assessment are of the highest possible quality

1.1.3 To provide clear minimum standards for UDS to those health care professionals with responsibilities for carrying out UDS

1.1.4 By providing a framework for best practice in the delivery of UDS, to ensure patient safety and maximize the benefits derived from these tests

1.1.5 To enable Commissioners to purchase a urodynamic service fit for purpose

1.2 Background

1.2.1 Urodynamics have developed in the UK since the early 1970s, thanks to the scientific efforts of a range of health care professionals (HCPs). These have included urologists, gynaecologists, clinical scientists, nurses, and technicians. Today in 2018, UDS are still performed by a range of HCPs, some of whom have received no formal UDS training, largely because they started urodynamic practice before there was any formal urodynamic training. However, today it is expected that all those starting to perform UDS should have received formal training and assessment

1.2.2 There are uncomfortable deficiencies in the regulation of UD services that undoubtedly harm patients. Indeed, there are currently no statutory requirements for the performance of urodynamic testing and little or no quality assurance, when compared to the essential regulations for treatment modalities from medicinal products to surgical procedures. The UK Continence Society (UKCS) believes that it is unacceptable that UDS, an invasive test and an important part of the patient pathway for many men, women and children, will, if inexpertly performed, lead to some patients being denied necessary treatment, and others being subjected to treatments they cannot, or are unlikely to, benefit from. The UKCS is the major multidisciplinary group of Health Care Professionals (HCPs), in the UK, dedicated to helping those suffering from LUTD such as urinary incontinence, and is determined to improve the care of patients. *However, even the NHS Improvements document does not outline a method by which UDS will be guaranteed to become part of a fully audited, quality controlled, clinical pathway (https://improvement.nhs.uk/ accessed 19.10. 2018).*

1.2.3 *The climate is changing, and the situation should be improved by the Improving Quality in Physiological Services (IQIPS) accreditation scheme, which will lead to increased audit activity. The GIRFT (Getting It Right First Time) initiative from the UK Department of Health, coupled with Central Commissioning offers some hope of better integration in regional networks, ensuring that patients are assessed and managed in those with appropriate expertise in those patients with complex problems.*

1.3 More detailed aims

1.3.1 The principal aims are to ensure that the patient who is referred for UDS:

1.3.1.1 Is appropriately referred, with adequate clinical information, and a statement as to how urodynamic testing would benefit the patient: "these are the question(s) I want the UDS to answer"

1.3.1.2 Receives clear and unambiguous information about the investigation, to allow fully informed consent

1.3.1.3 Has a test that is safe and of high technical quality

1.3.1.4 Has a test that is interpreted to a high clinical standard

1.3.1.5 Benefits from the information from the test which can be used by the multidis-

ciplinary team to optimize the patient's management

1.3.2 Secondary aims are to:

1.3.2.1 Provide guidance on the training and CPD requirements for all UD staff, in order to achieve technical and clinical excellence in the performance and interpretation of urodynamic testing

1.3.2.2 Provide recommended minimum standards for the performance of UDS

1.3.2.3 Provide audit standards for urodynamic units

1.3.2.4 Provide example documentation for all parts of the patient pathway

1.3.2.5 Provide the information on UDS that will guide providers by detailing the minimum standards for the UDS that they seek to provide, and commissioners to know what standards to expect when purchasing a urodynamic service.

1.3.3 Methodology

1.3.3.1 The document was developed through a consensus approach predominantly via membership of the UKCS Working Group. Any conflicts of interests were managed and agreement reached via discussion.

2 Principal indications for UDS in children, women, men and neurological patients

2.1 Background

2.1.1 The section does not seek to provide an exhaustive list that includes every possible indication, but to list those indications that include perhaps 90% of those having UDS. If the patient does not fit into these categories, then there should be a discussion between the referring clinician and the consultant urologist, consultant urogynaecologist, consultant nurse, or clinical scientist (*Band 8*) (*with skills and responsibilities as defined in 2018*) who is the Director of the Urodynamic Unit (UDU), and responsible for urodynamic services, before requesting UDS.

2.1.2 In general, urodynamics are only used if:

2.1.2.1 Lifestyle changes and drug therapy have not provided adequate improvement in the individual's quality of life, and further therapy such as surgery is being contemplated after discussion with the patient, and/or carer

2.1.2.2 There are factors that might lead to deterioration in lower urinary tract

(LUT) function with possible consequences for the upper urinary tract, particularly in children and some patients with neurogenic LUT dysfunction

2.1.3 Therefore it follows that UDS are not indicated when:

2.1.3.1 The patient has not been treated using lifestyle changes and drug therapy, when appropriate

2.1.3.2 The patient does not wish to consider surgical management after failed conservative treatment

2.1.3.3 UDS is not likely to provide information that will change the management of that patient

2.2. The most frequent indications for UDS are:

2.2.1 Children

2.2.1.1 Congenital neurological conditions, including spina bifida, and sacral agenesis

2.2.1.2 Congenital structural conditions, including posterior urethral valves, anorectal malformations, and bladder exstrophy

2.2.1.3 Dysfunctional voiding

2.2.1.4 Failed overactive bladder (OAB) treatment prior to Botulinum toxin type A (BTXA) or sacral nerve stimulation

2.2.2 Women

2.2.2.1 Prior to surgery for bothersome stress incontinence

2.2.2.2 Women with pelvic organ prolapse (POP) and urinary symptoms considering surgery and women with new onset lower urinary tract symptoms (LUTS) post pelvic floor surgery

2.2.2.3 Idiopathic voiding dysfunction/urinary retention

2.2.2.4 Failed OAB treatment prior to BTXA or sacral nerve stimulation

2.2.3 Men

2.2.3.1 Prior to possible surgery for suspected prostatic obstruction

2.2.3.2 Post-prostatectomy stress incontinence

2.2.3.3 In the younger man (eg, <45 years) with voiding symptoms/history of retention

2.2.3.4 Failed OAB treatment prior to BTXA or sacral nerve stimulation

2.2.4 Neurological patients

2.2.4.1 Congenital or acquired neurological conditions with a risk of upper tract deterioration (eg, spinal cord injured patient and spina bifida)

2.2.4.2 Significant LUTS, including incontinence, that have not responded to conservative management

3 Minimum standards for a urodynamic unit

The key features of a urodynamic unit (UDU) include:

3.1 Director of the UDU: A director should be appointed who is usually a consultant urologist specializing in functional urology or a consultant urogynaecologist. However, the Director may be a consultant nurse or clinical scientist (*Band 8*). He or she will be responsible for:

3.1.1 Determining the Scope of the UDU defined by whether the UDU has a secondary, tertiary, or specialist referral pattern

3.1.2 Integrating the UDU into the Hospital Environment

3.1.3 The UDU environment

3.1.4 Appointment of UDU staff

3.1.5 Ensuring that the necessary skill sets exist to ensure high quality UDS

3.1.6 Ensuring that urodynamic equipment is fit for purpose and maintained

3.1.7 Ensuring that Education, Training and CPD needs are met

3.1.8 Urodynamic MDT process

3.1.9 Regular UDU audits

3.2 UDU referral patterns: the patients to be investigated will depend on the type of Unit. There should not be a "drift expansion" of the type of patients seen, or the service, without transparent discussion *with the clinical and urodynamic networks and the Commissioners of clinical services*

3.2.1 Secondary care units offer a local service with basic UDS for men and/or women, without complex problems

3.2.2 Tertiary care unit offer a service that also includes video UDS, urethral function studies and ambulatory UDS for men and/or women with complex problems, from a wider geographical area

3.2.3 Specialist regional units offer the full range of UD tests to a well-defined population, such as children, or spinal cord injury patients.

3.3. Integration in the Hospital Environment:

3.3.1 Ensure that the UDU has support from the organization's Radiology, Information Technology (IT), and Medical Physics departments

3.3.2 Ensure that the UDU develops any business case development to secure funding, and purchases equipment and consumables in line with local policies

3.3.3 Ensure the security of patient sensitive data and system security in the UDU according to local policies

3.4 UDU clinical environment

3.4.1 The clinical space required will be determined by the type of UDU, the UD tests to be offered and, to some extent, by the numbers of patients to be seen. However the following need to be ensured:

3.4.1.1 Space for equipment/consumable storage, and consultation, as well as accessibility for wheelchairs/hoists etc.

3.4.1.2 Patient changing area

3.4.1.3 Toileting facilities

3.4.1.4 Waiting area with access to water for patients

3.4.1.5 Appropriate disposal facility for body fluids

3.4.1.6 Appropriate UD couch or UD chair

3.4.1.7 Maintenance of privacy and dignity

3.4.1.8 Emergency planning

3.4.2 Risk assessments should be carried out for infection control, radiation, lone worker and manual handling

3.4.3 Administrative requirements for service provision:

3.4.3.1 Patient information leaflets, ensuring the supply of up to date material

3.4.3.2 Booking of UD appointments of appropriate length

3.4.3.3 Ensuring that the number of sessions per week/month meet the service demands/workload

3.4.3.4 Adequate staffing to include contingency planning/continuity of service

3.4.3.5 Availability of chaperones

3.4.3.6 The local policy for safeguarding children should be followed

3.4.3.7 Administration, including processing of clinical notes and dictation on patients, and establishment and maintenance of a UD database

3.4.3.8 Monitoring adherence to quality control criteria such as diagnostic targets, for example, waiting times, and management of "long waiters" and those who did not attend (DNAs)

3.4.3.9 *Patients placed on an active waiting list for urodynamics should not have to wait longer than 6 weeks from referral in the UK (2018). UDS may be planned in children and neurological patients in which case*

referral to treatment (RTT) targets do not apply

3.4.3.10 Supporting the MDT pathway

3.4.3.11 Clinic coding

3.4.3.12 Management of materials/consumables

3.4.3.13 Facilitation of audit/service evaluation

3.5 UDU staffing

UDS in the UK are delivered in a variety of models, but all have the same common principles:

3.5.1 Patient safety and well-being necessitates there being two HCPs at each UDS. In general, this allows one to concentrate on the technical aspects of the test whilst the second person talks with the patient and interprets symptoms with urodynamic findings, during the test. In addition, if there is an unexpected event, such as a syncopal attack (fainting) then the patient can be properly cared for

3.5.2 All staff need to be aware of local policies including infection control, manual handling, intimate examination, and chaperoning

3.5.3 The technical aspects, can be provided by a nurse, technologist or other HCP *with a minimum grade of Band 5*, or a suitably trained doctor

3.5.4 The clinical aspects of UDS can also be provided by a nurse, clinical scientist or other HCP *with a minimum grade of Band 6* (*with skills and responsibilities as defined in 2018*), or a suitably trained doctor

3.5.5 During video UDS it may also be necessary to have radiology staff present

3.5.6 *The UD unit and staff should be certified by UKCS.*

3.6 Training and CPD for UD staff

3.6.1 The UKCS takes the view that those who have been formally trained best serve patients. Training should be based on indicative minimum numbers of UDS performed, combined with structured competence assessments which document the trainee's progress until he/she has acquired the competence needed to work independently. Assessment of competence varies with specialty *but will include a log of cases, objective structured assessments of training (OSATs), direct observations of procedure (DOPs), mini clinical examination (mini-CEX), and case-based discussions (CBDs), including analyses of traces. In addition, trainees will be expected to perform a relevant audit. Ensuring that proper training occurs is the*

good quality equipment. Table 1 lists the equipment recommended for different levels of urodynamic service. A guide to the specifications for this equipment can be found in the ICS guidelines for urodynamic equipment performance.

3.9.2 Maintenance routines and regular checks: maintenance of urodynamic equipment and checks of its proper calibration are essential, not just for patient safety but also for reliable urodynamic measurement. Responsibility for this is equally that of the UD HCPs, as well as the technical support. These checks should be planned and recorded and include:

3.9.2.1 regular check of calibration of the flowmeter (checking the accuracy of a known volume)

3.9.2.2 regular check of calibration of pressure transducers (checking eg, 0-50 cmH$_2$O is registered correctly)

3.9.2.3 computer software and hardware updates and maintenance

3.9.2.4 electrical safety tests, normally every year or two

3.9.2.5 additional technical support from Medical Physics or Clinical Engineering department, or from manufacturer, under contract if necessary

3.9.3 **Procurement:** a specification should clearly state what function is required, including the environment of use, numbers of pressure channels, accessories and software features required, the physical layout needed, electrical supply requirements, documentation and:

3.9.3.1 User training needed and the details of maintenance and service contracts necessary should be specified

3.9.3.2 Adequate data security, data backup and compatibility with IT networks are essential

3.9.3.3 Thought should also be made towards provision of replacement equipment in case of machine failure

3.9.3.4 Detailed technical and operational considerations are outlined in the "Buyers' guide for urodynamic equipment," published by the Department of Health (www.nhscep.useconnect.co.uk)

3.10 **Effective Multi Disciplinary Team (MDT) process**

3.10.1 Patients who have had UDS should be discussed in the MDT prior to invasive treatment. At present NICE has only considered MDTs in women with incontinence. The MDT should include nurses and clinical scientists performing UDS (NICE Urinary incontinence in women: management Clinical guideline [CG171] Published date: September 2013 Last updated: November 2015, Section 1.8.4). A paediatric MDT is not mandated but is generally regarded as best practice.

3.10.2 NICE stipulates that the MDT for urinary incontinence should include the following staff:

3.10.2.1 urogynaecologist

3.10.2.2 urologist with a sub-specialist interest in female urology

3.10.2.3 specialist nurse or clinical scientist

3.10.2.4 specialist physiotherapist

3.10.2.5 colorectal surgeon with a sub-specialist interest in functional bowel problems, for women with coexisting bowel problems

3.10.2.6 member of the care of the elderly team and/or occupational therapist,

TABLE 1 Recommended equipment for different urodynamic investigations

Type of service	Equipment required
Urine flow recording	Uroflowmeter Commode (female)/stand (male) Ultrasound machine for measurement of post-void residual volume
Standard UDS: Filling Cystometry and Pressure-Flow Study of Voiding	Uroflowmeter Commode (female)/stand (male) Pressure transducer mounting stand Urodynamic equipment with two pressure transducers and infusion pump, and, if required, Electromyography (EMG) recording channel
Video UDS (Additional requirements to above)	Imaging apparatus (image intensifier, fixed X-ray unit or ultrasound machine) Urodynamic equipment with video capture included.
Urethral Function Studies	Motorized withdrawal unit and pump for urethral pressure profilometry Three pressure channels required if urethral pressure is also measured while filling/voiding.
Ambulatory UDS	Ambulatory urodynamic equipment (two pressure channels, data logger, linked flowmeter, computer for data download and analysis)

for women with functional impairment

3.11 Regular audit

3.11.1 *Departments can be accredited under the Department of Health IQIPS scheme, which assesses quality in every aspect of service delivery. IQIPS accreditation is used as a mark of assurance, for instance, by the Care Quality Commission. IQIPS includes references to audit in the areas of: patient referrals, reporting to referrers, adherence to local protocol, and good practice, access to patient data, and safety.*

3.11.2 The UKCS Working Group therefore recommends regular audits on:

3.11.2.1 The appropriateness of UD referrals (*IQIPS patient referrals*)

3.11.2.2 Post UDS urinary tract infection (UTIs) (*IQIPS safety*)

3.11.2.3 Quality Control of UD traces (*IQIPS good practice*): see Table 2 , Section 5

3.11.2.4 Outcome of UDS in terms of whether the patient's symptoms were reproduced, and the defined urodynamic questions answered (*IQIPS good practice*)

3.11.2.5 Effect of UDS on clinical outcome (*IQIPS reporting to referrers and good practice*)

3.11.2.6 Patient experience/satisfaction (*IQIPS reporting to referrers and good practice*)

4 The urodynamic patient pathway

There are a number of important aspects that help to ensure that the patient has a satisfactory experience:

4.1 Patient referral: each referral must include:

4.1.1 The "Urodynamic Questions" that the referring clinician wants answered, for example, "this man has a reduced urine flow rate and has persistent bothersome LUTS and wishes to be considered for trans-urethral resection of prostate (TURP), can you confirm the presence of obstruction?" or "This woman has bothersome stress incontinence despite weight loss and a course of pelvic floor exercises and wishes to consider a surgical solution, can you confirm urodynamic stress incontinence, and no negative factors with respect to likely outcome?"

TABLE 2 Checklist for assessing quality in UD recordings

Display	Are intravesical pressure (p_{ves}), abdominal pressure (p_{abd}.) and detrusor pressure (p_{det}) and flow traces all present, scaled and labeled?
	Are infused and voided volume figures or graph displayed?
	Do the printing scales permit clear display of all trace features?
Quality Control	Are p_{ves} and p_{abd} zeroed to atmosphere (both >0 cmH$_2$O after zeroing & connection to patient)?
	Are resting p_{ves} and p_{abd} in the range 5-20 cmH$_2$O (supine), 15-40 cmH$_2$O (seated), and 30-50 cmH$_2$O (standing)?
	Is the resting p_{det} between -5 and $+5$ cmH$_2$O?
	Are live signals visible throughout the test (or after any correction) on p_{abd} and p_{ves}, but not visible on p_{det}?
	Are cough tests done: before filling, regularly during filling, before and after voiding?
	Are the smaller cough test peaks $\geq 70\%$ of the larger peaks in both p_{ves} and p_{abd} traces, or corrected if not?
	Is poor compliance seen, and if so, was the pump stopped until pressure stabilised?
	Is there abnormal steady pressure descent and was it corrected?
Flows (both pressure-flows and free flows)	Is the point of maximum flow (Q_{max}) marked or reported on all traces where flow occurs?
	Is the Q_{max} marker moved away from artefacts?
	Are voided volume, post-void residual, flow time and voiding time recorded, being corrected for any involuntary leakage during filling?
Markers	Are any involuntary detrusor contractions (DO), leaks, position changes, VLPP or stress tests marked as such?
	Is "permission to void" marked?
	Are all values at markers clear, either from the trace or the table of events?
	Are all values used in diagnosis free from artefact?

4.1.2 A summary of other important factors, including:

    4.1.2.1 Current medication for LUTD with drug dosage and length of treatment. Opinions vary as to whether patients should stop LUTD drugs before UDS, and there is no clear evidence to guide this decision. This emphasizes the importance of knowing which drugs a patient is taking at the time of UDS

    4.1.2.2 Relevant physical findings: in women, the results of a vaginal examination to exclude pelvic abnormalities, including details of any pelvic organ prolapse and oestrogenization of the vagina should be noted. However, the urodynamic HCP may be a clinical scientist who would not be expected to do a pelvic examination where appropriate: this issue needs to be resolved locally.

    4.1.2.3 Results of screening urine flow studies (UFS), with post void residual (PVR) measurement, which should be done prior to UDS in all men, and in women with voiding symptoms. Furthermore, the data from UFS are important for comparison with the flow measurements during the UD pressure-flow study (PFS)

    4.1.2.4 A statement as to whether the patient is one at high risk of getting a urinary tract infection (UTI) from the UDS. If so, then the local urodynamic antibiotic policy should be followed: see Appendix 8.1 for examples

    4.1.2.5 Indicate if an interpreter is required as it is essential that the interpreter is present at the UDS: experience shows that a telephone service is inadequate and compromises the UDS

4.1.3 Triaging referrals: referrals which fall outside the scope of the UDU should be referred elsewhere in the network, as appropriate, so that all patients are investigated by those with the necessary training and expertise. In broad terms, patients with complex problems need to be investigated in tertiary care centres with specialist consultant input. *This process is likely to become mandatory with Central Commissioning for complex cases*

4.2 Patient preparation

4.2.1 Written patient Information: it has been shown that good patient information about what he/she can expect during UDS maximizes patient satisfaction with the process. Patient information leaflets that include all the important elements can be found in Appendix 8.2

4.2.2 Bladder diary: the patient should be asked to complete a three-day diary and bring it to the UD appointment, unless a diary was recently completed. This is vital when interpreting the patient's LUTS and forms the basis for management of many patients' symptoms. It is also important in determining how full to fill the bladder during UDS. The ICIQ-Bladder Diary is the only fully validated diary that exists and is shown in Appendix 8.3

4.2.3 Symptom questionnaires: it is useful to ask the patient to complete a validated symptom questionnaire and bring this to the UD appointment. The ICIQ-FLUTS for women and the ICIQ-MLUTS for men are recommended, and are shown in Appendix 8.3. The Electronic Personal Assessment Questionnaire (EPAQ) is a commercially available package but only validated for use in women

4.2.4 Antibiotic prophylaxis should be arranged, if needed, according to the local urodynamic antibiotic policy (Appendix 8.1). Furthermore, the Working Group support the findings and recommendations of a Cochrane Systematic Review, which does not recommend the routine use of prophylactic antibiotics as there is no evidence that routine antibiotic prophylaxis reduces the incidence of UTIs or fever following UDS (Prophylactic antibiotics to reduce the risk of urinary tract infections after UDS. Foon R, Toozs-Hobson P, Latthe P. Cochrane Database of Systematic Reviews 2012, Issue 10. Art. No.: CD008224). They also recommended regular audit in every UDU to determine their incidence of UTI.

4.3 Day of the urodynamic study

  4.3.1 Safeguarding the Patient

    4.3.1.1 Staff introduce themselves wearing a clear ID, and welcome the patient (or child and their parent or responsible adult), and make sure she/he is not desperate to pass urine

    4.3.1.2 Review the referral letter with the patient/parent: confirm that the patient has received the appropriate conservative treatment/drug therapy according to guidelines and remains bothered by symptoms and wishes to have further treatment. Should there be no valid indication for UDS this should be discussed with the patient/parent and if necessary the UDS cancelled and/or the referring clinician contacted by phone

4.3.1.3 Receive and review the bladder diary, and patient completed questionnaires. Use the bladder diary and questionnaires to determine the patient's most bothersome symptoms

4.3.1.4 After review, the urodynamic clinician will decide which urodynamic tests are required to answer the urodynamic questions

4.3.1.5 Check that the patient knows what to expect during UDS

4.3.1.6 Ensure that any necessary antibiotic prophylaxis has been taken appropriately

4.3.1.7 Record verbal consent or take written consent (according to local policy) and document any risk factors

4.3.1.8 Provide an appropriate chaperone, and for a child, ensure that the local policy for safeguarding children is followed

4.3.1.9 Ensure that the clinical environment maintains the maximum possible privacy and dignity, with screens for changing, and availability of single sex changing areas/toilets in line with local policy.

4.3.2 Initial testing and physical examination

4.3.2.1 Ask the patient to empty their bladder and do a flow study, recording maximum urine flow rate (Q_{max}), volume voided (VV) and post-void residual urine volume (PVR)

4.3.2.2 Perform dipstick test on voided urine to exclude infection, and if positive follow the local Urodynamic Antibiotics Policy (Appendix 8.1)

4.3.2.3 Examine the patient: **Abdominal,** to exclude a palpable bladder after voiding and obvious masses; **Perineal** inspection for sensation, skin condition, and visible pelvic floor contraction; **Rectal** examination to assess anal tone, pelvic floor contraction and to exclude faecal loading; **In women**, if not previously examined and if trained to do so, perform vaginal examination for pelvic abnormalities and record details of any pelvic organ prolapse (POP) and oes-

trogenization of the vagina; Simple **neurological** testing of lower limbs to assess sensation, muscle strength, and reflexes, may be indicated

4.3.3 Urodynamic Studies

4.3.3.1 UDS vary in their complexity and their frequency of use. "Standard UDS" include filling cystometry and a pressure-flow study of voiding, and are applicable for the large majority of men and women coming to a UDU. The largest patient group in whom UDS is indicated are women with urinary symptoms. Men with urinary symptoms comprise the second largest group of patients referred for UDS, with significantly smaller numbers of patients with neurological disease and children undergoing this test. Video and Ambulatory UDS are indicated in much smaller sub-groups of patients

4.3.3.2 As a general rule, UDS are indicated in patients when lifestyle interventions and drug therapy have failed to alleviate bothersome symptoms, and invasive surgical treatment is being considered. In an important minority of patients, UDS are indicated if there is the possibility of the bladder being "unsafe" and there is a risk of deterioration in kidney function

4.3.3.3 UDS should be performed according to ICS Good Urodynamic Practice 2016 (see section 3.6.6.4 above), with constant communication with the patient to determine whether his/her everyday LUTS are reproduced and to correlate sensation with urodynamic findings and using the event marker on the urodynamic machine

4.3.3.4 An established methodology should be used. Currently this involves the use of water-filled catheters during pressure recording. The Working Group members have looked at the evidence for the clinical effectiveness of air-filled catheters, and do not recommend their use until there is an adequate evidence base of validation of the recordings obtained by this methodology

4.3.3.5 Perform those tests needed according to the individual patient and the clinical questions that have been asked. Tests may include urine flow study and measurement of PVR; filling cystometry; pressure-flow studies of voiding; urethral function studies; video UDS; and ambulatory UDS

4.3.4 Urodynamic report: the trace should be analyzed and the main urodynamic pressure and flow findings documented. Appendix 8.4 contains a specimen UD report. Any report should include the following:

4.3.4.1 Name of referring clinician

4.3.4.2 Patient history, including last menstrual period, pregnancy status, and allergies

4.3.4.3 UDS urinalysis result

4.3.4.4 Name and title of person performing the test

4.3.4.5 Findings on physical examination

4.3.4.6 Free flow data and any initial PVR

4.3.4.7 Catheters used including size, and the filling rate and position of patient during filling and voiding

4.3.4.8 Details of pressures recorded during both filling and voiding

4.3.4.9 LUT sensation, cystometric capacity, detrusor, and urethral function during filling

4.3.4.10 Type of any leakage seen during filling

4.3.4.11 Detrusor and urethral function during voiding

4.3.4.12 Urine flow as part of the pressure-flow study of voiding, voided volume, and PVR

4.3.4.13 The urodynamic diagnoses during filling and voiding, whether normal or abnormal

4.3.4.14 In every patient, it should be documented whether their everyday symptoms were reproduced, either fully or partly, or were not reproduced, and if the UD questions were answered

4.4 Ongoing care after UDS includes:

4.4.1 Advice to drink 500 mL – 1 litre of fluid as soon as he/she gets home, and to maintain a high fluid intake for 24 h, with aim of minimizing the chance of a UTI. It is useful to give written advice for the patient to take home: an example is given in Appendix 8.2

4.4.2 A statement as to the next step in their management

4.4.3 Patients appreciate a copy of both the urodynamic report and the letter to the referring consultant and their GP

4.4.4 Seek service users' (patients') experience where possible after UDS.

5 Urodynamic Techniques

This section sets out the skills that are required to deliver safe and effective UDS that benefit the patient by providing information, not otherwise available, to guide their future effective management. These skills are both **technical** (see section 3.7) and **clinical** (see section 3.8) and are needed to deliver an individualized test whilst assuring quality standards are met leading to the accurate, clinically relevant, interpretation of the test.

Quality of urodynamic recordings is of fundamental importance, because a poor quality study is of no use and at worst, might be interpreted wrongly and the patient's treatment misdirected. The table below gives the key measures by which quality can be assessed.

5.1 Urine flow studies and the measurement of post-void residual urine

5.1.1 Introduction: Introduction: Urine flow studies (UFS) are the simplest studies of voiding function, and it is considered mandatory to include the measurement of PVR. Patients presenting to the out-patient clinic with bothersome LUTS are usually asked to provide a urine sample for dipstick testing as a first-line basic screening assessment. This can mean that it is difficult for the patient to have an adequately filled bladder for UFS at the same clinic appointment. For this reason, many urological departments run a dedicated flow clinic. The largest group of patients undergoing UFS is men with LUTS presumed secondary to Benign Prostatic Obstruction (BPO), however this study is also an important initial investigation in females with voiding symptoms.

UFS are screening studies, without high diagnostic specificity. Their limitations are due to urine flow being a product of the propulsive forces generated by the bladder and the resistance to flow from the bladder outlet. Hence, low flow may be due to bladder outlet obstruction, or to detrusor muscle underactivity, or to a combination of the two.

5.1.2 Indications:

5.1.2.1 To screen for dysfunctional voiding in children

5.1.2.2 To screen for low flow prior to SUI surgery in women with voiding symptoms

5.1.2.3 To screen for voiding difficulties in women, including women with possible obstruction due to pelvic organ prolapse

5.1.2.4 To screen for low flow in men with LUTS possibly due to Bladder Outlet Obstruction (BOO)

5.1.3 Technical skill requirements:

5.1.3.1 To understand the principles by which uroflowmeters and ultrasound (US) scanners work

5.1.3.2 To be able to clean and maintain uroflowmeters and ultrasound machines

5.1.3.3 To be able to carry out calibration checks on the uroflowmeter

5.1.3.4 To recognize uroflowmetry trace artefacts

5.1.3.5 To understand the relevant measurements which must be made and documented to ensure complete information is acquired

5.1.4 Clinical skill requirements:

5.1.4.1 To know the indications for uroflowmetry and PVR measurement

5.1.4.2 To be able to provide clear instructions to the patient regarding the performance of the test

5.1.4.3 To understand how the uroflowmeter and ultrasound (US) machine function, and the principles of calibration

5.1.4.4 To understand the cause of, and prevent where possible, uroflowmetry trace artefacts

5.1.4.5 To try to ensure that an adequate voided volume is passed during uroflowmetry

5.1.4.6 To understand the importance of bladder diary data in interpreting the UFS

5.1.4.7 To establish whether the UFS was typical for the patient

5.1.4.8 To broadly categorize flow studies into normal, characteristic of urethral stricture, suggestive of bladder outlet obstruction or detrusor underactivity, or other abnormal pattern

5.1.4.9 To be able to issue a report detailing relevant history, any relevant physical findings, the measurements from the UFS, and the interpretation of the investigation together with any shortcomings of the individual's test, such as low voided volumes when there is no significant PVR

5.1.5 Special considerations in:

5.1.5.1 Children: often attend flow clinics with incompletely filled bladders, and pre-

scanning with the handheld bladder scanner is useful to document the bladder size before asking the child to void. If the bladder is under-filled, some degree of flexibility is then required to allow the child to drink and then undertake the study quickly if/when the child has a strong desire to void. ICCS guidelines are followed. Voided volumes should be greater than 50% of functional bladder capacity. As a general rule, the square of the maximum flow rate (Q_{max}^2) should be greater than the voided volume.

5.1.5.2 Women: in women with POP, consider reducing the prolapse to assess voiding

5.1.5.3 Men: clear instructions should be given to men prior to uroflowmetry in order to avoid potential artefacts arising from excessive movement of the urinary stream across the collecting funnel

5.1.5.4 Neurological: many neurological patients are unable to void voluntarily and therefore are unable to do UFS

5.2 Standard UDS: filling cystometry and pressure-flow studies of voiding

5.2.1 Introduction:

5.2.1.1 Standard UDS are the most frequently indicated type of UDS performed and assess both the filling and the voiding phases of the micturition cycle

5.2.1.2 The principal aims are to define detrusor and urethral function during both filling and voiding phases

5.2.1.3 The bladder is almost always filled through a urethral catheter, whilst the pressures in both the bladder and the rectum (or vagina) are measured

5.2.1.4 Standard UDS are used when simultaneous imaging of anatomy is unlikely to be relevant

5.2.2 Common indications:

5.2.2.1 In women prior to stress urinary incontinence (SUI) surgery, to confirm the diagnosis and to establish whether there are any factors that may mitigate against an optimal outcome

5.2.2.2 In women with bothersome voiding symptoms, in order to establish, if possible, the cause

5.2.2.3 In men with bothersome voiding symptoms, in order to establish the potential diagnosis of bladder outlet obstruction, particularly if LUTS persist despite non-surgical therapies, and when surgical treatment for BPO is being considered

5.2.2.4 In both men and women with persistent storage LUTS despite non-surgical therapies, most commonly for OAB when surgical treatment is being considered, such as sacral nerve stimulation or injection of botulinum toxin

5.2.2.5 Patients refractory to conservative and medical therapies but remain bothered by symptoms and who are willing to consider invasive therapy

5.2.2.6 In general, videourodynamics are the preferred UD test in children and neurological patients

5.2.3 Technical skill requirements:

5.2.3.1 To understand the principles of how the uroflowmeter, and urodynamic equipment functions, and their vulnerabilities, for example excess pressure on a pressure transducer

5.2.3.2 To be able to clean and maintain the uroflowmeter and urodynamic equipment

5.2.3.3 To be able to perform calibration checks on the uroflowmeter, the pressure transducers and the bladder filling pump

5.2.3.4 To assess the quality of the urodynamic recording during the test and to improve the quality if necessary

5.2.3.5 To recognise and know the cause of, and prevent where possible, artefacts on the UD trace

5.2.3.6 To be able to read the tracing, and analyse and record the urodynamic measurements of flow pressure and bladder capacity, in the UD report (see Appendix 8.4)

5.2.4 Clinical skill requirements:

5.2.4.1 To know the indications for standard UDS

5.2.4.2 To be able to take a detailed history from the patient

5.2.4.3 To confirm and document that the relevant physical examinations have taken place, and if competent, to carry out any examination that has not been previously recorded. If not competent to do this, to clearly state to the referring clinician, in the UD report, the examination that is still required

5.2.4.4 To be able to provide clear instructions to the patient regarding the performance of the test

5.2.4.5 To be able to pass the urodynamic catheters

5.2.4.6 To understand how the uroflowmeter, urodynamic machine, and the bladder filling pump function, and the principles of calibration for each

5.2.4.7 To recognise and know the cause of urodynamic trace artefacts

5.2.4.8 To know when and how to change the UD technique during the test, if indicated, for example, provocation testing or altering filling rate

5.2.4.9 To understand the importance of bladder diary data in interpreting the UDS

5.2.4.10 To establish whether the patient's experience of both the filling and voiding phases of their UDS was typical for them

5.2.4.11 To be able to interpret, and validate the urodynamic data from the UDS, and issue a report detailing relevant history, any relevant physical findings, and the measurements and diagnoses from the UDS, for example using the Bladder Outlet Obstruction Index and the Bladder Contractility Index in men

5.2.4.12 Interpretation of the investigation in the light of the patient's symptoms, mentioning any shortcomings or quality issues of the individual's test.

5.2.4.13 To manage any adverse reactions during the test and in the post procedure period for example, vasovagal attack

5.2.4.14 Compliance with local infection control best practice

5.2.5 Special considerations in:

5.2.5.1 Children: standard UDS are rarely performed in children. The majority undergo video UDS to allow maximum information to be obtained from the study

5.2.5.2 Women: if there is POP prolapse, reduction during urodynamics may be needed

5.2.5.3 Men: the voiding phase of the urodynamic study should be carried out with the man in his usual voiding position. For most men this is in the standing position, but this may not always be the case and the preferred voiding position should be established before the study

5.2.5.4 Neurological: standard UDS may be used when anatomical abnormalities and upper tract deterioration is unlikely, for example in multiple sclerosis, however, many do require video UDS

5.3 Urethral Function Studies

5.3.1 Introduction

5.3.1.1 Urethral function studies are not widely used. The most frequently used tests are urethral pressure profilometry (UPP) and abdominal/valsalva leak point pressure (ALPP/VLPP) measurement in patients with stress incontinence. There is no clear evidence as to which test is most useful: the principal aim is to assess urethral function during storage

5.3.1.2 Detrusor leak point pressures (DLPP) are also occasionally measured

5.3.2 Common indications:

5.3.2.1 In women, prior to surgery for recurrent or persistent bothersome stress incontinence

5.3.2.2 In women with bothersome voiding symptoms and or idiopathic urinary retention, to assess possible urethral sphincter overactivity

5.3.2.3 In women with suspected urethral relaxation incontinence

5.3.2.4 In younger men with voiding symptoms and low flow rates, who are unlikely to have prostatic obstruction, in order to identify the site of any obstruction and to assess possible urethral sphincter overactivity

5.3.2.5 In men with post-prostatectomy stress incontinence to assess the degree of urethral sphincter weakness prior to possible incontinence surgery

5.3.2.6 In men with possible BOO to assess possible BPO

5.3.2.7 In patients with poorly functioning artificial sphincters, to assess their function

5.3.2.8 In patients with neurological disease or those with poor bladder compliance whose upper urinary tracts may be at risk from high-pressure bladder filling ("unsafe bladders"). Detrusor leak point pressure (DLPP) measurement may be required

5.3.3 Technical skill requirements:

5.3.3.1 To understand the principles of urethral function studies and equipment

5.3.3.2 To be able to clean and maintain perfusion pump and withdrawal machine (profilometer)

5.3.3.3 To be able to check the calibration of the equipment

5.3.3.4 To understand different types of pressure measurement (solid state or water perfused) and their differences if more than one method is used

5.3.3.5 To be able to undertake static and dynamic UPP

5.3.3.6 To recognize and know the cause of, and prevent where possible, urethral function study artefacts

5.3.3.7 To know the standard measurements to make and to document for example, functional profile length and maximum urethral closure pressure

5.3.3.8 For fluid filled catheter UPP, to understand the relationship between withdrawal rate, infusion rate, system compliance, and the concomitant constraints

5.3.4 Clinical skill requirements:

5.3.4.1 To know the indications for urethral function studies

5.3.4.1 To understand the principles of urethral function studies

5.3.4.1 To know how the profilometer functions

5.3.4.1 To have a knowledge of the characteristic normal traces obtained in men and women

5.3.4.1 To recognize and know the cause of, and prevent where possible, urethral function study artefacts

5.3.5 Special considerations in:

5.3.5.1 Children: urethral function studies are not performed in children

5.3.5.2 Men: it is important to know the previous medical history for the male patient undergoing UPP. If radical prostate surgery has previously been undertaken then this will affect the shape of the UPP trace obtained

5.4 Video UDS (VUDS)

5.4.1 Introduction

5.4.1.1 Video UDS are performed when there is a likely patient benefit in having anatomical information during the UD test, as that information may make a difference to the decisions made for future management

5.4.1.2 The benefits of video UDS must be judged to be greater than the risks of irradiation to patients and staff, and the additional cost involved

5.4.1.3 Video UDS usually use X-ray fluoroscopic imaging although ultrasound can be used

5.4.1.4 *Units should perform in line with Ionising Radiation Medical Exposure Regulations (IRMER) regulations on safety, and follow "As Low As Reasonably Achievable" (ALARA) principles, with an appropriate audit trail*

5.4.2 Common indications:

5.4.2.1 In children with congenital neurological conditions (eg, spina bifida and sacral agenesis), congenital structural conditions (eg, posterior urethral valves, bladder exstrophy), dysfunctional voiding, and for failed OAB treatment prior to sacral nerve stimulation or BTXA

5.4.2.2 In women, prior to possible repeat surgery for recurrent or persistent bothersome stress incontinence

5.4.2.3 In women with urinary retention/incomplete emptying to provide information regarding the site of obstruction at bladder neck/mid-urethra/pelvic floor

5.4.2.4 In younger men with voiding symptoms and low flow rates, who are less likely to have prostatic obstruction, in order to identify the site of any obstruction

5.4.2.5 In men with post-prostatectomy stress incontinence prior to possible incontinence surgery

5.4.2.6 In neurological patients where the upper tract is potentially at risk, due to an "unsafe bladder," for example, in spinal cord injury and spina bifida

5.4.3 Technical skill requirements: Video UDS requires the same technical skill set needed for standard UDS (see 5.3.3 above), and in addition, staff should:

5.4.3.1 Have had the radiological training in order to use the X-ray equipment, unless this is a responsibility of radiology staff

5.4.3.2 Have an understanding of the safety issues arising from video UDS using X-ray imaging

5.4.3.3 Know when and how to obtain the necessary images

5.4.3.4 Be able to reset the UD software to allow for the increased fluid density of contrast medium

5.4.4 Clinical skill requirements: Video UDS requires the same clinical skill set needed for standard UDS (see 5.3.4 above), and in addition, staff should:

5.4.4.1 Have an understanding of the safety issues arising from video UDS using X-ray imaging

5.4.4.2 Ensure that all women under 55 have an assessment of pregnancy/breast feeding status

5.4.4.3 Know when and how to obtain the necessary images

5.4.4.4 Have a detailed knowledge of the anatomy of the pelvic region

5.4.4.5 Know how to manage a reaction to contrast media

5.4.5 Special considerations in children:

5.4.5.1 The child must be prepared for the process of urethral (and rectal) catheterisation prior to the study. If the child has neurogenic LUTD, intermittent self-catheterisation (ISC) is likely to have been established already, and the urodynamics is generally well tolerated. If the child has idiopathic LUTD, then it is likely that they will need to undertake ISC in the future. In that situation, the urology nurse specialist will need to be closely involved with the family and home/hospital visits organized to try to establish ISC. If this proves impossible, then suprapubic urodynamic lines may need to be placed under general anaesthetic 24h prior to the study.

5.4.5.2 Most children prefer to sit for the study

5.4.5.3 Distracting the child with cartoons/videos/games on iPad/tablet/phone may be useful

5.4.5.4 Bladder capacity must be considered prior to starting the study (either functional from a bladder diary, or expected using standard formulae for example, capacity (mL) = (age in years × 30) + 30)

5.4.5.5 Fill rates should be low, generally 5-10 mL/min with an absolute maximum of 10% of bladder capacity per minute

5.4.5.6 Video images should be taken regularly during the study

5.4.5.7 The voiding phase may provide limited information in children, as children with neurogenic LUTD are generally unable to empty, and children with idiopathic LUTD may be unhappy to void with the urethral catheter in situ

5.4.6 Special considerations in women: the benefits of video must be clearly established in women of reproductive age. Local policy will likely require a pregnancy test, and if positive, will prevent X-ray from being used

5.4.7 Special considerations in men:

5.4.7.1 When anatomical detail of the bladder neck and urethra are required, it may be necessary to position the male patient in the 30 degrees oblique position in order to avoid any potential artefact from the bony pelvis

5.4.7.2 During provocation for suspected stress urinary incontinence in males it is often necessary to carry out a second fill, following which the urodynamic catheters should be removed and the provocation repeated: the increase in outlet resistance, due to the presence of urodynamic catheters, can sometimes prevent the demonstration of mild urodynamic stress incontinence

5.4.8 Special considerations in neurological patients:

5.4.8.1 Health-care professionals should only undertake urodynamics on neurological patients if they understand the patient's condition, including hand function, and mobility and cognition, and the potential effects these will have on the management of the patient's bladder and bowel function. They also need to understand the potential for progression and change to make the urodynamics meaningful. Neurological patients need an individualized study according to the urodynamic questions that need to be answered

5.4.8.2 Spinal injury patients with a level of T6 or above are at risk of autonomic dysreflexia and should only undergo urodynamics in a unit that is familiar with recognising and managing this condition

5.4.8.3 Safety issues that are most important in spinal cord injured patients: higher risk of latex allergy – the UDU should have a latex free policy; attention needs to be paid to skin areas, particularly if the patient has a lack of sensation or skin breakage; assess the risk of autonomic dysreflexia – staff should know when to use prophylaxis and how to treat if it occurs

5.4.8.4 Practical issues include: mobility is often reduced and therefore the patient may need hoisting onto the UD table and positioning on the table may be difficult; recording flow in the voiding phase may not be possible, although, in men, a drainpipe may need to be used to measure leakage and collect voided urine; although most VUDS are done supine, some patients can stand

5.4.8.5 Urodynamic technique adaptations include: the bladder should be emptied if that patient would normally do so; those with a suprapubic catheter (SPC) should be filled, and pressure recorded, through the SPC; bladder filling should be done slowly, usually commencing at a rate of 20 mL/min; the rectum should be emptied if found to be loaded, as this can affect the recording of rectal (abdominal) pressure and detrusor function during voiding; and DLPP may need to be measured, and the effect that VUR may have on DLPP appreciated

5.4.8.6 If incontinence surgery is being considered, the bladder needs to be filled to the appropriate volume for that patient, and it may be necessary to obstruct the urethra to achieve this: in men this can be performed by a penile clamp, and in women urethral compression may be needed

5.5 Ambulatory UDS (AUDS)

5.5.1 Introduction

5.5.1.1 The aim of AUDS is to reproduce the patient's symptoms by allowing the patient to do those activities that cause the symptoms. During AUDS the patient can move freely and leave the UDU returning to void

5.5.1.2 Instead of artificial bladder filling, the bladder is filled naturally (physiologically) by the patient's own urine.

Therefore, the average bladder filling rate is 60-120 mL per hour (1–2 mL/min). As with other UD techniques, both bladder and rectal or vaginal pressure are recorded throughout filling and voiding phases

5.5.1.3 AUDS are performed in regional centres in a highly selected group of patients and require considerable additional time, resources, and equipment which is specifically designed for this purpose

5.5.2 Common indications:

5.5.2.1 Those patients with bothersome LUTS who have failed non-surgical treatments, but whose standard or video UDS have failed to reproduce the patient's symptoms, and therefore further treatment is being delayed whilst a clear cause for the LUTS is established

5.5.3 Technical skill requirements: Ambulatory UDS requires the same technical skill set needed for standard UDS (see 5.3.3 above), and in addition, staff should:

5.5.3.1 Understand how the AUDS equipment functions, including use of solid state, air filled or water filled catheters, including any sterilization issues

5.5.3.2 Be able to clean and maintain the AUDS equipment

5.5.3.3 Be able to check calibration of the transducers and the AUDS machine

5.5.3.4 Recognize and know the cause of, and prevent where possible, AUDS artefacts

5.5.4 Clinical skill requirements: Ambulatory UDS requires the same clinical skill set needed for standard UDS (see 5.3.4 above), and in addition, staff should:

5.5.4.1 Know the indications for ambulatory UDS.

5.5.4.2 Be able to adapt the test and the clinical environment to ensure the patient's symptoms/exacerbating conditions are recreated

5.5.4.3 Be able to download and to analyse the AUDS recording

5.5.4.4 Be able to use the urodynamic data from the AUDS, and issue a report detailing relevant history, any relevant physical findings, the measurements from the UDS, and the interpretation of the investigation together with any shortcomings of the individual's test

5.5.5 Special considerations in:

5.5.5.1 Children: although ambulatory UDS and natural bladder filling offer potential benefit in children, the equipment and expertise is only available in a very limited number of tertiary centres and as a result the technique has not been widely adopted.

6 Guidance for commissioners and providers of urodynamic services

6.1. Guidance for Providers: Section 3 provides detail in "Minimum Standards for a Urodynamic Unit" of the issues that are important and give the details which providers of UD services should include when describing the UD Services they wish to offer to patients. In the UK NHS the provider is usually a hospital.

6.2 *Guidance for Commissioners:* In England, the NHS commissioners are known as the Clinical Commissioning Group, and "purchase" urodynamic services from a hospital which is the provider. Section 3 in "Minimum Standards for a Urodynamic Unit" provides the details of the urodynamic services that the commissioners can expect from the providers of UD services.

7 General recommendations

7.1 Urodynamic studies (UDS) have become widely accepted as an essential investigation into lower urinary tract dysfunction over the last 40 years. However, there is no regulation with respect to the training of staff or assessment of quality in the performance of UDS. Hence patients are at risk from sub-standard UD assessment, and are not aware of this regrettable omission.

7.2 The UKCS considers that all UD staff should undergo formal training, and fulfill set CPD requirements in order to maintain their skills.

7.3 *The UKCS considers that all UDUs should be accredited to UKCS standards and would hope to work with NHS England to achieve this through IQIPS*

7.4 It is hoped that Central Commissioning will allow this system to be developed so that patients are investigated at the most appropriate UDU

7.5 All UDUs should have a designated suitably qualified director responsible for UD quality assurance including UD audit, staff appointment and training, and the MDT process

7.6 High quality UDS demand that the UD HCPs possess two essential skill sets, technical and clinical and these are defined for the first time.

7.7 The patient's UD pathway is defined, and integral to this is an appropriate UD referral and the systematic provision of full information to all patients

7.8 The requirements for the range of UD tests is defined, and the skill sets required to deliver a high quality UDS are listed

7.9 This report provides the details required to ensure that the Commissioners know the necessary specification of the UD services that they are purchasing, and that the providers know the criteria they must meet when offering to provide a urodynamic service.

8 Appendix

This appendix includes examples of practice and documents required in every UDU. Individual organizations may wish to develop their own versions according to the needs of their patients in general and specific patient groups, in particular, and local factors.

The documents listed can be accessed through the UKCS website www.ukcs.uk.net

8.1 Urodynamics antibiotic policies:
  8.1.1 Adult UDU Bristol Urological Institute
  8.1.2 Paediatric, Bristol Children's Hospital
8.2 Urodynamic Patient Leaflets
  8.2.1 Adults, Bristol Urological Institute
  8.2.2 Children, Bristol Children's Hospital
  8.2.3 Neurological patients, Sheffield Spinal Cord Injury Unit
  8.2.4 Women, Leaflets from Birmingham Women's Hospital, and St Mary's Hospital Manchester
  8.2.5 "After your test", Queen Elizabeth Hospital, Glasgow
8.3 Bladder Diary and Male and Female Symptom Questionnaires
  8.3.1 International Consultation on Incontinence Questionnaire – bladder diary (ICIQ-BD)
  8.3.2 International Consultation on Incontinence Questionnaire – male lower urinary tract symptoms (ICIQ-MLUTS)
  8.3.3 International Consultation on Incontinence Questionnaire – female lower urinary tract symptoms (ICIQ-FLUTS)
8.4 Urodynamic reports for men and women, Bristol Urological Institute
8.5 Skills for health competencies: www.tools.skillsforhealth.org.uk

8.6 Training and CPD details for Urodynamic Staff
  8.6.1 Adult Urology
  8.6.2 Paediatric Urology
  8.6.3 Urogynaecology
  8.6.4 Nurses
  8.6.5 Clinical scientists
  8.6.6 Clinical technologists
8.7 Working Group Members
  Abrams P Professor of Urology
  Eustice S Nurse Consultant
  Gammie A Clinical Engineer
  Harding C Consultant Urological Surgeon
  Kearney R Consultant Urogynaecologist
  Rantell A Lead Nurse Urogynaecology
  Reid S Consultant Urological Surgeon, Spinal Cord Injury Centre
  Small D Clinical Scientist
  Toozs-Hobson P Consultant Urogynaecologist
  Woodward MN Consultant Paediatric Urologist

ORCID

Paul Abrams (iD) http://orcid.org/0000-0003-2776-2200
Sharon Eustice (iD) http://orcid.org/0000-0002-1538-5594
Andrew Gammie (iD) http://orcid.org/0000-0001-5546-357X
Christopher Harding (iD) http://orcid.org/0000-0002-9407-382X
Rohna Kearney (iD) http://orcid.org/0000-0002-1489-4397
Angie Rantell (iD) http://orcid.org/0000-0002-9123-5352
Sheilagh Reid (iD) http://orcid.org/0000-0002-8050-7332
Douglas Small (iD) http://orcid.org/0000-0002-6952-2427
Philip Toozs-Hobson (iD) http://orcid.org/0000-0002-1859-9934
Mark Woodward (iD) http://orcid.org/0000-0002-9808-8842

How to cite this article: Abrams P, Eustice S, Gammie A, et al. United Kingdom Continence Society: Minimum standards for urodynamic studies, 2018. *Neurourology and Urodynamics.* 2019;38:838–856. https://doi.org/10.1002/nau.23909

NHS
Purchasing and Supply Agency

Centre for Evidence-based Purchasing

Buyers' guide

Urodynamic systems

CEP09037

December 2009

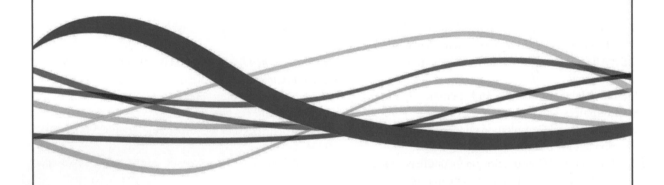

Informing procurement - Encouraging innovation

Contents

2

CEP09037: December 2009

Introduction

CEP buyers' guides are intended to provide prospective purchasers of healthcare products on the UK market with general guidance on the technical, operational, and economic considerations to be taken into account in selecting the most appropriate product where a range of similar products exists. They do not include product-specific information, which is published separately via market reviews (which contain product specifications and expert commentary) or evaluation reports (which contain additional technical and / or user evaluation data). Readers are encouraged to check CEP's web site for updates.

Scope

Urodynamics is the term used to describe the investigation of bladder and urethral function by means of pressure and flow measurements. In the UK, urodynamic investigations are performed widely and several companies produce urodynamic equipment. There have been reviews of urodynamic equipment in the UK in the past [1], but none recently, except CEP Guide 08045 of which this is an update.

This buyers' guide offers a comprehensive overview of urodynamic equipment available in the UK. It discusses the technical, operational, economic and purchasing considerations which might influence purchasing decisions, and provides comparative product specifications. Urine flow testing (uroflowmetry) is an integral part of urodynamic assessment, but 'stand-alone' flow meters, sold separately from urodynamic equipment, are beyond the scope of this guide. Ambulatory urodynamic systems and non-invasive urodynamic systems are also beyond the scope of this guide.

Urodynamic investigations

A number of different tests are included under the umbrella term of urodynamics:

- uroflowmetry (urine free flow tests)
- filling and voiding cystometry (bladder pressure and urine flow measurement, with or without X-ray imaging)
- urethral pressure measurements (by withdrawing a catheter slowly through the urethra)
- ambulatory monitoring (cystometry studies using portable equipment)

The range of urodynamic tests offered by any centre will vary according to referral patterns. A district general hospital will generally only offer flow studies and filling and voiding cystometry, whereas a regional centre receiving tertiary referrals may offer videocystometry and perhaps ambulatory monitoring in addition to the more routine tests.

Introduction

4

Clinical background

Lower urinary tract symptoms (LUTS) is the collective term for symptoms suggestive of bladder or urethral dysfunction. Symptoms include frequent urination, incontinence and difficulties in bladder emptying.

Men

In men, difficulty in voiding is the most common symptom investigated using urodynamics. The first urodynamic test performed is usually a flow study (uroflowmetry). Flow studies are commonly used in isolation to investigate voiding problems. In addition voiding cystometry (pressure/flow study) is performed to differentiate between obstruction and detrusor underactivity as a cause for voiding difficulties [2;3]. The International Continence Society (ICS) uses pressure/flow study measurements to define whether urinary flow is obstructed [4].

Women

In women, incontinence is more common than voiding difficulties. Filling and voiding cystometry, and sometimes urethral pressure monitoring, are the main urodynamic investigations.

Children and patients with complex conditions

It is often difficult to predict the underlying bladder pathology from knowledge of the disease alone, and symptoms are not always helpful when sensation may be impaired [5]. Urodynamic testing, usually by means of videocystometry, is recognised as having an important role in the management of children and adults with complex urological and neurological problems.

Development of urodynamics

Historically, the diagnosis and management of women with LUTS has been based on careful history taking and physical examination. These methods are useful but not entirely accurate; studies have demonstrated an improvement in diagnostic accuracy when urodynamic testing is used in addition to history and examination [6;7].

Developments in electronics, allowing more accurate measurement of bladder pressure, and a greater awareness of the clinical and economic benefits of a reliable diagnosis prior to surgical intervention have led to the widespread uptake of urodynamics as a clinical investigation.

The need for standardisation was recognised early, and the International Continence Society (ICS) was founded in 1971 to encourage a uniform approach to urodynamic testing.

Introduction

National guidance

A Cochrane review has considered whether treatment based on urodynamic diagnosis was more likely to be successful than treatment based on presumptive diagnosis. This review recommended that a larger definitive trial was needed, as the numbers in published randomised controlled trials were too small to draw a conclusion [8].

The National Institute for Health and Clinical Excellence (NICE) recently published guidelines on the role of urodynamics in women with incontinence [9]. Cystometry is recommended before surgery to treat incontinence if:

- there is a suspicion of bladder muscle over-activity (spontaneous bladder contractions associated with urgency),
- there has been previous surgery for stress incontinence or prolapse, or
- there are voiding difficulties.

The guidelines recommend that cystometry is not necessary before starting conservative treatment (such as pelvic floor exercises) or before surgery for the "small group of women with a clearly defined clinical diagnosis of pure stress urinary incontinence" [9].

There have been no published Cochrane reviews or NICE guidelines concerning the role of urodynamic investigations in men.

Technical considerations

Urodynamic investigations

Uroflowmetry

Urodynamic equipment includes a flow meter so that pressure/flow studies can be performed. For urine free flow study (uroflowmetry) the patient voids into a machine that measures the rate and pattern of urinary flow. There are two types of urine flow meters: spinning disc and weight transducer. In addition, the perineal electromyographic (EMG) signal within muscles is sometimes measured during voiding.

The parameters for the uroflowmetry equipment are specified by the ICS and are recommended to be in the following range: flow rate 0 to 50 ml/s, volume up to 1000 ml, maximum time constant 0.75 s, and accuracy of ± 5% full scale [10].

Filling and voiding cystometry

During filling cystometry, vesical (bladder) pressure (p_{ves}) and abdominal pressure (p_{abd}) are measured. The detrusor is the muscle that is present in the bladder wall and detrusor pressure (p_{det}) is calculated by subtracting the abdominal pressure from the vesical pressure (p_{ves}-p_{abd} = p_{det}). Abdominal pressure is recorded to allow for any changes, such as straining or talking, which might influence bladder pressure but not detrusor pressure. The calculated p_{det} thus reflects true changes in vesical / detrusor pressures caused by detrusor muscle activity

To conduct filling and voiding cystometry the bladder must first be filled actively by an infusion of normal saline or X-ray contrast medium. During filling cystometry, bladder and abdominal pressures are measured constantly using inserted catheters. After filling, voiding cystometry - also known as a pressure/flow study - is performed as the patient urinates, recording bladder and abdominal pressures together with urine flow rate. Data are analysed and pressure/flow graphs are generated to determine whether or not a patient has an obstructed (high pressure/low flow) or underactive (low pressure/low flow) void. Videocystometry will require additional computer hardware to capture X-ray images from an image intensifier. EMG recording is also an option usually available, although the requirement for it varies between departments.

The ICS recommends the use of water-filled catheters, although air-filled and microtip catheters are also acceptable, provided precaution is taken with initial setting of zero pressure levels. The recommended accuracies are: ± 1cmH$_2$O for pressure and ± 5% full scale for flow and volume. The recommended ranges for operational measurements are: 0 - 250 cmH$_2$O, 0 - 25 ml/s (with 50 ml/s option), and 1000 ml for pressure, urine flow rate and volume respectively. The rate of data acquisition should be at least 10 Hz [10].

Technical considerations

Urethral pressure profile (UPP) measurement

A special catheter is withdrawn slowly through the urethra while fluid is slowly infused through it, and urethral pressure at the catheter tip is recorded continuously. The resulting graph can give information on sphincter strength and prostate length and pressure. Machines normally use a small motorised arm (also called profilometer) to withdraw the catheter at a fixed rate. Many UK departments do not use UPPs on a regular basis.

Ambulatory monitoring

During ambulatory monitoring bladder and abdominal pressures are recorded as for cystometry, but the bladder is allowed to fill naturally and a portable recording device is used. It is particularly useful if the patient's symptoms were not reproduced (for whatever reason) during a standard urodynamic test. Ambulatory monitoring is normally carried out at specialist urodynamics centres using microtip rather than water-filled pressure measurement catheters.

Types of urodynamic systems

Portable or pole-mounted systems

These systems are designed for mobile clinic use or for easy portability within a department. They tend to use laptop computers and wireless links and occupy only a small floor area. They tend to have limited functionality as a result but are generally adequate for routine urodynamic testing.

Trolley mounted systems

The majority of equipment sold in the UK is mounted on a dedicated trolley, which often holds the pump and pressure transducers as well as the desktop computer. They can be moved around a hospital fairly easily but occupy a little more floor space than a portable system and are best kept on the trolley once assembled.

Operational considerations

8

Specifications

Transducers

Bladder and abdominal pressure can be measured with several types of pressure sensor. The ICS recommends water-filled catheters connected to an external pressure sensor, but solid state (microtip) or air-filled catheters may also be used. Water-filled systems give more reliable resting pressures but are more susceptible to movement artefacts when for instance the tube is knocked. The reverse is true for other sensor types. In all cases, it is vital for good quality urodynamic traces that appropriate calibration and measurement protocols are followed [10]. It is possible to use different types of sensor for different pressure channels. The department should be clear before purchase which method is preferred as all manufacturers offer a choice of pressure transducers.

Other types of transducers will also need to be considered. Fluid infused is usually measured by a weight transducer holding the saline bag, although in practice a carefully calibrated pump will give a measure of infused fluid accurate enough for clinical purposes. Urine flow is measured by either a weight sensor measuring rate of change of urine weight, or a spinning disc flowmeter that calculates volume from direct measures of flow. There is no clinically significant difference in the accuracy of the flowmeter types [11], so considerations may only rest on, for example, compatibility with existing equipment or cleaning requirements.

Ergonomics and physical arrangements

One of the most important considerations for the department will be the physical layout of the machine. A department that has a dedicated room will not need to move the equipment much, but one that shares space will need to consider issues such as how easy the unit is to take in and out of store, the presence of trailing wires, and whether the unit will restrict patient or staff access. A department that is either mobile or is very constrained for space will need to consider the smaller, portable models, all of which connect to laptop computers. In addition, if videocystometry is intended, it will be vital to check the range of movement of the fluoroscopy unit and how this matches the layout of the urodynamic machine and height of commode.

Another important parameter to consider is the location of the pump and volume transducer. Some machines have these rather low which hampers inspection of the drop chamber and increases difficulty of bag loading. During evaluation, staff should check the comfort of the access and ease of setting up the infusion set in the pump. The range of movement of keyboard and screen should also be noted during assessment, to ensure suitable ergonomics. If UPPs are used regularly, checks should also be made of the method used to deliver slow infusion. Roller pumps have the disadvantage of giving large pressure waves on the UPP trace, whereas machines that use compression bags wrapped around the saline have steady pressure but require careful attention to maintain the bag's inflation.

Operational considerations

Consumables

The supply of consumables should also be investigated during purchase. In addition to a standard cost comparison, the number of supply sources available should also be considered. A greater choice will give better backup if one supplier fails. The configuration of consumables can also boost efficiency. For instance, the use of combined tube, tap and pressure dome set would result in lowering stock requirements and increasing clinic speed.

Infection control

During equipment evaluations, the ease of cleaning according to department protocol between tests should be considered. Equipment that has cloth-covered or inaccessible surfaces should be shielded or modified. The MHRA recommends that water filled domes are disposed between tests to reduce the risk of cross infection [12], a practice that should be factored into the costing of consumables.

Software

While the complexity of urodynamic equipment varies between systems, it does not always correlate with clinical usefulness. There may be a tendency for the operator to rely overly on automated results [13]. Since the acceptability of many software features is essentially subjective, purchasers should assess software suitability as part of their evaluations. Listed below are particular features that should be scrutinised before purchase:

Area	Considerations
Urine flow	• Is the signal filtered, smoothed or analysed excessively before display?
UPPs	• What automatic features are available? • Are they necessary and helpful to us?
Cystometry	• What automatic analysis occurs at the end of the test? • Do we need it? • What points are taken for compliance measurements? • Are flow and pressure signals excessively processed before display? • Do volume calculations allow the user to incorporate leakage and residuals?
Calibration	• Does the department prefer calibration by their own personnel or by the supplier?
On-screen prompts and information	• Are these helpful or do they reduce clarity? • Do they improve clinic operation?
Connectivity	• Is a network connection required and if so will it affect system reliability?
Reporting	• What formats are required for patient records? • Is recalling and printing a report straightforward? • Can reports and data analyses be manually edited?
Data archiving	• Are the data storage and transfer methods compatible with IT policies and hardware?

Operational considerations

Other considerations

The specifying department should consider carefully which tests are essential for their clinical use and which tests are merely desirable, as each option will add not just cost but also complexity to the machine. The following issues were highlighted as key to the acceptability and usability of a given device:

- size and layout of the machine
- level of complexity relative to required functionality
- training programme during the early days of use
- availability of disposables (standard type or single source)
- ease of printing and post-test analysis
- personal, subjective acceptability of software interface, therefore trialling equipment prior to purchase is essential

Staff requirements and training

In order to operate a urodynamic clinic, it is necessary to have adequately trained staff. At present in the UK, there are no specific training or certification requirements for operators of urodynamic equipment. A joint statement on minimum standards for urodynamic practice in the UK was published in April 2009 by the UK Continence Society in discussion with the Royal College of Obstetricians and Gynaecologists, Royal College of Surgeons, Royal College of Nursing, British Association of Paediatric Urologists and the Chartered Society of Physiotherapy. Certificate courses are available under the auspices of the ICS and it is probable that these will be incorporated into the training requirements. All manufacturers give user training upon purchase of the equipment. The department will find additional training of value once some experience on the equipment has been gained.

Levels of staffing for a particular clinic will vary depending on the range and type of tests that are offered. For example, a centre that sees mainly patients from one specialty for standard cystometry may be nurse led, whereas a centre that offers a wide range of tests will need levels of staffing that reflect that. The use of fluoroscopy in video urodynamics will necessitate input from medical physics and radiology.

Servicing and maintenance

Service contracts, proximity for repair calls and technical staff support levels will also need to be considered. In-house biomedical or clinical engineering departments will be able to offer safety testing, regular maintenance and calibration checks. Specific training on particular equipment is not generally offered by suppliers as they have their own maintenance services available under contract, but such training is not essential for routine preventative maintenance. Detailed repair work and the purchase of parts will, of course, require supplier services. Monthly equipment calibration checks should be part of the in-house clinical routine.

Operational considerations

Setting up clinics

Clinics are most commonly run from a fixed location, such as a hospital. Not all urodynamic clinics have dedicated facilities, but this might be justified for those dealing with large numbers of patients. Mobile clinics providing more basic investigations are feasible.

Range of tests

The range of tests offered will vary depending upon local requirements and clinical expertise. For example, a particular gynaecologist or urologist might run a clinic performing standard cystometry on their own patients prior to intervention. In contrast, regional centres, where referrals are often tertiary, might choose to offer a more comprehensive range of tests, including urethral pressure profilometry and videocystometry in addition to standard cystometry.

Choice of equipment

The choice of equipment for any centre will be determined by the planned clinic location, as well as by the range of investigations that will be offered. For example, a mobile unit will require a more portable piece of equipment, even if that means giving up some functionality. A tertiary referral centre will need a piece of equipment with software capable of performing videocystometry.

All manufacturers offer a variety of options for each device, such as increased computer memory (RAM) for faster performance, extra software modules for automatic processing or reporting, backup hardware options for data storage, larger screen if required, etc. The purchasing department should consider carefully what performance features are clinical requirements in compiling the specification for potential suppliers. It should be noted that all machines currently available on the market have the option of network operation, include training packages with the supplier, and have acceptable parameter ranges for normal clinical use.

Economic considerations

Whole-life costing

The purchaser should bear in mind that the capital cost of a device is only a fraction of the total cost of running a urodynamic machine. Other costs include equipment maintenance costs, staff time costs, consumables, laundry, room cleaning and facility depreciation. For a practical comparison, some of these costs are used below to demonstrate the use of the whole-life costing method in determining the total cost of a purchase. For simplicity, inflation affecting both costs and cash value has been ignored.

If we consider the consumables used over the average seven year lifetime of a machine, assume a two-year warranty followed by a five-year service contract, but ignore facility and staff costs as these are the same for each device, the following equation can be suggested to calculate the whole life cycle cost of a urodynamic machine:

$$\text{Whole-life cost} = P + (C \times N \times 7) + (M \times 5)$$

where:

P = initial purchase cost
C = consumable cost per test
N = number of tests carried out per year
M = maintenance contract annual fee

The initial purchasing cost is based on the list price provided by a supplier, which is often given as a range of list prices. This range reflects the various hardware and software options available on a machine.

The typical cost for consumables per test is roughly the same for water-filled catheters on any machine, and is £30 (or £73 for video urodynamics). This includes the cost of a pump tube set, syringes and taps, 500ml bag of normal saline, sterile water, bladder and rectal catheters, disposable transducer domes, lignocaine and a catheter pack. For video urodynamics a more expensive contrast medium instead of saline fluid would be required. Many urodynamic systems use standard consumables available from multiple sources. As prices can vary significantly between suppliers, future price differences may be exploited. If a single supplier or proprietary consumable is used, the department should ensure there are clear benefits from choosing that route.

The average department might carry out 250 tests per year with typical duration of a test being 60 minutes with the cost per person per hour being £40 (North Bristol NHS Trust funding office).

Glossary

BUI	Bristol Urological Institute (www.bui.ac.uk)
BIME	Bath Institute of Medical Engineering (www.bime.org.uk)
Cystometry	the study of bladder pressure and volume
Detrusor	the muscle found in the bladder wall
EMG	electromyographic signal, the electrical signal within muscles
ICS	International Continence Society (www.icsoffice.org)
LUTS	lower urinary tract symptoms
MHRA	Medicines and Healthcare products Regulatory Agency
NICE	National Institute for Health and Clinical Excellence
N/A	Not Available - the data not provided by the supplier
p_{abd}	abdominal pressure, measured usually rectally or vaginally
p_{det}	detrusor pressure (= p_{ves} - p_{abd})
p_{ves}	vesical pressure, the pressure inside the bladder lumen
Pressure/flow	or voiding cystometry, the study of bladder pressure and urine flow
UPP	urethral pressure profile
Vesical	within the bladder

References

[1] Barnes DG, Ralph D, Hill PD, et al. A consumer's guide to commercially available urodynamic equipment. British Journal of Urology 1991 Aug;68(2):138-43.

[2] Abrams PH, Farrar DJ, Turner-Warwick RT, et al. The results of prostatectomy: a symptomatic and urodynamic analysis of 152 patients. Journal of Urology 1979;121(5):640-2.

[3] Abrams P. Objective evaluation of bladder outlet obstruction. British Journal of Urology 1995;76(Suppl 1):11-5.

[4] Abrams P. Bladder outlet obstruction index, bladder contractility index and bladder voiding efficiency: three simple indices to define bladder voiding function. BJU International 1999 Jul;84(1):14-5.

[5] McGuire EJ, Woodside JR, Borden TA, et al. Prognostic value of urodynamic testing in myelodysplastic patients. Journal of Urology 1981;126(2):205-9.

[6] Clarke B. The role of urodynamic assessment in the diagnosis of lower urinary tract disorders. Int Urogynecol J Pelvic Floor Dysfunct 1997;8(4):196-9.

[7] Fitzgerald MP, Brubaker L. Urinary incontinence symptom scores and urodynamic diagnoses. Neurourology and Urodynamics 2002;21(1):30-5.

[8] Glazener CMA, Lapitan MC. Urodynamic investigations for management of urinary incontinence in children and adults. 2002. Report No.: Issue 3. Art. No: CD003195.

[9] National Institute for Health and Clinical Excellence. Urinary incontinence: the management of urinary incontinence in women. 2006 Oct.

[10] Schäfer W, Abrams P, Liao LM, et al. Good Urodynamic Practices: Uroflowmetry, Filling Cystometry and Pressure-Flow Studies. Neurourology and Urodynamics 2002;21(3):261-74.

[11] Gammie et al. UKCS ASM 2007, Birmingham. 2007.

[12] Medical Devices Agency. MDA Safety notice: SN 2000(09) Pressure transducer cover (SensoNor Pressure Dome) for urodynamic system of bladder pressure measurement. 11-5-2000.
Ref Type: Generic

[13] Lewis P, Howell S, Shepherd A, et al. Computerised urodynamics: help or hindrance? Neurourology and Urodynamics 1997;16(5):508-9.

Received: 12 May 2016 | Accepted: 13 May 2016

DOI 10.1002/nau.23124

REVIEW ARTICLE

WILEY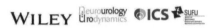

International Continence Society Good Urodynamic Practices and Terms 2016: Urodynamics, uroflowmetry, cystometry, and pressure-flow study

Peter F.W.M Rosier[1]* | Werner Schaefer[2] | Gunnar Lose[3] |
Howard B. Goldman[4] | Michael Guralnick[5] | Sharon Eustice[6] |
Tamara Dickinson[7] | Hashim Hashim[8]

[1] Department of Urology, University Medical Center Utrecht, Utrecht, The Netherlands

[2] Department of Medicine (Geriatrics), University of Pittsburgh, Pittsburgh, Pennsylvania

[3] University of Copenhagen Herlev Hospital, Herlev, Denmark

[4] Glickman Urologic and Kidney Institute Cleveland Clinic, Lerner College of Medicine, Cleveland, Ohio

[5] Medical College of Wisconsin, Milwaukee, Wisconsin

[6] Peninsula Community Health, Cornwall, UK

[7] UT Southwestern Medical Center, Dallas, Texas

[8] Bristol Urological Institute, Bristol, UK

*Correspondence
Peter F.W.M Rosier, MD, PhD, Department of Urology, University Medical Centre Utrecht, C04.236, Heidelberglaan 100 PoBox 85500, 3508GA Utrecht, The Netherlands
Email: p.f.w.m.rosier@umcutrecht.nl

Aims: The working group initiated by the ICS Standardisation Steering Committee has updated the International Continence Society Standard "Good Urodynamic Practice" published in 2002.

Methods: On the basis of the manuscript: "ICS standard to develop evidence-based standards," a new ICS Standard was developed in the period from December 2013 to December 2015. In July, a draft was posted on the ICS website for membership comments and discussed at the ICS 2015 annual meeting. The input of ICS membership was included in the final draft before ICS approval and subsequent peer review (for this journal).

Results: This evidence-based ICS-GUP2016 has newly or more precisely defined more than 30 terms and provides standards for the practice, quality control, interpretation, and reporting of urodynamics; cystometry and pressure-flow analysis. Furthermore, the working group has included recommendations for pre-testing information and for patient information and preparation. On the basis of earlier ICS standardisations and updating according to available evidence, the practice of uroflowmetry, cystometry, and pressure-flow studies are further detailed.

Conclusion: ICS-GUP2016 updates and adds on to ICS-GUP2002 to improve urodynamic testing and reporting both for individual care and scientific purposes.

KEYWORDS

clinical practice standard and quality, cystometry, incontinence, lower urinary tract dysfunction, pressure-flow study, urodynamic, uroflowmetry

1 | INTRODUCTION

The ICS Standardisation Steering Committee has initiated a working group (WG) to update the International Continence Society's Good Urodynamic Practice 2002[1] (GUP2002) with the aim of including new evidence and information on urodynamic practice and urodynamic quality control and the revised ICS standard on urodynamic equipment.[2] Following the traditional ICS Standardisation style, while including the new method and structure,[3] changes of current standards are recommended and arguments provided for making these changes.

This report provides evidence-based specific recommendations for routine clinical urodynamic testing, and includes expert consensus where evidence is lacking.

Dr. Roger Dmochowski led the peer-review process as the Associate Editor responsible for the paper

Conclusions and recommendations are highlighted in the text and can be used for summary and express reading. We define "ICS standard" as: "Best practice, based on evidence, with the use of standard terms and standard techniques, evaluated and reported clinically or scientifically, in a complete and validated manner." In individual cases and/or in research settings, the decision may be made not to adhere to this standard, but any deviation from the standard should be specified.

The ICS standard is particularly intended for evaluation of the function of the lower urinary tract (LUT) of adult persons without relevant neurological abnormalities and with intact "normal" anatomy of the LUT. Many of the recommendations in this document may, however, also be considered relevant, generalizable, or applicable for patients with neurological abnormalities, for Video-urodynamics or for urodynamics in research settings and/or also for patients with neobladders, augmented bladders, or diversions. The recommendations may also be helpful for performing urodynamics in children.[4]

2 | DEFINITIONS OF TERMS FOR URODYNAMIC TESTS

2.1 | Introduction and evidence base

Over the years, a variety of terms have been developed for the group of diagnostic tests that evaluate LUT function. The WG has constructed a table with terms and has provided their frequencies of use, both in PubMed (searching in title and abstract) and in Google (Table S1). Uroflowmetry, Post Void Residual (PVR), Cystometry, Pressure-flow study, Electro-myography (EMG), Urethral Pressure Profile, and Video urodynamics are the terms most frequently used in the scientific literature. The ICS Standardisation of Terminology of LUT Function (ST2002)[5] (re-) introduced or used many of these terms, and the AUA-SUFU has also provided definitions of some terms.[6]

2.2 | Conclusions

Many terms have been introduced in earlier standardizations, without providing a precise definition.

A significant variety of synonyms are used for urodynamic tests and studies in the scientific literature as well as in lay texts and we conclude that the use of currently existing terms is not yet without variation in scientific literature.

2.3 | Discussion

Variations in the application of terms may bias communication, in science and also in communication with patients. The following terms are not really new and many were introduced earlier, sometimes long ago.

2.4 | Recommendation

For the purpose of uniformity, particularly in research we recommend and define the following as ICS standard terms:

Urodynamics: The general term to describe all the measurements that assess the function and dysfunction of the LUT by any appropriate method. Urodynamics allows direct assessment of LUT function by the measurement of relevant physiological parameters. (GUP2002 not changed).

Invasive urodynamics: Any test that is invasive, as it involves insertion of one or more catheters or any other transducers into the bladder and/or other body cavities, or insertion of probes or needles, for example for EMG measurement.

Non-invasive urodynamics: All urodynamics done without the insertion of catheters: for example, uroflowmetry, PVR, penile compression-release test, penile cuff, urethral connector, condom catheter, or sonography.

Ambulatory urodynamics: See the applicable ICS Standard.[7] (Not further discussed in this standard.)

ICS standard urodynamics protocol (NEW): a patient undergoing collection of a clinical history (should include (a) valid symptom and bother score(s) and medication list), relevant clinical examination, (3 days) bladder diary, representative uroflowmetry with post-void residual (PVR) and a complete ICS standard urodynamic test (see below), is referred to as having had the "ICS standard urodynamics protocol (ICS-SUP)."

ICS standard urodynamic test (NEW): Uroflowmetry and PVR plus transurethral cystometry and pressure-flow study (see below): all tests are performed in the patient's preferred or most usual position: comfortably seated and/or standing, if physically possible. The patient(s) is reported as having had an ICS standard urodynamic test (ICS-SUT).

ICS supplementary urodynamic tests: ICS-SUT may be supplemented with EMG, with imaging, with continuous urethral pressure(s) and/or with urethral pressure profile measurement. Cystometry may be done via a suprapubic catheter (specify supplements).

> **Recommendation**: The WG suggests all ICS-SUT-data as a minimum, and preferably complete ICS-SUP data should be specifically reported or summarized for the total cohort of patients in all research reports that contain (invasive) urodynamic results.
>
> Furthermore, the WG suggests referring to the current manuscript when research is reported as "... according to ICS Standard Good Urodynamic Practices (ICS-GUP2016)," when complete ICS-SUT or SUP data are reported.

Uroflowmetry: A test that produces the [Citation from GUP2002]: "... flow rate of the external urinary stream as

recommends that three sensation parameters be recorded during cystometry: first sensation of filling (FSF), first desire to void (FDV) and SDV. In addition, the patient may report sensation(s) that are considered to represent "urgency" (ST2002) which can be marked specifically. These sensory parameters have been confirmed as applicable, consistent, and reproducible in healthy persons and in patients with overactive bladder (OAB) syndrome.[52–54,57,58] There is, however, conflicting data regarding the reliability and/or representativeness of bladder sensation reporting during cystometry.[55–57,59,60] The use of a visual analogue scale (VAS) to grade the level of sensation has been shown to correlate well with some of the standard sensation parameters.[61] Similarly, a keypad, allowing patients to indicate differing levels of sensation, had a good and reproducible association with filling volume.[62]

7.3.1 | Conclusions

The ST2002 expert-based recommendation for the assessment of sensations during cystometry is reasonable and applicable as is demonstrated in various study reports.

7.3.2 | Discussion

The WG has decided not to change the ICS standard in favor of the use of VAS. However, despite introduction of standard terms in 2002, few studies published have reported cystometry filling sensations and the WG feels the need to reintroduce these and to add practice recommendations. It should be noted that the WG has not evaluated the relevance of the filling sensation parameters.

FSF should, at the beginning of the cystometry, be separated from the (urethral) sensations caused by the catheterization. The explanation to the patient may be that FSF is "Tell me the moment when you perceive that your bladder is not empty anymore"; FDV is (if little or no chronic PVR exists) usually roughly associated with FVC-BD "typical voided" volumes and can be asked as "Tell me when you have the sensation that normally tells you to go to the toilet, without any hurry, at the next convenient moment." SDV is "... the moment that you, without any pain or any fear of losing urine, will not postpone the voiding; you will visit the nearest restroom also, for example, while shopping." SDV may however occur suddenly and include the fear of leaking (or actual urine loss) in specific patients and patients should report this also. Correlating the results of cystometry volume and sensations with FVC-BD may provide background information regarding day-to-day sensory findings and bladder volumes and may also limit the risk of overfilling.

Fear of leakage, pain, or other signs or symptoms during the test should be specifically marked on the urodynamic graph.

7.3.3 | Recommendations

The WG recommends marking FSF, FDV, and SDV, during cystometry as recommended by ST2002, on the basis of explicit verbal instructions and communication before and during the test specified in this GUP, and reporting the results.

7.4 | Fluid-filled external transducers and catheter system

Current ICS standard cystometry and pressure-flow study requires fluid-filled catheters with external pressure transducers to be leveled at the height of the upper edge of symphysis pubis. (GUP2002, ST2002). The urodynamic pressure is therefore the excess pressure above atmospheric pressure at the hydrostatic level of the upper edge of the symphysis pubis. Some studies that have compared fluid-filled catheters with microtip sensor catheters or air-filled catheters have shown that the results of the cystometry using these alternative systems are not interchangeable with the current ICS standard.[63–65]

7.4.1 | Conclusions

ICS standard urodynamic intravesical pressure (p_{ves}), abdominal pressure (p_{abd}) or other urodynamic pressure is the excess pressure above atmosphere at the hydrostatic level of the upper edge of the symphysis pubis. This is valid for all pressures recorded with fluid-filled lines.

The WG concludes that comparisons of micro-tip catheter systems (multicenter group averages) or air-filled catheters in vitro or in vivo (pairwise averages of two measurements) with ICS standard fluid-filled systems demonstrated that both systems give different results. The reports of these studies have concluded that systems are not interchangeable.

7.4.2 | Discussion

Fluid-filled external pressure systems referenced to the symphysis pubis are fundamentally different from the micro-tip or air-filled catheter systems, as the latter record pressure without a clear reference level. The use of ICS standard urodynamic pressures allows pressure related data to be comparable between patients and centers. Systematically obtained clinical evidence for the clinical reliability of micro-tip or air-filled catheter systems is scarce. Every urodynamic laboratory should be familiar with the potential artefacts of the specific system used for pressure measurement, and take the possibility of system- differences of up to 10 cm H_2O into account.[66] The WG considers that the availability of alternative systems has consequences for multi-center studies. Also the WG has considered generalizability of pressure values published in studies using other than fluid-filled external pressure systems is undecided.

ICS guidelines on equipment performance provide minimum system requirements for pressure responses and calibration.[2,66] Centers that utilize other pressure systems should provide reference values for their data.

7.4.3 | Recommendations

ICS standard cystometry is performed with a fluid-filled system with external transducers at the reference level of the upper edge of the symphysis pubis.

Urodynamic laboratories should ensure that the equipment, including the catheters and transducers, meet the requirements as explained in the ICS guideline on equipment performance.[2,66]

Urodynamic laboratories should check the performance of their system at regular intervals and calibrate according to manufacturer recommendation, and as advised in the ICS guideline on equipment performance.[66]

7.5 | Transurethral catheter

ICS standard invasive urodynamics is done with the thinnest possible (6–7F) transurethral double or triple lumen catheter or a suprapubic catheter on the basis of ST2002 and GUP2002.

7.5.1 | Discussion

The ICS recommendation, reiterated here above, is based on expert opinion and consensus. GUP2002 notes that the use of two separate catheters is "less convenient." However, many studies since 2002 report the use of separate filling and pressure catheters and the removal of the filling catheter for stress provocation and/or for the pressure-flow study. Reported practice includes the range from 5 to 8F for the pressure recording catheter and usually ±10F for the filling catheter. The WG has no arguments for discarding the use of double catheter systems at present but has again (after GUP2002) discussed the need to re-catheterize if the test needs to be repeated and also the necessity to interfere with the patient at the moment of SDV, just before the voiding. However, the excess cost of the double or triple lumen catheter is a disadvantage. No head to head comparisons have been performed and no new evidence has been published on the spectrum of advantages and disadvantages of two catheter technique versus the recommendations in GUP2002.

Publications applying results of invasive urodynamics sometimes report a high rate of expelled catheters and it is the WG's opinion that advice on catheter fixation, applicable for both intravesical (shown here for double lumen) and rectal catheters, will reduce that problem:

> Men (left picture): Catheter is taped in the length of the penis over the catheter, without obstructing the meatus.

> Women (right picture): Catheter is taped to the inner side of the labia or (similar in men and women) adjacent to the anus.

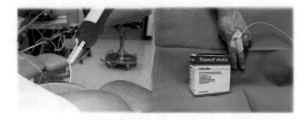

7.5.2 | Recommendation

ICS standard invasive urodynamics is done with the thinnest possible double lumen catheter. However, on the basis of the lack of evidence for inferiority of two catheter techniques, this alternative is considered acceptable.

The WG recommends finding evidence with specific studies to direct practice standardization and harmonization for the catheters used for invasive urodynamics.

The WG recommends fixation of the catheters as adjacent as possible to the anus and the urethral meatus with tape, without blocking the urinary meatus.

7.6 | Abdominal pressure catheter placement: rectal versus vaginal

Flaccid filled balloon which may be punctured or slowly perfused open end catheters in the rectal ampulla are used to measure abdominal ("perivesical") pressure (GUP2002). The WG has discussed that "slowly perfused open end" should not be used because rectal filling may cause a sensation of need to defecate and may influence the result of urodynamics, though there is no research evidence on this topic.

In a prospective, randomized trial comparing open (without balloon) vaginal versus open rectal abdominal pressure 6F catheters in women undergoing external sensor, fluid fill cystometry, the authors noted no differences in discomfort or patient acceptability, however it was reported that women declined randomization on the basis of a preference for a vaginal catheter. Set-up time, catheter events affecting signal quality (including during provocation), or alteration in patients with vaginal prolapse were also not different. The report states that despite quality control measures (catheter repositioning and flushing of air bubbles, checking signal quality during and at end of study) only 13% of graphs all had optimum quality and a significant number of catheters was lost during the tests.[67]

7.6.1 | Conclusions

Although limited evidence suggests that women may prefer vaginal reference catheter placement, the WG concludes that this is insufficient to demonstrate that this is a reliable alternative to rectal catheterization.

but advises that the term should be preferred for both genders and all ages).

ST1997 also stated that the urethral function during voiding can be overactive, without further definition or specification. There is a lack of terminology with regard to specific diagnosis of voiding dysfunction, also here the here above mentioned specific new ICS standard is needed.

The WG suggests already now: (NEW) **Normal voiding function**: flow rate (and pressure-rise) are within normal limits, begin more or less directly after permission to void and ends with an empty bladder.

Bladder outflow physical properties may vary during one course of voiding and the WG suggests that new terms are introduced when analysis methods and cut-off values or pattern descriptions are provided to describe (as introduced in ST1997) "overactive urethral function during voiding." We conclude that no commonly agreed parameter or pattern description exists to clinically quantify or qualify "(over-) active urethral function" (if) outflow properties vary during a voiding.

"Underactive detrusor" and "acontractile detrusor" are defined in ST1997 and ST2002 as different from "normal detrusor" during micturition. GUP 2002 has also introduced that contraction during micturition may vary, or may be variable. Within this context, the WG discussed that voiding may be influenced by mental state and, although evidence is lacking in the neuro–gyneco–urological literature, anxiety in the test situation for the patient may plausibly influence initiation of the voiding reflex[83–85] and consequently affect detrusor function. The WG suggests (NEW) **"Situational inability to void"** and **"Situational inability to void as usual"** when in the opinion of the person performing the test, in communication with the patient, the attempted voiding has been not representative.

The WG here introduces the term **"detrusor voiding contraction"** for any analysis of combined pressure and flow (± other variables) that qualifies or quantifies the actual observed voiding. Following on to this: **"detrusor contractility"** is now suggested for any method that aims to quantify "intrinsic" detrusor muscle properties (eg, potential-maximum-force or velocity) by any method. We refer to, for example, stop-flow or interrupted-voiding tests and mathematical (extrapolation) or graphical analysis methods of pressure, flow and/or other parameters, such as, for example, the bladder working function.

Acknowledging the GUP2002, we suggest that the terms **"unsustained contraction"** (when waxing and waning) or **"fading contraction"** may be used when analysis methods and cut-off values or pattern descriptions are provided. We also acknowledge that no parameters to clinically demarcate normal, stable, or sustained detrusor contraction are available as yet.

8.5 | Recommendations

The WG has suggested some terms with the aim of improving communication with regard to pressure-flow analysis. However, the WG strongly recommends an updated ICS standard for pressure-flow analysis to ensure optimal ICS standardization of quantitative analysis (and standardization of diagnosis) of bladder outflow function as well as of detrusor voiding contraction diagnosis and/or detrusor contractility analysis for all patient groups.

9 | TECHNICAL AND CLINICAL QUALITY CONTROL DURING INVASIVE URODYNAMICS

9.1 | Introduction and evidence base

Quality control and standardization are an important part of urodynamics. Without training and standardization of equipment, and adherence to quality control and standards of urodynamic practice has been shown to be difficult.[17] The consequence is a large inter-site variability.[18] One national board has argued that maintaining expertize requires performing at least 30 urodynamic tests a year per urodynamicist and 200 tests in a department.[19,20]

A number of recommendations for control during urodynamics has been provided in the GUP2002 and a number are renewed or added, in the recently published "ICS guidelines on urodynamic equipment performance."[2] Furthermore, an overview of common features errors and artefacts has been published.[66,86]

The WG has found no new evidence necessitating re-discussion of equipment requirements, labelling and scaling of traces in the graph and refers to earlier documents in this regard.[1,2,5,79]

Typical signal patterns, such as straining, rectal contractions, coughing and DO are important in quality control and everyone who performs or evaluates urodynamic tests should be able to recognize these during the test.[66,87,96–100] In diverse retrospective single and multicenter evaluations, it was demonstrated that the expert recognition and identification of specific patterns occurring in the urodynamic traces has required adaption or correction of the—initial—diagnoses.[19,87–100]

9.2 | Conclusions

Expert evidence confirms that prevention, recognition and management of errors and recognition of artefacts are important elements of urodynamic quality control. Systematic urodynamic quality management, including plausibility analysis, is relevant before, during and after the test as well as while reporting the results of the test.

9.3 | Discussion

The WG considers that regular calibration of pressure measurement systems should be documented in each urodynamic laboratory and that, in general, new technologies need to prove their usefulness as well as accuracy compared to existing standards before clinical application.

9.4 | Recommendations

The WG recommends that everyone performing or evaluating urodynamics should be able to recognize usual pressure patterns and be able to perform continuous quality control during the test.

The WG recommends that training and a process of continuous knowledge maintenance as the basis for performing urodynamic tests should be established.

Terms related to the cystometry observations and evaluation.

Adequate set-up of the system and continuous quality monitoring are mandatory and all patterns and features occurring during the test should be recognized. Typical patterns may lead to recognition of pathophysiology or explain the perceived dysfunction. However, when an error or an artefact is observed during the test,[59] the person performing the test should act accordingly and prevent continuation in case of an error. The WG explains here for clarity that artefacts are, like rectal activity, in analogy with, for example, scattering on ultrasound imaging, more or less unavoidable. Errors are usually preventable or correctable.

Recommended terms to describe most common features, artefacts, and errors during invasive urodynamics: A fluid-filled pressure measuring system shows patient movement and external manipulation of the catheter. This causes signals or signal patterns that should be recognized during the test and at (re-) evaluation of graphs. Prevention of fluid leaks and air bubbles in the pressure tubing system is needed (GUP2002). This already starts before beginning the test while setting up the equipment. However, the effects of fluid leaks and air in the system on the pressures should be recognized at the beginning of the test and during the test also and should be corrected (GUP2002). Furthermore, they should also be recognized and reported during post-test analysis, if recognition and correction during the procedure has failed, to prevent mis-diagnosis.[66]

Urodynamic laboratories should apply standard practice and therefore be aware of all potential features, errors, and artefacts that may occur when measuring with the fluid-filled system. Whoever is performing tests should be able to recognize artefacts and prevent, recognize, and correct errors.

The WG has listed terms here that are considered to be of use during the test and its evaluation. Many of the terms have been used in earlier ICS standardization documents, but usually not with precise definitions. While many terms refer to preventable or correctable problems, these features including artefacts should nevertheless also be recognized during evaluation after the test. The WG has opted for terms that are as descriptive as possible and is convinced that better definition and description of these errors and artefacts is a tool to improve practice. The features, patterns or events terms mentioned here should also be used in the ICS standard urodynamics report (see below).

Initial resting pressure (NEW) is the p_{ves} and the p_{abd} pressure at the beginning of the cystometry. To prevent reading measurements from a kinked catheter in an empty bladder with the catheter holes blocked with (insertion) gel and/or pushed against the bladder surface, the WG recommends (GUP2002) gentle flushing of both catheter channels and/or filling 20–30 mL of the bladder, before the initial resting intravesical pressures are considered to be "established." Initial resting pressures should be within the physiological limits specified in previous manuscripts[96,97] and GUP2002.

Dead signal (NEW): A signal that is not showing small pressure fluctuations and is not adequately responding on straining, patient movements, or coughing is reported as a dead signal.

Previously (GUP2002): "In principle, a good p_{det} signal requires only that p_{ves} and p_{abd} show the same fine structure and quality of signals before filling, during filling, and after voiding."

Pressure drift (NEW): Continuous slow fall or rise in pressure, that is physiologically inexplicable.

Poor pressure transmission (NEW): Poor pressure transmission has occurred when the cough/effort pressure peak signals on p_{ves} and p_{abd} are not nearly equal.

Note: The WG does not define a new limit for not "nearly equal."

Expelled catheter (NEW): When a catheter is expelled, this is observed as a sudden drop in either p_{ves} or p_{abd}, usually below zero.

Earlier ICS description: "If a sudden drop or increase occurs in either p_{ves} or p_{abd} signal, the usual cause is movement, blockage, or disconnection of a catheter."

Expelled catheter is usually simply visible during the test and should provoke correction or repetition of the test. However, this term should also be used in post-test evaluation.

Catheter flush (NEW): When one of the catheters is flushed during the test a steep pressure rise is observed in that pressure line for one or two seconds followed by an immediate fall to resting pressure.

A catheter flush is not always necessary after a carefully performed set-up but is suggested in GUP2002.

REFERENCES

1. Schäfer W, Abrams P, Liao L, et al. International Continence Society. Good urodynamic practices: uroflowmetry, filling cystometry, and pressure-flow studies. *Neurourol Urodyn.* 2002;21:261–274.

2. Gammie A, Clarkson B, Constantinou C, et al. International continence society guidelines on urodynamic equipment performance. *Neurourol Urodyn.* 2014;33:370–379.

3. Rosier PF, de Ridder D, Meijlink J, Webb R, Whitmore K, Drake MJ. Developing evidence-based standards for diagnosis and management of lower urinary tract or pelvic floor dysfunction. *Neurourol Urodyn.* 2012;31:621–624.

4. Bauer SB, Nijman RJ, Drzewiecki BA, Sillen U, Hoebeke P. International Children's Continence Society standardization report on urodynamic studies of the lower urinary tract in children. *Neurourol Urodyn.* 2015;34:640–647.

5. Abrams P, Cardozo L, Fall M, et al. Standardisation sub-mommittee of the International Continence Society. The standardisation of terminology in lower urinary tract function: report from the standardisation sub-committee of the International Continence Society. *Urology.* 2003;61: 37–49.

6. Winters JC, Dmochowski RR, Goldman HB, et al. American Urological Association; Society of Urodynamics Female Pelvic Medicine & Urogenital Reconstruction. Urodynamic studies in adults: AUA/SUFU guideline. *J Urol.* 2012;188: 2464–2472.

7. van Waalwijk van Doorn E, Anders K, Khullar V, et al. Standardisation of ambulatory urodynamic monitoring: report of the sandardisation sub-committee of the International Continence Society for Ambulatory Urodynamic Studies. *Neurourol Urodyn.* 2000;19:113–125.

8. Lose G, Griffiths D, Hosker G, et al. Standardisation of urethral pressure measurement: report from the standardisation sub-committee of the International Continence Society. *Neurourol Urodyn.* 2002;21:258–260.

9. Yiou R, Audureau E, Loche CM, Dussaud M, Lingombet O, Binhas M. Comprehensive evaluation of embarrassment and pain associated with invasive urodynamics. *Neurourol Urodyn.* 2015;34:156–160.

10. Yeung JY, Eschenbacher MA, Pauls RN. Pain and embarrassment associated with urodynamic testing in women. *Int Urogynecol J.* 2014;25:645–650.

11. Scarpero HM, Padmanabhan P, Xue X, Nitti VW. Patient perception of videourodynamic testing: a questionnaire based study. *J Urol.* 2005;173:555–559.

12. Hadjipavlou M, Khan S, Rane A. Readability of patient information leaflets for urological conditions and treatments. *J Clin Urol.* 2013;6:302.

13. Garner M, Ning Z, Francis J. A framework for the evaluation of patient information leaflets. *Health Expect.* 2012;15:283–294.

14. Bright E, Parsons BA, Swithinbank L. Increased patient information does not reduce patient anxiety regarding urodynamic studies. *Urol Int.* 2011;87:314–318.

15. Hougardy V, Vandeweerd JM, Reda AA, Foidart JM. The impact of detailed explanatory leaflets on patient satisfaction with urodynamic consultation: a double-blind randomized controlled trial. *Neurourol Urodyn.* 2009;28:374–379.

16. Smith AL, Nissim HA, Le TX, et al. Misconceptions and miscommunication among aging women with overactive bladder symptoms. *Urology.* 2011;77:55–59.

17. Singh G, Lucas M, Dolan L, Knight S, Ramage C, Hobson PT. Minimum standards for urodynamic practice in the UK. United Kingdom Continence Society. 3. *Neurourol Urodyn.* 2010;29: 1365–1372.

18. Moore KC, Emery SJ, Lucas MG. Quality and quantity: an audit of urodynamics practice in relation to newly published National Standards. *Neurourol Urodyn.* 2011;30:38–42.

19. Sullivan J, Lewis P, Howell S, Williams T, Shepherd AM, Abrams P. Quality control in urodynamics: a review of urodynamic traces from one centre. *BJU Int.* 2003;91:201–207.

20. Sriram R, (1), Ojha H, Farrar DJ. An audit of urodynamic standardization in the West Midlands, UK. *BJU Int.* 2002;90:537–539. Comment in BJU Int. 2003 Mar;91(4):430. An audit of urodynamic standardization in the West Midlands, UK. Sullivan J, Swithinbank L, Abrams P. 2. *BJU Int.* 2003;91: 430.

21. Peters DH, Adam T, Alonge O, Agyepong IA, Tran N. Implementation research: what it is and how to do it. *BMJ.* 2013;347:f6753.

22. Brouwers MC, Kho ME, Browman GP, et al. AGREE Next Steps Consortium. AGREE II: advancing guideline development, reporting and evaluation in health care. *CMAJ.* 2010;182: E839–E842.

23. Curran GM, Bauer M, Mittman B, Pyne JM, Stetler C. Effectiveness-implementation hybrid designs: combining elements of clinical effectiveness and implementation research to enhance public health impact. *Med Care.* 2012;50:217–226.

24. Winters JC, Dmochowski RR, Goldman HB, et al. American Urological Association Society of Urodynamics Female Pelvic Medicine Urogenital Reconstruction. Urodynamic studies in adults: AUA/SUFU guideline. *J Urol.* 2012;188: 2464–2472.

25. McNanley AR, Duecy EE, Buchsbaum GM. Symptom-based, clinical, and urodynamic diagnoses of urinary incontinence: how well do they correlate in postmenopausal women? *Female Pelvic Med Reconstr Surg.* 2010;16:97–101.

26. Lenherr SM, Clemens JQ. Urodynamics: with a focus on appropriate indications. *Urol Clin North Am.* 2013;40:545–557.

27. Lucas MG, Bosch RJ, Burkhard FC, et al. European Association of Urology. EAU guidelines on assessment and nonsurgical management of urinary incontinence. *Eur Urol.* 2012;62: 1130–1142.

28. Rosier P.F.W.M., Kuo H-C, De Gennaro M, et al.: Urodynamic testing, Chapter 6. In Incontinence. Ed: Abrams P, Cardozo L, Khoury S, Wein A. 5th Edition. 2013. International Consultation on Urologic Disease. 5th International Consultation on Incontinence; Recommendations of the International Scientific Committee: Evaluation and Treatment of Urinary Incontinence, Pelvic Organ Prolapse and Faecal Incontinence. Abrams et al In Incontinence. Abrams P Cardozo L Khoury S and Wein A, eds. Paris: ICUD-EAU2013 (ISBN 978-9953-493-21-3); 2013:1895–1955.

29. Haylen BT, de Ridder D, Freeman RM, et al. International Urogynecological Association; International Continence Society. An International Urogynecological Association (IUGA)/International Continence Society (ICS) joint report on the terminology for female pelvic floor dysfunction. *Neurourol Urodyn.* 2010;29:4–20.

30. Messelink B, Benson T, Berghmans B, et al. Standardization of terminology of pelvic floor muscle function and dysfunction: report from the pelvic floor clinical assessment group of the International Continence Society. *Neurourol Urodyn.* 2005;24: 374–380.

31. Grino PB, Bruskewitz R, Blaivas JG, et al. Maximum urinary flow rate by uroflowmetry: automatic or visual interpretation. *J Urol.* 1993;149:339–341.

32. Choudhury S, Agarwal MM, Mandal AK, et al. Which voiding position is associated with lowest flow rates in healthy adult men? Role of natural voiding position. *Neurourol Urodyn.* 2010;29:413–417.

33. El-Bahnasawy MS, Fadl FA. Uroflowmetric differences between standing and sitting positions for men used to void in the sitting position. *Urology.* 2008;71:465–468.

34. Aghamir SM, Mohseni M, Arasteh S. The effect of voiding position on uroflowmetry findings of healthy men and patients with benign prostatic hyperplasia. *Urol J.* 2005;2:216–221.

35. Amjadi M, Madaen SK, Pour-Moazen H. Uroflowmetry findings in patients with bladder outlet obstruction symptoms in standing and crouching positions. *Urol J.* 2006;3:49–53.

36. Eryildirim B, Tarhan F, Kuyumcuoğlu U, Erbay E, Pembegül N. Position-related changes in uroflowmetric parameters in healthy young men. *Neurourol Urodyn.* 2006;25:249–251.

37. Unsal A, Cimentepe E. Voiding position does not affect uroflowmetric parameters and post-void residual urine volume in healthy volunteers. *Scand J Urol Nephrol.* 2004;38: 469–471.

38. Unsal A, Cimentepe E. Effect of voiding position on uroflowmetric parameters and post-void residual urine volume in patients with benign prostatic hyperplasia. *Scand J Urol Nephrol.* 2004;38:240–242.

39. Yamanishi T, Yasuda K, Sakakibara R, et al. Variation in urinary flow according to voiding position in normal males. *Neurourol Urodyn.* 1999;18:553–557.

40. Riehmann M, Bayer WH, Drinka PJ, et al. Position-related changes in voiding dynamics in men. *Urology.* 1998;52:625–630.

41. Moore KH, Richmond DH, Sutherst JR, Imrie AH, Hutton JL. Crouching over the toilet seat: prevalence among British gynaecological outpatients and its effect upon micturition. *Br J Obstet Gynaecol.* 1991;98:569–572.

42. Devreese AM, Nuyens G, Staes F, Vereecken RL, De Weerdt W, Stappaerts K. Do posture and straining influence urinary-flow parameters in normal women? *Neurourol Urodyn.* 2000;19:3–8.

43. Gupta NP, Kumar A, Kumar R. Does position affect uroflowmetry parameters in women? *Urol Int.* 2008;80:37–40.

44. Yang KN, Chen SC, Chen SY, Chang CH, Wu HC, Chou EC. Female voiding postures and their effects on micturition. *Int Urogynecol J.* 2010;21:1371–1376.

45. Rane A, Corstiaans A. Does leaning forward improve micturition? *J Obstet Gynaecol.* 2000;20:628–629.

46. Rane A, Corstiaans A. Does micturition improve in the squatting position? *J Obstet Gynaecol.* 2008;28:317–319.

47. Sonke GS, Kiemeney LA, Verbeek AL, Kortmann BB, Debruyne FM, de la Rosette JJ. Low reproducibility of maximum urinary flow rate determined by portable flowmetry. *Neurourol Urodyn.* 1999;18:183–191.

48. Robertson AS, Griffiths CJ, Ramsden PD, Neal DE. Bladder function in healthy volunteers: ambulatory monitoring and conventional urodynamic studies. *Br J Urol.* 1994;73: 242–249.

49. Ko HY, Lee JZ, Park HJ, Kim H, Park JH. Comparison between conventional cystometry and stimulated filling cystometry by diuretics in a neurogenic bladder after spinal cord injury. *Am J Phys Med Rehabil.* 2002;81:731–735.

50. Heesakkers JP, Vandoninck V, van Balken MR, Bemelmans BL. Bladder filling by autologous urine production during cystometry: a urodynamic pitfall! *Neurourol Urodyn.* 2003; 22:243–245.

51. Lee SW, Kim JH. The significance of natural bladder filling by the production of urine during cystometry. *Neurourol Urodyn.* 2008;27:772–774.

52. Bradley WE, Timm GW, Scott FB. Cystometry. V. Bladder sensation. *Urology.* 1975;6:654–658.

53. Nathan PW. Sensations associated with micturition. *Br J Urol.* 1956;28:126.

54. Erdem E, Akbay E, Doruk E, Cayan S, Acar D, Ulusoy E. How reliable are bladder perceptions during cystometry? *Neurourol Urodyn.* 2004;23:306–309.

55. Erdem E, Tunçkiran A, Acar D, Kanik EA, Akbay E, Ulusoy E. Is catheter cause of subjectivity in sensations perceived during filling cystometry? *Urology.* 2005;66:1000–1003.

56. De Wachter S, Wyndaele JJ. Frequency-volume charts: a tool to evaluate bladder sensation. *Neurourol Urodyn.* 2003;22: 638–642.

57. De Wachter S, Van Meel TD, Wyndaele JJ. Can a faked cystometry deceive patients in their perception of filling sensations? A study on the reliability of spontaneously reported cystometric filling sensations in patients with non-neurogenic lower urinary tract dysfunction. *Neurourol Urodyn.* 2008;27:395–398.

58. Naoemova I, Van Meel T, De Wachter S, Wyndaele JJ. Does sensory bladder function during cystometry differ from that in daily life? A study in incontinent women. *Neurourol Urodyn.* 2009;28:309–312.

59. Van Meel TD, Wyndaele JJ. Reproducibility of urodynamic filling sensation at weekly interval in healthy volunteers and in women with detrusor overactivity. *Neurourol Urodyn.* 2011;30:1586–1590.

60. Dmochowski RR, FitzGerald MP, Wyndaele JJ. Measuring urgency in clinical practice. *World J Urol.* 2009;27:739–45.

61. Dompeyre P, Fritel X, Bader G, Delmas V, Fauconnier A. Bladder sensitivity testing using a visual analogue scale: comparative cystometric study on women. *Neurourol Urodyn.* 2007;26: 350–355.

Neurourology and Urodynamics 21:261–274 (2002)

Good Urodynamic Practices: Uroflowmetry, Filling Cystometry, and Pressure-Flow Studies

Werner Schäfer,* Paul Abrams, Limin Liao, Anders Mattiasson, Francesco Pesce, Anders Spangberg, Arthur M. Sterling, Norman R. Zinner, and Philip van Kerrebroeck

International Continence Society Office, Southme Hospital, Bristol, BSIO 5NB, United Kingdom

This is the first report of the International Continence Society (ICS) on the development of comprehensive guidelines for Good Urodynamic Practice for the measurement, quality control, and documentation of urodynamic investigations in both clinical and research environments. This report focuses on the most common urodynamics examinations; uroflowmetry, pressure recording during filling cystometry, and combined pressure–flow studies. The basic aspects of good urodynamic practice are discussed and a strategy for urodynamic measurement, equipment set-up and configuration, signal testing, plausibility controls, pattern recognition, and artifact correction are proposed. The problems of data analysis are mentioned only when they are relevant in the judgment of data quality. In general, recommendations are made for one specific technique. This does not imply that this technique is the only one possible. Rather, it means that this technique is well-established, and gives good results when used with the suggested standards of good urodynamic practice. *Neurourol. Urodynam. 21:261–274, 2002.* © 2002 Wiley-Liss, Inc.

Key words: urodynamics; standardisation; uroflowmetry; cystometry; pressure-flow studies

INTRODUCTION

A Good Urodynamic Practice comprises three main elements:

- A clear indication for and appropriate selection of, relevant test measurements and procedures
- Precise measurement with data quality control and complete documentation
- Accurate analysis and critical reporting of results

The aim of clinical urodynamics is to reproduce symptoms whilst making precise measurements in order to identify the underlying causes for the symptoms, and to quantify the related pathophysiological processes. By doing so, it should be possible to establish objectively the presence of a dysfunction and understand its clinical implications. Thus, we may either confirm a diagnosis or give a new, specifically urodynamic, diagnosis. The quantitative measurement may be supplemented by imaging (videourodynamics).

Urodynamic measurements cannot yet be completely automated, except for the most simple urodynamic procedure, uroflowmetry. This is not an inherent problem of the measurement itself, but is due to the current limitations of urodynamic equipment and the lack of a consensus on the precise method of measurement, signal processing, quantification, documentation, and interpretation. With the publication of this ICS Standardisation document on good urodynamic practice, it

is expected that the necessary technological developments in automation will follow.

Urodynamics allows direct assessment of lower urinary tract (LUT) function by the measurement of relevant physiological parameters. The first step is to formulate the 'urodynamic question or questions' from a careful history, physical examination, and standard urological investigations. The patient's recordings of micturitions and symptoms on a frequency volume chart, and repeated free uroflowmetry with determination of post-void residual volume provide important

---

Urodynamic techniques were performed according to the 'Good Urodynamic Practice' recommended by the International Continence Society.

This report is from the Standardization Committee of the International Continence Society.

*Correspondence to: Werner Schäfer, International Continence Society Office, Southme Hospital, Bristol, BSIO 5NB, United Kingdom. E-mail: Vicky@icsoffice.org

DOI 10.1002/nau.10066

Published online in Wiley InterScience (www.interscience.wiley.com).

262   Schäfer et al.

noninvasive, objective information that helps to define the specific 'urodynamic question' or questions, prior to invasive urodynamics such as filling cystometry and pressure-flow studies.

Recommendations for good urodynamic practice are bullet pointed, inset, and printed in bold.

RECORDING MICTURITIONS AND SYMPTOMS

A *Micturition Time Chart* records the time of each micturition. The usefulness of such a record is significantly enhanced when the voided volumes are recorded in a *Frequency Volume Chart*. The *Bladder Diary* adds to this the relevant symptoms and events such as urgency, pain, incontinence episodes, and pad usage. Recording for a minimum of 2 days is recommended. From the recordings, the average voided volume, voiding frequency, and if, the patient's time in bed is recorded, day/night urine production and nocturia can be determined. This information provides objective verification of the patient's symptoms, and furthermore, key values for plausibility control of subsequent urodynamic studies, for example, in order to prevent over-filling of the patient's bladder.

UROFLOWMETRY

Uroflowmetry is noninvasive and relatively inexpensive. Therefore, it is an indispensable, first-line screening test for most patients with suspected LUT dysfunction. Objective and quantitative information, which helps one to understand both storage and voiding symptoms are provided by this simple urodynamic measurement.

Adequate privacy should be provided and patients should be asked to void when they feel a "normal" desire to void. Patients should be asked if their voiding was representative of their usual voiding and their view should be documented. Automated data analysis must be verified by inspection of the flow curve, artifacts must be excluded, and verification must be documented. The results from uroflowmetry should be compared with the data from the patient's own recording on a frequency/volume chart. Sonographic estimation of postvoid residual volume completes the noninvasive assessment of voiding function.

Normal Uroflow

Normal voiding occurs when the bladder outlet relaxes (is passive) and the detrusor contracts (is active). An easily distensible bladder outlet with a normal detrusor contraction results in a smooth arc-shaped flow rate curve with high amplitude. Any other shapes, such as curves that are flat, asymmetric, or have multiple peaks (fluctuating and/or intermittent), indicate abnormal voiding, but are not specific for it's cause.

It is assumed that it is normal for the mechanical properties of a relaxed outlet to be constant, and that the properties can be defined by the dependency of the cross-sectional area of the

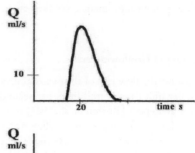

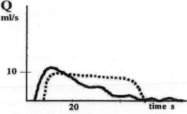

Fig. 1. Typical normal flow (**top**), constrictive flow (**bottom**, dotted line), compressive flow curve (bottom).

urethral lumen on the intraurethral pressure at the flow rate controlling zone (FRCZ). Typically, below the minimum urethral opening pressure (pmuo), the urethral lumen is closed. The lumen then opens widely with little additional pressure increase. With normal detrusor contractility and low intraurethral pressure, the normal flow curve is arc-shaped with a high maximum flowrate. (Fig. 1, top).

A normal flow curve is a smooth curve without any rapid changes in amplitude, because the shape of the flow curve is determined by the kinetics of the detrusor contraction, which arising from smooth muscle, does not show rapid variations. A decreased detrusor power and/or a constant increased urethral pressure will both result in a lower flowrate and a smooth flat flow curve. A constrictive obstruction (e.g., urethral stricture), with reduced lumen size results in a plateaulike flow curve. (Fig. 1, broken line).

A compressive obstruction with increased urethral opening pressure (e.g., benign prostatic obstruction) shows a flattened asymmetric flow curve with a slowly declining end part. (Fig. 1, bottom).

The same pattern may also originate from a weak detrusor in aging males and females. Fluctuations in detrusor contractility or abdominal straining, as well as variable outlet conditions, (e.g., intermittent sphincter activity) will lead to complex flow rate patterns.

Rapid changes in flowrate may have physiological or physical causes that owe to either changes in outlet resistance, for example, sphincter/pelvic floor contraction or relaxation, mechanical compression of the urethral lumen, or interference at the meatus, or to changes in driving energy, for example, abdominal straining. These intracorporeal causes lead to true flowrate changes. Rapid changes in flowrate may also be artifacts, when the flowrate signal is extracorporeally modified through interference between the stream and the collecting funnel, the flowmeter, movement of the stream across the surface of the funnel, or patient movements. (see flow-curves in Figs. 3–8).

Accuracy of Uroflowmeters

Uroflowmetry measures the flow rate of the external urinary stream as volume per unit time in milliliters per second, (ml/s). The ICS Technical Report [Rowon et al., 1984] made technical recommendations with respect to uroflowmetry, but did not compare different flowmeters by specific testing. There are, however, differences in the accuracy and precision of the flow rate signals that depend on the type of flowmeter, on internal signal processing, and on the proper use and calibration of the flowmeter. The desired and actual accuracy of uroflowmetry should be assessed in relation to the potential information that could be obtained from the urinary stream compared to the information actually abstracted for clinical and research purposes. Some relevant aspects of the physiological and physical information contained in the urinary stream are outlined here.

The desired clinical accuracy may differ from the technical accuracy of a flow meter. The ICS Technical report recommended the following standards: a range of 0–50 ml/s for Q_{max}, and 0–1,000 ml for voided volume, maximum time constant of 0.75 s; an accuracy of $\pm 5\%$ relative to full scale, although a calibration curve representing the percentage error over the entire range of measurement should be made available. However, technical specifications from the manufacturers are rare and often not in accordance with ICS recommendations: this situation should be rectified.

Furthermore, as most flowmeters are mass flow meters (e.g., a weight transducer or rotating disk), variations in the specific gravity of the fluid will have a direct influence on the measured flow rate. For example, urine of high concentration may increase apparent flow rate by 3%. With X-ray medium, the flow rate may be overestimated by as much as 10%. These effects should be corrected by calibration software.

Thus, since the overall accuracy of flow rate signals will not be better than $\pm 5\%$, it would not be meaningful to report a maximum flow rate to a resolution better than a full milliliter per second (ml/s). Under carefully controlled research conditions, a better resolution may be possible by flowmeter calibration and instrument selection. However, such improvements in resolution may not be required for routine clinical applications. The dynamic properties of most flowmeters will be good enough for free uroflowmetry. When pressure flow data are analyzed, however, the limitation in signal dynamics should be taken into account because they will be different for pressure than for flow. Flow signals have a much slower response, and are less accurate than pressure signals.

Problems in Urine Flow Rate Measurement

The problems in measurement, as well as the information that can be abstracted from the flow rate signal are rather dif-

ferent for free uroflowmetry compared to combined pressure/flow recordings.

In free uroflowmetry, the shape of the flow curve may suggest specific types of abnormality, but reliable, specific, and detailed information about the cause for abnormal voiding cannot be derived from a flow curve alone. Only when uroflowmetry is combined with intravesical and abdominal pressure recordings does it become possible, from the pressure–flow relationship, to analyze separately the contributions of detrusor contractility and bladder outlet function to the overall voiding pattern. (Figs. 3–8)

Urine flow rate measurement is affected by a number of important factors.

Detrusor Contractility

As the voiding function reflects the interaction between the relaxed outlet and the contracting detrusor, variation of both will affect the flow. For steady outflow conditions, all variations in flowrate are related to changes in detrusor activity alone. The detrusor contraction strength varies neurogenically and myogenically, and can cause significant variability in urine flow rate measurements. (Fig. 5).

Bladder Outflow Resistance

If detrusor, contractility is constant, then changes in outflow resistance will lead to changes in flow rate, for example, in patients with detrusor–sphincter dyssynergia (Figs. 3, 7, 8).

Bladder Volume

As the bladder volume increases and the detrusor muscle fibers become more stretched, there is an increase in the potential bladder power and work associated with a contraction. This is most pronounced in the range from empty up to 150–250 ml bladder filling volume. It appears that at volumes higher than 400–500 ml, the detrusor may become overstretched and contractility may decrease again. Therefore, Q_{max} is physiologically dependent on the bladder volume. This dependency will vary between individuals and with the type and degree of pathology, for example, in constrictive obstruction, Q_{max} is almost independent of volume, and in compressive obstruction, the dependency becomes weaker with increasingly obstructed outlet conditions and lower flow rate.

Technical Considerations

The flow rate signal is influenced by the technique of measurement and by signal processing. The external urinary stream should reach the flowmeter unaltered and with minimal delay. However, any funnel or collecting device, as well as the flowmeter, will inevitably introduce modifications to the flow rate recording. Physically, the external urinary stream breaks into drops not far from the meatus. This fine structure of the stream has a high frequency, which can be assessed by drop spectrometry, and contains interesting information. For standard uroflowmetry, however, such high frequencies should be eliminated by signal processing.

For free uroflowmetry, all intracorporeal modulations of the flow rate are physiological artifacts and should be minimized, for example by asking the patient to relax and not to strain. Nevertheless, certain dynamic patterns of intracorporeal modulations can provide information about functional obstruction, for example, typical patterns of the detrusor–sphincter dyssynergia, or abnormal straining. This information may be lost by excessive filtering or during analog to digital A/D conversion with a filter speed of less than 10 Hz. The precise interpretation of dynamic variations in the flow rate signal is only possible when the flow rate is viewed together with the simultaneously recorded pressure signals. Thus, only in combined pressure–flow recordings can the details of the flow signal be fully understood.

For the determination of the 'true' maximum flow rate value, particularly during free flow, such high frequency signal variations are more likely to be misleading, and consequently they should be suppressed electronically.

Recommendations for Uroflowmetry

In order to facilitate the recording of urine flow rate and pattern recognition of flow curves, it is recommended that graphical scaling should be standardized as follows:

- one millimeter should equal 1 s on the x-axis and 1 ml/s and 10 ml voided volume on the y-axis.

With respect to the technical accuracy of uroflowmeters, it is meaningful for routine clinical measurements to read flowrate values only to the nearest full ml/s and volumes to the nearest 10 ml.

In order to make electronically-read Q_{max} values more reliable, comparable, and clinically useful, we recommend internal electronic smoothing of the flow rate curve. It is recommended that:

- a sliding average over 2 s should be used to remove positive and negative spike artifacts.

If curves are smoothed by hand, the same concept should be applied. That is, when reading Q_{max} graphically, the line should be smoothed by eye into a continuous curve so that in each period of 2 s, there are no rapid changes. Such a smoothed, clinically-meaningful maximum free flow Q_{max} will be different (lower) from the peak value in the flow rate recording of electronic instruments currently available. (see Figs. 2, 5, 6, 8).

It is recommended that:

- only flow rate values, which have been 'smoothed', either electronically or manually, should be reported.

If a maximum flow value is determined electronically by simple signal peak detection without the recommended electronic smoothing, it should be labeled differently, $Q_{max.raw}$. Such raw data has meaning only if a detailed specification of the type of flowmeter used is given.

The interpretation of any dynamic variation (signal patterns) in free flow will rely on personal experience, can be only descriptive, and in general will remain speculative.

For the documentation of the results of uroflowmetry, the following recommendations are made:

- Maximum (smoothed) urine flow rate should be rounded to the nearest whole number (a recording of 10.25 ml/s would be recorded as 10 ml/s);
- Voided volume and post void residual volume should be rounded to the nearest 10 ml (a recording of a voided volume of 342 ml would be recorded as 340 ml);
- The maximum flow rate should always be documented together with voided volume and post void residual volume using a standard format: VOID: Maximum Flow Rate/Volume Voided/Post Void Residual Volume.

For example, the automatically detected flows, $Q_{max.raw}$, are 16.6 and 21.3 ml/s with voided volumes 86 and 182 ml, respectively. The smoothed Q_{max} values are 8 and 17 ml/s and should be reported with voided volumes of 90 and 180, respectively, and the estimated residuals as VOID1 = 8/90/0 and VOID2 = 17/180/20 (see Figs. 2, 5, 6).

The adoption of these standards will aid the interpretation of uroflowmetry results. If data are not available, then a hyphen should be used, for example, if only the voided volume is known, VOID:—/340/—or if the voided volume was missing, VOID: 10/—/90.

- If a flow/volume nomogram is used, this should be stated and referenced.

Uroflowmetry data from other than free flow, for example, measured in combination with intravesical pressure should be reported with an additional descriptive index, p, i.e., $Q_{max.p}$, for pressure–flow recording.

INVASIVE URODYNAMICS: FILLING CYSTOMETRY, PRESSURE–FLOW STUDY OF VOIDING

Introduction

Invasive urodynamic procedures should not be performed without clear indications and the formulation of specific urodynamic question(s). This process will usually be aided by the a priori completion of a frequency volume chart and free uroflowmetry. There are certain key recommendations, which will lead to the performance of a successful urodynamic study.

- A good urodynamic investigation should be performed interactively with the patient. It should be established by

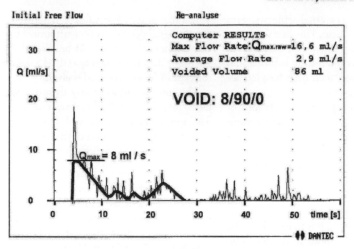

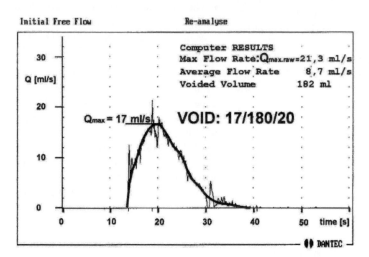

Fig. 2. Exclusion of artifactual spikes in the flow curve, $Q_{max.raw}$, and determination of a clinically relevant maximum flow rate, Q_{max}, by manual smoothing. The results from uroflowmetry should be reported in the standard format: $Q_{max}/V_{void}/V_{res}$.

discussion with the patient that the patient's symptoms have been reproduced during the test;
- There should be continuous and careful observation of the signals as they are collected, and the continuous assessment of the qualitative and quantitative plausibility of all signals;
- Artifacts should be avoided, and any artifacts that occur should be corrected immediately. It is always difficult and is often impossible to correct artifacts during a retrospective analysis. Furthermore, it is more time consuming than if the signals are continuously observed and tested at regular intervals and artifacts recognized during the urodynamic study and corrected.

At present, ambulatory urodynamic monitoring has to rely on retrospective quality control and artifact corrections. However, in principle, the same quality criteria apply for ambulatory urodynamic monitoring as for standard urody-

namics [van Waalwijk et al., 2000]. This makes a consensus on quality even more important, because only when such criteria are precisely defined can they be implemented in an "automated intelligent" ambulatory system.

Quality control relies on pattern recognition and a knowledge of normal values as well as prior identification of useful information obtained from noninvasive urodynamics and all other sources relevant for the urodynamic question. Thus, before invasive urodynamics, a frequency volume chart should be completed and multiple free flows should be evaluated. Useful information obtained from noninvasive testing includes typical voided volumes and post-void residual volumes as well as the expected values for Q_{max}. This information should be used for the control of subsequent invasive studies. Only by good preparation can it be assured that (a) the proper answers to the urodynamic questions will be obtained before the study is terminated and (b) necessary modifica-

266   Schäfer et al.

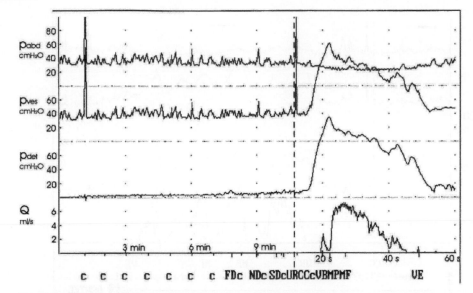

Fig. 3. Full recording of filling and voiding. Starting with initial values for p_{ves}, p_{abd} of 32 cmH$_2$O in the typical range for a standing patient with zero p_{det}; testing signal quality with a vigorous cough at beginning, and regularly repeated (here less strong) coughs. Additionally, the pressure recordings show the typical pattern of a talking patient, while the p_{det} trace is unaffected; a weak contraction at first desire FD; another vigorous cough before voiding; beginning of flow shows dyssynergic sphincter activity as proven by decrease in flow with increase in p_{det}.

tions, additions, or repetitions of measurements will have been performed in order to derive the necessary information.

The effective practice of urodynamics requires: (a) a theoretical understanding of the underlying physics of the measurement, (b) practical experience with urodynamic equipment and procedures, (c) an understanding of how to assure quality control of urodynamic signals, and (d) the ability to analyze critically the results of the measurements. Because urodynamics deals largely with mechanical measurements such as pressure and volume and their related changes in time, and

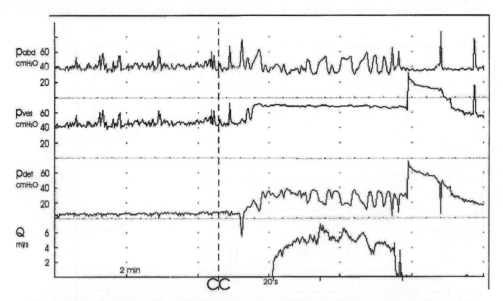

Fig. 4. Good recording quality until cystometric capacity CC is reached; at second cough before voiding the intravesical signal is lost (no response in p_{ves}, negative spike in p_{det}). Dead p_{ves} − signal during voiding, which is "live" again only at second cough after voiding. Thus, pressure–flow study is lost. Careful observation of signals would have made it possible to interrupt the study immediately when signal failed and correct this problem before voiding starts.

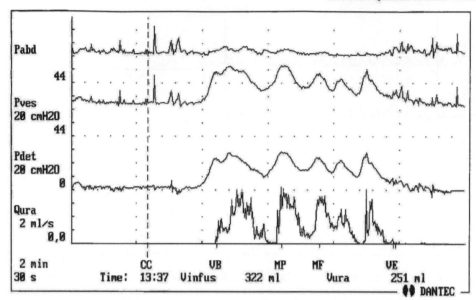

Fig. 5. Variable flowrate due to varying detrusor contraction strength. VOID: 7/250/70.

because many analytical models use mechanical concepts such as resistance to flow or contraction power, it is essential that the nature of these measurements and concepts, in particular for pressure and flowrate, are understood. Therefore, in addition to a comprehensive understanding of anatomy and physiology, some basic knowledge of biomechanics and physics is required.

The quality control of urodynamic measurements must be approached on a holistic basis. Different types and levels of data quality and plausibility control should be used: (a) on a physical and technical level, (b) on a biomechanical level, and (c) on a pathophysiological clinical level. A common problem in urodynamics is that clinicians often proceed immediately to a clinical interpretation, i.e., to level c without a critical analysis of the potential pathophysiological information content, without considering the plausibility of the signals (level a), without considering the biomechanical context of the measurements (level b), and without taking into account the physical properties of the

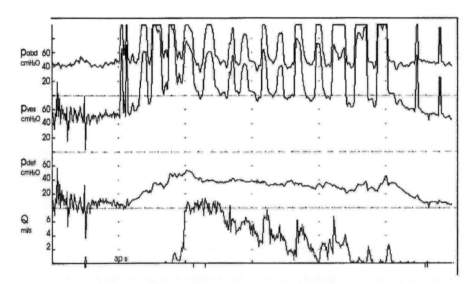

Fig. 6. The first part of the traces shows typical bi-phasic movement artifacts. The two coughs before voiding prove good recording quality. The typical picture of a unobstructed voiding: a weak detrusor contraction with p_{det} of 40 cmH$_2$O and a Q_{max} of 9 ml/s is supported by vigorous straining, which causes some variability in flow (VOID: 9/380/100).

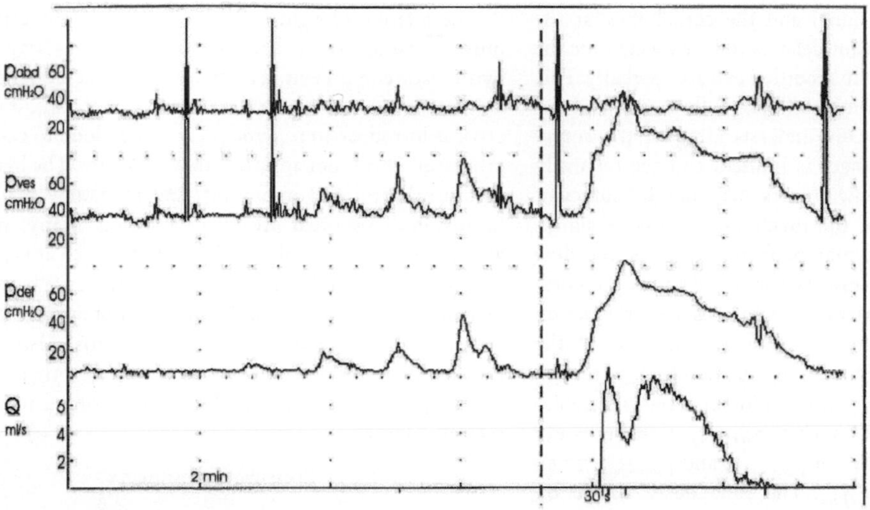

268   Schäfer et al.

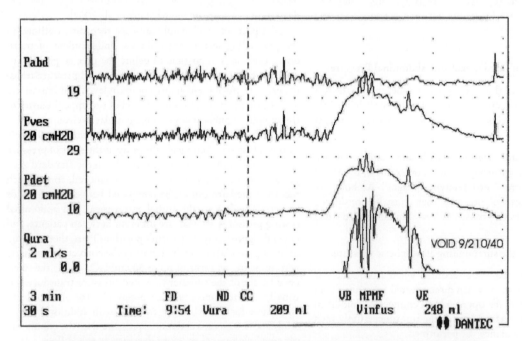

Fig. 7. A good recording showing the typical pattern of increasing detrusor overactivity and a dyssynergic event during voiding.

parameters, technical limitations, and accuracy of the signals. Therefore, it is recommended that:

- Invasive urodynamics should not be performed without precise indications and well-defined 'urodynamic questions' that are to be answered by the results of the urodynamic study.

Measurement of Urine Flow Rate During Pressure–Flow Studies

The usefulness of the concept of a FRCZ for data analysis requires that the recorded pressure and flow rate signal be synchronized with respect to the FRCZ [Griffiths et al. 1997]. Normally, no measurable time delay will exist between

Fig. 8. High quality recordings allow detailed interpretation. The typical pattern of rectal activity becomes clearly visible in p_{det}. The flow artifacts can identified as dyssynergic events and manually corrected from $Q_{max.raw} = 11.2$ ml/s to $Q_{max} = 9$ ml/s.

the intravesical pressure signal and the actual flow at the FRCZ. However, a significant delay is to be expected for the typical urodynamic flow rate recorded extracorporeally. This delay will vary with anatomy, pathology, flow rate, and the set-up for measurement. Our understanding of the actual dynamics of flow rate changes is limited, and the relatively slow response of most flow meters may not be sufficient to match the dynamics of the much-faster pressure signal. The actual time difference may be from 0.5 to 2 s; the time delay between urethral closure and the end of any flow recording may be much longer, particularly in prostatic obstruction and terminal dribbling than between the opening of the urethra and the start of a flow rate signal. Therefore, we recommend the use of more descriptive terminology for synchronizing pressure and flow values, such as $p_{det.Qbeg}$ for the pressure at which flow begins instead of $p_{det.open}$, and $p_{det.Qend}$ when flow ends instead of $p_{det.close}$. The time delay correction needs to be considered when analyzing pressure flow studies [Griffiths et al. 1997].

In average, the maximum flow rate Q_{max} recorded during PF studies, ($Q_{max.p}$), is lower than during free flow (Q_{max}). This, however, is not due simply to a mechanical increase of outflow resistance by the intraurethral catheter, because such a difference is also found in suprapubic PF studies. A difference has also been reported between $Q_{max.p}$ during conventional and ambulatory urodynamics. This indicates more complex causes, possible psychogenic, but also physiologic, for example, that a difference in detrusor contraction strength may be involved, and that the fast filling rate used in clinical studies may lead to reduced contractility. This could also explain the difference in results between conventional and ambulatory studies.

Measurement of Intravesical and Abdominal Pressure

- It is recommended that there is strict adherence to the ICS standardization of zero pressure and reference height. Only then can pressure recordings be compared between patients and centers.

Zero pressure and reference height are concepts which are often confused in urodynamics. For example, by use of the misleading term "zero reference height". As both are independent features of pressure, they must be considered separately, and both must follow recommended ICS methodology.

- Zero pressure is the surrounding atmospheric pressure.

Zero pressure is the value recorded when a transducer is open to the environment when disconnected from any tubes or catheters, or when the open end of a connected, fluid-filled tube is at the same vertical level as the transducer. Only then can a "set zero" or "balance" be performed.

- The reference height is defined as the upper edge of the symphysis pubis.

The reference height is the level at which the transducers must be placed so that all urodynamic pressures have the same hydrostatic component. It is often argued that it does not make a difference for the most relevant parameter, p_{det}, if the same error is introduce to p_{ves} and p_{abd}, as they tend to cancel each other out. This is not an acceptable argument. The hydrostatic pressure is real and important, and inevitably plays a role in any intracorporeal pressure recording. Many important aspects of quality and plausibility control, such as typical resting value ranges at different patient position, are based on the proper recording of pressures, and will not apply if pressures are not recorded according to ICS standards. Also, it is only meaningful to subtract one pressure from the other, for example ($p_{ves} - p_{abd} = p_{det}$), when both are recorded to the same reference level.

Pressure Transducers

Urodynamic techniques were developed using external pressure transducers connected to the patient with fluid-filled lines, allowing easier compliance with the standards of correct zero and reference height. Catheter mounted pressure transducers, so-called microtip transducer catheters have become popular due to their apparent higher accuracy, better dynamic resolution, and their apparent independence from hydrostatic pressure. A catheter mounted pressure transducer is an advantage for dynamic recordings of urethral pressures during coughing (stress profiles) as well as for ambulatory urodynamics in mobile patients. Here only the application of catheter mounted pressure transducers for intravesical and abdominal pressure recordings will be discussed as urethral pressures are dealt with in a separate report [Lose et al., 2002].

All aspects of urodynamic pressure recording outlined in the preceeding section are valid and independent of transducer type. It is impossible to define the precise position of an intravesical and a rectal catheter mounted pressure transducers at to place them at any common level, and impossible to position them at the standard level of the upper boarder of the symphysis pubis. It has become popular to circumvent this problem by setting the catheter mounted pressure transducers to zero pressure when inside the body at the start of pressure recording. This, however, means that both the standard zero pressure as well the reference level are ignored, so that such recorded pressure cannot be compared between patients or centers. The fact is, the initial intravesical and abdominal resting pressures are real, are different between patients, and depend significantly on patient's position. Thus, there are significant potential errors; by ignoring the correct atmospheric zero pressure, an error of up to 50 cmH$_2$O, and as the reference height of the catheter mounted pressure transducers is usually undetermined, another potential error of 10 cmH$_2$O is possible for a full bladder can occur. In addition, when a study starts with zero abdominal pressure then the commonly observed abdominal pressure decrease at pelvic floor relaxation during voiding will evidently result in negative abdominal pressure values, and thus in p_{det} being higher than p_{ves}.

The same problems of apparent independence from the existing hydrostatic pressure also applies to air-filled catheters and/or connection tubings. Due to the absence of a water column between the balloon-covered opening on the catheter and the external transducer, the reference height in an air-filled system will refer to the position of the sensing balloon on the catheter and not to the external transducer.

- It is recommended that for intravesical and abdominal pressure recording external transducers connected to fluid-filled tubings and catheters be used. If microtip or air-filled catheters are used, any deviation from standard zero and reference level should be minimized and taken into account at the time of data analysis.

Urodynamic Catheters

Comparison between patients and urodynamic studies performed in different centers would be facilitated by the use of standard catheters. It is recommended that:

- For the measurement of intravesical pressure and for bladder filling, the standard catheter for routine urodynamics is a transurethral double-lumen catheter.

Only in small children and patients with severe constrictive obstruction (stricture) does suprapubic pressure recording have clear advantages. Intraurethral catheters should be as thin as possible, limited only by the practicality of insertion and by internal lumen sizes, which should be sufficiently large to avoid excessive damping of pressure transmission and to achieve the desired filling rate with standard pumps. A 6-Fr double lumen catheter is the smallest practical size at present.

The major advantage of a double lumen catheter is that the fill/void sequence can be repeated without the need for re-catheterization. Note that the use of a 6-Fr double lumen catheter can limit the infusion rate during cystometry to 20–30 ml/min, as a typical roller pump may not manage to transport a higher perfusion rate through such a small lumen. This can result in a incorrect filling volume being indicated by the machine, when the filling volume is calculated from the pump setting. For example, with a filling rate set at 60 ml/min and an actually achieved filling rate of 30 ml/min, the machine will show double the filling volume. Thus after voiding, a high calculated residual will occur. With some equipment, higher filling rates are possible; it is essential that any system should be critically tested to (a) measure the maximum filling rate that can be achieved by a particular catheter attached to an individual pump and (b) correct or calibrate the indicated infused volume.

The use of two separate tubes for filling and recording is less convenient. Removing the larger filling tube for voiding may appear to be an advantage because only a single small tube is left in the urethra. However, there are no data to suggest that, for example, in a compressive obstruction such as BPO, a 6-F catheter has detrimental influence on the pressure or flow data. There are, however, data suggesting that results from a single study may be misleading. A double lumen catheter facilitates a second fill/void study to establish reproducibility. Re-introduction of the separate filling tube for a repeated study is more invasive and complicated.

- The use of a rectal balloon catheter is recommended for the measurement of abdominal pressure, p_{abd}.

Although there are various methods for the successful recording of abdominal pressures, a flaccid, air-free balloon in the rectal ampulla gives a suitable signal for p_{abd} to determine a meaningful p_{det} when p_{ves} is measured synchronously ($p_{det} = p_{ves} - p_{abd}$). In females, vaginal recording may be more acceptable and provides comparable results. The recording of p_{abd} allows the measurement of any abdominal (i.e., perivesical) pressure component during changes in intravesical pressure. The role of the balloon is to maintain a small fluid volume at the catheter opening and to avoid fecal blockage, which can prevent or impair pressure transmission to the transducer. Additionally, as the rectal ampulla and the vagina are not homogeneously fluid filled spaces, the balloon prevents pressure artifacts arising from contact between the catheter opening and the wall tissue. The balloon serves this function best when it is filled only to 10–20% of its unstretched capacity. Overfilling and elastic distention of the balloon is the most common mistake in abdominal pressure recording. The resultant high balloon (not abdominal) pressure will produce a misleading pressure reading. Such an artificially-elevated balloon distention pressure can be avoided by making a small hole in the balloon, although this is unnecessary if the balloon is filled properly as described above. It is also possible to record reliable abdominal pressure with a very slowly perfused (<2 ml/min) open ended catheter. However, excessive fluid volume in the rectal ampulla may cause problems.

Equipment: Minimum Requirements for Filling Cystometry and Pressure–Flow Studies of Voiding

The ICS has not yet specified definite technical standards in respect of minimum requirements for filling cystometry and pressure flow studies beyond the ICS Technical Equipment Report [Rowan et al. 1997] and the appendix to the ICS document on pressure flow [Griffiths et al., 1997], where an data exchange software standard is recommended. Some further aspects will be discussed in more detail here.

Equipment Recommendations

The minimum recommended requirements for a urodynamic system are:

- three measurement channels, two for pressure and one for flow;
- a display (on printer and/or monitor) and secure storage of three pressures (p_{abd}, p_{ves}, p_{det}) and flow (Q) as tracings against time;

- infused volume and voided volume may be shown graphically or numerically;
- on-line display of pressures and flow, with adequate scale and resolution; scales must be clearly given on all axes; no information should be lost electronically when tracings go off-scale on display;
- possibilities to record standard information about sensation and additional comments (event recording).

Meaningful plausibility assessment and quality control is possible only when the measured and derived signals are displayed continuously as curves over time, without delay (in real time), as the examination proceeds. Each displayed curve and number should be labeled according to ICS standards with clear scaling of amplitudes and the time axis. The following sequential position of tracings is suggested: p_{abd} at the top, then p_{ves}, p_{det} and Q (see Figs. 3–8). It is least important when p_{abd} goes off-scale and is cut off (Fig. 6). Additional parameters such as EMG, bladder filling, and voided volumes can be displayed either as curves or digitally as numbers.

The following minimum technical specifications are recommended:

- Minimum accuracy should be ± 1 cmH$_2$O for pressure and $\pm 5\%$ full scale for flow and volume;
- Ranges of 0–250 cmH$_2$O, 0–25(50) ml/s, and 1,000 ml for pressure, flow, and volume, respectively;
- The software must ensure that no information for pressures up to 250 cmH$_2$O and for flow rates up to 50 ml/s is lost internally even when not displayed and that off-scale values are clearly identified;
- An analog/digital (A/D) frequency of 10 Hz per channel as the lower limit for pressure and flow;
- A higher frequency (minimum 20 kHz) is necessary for recording EMG;
- Calibration of all measurements should be possible.

The scalings should be kept unchanged as much as possible, because urodynamic data quality control is based on pattern recognition, and the recognition of patterns depend on scaling. Therefore, it is recommended that:

- During recording and for analysis, minimum scaling for pressure be of 50 cmH$_2$O per cm, for flow 10 ml/s per cm, and for the time axis 1 min/cm or 5 s/mm during filling and 2 s/mm during voiding.

To enable a retrospective judgment of the curves, urodynamic measurements should be documented as curves over time with comments and explanations. It is usually insufficient to document urodynamic measurements by a few numerical values alone. The same amplitude of scaling should be used for all documentation, although the time axis may be compressed. Only if there is no relevant information to be lost by reducing resolution, for example, during filling, the time scale can be compressed.

For a print-out, maximum full scale deflections of 200 cmH$_2$O, 50 ml/s, and 1,000 ml are sufficient for pressure, flow and volume, respectively. In most cases, half the maximum full scale will be sufficient to show all relevant parts of curves. Line resolution should be better than 0.10 mm.

During interventions, for example, interruption of bladder filling or manipulation of catheters, the continuation of both measurement and recording must always be possible.

On-line recording of comments should be possible, to complete the documentation.

Calibration of Equipment

The need to calibrate pressure transducers, flowmeters, and pumps cannot be stated; simply "yes" if there is a need or "no" there is not. The specification of the manufacturer should be studied. Two aspects must be considered: the intended accuracy of the system and the investigator's experience with the system. If a new system is installed or new transducers are being used, it is recommended that regular calibration be carried out. If experience with daily calibration shows that the potential error is small (e.g., <2 cmH$_2$O), then it will be sufficient to calibrate once a month. However, calibration should not be ignored and good urodynamic equipment makes it technically possible to perform a calibration. Calibration should not be confused with simple 'zero balancing', which is only one part of a calibration. In addition to setting the zero, it must possible to check and adjust the amplitudes of all measurement channels, i.e., to calibrate all signals.

Calibration of a flowmeter can be achieved by pouring a precisely measured volume at a constant flow into the flowmeter, typically 400 ml in 20–30 s (at 15–20 ml/s) and checking the recorded volume. Special constant-flowrate bottles are available for flow calibration. Similarly, one can test a pump by measuring the time to deliver a known volume, for example, 100 ml into a measuring cylinder. It is recommended that pump calibration be performed with the filling catheter connected. Such a pump calibration can only be as good as the cylinder used, which needs to have good resolution and be accurate. Some measuring beakers that are usually available in clinics are not accurate.

Pressure Signal Quality Control: Qualitative and Quantitative Plausibility

It is very important to observe and to test signals carefully and to correct any problems before starting the urodynamic study. If the signals are perfect at the beginning of the study, they usually remain so without the need for major intervention. If the signals are not perfect, remedial action must be taken. If a quality problem does not disappear at once, when filling commences, it will usually deteriorate further during the study.

Conscientious observation of the patient and of the signals, in particular p_{det}, during all parts of the study, together with

272   Schäfer et al.

continuous signal testing, are the keys to high quality urody-namics. The first aim is to avoid artifacts and the second to correct the source of all artifacts immediately when they occur.

The following three criteria form the minimum recommen-dations for ensuring quality control of pressure recordings:

- Resting values for abdominal, intravesical, and detrusor pressure are in a typical range (see below);
- The abdominal and intravesical pressure signals are 'live', with minor variations caused by breathing or talking being similar for both signals; these variations should not appear in p_{det};
- Coughs are used (every I min. or, for example, 50 ml filled volume) to ensure that the abdominal and intravesical pres-sure signals respond equally. Coughs immediately before voiding and immediately after voiding should be included.

When standards are followed, i.e., with the transducer zeros set to atmospheric pressure, and the transducers placed at the level of the upper edge of the symphysis, a typical range for initial resting pressures values for p_{ves} and p_{abd} is (Schäfer, unpublished communications):

- supine 5–20 cmH$_2$O.
- sitting 15–40 cmH$_2$O.
- standing 30–50 cmH$_2$O.

Usually both recorded pressures are almost identical, so that the initial p_{det} is zero, or close to zero, 0–6 cmH$_2$O in 80% of cases and in rare cases up to 10 cmH$_2$O [Liao et al., 1999].

All initial pressure values should be verified and patients' position should be documented on the urodynamics trace.

All negative pressure values, except when caused by rectal activity, should be corrected immediately. It should always be kept in mind that p_{abd} is recorded not to know the actual rec-tal pressure, but to eliminate the impact of (abdominal) pres-sure changes on p_{ves}. The principal aim is to determine the detrusor pressure, p_{det}, which is the pressure in the bladder without the influence of abdominal pressure. Therefore, p_{det} cannot be negative.

By talking to the patient during the study, the proper dynamic response in the pressure signals can be observed and is "automatically" documented (see Figs. 3, 4, 8).

Problem Solving

If either detrusor or rectal contractions occur, the recorded pressures in p_{ves} and in p_{abd} will be different. Such changes can be identified and interpreted with sufficient accuracy and reliability only when the patient is observed and the relation between signal changes and patient sensation/activity are checked for plausibility and documented. Any pressure change caused by smooth muscle contractions will show a "smooth" pattern, (Figs. 5, 7, 8) i.e., there should be no rapid ("stepwise") changes (Fig. 4). If pressures increase or decrease step-wise, or with a constant slope over a long period of time,

a nonphysiological cause, such as catheter movement, should be considered.

If a sudden drop or increase occurs in either the p_{ves} or p_{abd} signal, the usual cause is the movement, blockage (Fig. 4), or disconnection of a catheter. When the patient changes posi-tion, sudden changes in resting values occur and are seen equally in both pressure signals. If p_{ves} (without change in p_{abd}) increases slowly—as typical for a low compliance blad-der—it is important to test for any other possible cause for a slow pressure increase. One cause could be a problem with the intravesical catheter measurement, for example, the hole for the pressure conducting lumen is slowly moving into the blad-der neck region. This should be assessed by asking the patient to cough, if there is no other apparent artifact. Furthermore, it is recommended that bladder filling is stopped, if the filling rate was above a physiological limit of 10 ml/min. If the value of p_{ves} drops after filling is stopped, it is likely that 'low com-pliance' was, at least in part, related to fast filling.

There are several common problems that must be solved before the study is started or when observed during a study: *Problem: Initial resting p_{det} is negative, for example, −5 cmH$_2$O Possible explanations:*

- *because p_{abd} is too high*

  Solution: If p_{ves} is in the typical range, and both pressures are 'live', open the valve in the abdominal line and drain 1 or 2 drops from the rectal balloon filling volume. This will usually cause p_{abd} to fall to a proper value. If not, gently re-position the rectal balloon and/or make a small hole in the balloon.

- *because p_{ves} is too low*

  Solution: This may be due to air bubbles trapped in the cathe-ter, the catheter not being in the bladder, or the catheter being blocked/kinked. Gently flush through the p_{ves} line (max. 10 ml). It is very important to flush slowly while obser-ving the pressure signal because pressures above 300 cmH$_2$O may damage the transducer. If this does not solve the pro-blem, add some more volume to the bladder via the filling lumen. If resistance to filling is high and it does not drain easily when opened, it will be necessary to check catheter position, and to re-position the catheter, if necessary.

Problem: Initial p_{det} too high, for example, 15 cmH$_2$O Possible explanations:

The key problem here is indicated by the measurement of 15 cmH$_2$O. The situation is different from the clear state-ment that 'p_{det} cannot be negative', as we do not have a defi-nite upper limit for the normal maximum 'resting' value for p_{det}. Thus, we can only follow the present guidelines that in most tests, in an empty bladder p_{det} is between 0–5 cmH$_2$O, and in some 90% it is between 0–10 cmH$_2$O. For any higher value, stringent plausibility checking must be applied. If the patient has no detrusor overactivity, a p_{det} of 15 cmH$_2$O is unlikely to be valid and there may be a signal problem. First *check, if p_{abd} and p_{ves} are in the expected ranges. For example, if in a standing patient, initial p_{ves} is 30 cmH$_2$O and p_{abd} is 15 cmH$_2$O, then by experience the value of p_{abd} is too low (because p_{abd} is too low). If in a supine patient p_{abd} is 10 cmH$_2$O and p_{ves} is 25 cmH$_2$O, then the value of p_{ves} is too high (because p_{ves} is too high). Check the zero balance and proper signal response to coughing for both signals.*

- *because p_{abd} is too low*

  Solution to p_{abd} being too low: Very slowly flush the rectal balloon with 1 or 2 ml.

- *because p_{ves} is too high.*

  Solution to p_{ves} being too high: This problem can be related to a misplaced catheter, a kink in the catheter, or contact with the bladder wall in an empty bladder, which occludes the eyehole(s) of the catheter. Proceed according to the solution for p_{ves} being too high, in the first example above.

If no signal problem can be identified, the clinical study may be started, but the p_{det} signal deserves particular attention. If compliance is normal and the bladder normal at filling, then it is very important to record and check, for some period after the micturition, the post-voiding resting value of p_{det}. Only if an elevated p_{det} is perfectly reproducible for repeated filling and voiding studies can it be accepted. However, it is most likely that a high resting p_{det} will not be reproducible and will be corrected by the measures described above.

In summary, if any resting value or cough response does not fit the usual values or patterns, it should be corrected before bladder filling is started. If this is not possible, the signals must be observed even more carefully and every effort made to reveal the potential source of error or artifact during the study.

Retrospective Artifact Correction

In principle, a good p_{det} signal requires only that p_{ves} and p_{abd} show the same fine structure and quality of signals before filling, during filling, and after a voiding. (Figs. 3, 4, 7, 8) Both p_{ves} and p_{abd} must have the same zero and reference level. The most common mistake is to set *(balance)* the initial pressure values of p_{ves} and p_{abd} to zero with the catheters connected to the patient instead of setting zero to atmospheric pressure. This results in incorrect p_{ves} and p_{abd}. If this is done, urodynamic studies cannot be compared between centers and between patients. Although it may seem convenient and easy to start with a value of p_{det} as zero, this practice will lead to problems later in the test. As soon as pelvic floor relaxation occurs, which is particularly common during voiding, the value of p_{abd}, if starting at zero, becomes negative. With a negative p_{abd}, p_{det} will be higher than p_{ves}, a conceptually meaningless result. Furthermore, it will then be impossible to correct a negative p_{abd}. Cough tests at regular intervals, particularly before voiding and after voiding, document the dynamic response of the pressure channels and are fundamentally important.

A typical physiological artifact that can be easily recognized is a rectal contraction. Rectal contractions are usually of low amplitude and may or may not be felt by the patient (Fig. 8). The value of p_{abd} shows a phasic rise with no change in the p_{det} signal—a potentially confusing fall in p_{det} results from the electronic subtraction, but this is, of course, an artefact. Usually rectal contractions are relevant only because they may be misinterpreted as detrusor overactivity (Fig. 8): they have no relevance to voiding.

Biphasic spikes as a response to cough tests are another example of artifacts that are easy to correct. However, any other artifacts such as a signal which is nonresponding (dead), has stepwise changes in pressure, or has negative pressures, often cannot be corrected or can be corrected only with a lot of speculation about the underlying causes of the problem. Studies with such artefacts, should be repeated see the next section).

Retrospective corrections require the same strategies for plausibility control as during recording, but then they are much more difficult and less successful to perform.

A few common artifacts (e.g., rectal activity, biphasic spikes at cough tests, or insufficient p_{abd} response during straining) can be accepted during the study as they can be corrected retrospectively. Usually, this is easier to do manually than through a computerized system.

Urodynamic Computer Software

Computer applications should allow the easy use of even the most complicated analytical algorithms. However, most of the software offered by the urodynamic equipment industry is neither original nor validated. The software may, in fact, not do what the original developer(s) of the algorithm intended. Therefore, it is recommended that:

- When analytical urodynamic software is used to perform data analysis according to any published concept, the source of the software should be specified. It should also be clearly stated if the software has been validated, i.e., proven to provide results consistent with the algorithms to which the analyses are attributed.

STRATEGY FOR REPETITION OF URODYNAMIC TESTS

- It is recommended that a urodynamic test should be repeated if the initial test suggests an abnormality, leaves the cause of troublesome lower urinary tract symptoms unresolved, or if there are technical problems preventing proper analysis.

It may not be necessary, however, to repeat a study, which beyond any doubt, confirms the expected pathology, for example, detrusor overactivity which correlates with the patient's symptoms. However, if the study is inconclusive, then the

274   Schäfer et al.

consequences of not finding a clear answer to the urodynamic question(s) should be considered. If an invasive therapy is planned, the urodynamics should be repeated. Therefore, it is necessary to analyze the signals during the study and document the study immediately upon its conclusion. Only then is it possible to be sure that the urodynamic study is of a quality that answers the urodynamic question and provides an understanding about the patient's clinical problem. Therefore, it is recommended that:

- The urodynamic findings and the interpretation of the results should be documented immediately after the study is finished, i.e., before the patient has left the urodynamic laboratory. Doing so allows for a second test if required.

The analysis of a good study is easy and straight-forward. Indeed, an easy analysis actually is the key criterion for good urodynamics. A good study is one that is easy to read and one from which a any experienced urodynamicist will abstract the same results and come to the same conclusions. For computerized analyses, high data quality is even more important than for manual graphical data analysis. Efforts to achieve urodynamic data of high quality during the study will produce great benefits at the time of data analysis. The future development of urodynamic equipment and software should force investigators to conduct proper on-line data quality control. Analysis of ambulatory studies will remain problematic, as it is less easy to conduct on-line assessment of quality, and analysis is time consuming. Hence, it will be necessary to ask the patient to return, on another occasion, should the investigation require repeating, for whatever reason.

CONCLUSIONS

This is the first report of the ICS Standardization committee of Good Urodynamic Practice. The authors are well aware that this is just a first step and many more will have to follow. Only the essential aspects are considered, but if these basic standards are followed, the quality of urodynamic studies will be significantly improved.

ACKNOWLEDGMENTS

The Standardisation Committee is grateful for the extensive editing performed by Vicky Rees, ICS Administrator. The committee is also grateful for the detailed comments received from Linda Cardozo, Paul Dudgeon, Guus Kramer, Joseph Macaluso, Gerry Timm, and Alan Wein.

REFERENCES

Griffiths DJ, Höfner K, van Mastrigt R, Rollema HJ, Spangberg A, Gleason DM. 1997. Standardization of terminology of lower urinary tract function: pressure-flow studies of voiding, urethral resistance, and urethral obstruction. Neurourol Urodyn 16:1–18.

Liao L, Kirshner-Hermanns R, Schäfer W. 1999. Urodynamic quality control: quantitative plausibility control with typical value ranges. Neurourol Urodyn 18(abstract 99a):365–366.

Lose G, Griffiths DJ, Hosker G, Kulseng-Hansen S, Perucchini D, Schäfer W, Thind P, Versi E. 2002. Standardisation of urethral pressure measurement: Report of the sub-committee of the International Continence Society. Neurourol Urodyn 21:258–60.

Rowan D, James DE, Kramer AEJL, Sterling AM, Suhel PF. 1987. Urodynamic equipment: technical aspects. J Med Eng Tech 11:57–64.

van Waalwijk E, Anders K, Khullar V, Kulseng-Hanssen S, Pesce F, Robertson A, Rosario D, Schäfer W. 2000. Standardisation of ambulatory urodynamic monitoring: Report of the standardisation sub-committee of the International Continence Society. Neurourol Urodyn 19:113–125.

Index